Clinical Cases in
Periodontics

Clinical Cases Series

Wiley-Blackwell's Clinical Cases series is designed to recognize the centrality of clinical cases to the dental profession by providing actual cases with an academic backbone. This unique approach supports the new trend in case-based and problem-based learning. Highly illustrated in full color, the Clinical Cases series utilizes a format that fosters independent learning and prepares the reader for case-based examinations.

Clinical Cases in Pediatric Dentistry
by Amr M. Moursi and Amy L. Truesdale
February 2020

Clinical Cases in Dental Hygiene
by Cheryl M. Westphal Theile, Mea A. Weinberg, and Stuart L. Segelnick
January 2019

Clinical Cases in Endodontics
by Takashi Komabayashi
November 2017

Clinical Cases in Orofacial Pain
by Malin Ernberg and Per Alstergren
March 2017

Clinical Cases in Implant Dentistry
by Nadeem Karimbux and Hans-Peter Weber
December 2016

Clinical Cases in Orthodontics
by Martyn T. Cobourne, Padhraig S. Fleming, Andrew T. DiBiase, and Sofia Ahmad
June 2012

Clinical Cases in Prosthodontics
by Leila Jahangiri, Marjan Moghadam, Mijin Choi, and Michael Ferguson
October 2010

Clinical Cases in Restorative and Reconstructive Dentistry
by Gregory J. Tarantola
September 2010

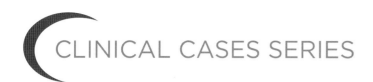
CLINICAL CASES SERIES

Clinical Cases in
Periodontics

SECOND EDITION

Edited by

Nadeem Karimbux, DMD, MMSc
Tufts University School of Dental Medicine
Boston, MA, USA

WILEY Blackwell

Registered Office
John Wiley & Sons, Inc., 111 River Street, Hoboken, NJ 07030, USA

Editorial Office
111 River Street, Hoboken, NJ 07030, USA

For details of our global editorial offices, customer services, and more information about Wiley products visit us at www.wiley.com.

Wiley also publishes its books in a variety of electronic formats and by print-on-demand. Some content that appears in standard print versions of this book may not be available in other formats.

Limit of Liability/Disclaimer of Warranty
The contents of this work are intended to further general scientific research, understanding, and discussion only and are not intended and should not be relied upon as recommending or promoting scientific method, diagnosis, or treatment by physicians for any particular patient. In view of ongoing research, equipment modifications, changes in governmental regulations, and the constant flow of information relating to the use of medicines, equipment, and devices, the reader is urged to review and evaluate the information provided in the package insert or instructions for each medicine, equipment, or device for, among other things, any changes in the instructions or indication of usage and for added warnings and precautions. While the publisher and authors have used their best efforts in preparing this work, they make no representations or warranties with respect to the accuracy or completeness of the contents of this work and specifically disclaim all warranties, including without limitation any implied warranties of merchantability or fitness for a particular purpose. No warranty may be created or extended by sales representatives, written sales materials or promotional statements for this work. The fact that an organization, website, or product is referred to in this work as a citation and/or potential source of further information does not mean that the publisher and authors endorse the information or services the organization, website, or product may provide or recommendations it may make. This work is sold with the understanding that the publisher is not engaged in rendering professional services. The advice and strategies contained herein may not be suitable for your situation. You should consult with a specialist where appropriate. Further, readers should be aware that websites listed in this work may have changed or disappeared between when this work was written and when it is read. Neither the publisher nor authors shall be liable for any loss of profit or any other commercial damages, including but not limited to special, incidental, consequential, or other damages.

Library of Congress Cataloging-in-Publication Data

Names: Karimbux, Nadeem, editor.
Title: Clinical cases in periodontics / edited by Nadeem Karimbux.
Other titles: Clinical cases (Ames, Iowa)
Description: Second edition. | Hoboken, NJ : Wiley-Blackwell, 2022. |
  Series: Clinical cases series | Includes bibliographical references and index.
Identifiers: LCCN 2021038707 (print) | LCCN 2021038708 (ebook) | ISBN
  9781119583950 (paperback) | ISBN 9781119583974 (adobe pdf) | ISBN
  9781119583943 (epub)
Subjects: MESH: Periodontal Diseases–therapy | Periodontics–methods |
  Case Reports
Classification: LCC RK450.P4 (print) | LCC RK450.P4 (ebook) | NLM WU 240 |
  DDC 617.6/32–dc23
LC record available at https://lccn.loc.gov/2021038707
LC ebook record available at https://lccn.loc.gov/2021038708

Cover Design: Wiley
Cover Images: Images on left and right side photo credit – Irina F. Dragan and Wael Att
Photo credit – Liran Levin and Tae Hyun Kwon

Set in 10/13 pt UniversLTStd-Light by Straive, Pondicherry, India

Printed in Singapore
M097278_030122

DEDICATION

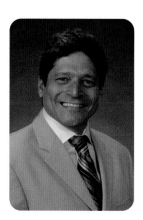

The authors would like to dedicate this book to Dr. Ricardo Teles. Dr. Teles was an excellent periodontist, an inspiring teacher, and a gifted clinical scientist. In fact, he was a teacher, mentor, colleague, and friend to many of the contributors to this publication. His charisma, passion, brilliance, and enthusiasm were at the core of his excellence.

Ricardo loved teaching periodontology and considered the students his colleagues, just with less experience, and was genuinely happy with the success of his students and peers. He really wanted to make an impact in the field and ultimately improve the way we treat patients. And he wanted to do that by better understanding the biology of periodontal diseases and shaping the next generation of periodontists. We hope that this book bring us one step closer to his goals.

Flavia Teles

CONTENTS

Contributors..xiii

Preface xvii

About the Companion Website xix

Chapter 1   Examination and Diagnosis   1

Case 1   Examination and Documentation........................ 2
Tae H. Kwon, DDS, MMSc, Howard H. Yen, DMD,
and Liran Levin, DMD, FRCD(C), FIADT, FICD

Case 2   Dental Plaque-Induced Gingivitis..................... 11
Nadeem Karimbux, DMD, MMSc , Ningyuan Sun, B.D.S, Ph.D,
and Satheesh Elangovan, BDS, DSc, DMSc

Case 3   Non-Plaque-Induced Gingivitis....................... 17
N. Joseph Laborde III, DDS, MMSc and Mark
A. Lerman, DMD

Case 4   Gingival Enlargement 23
T. Howard Howell, DDS, Maria Dona, DMD, MSD, DMSc,
and Thomas T. Nguyen, DMD, MSc, FRCD(C)

Case 5   Aggressive Periodontitis............................ 30
Nadeem Karimbux, DMD, MMSc and Martin Ming-Jen Fu,
BDS, MS, DMsc

Case 6   Chronic Periodontitis............................... 38
Flavia Teles, DDS, MS, DMSc, Ricardo Teles, DDS, DMSc,
Magda Feres, DDS, MSc, PhD, Belen Retamal-Valdes, DDS,
MSc, PhD, and Vinicius Souza Rodrigues, DDS, SDD, DMSc

Case 7   Local Anatomic Factors Contributing to Periodontal
Disease 48
Daniel Kuan-te Ho, DMD, DMSc, MSc and David M. Kim,
DDS, DMSc

Case 8   Oral–Systemic Links. 57
Lorenzo Mordini, DDS, MS, Carlos Parra, DDS, and Po Lee, DDS

Case 9   Developments in Diagnostics 73
Aruna Ramesh, BDS, MS, DMD and Hugo Campos, DDS, DMD

Chapter 2   Nonsurgical Periodontal Therapy   85

Case 1   Hand and Automated Instrumentation. 86
Helen Livson, DMD, MMSc

Case 2   Local Drug Delivery 92
Emilio I. Arguello, DDS, MSc and Naciye G. Uzel, DMD, DMSc

Case 3   Systemic Antibiotics 101
Flavia Teles, DDS, MS, DMSc, Ricardo Teles, DDS, DMSc, Magda Feres, DDS, MSc, PhD, Belen Retamal-Valdes, DDS, MSc, PhD, and Vinicius Souza Rodrigues, DDS, SDD, DMSc

Case 4   Use of Lasers in Periodontology. 114
Abiar Alwael, DDS, MS, Irina F. Dragan, DDS, DMD, MS, and Charles Hawley, DDS, PhD

Chapter 3   Resective Periodontal Therapy   119

Case 1   Gingivectomy. 120
T. Howard Howell, DDS, Maria Dona, DMD, MSD, DMSc, and Thomas T. Nguyen, DMD, MSc, FRCD(C)

Case 2   Preprosthetic Hard Tissue and Soft Tissue Crown
Lengthening 128
Guillaume Campard, DDS, MMSc, Emilio I. Arguello, DDS, MSc, and Naciye G. Uzel, DMD, DMSc

Case 3   Flap Osseous Surgery 138
Kevin Guze, DMD, DMSc, MSc, FRCD(C), FICOI

Case 4   Root Resection 145
Philip Walton, DDS, MMSc and Paul A. Levi, Jr., DMD

Chapter 4   Regenerative Therapy   155

Case 1   Treatment of Furcations. 156
Soo-Woo Kim, DMD, MS and Myron L. Nevins, DMD, MMSc

Case 2   Treatment of Intrabony Defects Using Allografts 164
Kevin Guze, DMD, DMSc, MSc, FRCD(C), FICOI

Case 3   Treatment of Intrabony Defects Using Growth Factors 174
          Marc L. Nevins, DMD, MMSc and Vinicius Souza Rodrigues,
          DDS, SDD, DMSc

Case 4   Treatment of Intrabony Defects Using Alloplastic Materials 181
          N. Joseph Laborde III, DDS, MMSc and Giuseppe Intini,
          DDS, MS, PhD

Case 5   Guided Bone Regeneration......................... 188
          Kevin Guze, DMD, DMSc, MSc, FRCD(C), FICOI and
          Mohamed A. Maksoud, DMD

Chapter 5   Mucogingival Therapy   199

Case 1   Pedicle Flaps................................. 200
          N. Joseph Laborde III, DDS and Kasumi Kuse
          Barouch, DDS, PhD, CAGS

Case 2   Connective Tissue Grafts........................ 206
          Ronny S. Taschner, DDS and Jennifer F. Taschner, DDS,
          MMSc

Case 3   Free Gingival Grafts............................ 214
          Ronald M. Fried, DMD, MMSc and Maria Dona, DMD,
          MSD, DMSc

Case 4   Allografts (Alloderm) for Mucogingival Therapy.......... 228
          Livia Valverde, DDS, MS, PhD, DMSc and Sarah D. Shih,
          DDS, MS, DMSc

Case 5   Frenectomy and Vestibuloplasty.................... 235
          Daniel Kuan-te Ho, DMD, DMSc, MSc, Satheesh Elangovan,
          BDS, DSc, DMSc, and Sarah D. Shih, DDS, MS, DMSc

Case 6   Minimally Invasive Coronally Advanced Flap Techniques 242
          Samar Shaikh, BDS, MS, Pooyan Refahi, DMD, MS,
          and Irina F. Dragan, DDS, DMD, MS

Chapter 6   Interdisciplinary Treatment   247

Case 1   Periodontics–Endodontics......................... 248
          Paul A. Levi Jr., DMD and Campo E. Perez Jr., DDS

Case 2   Periodontics–Prosthodontics...................... 260
          Kevin Guze, DMD, DMSc, MSc, FRCD(C), FICOI and
          Ryan D. Blissett, DMD, MMSc

Case 3   Periodontics–Orthodontics: Part I.................. 268
          Athbi Alqareer, BDM, DMSc, Shankar Rengasamy
          Venugopalan, BDS, DDS, PhD, DMSc, and Veerasathpurush
          Allareddy, BDS, MBA, MHA, PhD, MMSc

CONTENTS

Case 4   Periodontics–Orthodontics: Part II 276
Camille Neste Laboy, DDS, MPH, Sercan Akyalcin,
DDS, PhD, and Irina F. Dragan, DDS, DMD, MS

Case 5   Occlusion–Periodontology 284
Mohamed H. Hassan, BDS, DMD, MS, FICD, Irina F. Dragan,
DDS, DMD, MS, and Rory O'Neil, DMD, BDS, MSc

Case 6   Periodontics–Pediatric Dentistry. 289
Nadeem Karimbux, DMD, MMSc, Roslayn Sulyanto, DMD,
MS, and Soo-Woo Kim, DMD, MS

Chapter 7   Implant Site Preparation   297

Case 1   Sinus Grafting: Lateral. 298
Guillaume Campard, DDS, MMSc, Emilio I. Arguello, DDS,
MSc, and Naciye G. Uzel, DMD, DMSc

Case 2   Internal Sinus Lift Using the Crestal Window Technique . . . 307
Samuel Lee, DMD, DMSc, Nadeem Karimbux, DMD, MMSc,
and Y. Natalie Jeong, DMD, MA

Case 3   Alveolar Ridge Preservation 315
Satheesh Elangovan, BDS, DSc, DMSc

Case 4   Ridge Split and Osteotome Ridge Expansion Techniques 323
Emilio I. Arguello, DDS, MSc and Daniel Kuan-te Ho,
DMD, DMSc, MSc

Chapter 8   Dental Implants   337

Case 1   Conventional Implant Placement 338
Samuel Koo, DDS, MS

Case 2   Immediate Implant Placement 345
Mohamed A. Maksoud, DMD

Case 3   Sinus Lift and Immediate Implant Placement 350
Samuel Lee, DMD, DMSc, Nadeem Karimbux, DMD, MMSc,
Ningyuan Sun, B.D.S, Ph.D, and Irina F. Dragan, DDS, DMD, MS

Case 4   Implant Rehabilitation for Missing Adjacent Teeth
in the Maxillary Esthetic Zone. 357
Panos Papaspyridakos, DDS, PhD, MS, Behshid Bahraini,
DDS, MS, Aikaterini Papathanasiou, DDM, DMD, and Wael
Att, DDS, PhD, Dr Med Dent

Case 5   Combination of Implant Single Crowns and Porcelain
Veneers in the Esthetic Zone. 365
Aikaterini Papathanasiou, DDM, DMD, Rayyan A. Alfirdous,
BDS, MS, BMS-MS, Dip ABOP, Abiar Alwael, DDS, MS,
Panos Papaspyridakos, DDS, PhD, MS, and Wael Att, DDS,
PhD, Dr Med Dent

Chapter 9   Preventive Periodontal Therapy   373

Case 1   Plaque Removal 374
                Paul A. Levi Jr., DMD and Luca Gobbato, DDS, MS

Index **383**

CONTRIBUTORS

Sercan Akyalcin, DDS, PhD
Tufts University School of Dental Medicine
Boston, MA, USA

Rayyan A. Alfirdous, BDS, MS, BMS-MS, Dip ABOP
Prince Abdul Rahman Advanced Dental Institute
Riyadh, Kingdom of Saudi Arabia

Veerasathpurush Allareddy, BDS, MBA, MHA, PhD, MMSc
University of Illinois at Chicago, College of Dentistry
Chicago, IL, USA

Athbi Alqareer, BDM, DMSc
Faculty of Dentistry, Kuwait University
Kuwait City, Kuwait

Abiar Alwael, DDS, MS
Private Practice
Kuwait City, Kuwait

Emilio I. Arguello, DDS, MSc
Harvard School of Dental Medicine
Boston, MA, USA

Wael Att, DDS, PhD, Dr Med Dent
Tufts University School of Dental Medicine
Boston, MA, USA

Behshid Bahraini, DDS, MS
Private Practice
Houston, TX, USA

Kasumi Kuse Barouch, DDS, PhD, CAGS (in Periodontology)
Iman Abdulrahmen bin Al Faisal University
Dammam, Kingdom of Saudi Arabia;
Goldman School of Dental Medicine,
Boston University
Boston, MA, USA

Ryan D. Blissett, DMD, MMSc
Private Practice
Boston, MA, USA

Guillaume Campard, DDS, MMSc
Private Practice
Nantes, France

Hugo Campos, DDS, DMD
Tufts University School of Dental Medicine
Boston, MA, USA

Maria Dona, DMD, MSD, DMSc
Private Practice
Andover, MA, USA

Irina F. Dragan, DDS, DMD, MS
Tufts University School of Dental Medicine
Boston, MA, USA

Satheesh Elangovan, BDS, DSc, DMSc
University of Iowa College of Dentistry
Iowa City, IA, USA

CONTRIBUTORS

Magda Feres, DDS, MSc, PhD
Department of Periodontology, Guarulhos University
Guarulhos, São Paulo, Brazil

Ronald M. Fried, DMD, MMSc
Harvard School of Dental Medicine
Boston, MA, USA

Martin Ming-Jen Fu, BDS, MS, DMsc
National Defense Medical Center
Taipei, Taiwan

Luca Gobbato, DDS, MS
Harvard School of Dental Medicine
Boston, MA, USA

Kevin Guze, DMD, DMSc, MSc, FRCD(C), FICOI
Harvard School of Dental Medicine
Boston, MA, USA

Mohamed H. Hassan, BDS, DMD, MS, FICD
Harvard School of Dental Medicine
Boston, MA, USA

Charles Hawley, DDS, PhD
Tufts University School of Dental Medicine
Boston, MA, USA

Daniel Kuan-te Ho, DMD, DMSc, MSc
School of Dentistry, University of Texas at Houston
Houston, TX, USA

T. Howard Howell, DDS
Harvard School of Dental Medicine
Boston, MA, USA

Giuseppe Intini, DDS, MS, PhD
University of Pittsburgh School of Dental Medicine
Pittsburgh, PA, USA

Y. Natalie Jeong, DMD, MA
Tufts University School of Dental Medicine
Boston, MA, USA

Nadeem Karimbux, DMD, MMSc
Tufts University School of Dental Medicine
Boston, MA, USA

David M. Kim, DDS, DMSc
Harvard School of Dental Medicine
Boston, MA, USA

Soo-Woo Kim, DMD, MS
Harvard School of Dental Medicine
Boston, MA, USA

Samuel Koo, DDS, MS
Private Practice
Boston, MA, USA

Tae H. Kwon, DDS, MMSc
Private Practice
Keene, NH, USA

N. Joseph Laborde III, DDS, MMSc
Private Practice
Fort Worth, TX, USA

Camille Neste Laboy, DDS, MPH
Private Practice
Puerto Rico, USA

Po Lee, DDS, MS
Tufts University School of Dental Medicine
Boston, MA, USA

Samuel Lee, DMD, DMSc
Private Practice
San Diego, CA, USA

Mark A. Lerman, DMD
Tufts University School of Dental Medicine
Boston, MA, USA

Paul A. Levi, Jr., DMD
Tufts University School of Dental Medicine
Boston, MA, USA

Liran Levin, DMD, FRCD(C), FIADT, FICD
Faculty of Medicine and Dentistry, University of Alberta
Edmonton, Alberta, Canada

Helen Livson, DMD, MMSc
Private Practice
Wellesley, MA, USA

Mohamed A. Maksoud, DMD
Harvard University School of Dental Medicine
Boston, MA, USA

Lorenzo Mordini, DDS, MS
Tufts University School of Dental Medicine
Boston, MA, USA

Marc L. Nevins, DMD, MMSc
Harvard School of Dental Medicine
Boston, MA, USA

Myron L. Nevins, DMD, MMSc
Harvard School of Dental Medicine
Boston, MA, USA

Thomas T. Nguyen, DMD, MSc, FRCD(C)
Harvard School of Dental Medicine
Boston, MA, USA

Rory O'Neil, DMD, BDS, MSc
Tufts University School of Dental Medicine
Boston, MA, USA

Panos Papaspyridakos, DDS, PhD, MS
Tufts University School of Dental Medicine
Boston, MA, USA

Aikaterini Papathanasiou, DDM, DMD
Tufts University School of Dental Medicine
Boston, MA, USA

Carlos Parra, DDS
School of Dentistry, Texas A&M University
Dallas, TX, USA

Campo E. Perez, Jr., DDS
University of Pennsylvania School of Dental Medicine
Pennsylvania, PA, USA

Aruna Ramesh, BDS, MS, DMD
Tufts University School of Dental Medicine
Boston, MA, USA

Pooyan Refahi, DMD, MS
Tufts University School of Dental Medicine
Boston, MA, USA

Belen Retamal-Valdes, DDS, MSc, PhD
Department of Periodontology, Guarulhos University
Guarulhos, São Paulo, Brazil

Vinicius Souza Rodrigues, DDS, SDD, DMSc
University of Detroit Mercy Dental School
Detroit, MI, USA

Samar Shaikh, BDS, MS
Tufts University School of Dental Medicine
Boston, MA, USA

Sarah D. Shih, DDS, MS, DMSc
Private Practice
Boston, MA, USA

Roslayn Sulyanto, DMD, MS
Harvard School of Dental Medicine
Boston, MA, USA

Ningyuan Sun, B.D.S, Ph.D
Tufts University School of Dental Medicine
Boston, MA, USA

Jennifer F. Taschner, DDS, MMSc
Private Practice
Fort Myers, FL, USA

Ronny S. Taschner, DDS
Private Practice
Fort Myers, FL, USA

Flavia Teles, DDS, MS, DMSc
University of Pennsylvania School of Dental Medicine
Pennsylvania, PA, USA

Ricardo Teles, DDS, DMSc (Deceased)
Formerly University of Pennsylvania School of Dental
Medicine
Pennsylvania, PA, USA

Naciye G. Uzel, DMD, DMSc
Tufts University School of Dental Medicine
Boston, MA, USA

Livia Valverde, DDS, MS, PhD, DMSc
Tufts University School of Dental Medicine
Boston, MA, USA

**Shankar Rengasamy Venugopalan,
BDS, DDS, PhD, DMSc**
University of Iowa College of Dentistry and Dental
Clinics
Iowa City, IA, USA

Philip Walton, DDS, MMSc
Private Practice
Toronto, Ontario, Canada

Howard H. Yen, DMD
Private Practice
Keene, NH, USA

PREFACE

A dental student at Tufts University School of Dental Medicine (TUSDM) recently asked me about why I chose a career in "academics." I told the student that as I progressed through the early years of my education I was not only exposed to topics in medicine and dentistry (basic knowledge and clinical skills) but was also required to conduct a research project and obliged to present clinical cases to my fellow students. My research experiences honed skills that have served me throughout my career: the ability to ask questions (curiosity), the intellect to review the literature (interpreting the scientific evidence), and the background needed to apply research methods (quantitative and qualitative) to answer my questions. My early experiences in presenting cases to classmates and faculty allowed me the good fortune of teaching others and learning from others. It is these collective experiences that led to an academic career in clinical care, teaching and research.

As my career has progressed, that ability to balance all three aspects (the triple threat) is no longer viable in a world that is fast-paced and much more complex. As a Dean of TUSDM I find myself involved in much administration. However, it is efforts such as editor of the second edition of *Clinical Cases in Periodontology* that take me back to my roots: connecting with my fellow clinicians (faculty, colleagues, and residents), taking a problem-based approach to clinical cases, and using an evidence-based approach to answer the clinical questions posed by the clinical cases.

I thank my current and past faculty and residents for the care they provide to their patients and for allowing me to stay connected to my roots.

Nadeem Karimbux
Tufts University School of Dental Medicine

ABOUT THE COMPANION WEBSITE

The companion website for this book is at

www.wiley.com/go/karimbux/periodontics

The website contains –
- Videos from within the book as downloadable PowerPoint slides
- Figures from within the book as downloadable PowerPoint slides

1

Examination and Diagnosis

Case 1: Examination and Documentation 2
Tae H. Kwon, DDS, MMSc, Howard H. Yen, DMD, and Liran Levin, DMD, FRCD(C),
FIADT, FICD

Case 2: Dental Plaque-Induced Gingivitis 11
Nadeem Karimbux, DMD, MMSc, Ningyuan Sun, B.D.S, Ph.D and Satheesh Elangovan,
BDS, DSc, DMSc

Case 3: Non-Plaque-Induced Gingivitis 17
N. Joseph Laborde III, DDS, MMSc and Mark A. Lerman, DMD

Case 4: Gingival Enlargement 23
T. Howard Howell, DDS, Maria Dona, DMD, MSD, DMSc, and Thomas T. Nguyen, DMD, MSc,
FRCD(C)

Case 5: Aggressive Periodontitis 30
Nadeem Karimbux, DMD, MMSc and Martin Ming-Jen Fu, BDS, MS, DMsc

Case 6: Chronic Periodontitis 38
Flavia Teles, DDS, MS, DMSc, Ricardo Teles†, DDS, DMSc, Magda Feres, DDS, MSc, PhD, Belen
Retamal-Valdes, DDS, MSc, PhD, and Vinicius Souza Rodrigues, DDS, SDD, DMSc

Case 7: Local Anatomic Factors Contributing to Periodontal Disease 48
Daniel Kuan-te Ho, DMD, DMSc, MSc and David M. Kim, DDS, DMSc

Case 8: Oral–Systemic Links 57
Lorenzo Mordini, DDS, MS, Carlos Parra, DDS, and Po Lee, DDS

Case 9: Developments in Diagnostics 73
Aruna Ramesh, BDS, MS, DMD and Hugo Campos, DDS, DMD

†Deceased

Case 1

Examination and Documentation

CASE STORY

A 44-year-old Caucasian female presented with chief concern "I have pain on my upper left molar, which has gradually increased. I would like to fix my gum diseases. I would like to receive dental implants to replace my missing teeth also."

LEARNING GOALS AND OBJECTIVES

- The patient's chief complaint
- Medical and dental history
- Soft tissue and gingival examination
- Periodontal charting
- Radiographic interpretations
- Periodontal diagnosis

Medical History

- ASA classification 1
- Vital signs: blood pressure 130/80 mmHg
- Medication: none
- Supplement: daily multivitamin
- Allergy: none

Dental History

- The patient brushed three times daily and flosses daily.
- The patient had received routine dental prophylaxis at her general dental practitioner's office. Recently, the patient underwent extraction of her mandibular left first and second molars due to severe periodontal disease, and she would like to replace them with dental implants.
- The patient denied any smoking habit and had never smoked.
- The patient's father suffered from periodontal disease and ended up receiving complete maxillary and mandibular removable dentures.
- Patient was extremely motivated for dental treatment.

Soft Tissue and Gingival Examination

Extraoral examination did not reveal any significant findings. Intraorally, generalized gingival edema and erythema were noted (Figure 1.1.1), which were more pronounced on #3 buccal, #8 buccal, #8 palatal, interproximal papilla between #8 and #9, interproximal papilla between #9 and #10, buccal gingival margin and interproximal papillae in mandibular incisors; rolled buccal gingival margins were noted on #3 mesiobuccal and #8 mesiobuccal aspect.

Comprehensive Periodontal Examination

A comprehensive periodontal examination (Figure 1.1.2) revealed localized deep probing depths of 10–12 mm on tooth #3 mesial aspect with grade I mobility and grade II mesiopalatal furcation involvement. Tooth #14 exhibited localized deep probing depths of 7 mm on its distal aspect with grade II distopalatal furcation involvement. Teeth #2, #8, #10, and #15 also exhibited localized probing depths of 5 mm. Teeth #2 and #15 exhibited Class I mesiopalatal furcation involvement. Otherwise, the remaining dentitions exhibited generalized probing depths of 1–4 mm. There was generalized bleeding on probing. Furthermore, localized areas with gingival recession were noted in some posterior teeth.

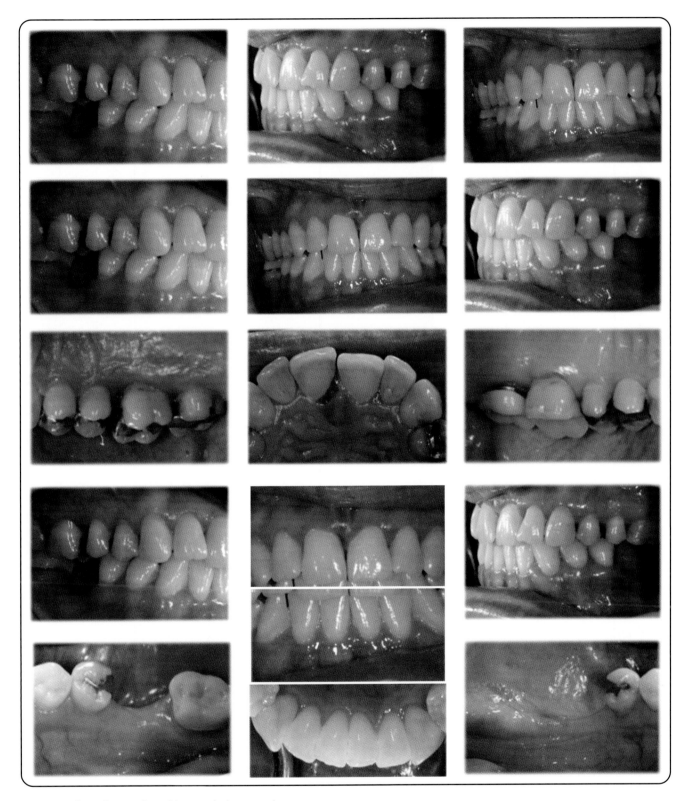

Figure 1.1.1 Complete series of intraoral photographs.

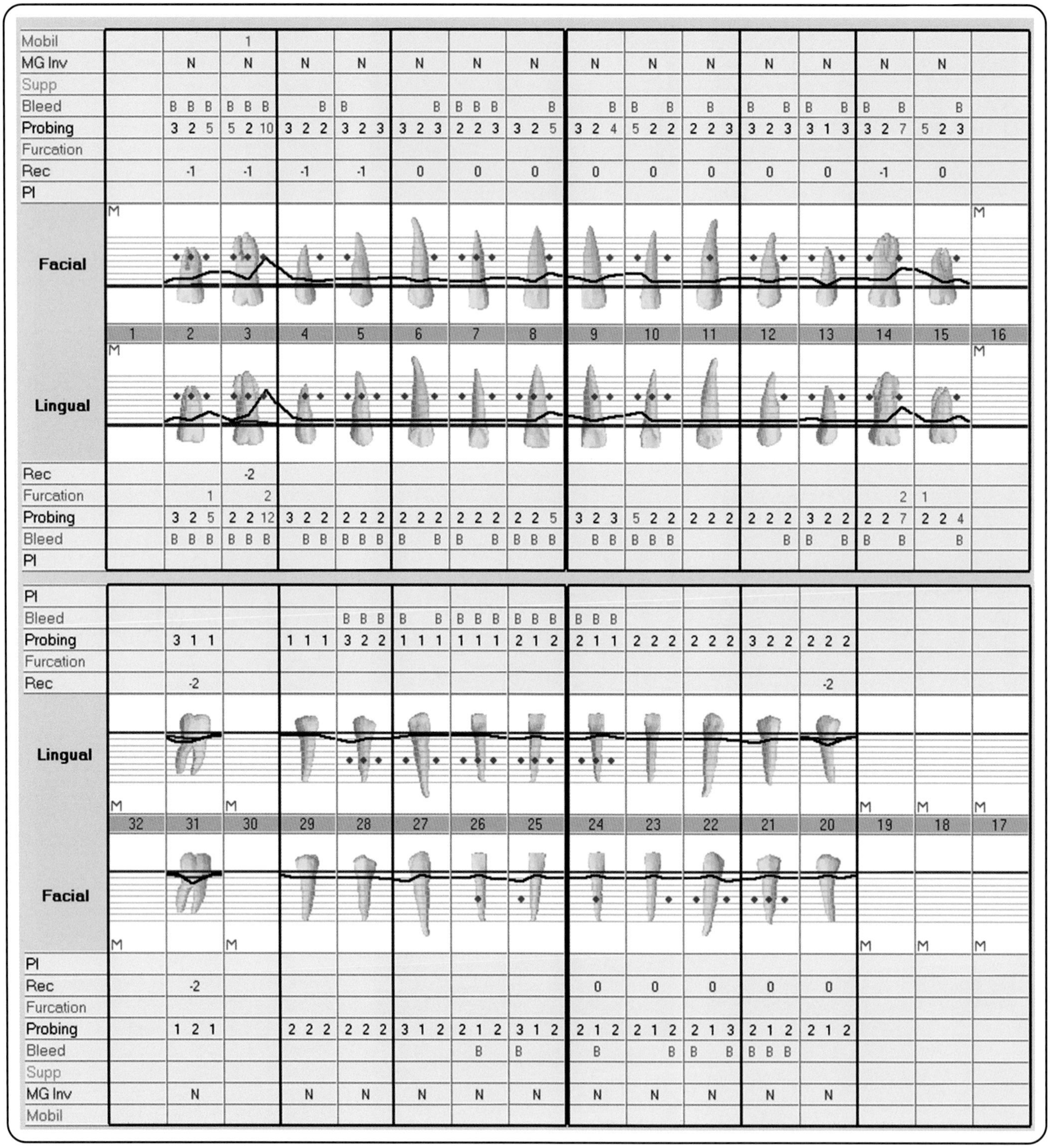

Maxillary arch (teeth 1–16)

	1	2	3	4	5	6	7	8	9	10	11	12	13	14	15	16
Mobil			1													
MG Inv		N	N	N	N	N	N	N	N	N	N	N	N	N	N	
Supp																
Bleed		B B B	B B B	B	B	B	B B B	B		B B	B	B B	B B	B B	B	
Probing		3 2 5	5 2 10	3 2 2	3 2 3	3 2 3	2 2 3	3 2 5	3 2 4	5 2 2	2 2 3	3 2 3	3 1 3	3 2 7	5 2 3	
Furcation																
Rec		-1	-1	-1	-1	0	0	0	0	0	0	0	0	-1	0	
Pl																

Facial

(tooth numbers: 1 2 3 4 5 6 7 8 9 10 11 12 13 14 15 16)

Lingual

	1	2	3	4	5	6	7	8	9	10	11	12	13	14	15	16
Rec			-2													
Furcation		1	2											2	1	
Probing		3 2 5	2 2 12	3 2 2	2 2 2	2 2 2	2 2 2	2 2 5	3 2 3	5 2 2	2 2 2	2 2 2	3 2 2	2 2 7	2 2 4	
Bleed		B B B	B B B	B B	B B B	B	B	B	B B B	B B	B B B		B B	B B	B	
Pl																

Mandibular arch (teeth 32–17)

	32	31	30	29	28	27	26	25	24	23	22	21	20	19	18	17
Pl																
Bleed					B B B	B	B	B B B	B B B	B B B						
Probing		3 1 1		1 1 1	3 2 2	1 1 1	1 1 1	2 1 2	2 1 1	2 2 2	2 2 2	3 2 2	2 2 2			
Furcation																
Rec		-2										-2				

Lingual

(tooth numbers: 32 31 30 29 28 27 26 25 24 23 22 21 20 19 18 17)

Facial

	32	31	30	29	28	27	26	25	24	23	22	21	20	19	18	17
Pl																
Rec		-2							0	0	0	0	0			
Furcation																
Probing		1 2 1		2 2 2	2 2 2	3 1 2	2 1 2	3 1 2	2 1 2	2 1 2	2 1 3	2 1 2	2 1 2			
Bleed							B	B	B		B B	B	B B B			
Supp																
MG Inv		N		N	N	N	N	N	N	N	N	N	N			
Mobil																

Figure 1.1.2 Complete periodontal charting.

Radiographic Examination

A full-mouth series of intraoral radiographs revealed generalized horizontal bone loss (Figure 1.1.3). There was localized moderate horizontal bone loss on teeth #2 and #15. Tooth #3 exhibited vertical bone loss on its mesial aspect while tooth #4 exhibited vertical bone loss on its distal aspect. An open interproximal contact was evident on #3 mesial aspect. Vertical ridge deficiency was noted on edentulous teeth #18, #19 and #30, areas with slight radiolucency indicating possible horizontal ridge deficiency as well.

Diagnosis

According to the 2017 World Workshop on the Classification of Periodontal and Peri-Implant Diseases and Conditions by the American Academy of Periodontology and the European Federation of Periodontology [1], the patient exhibited stage III grade C periodontitis (localized).

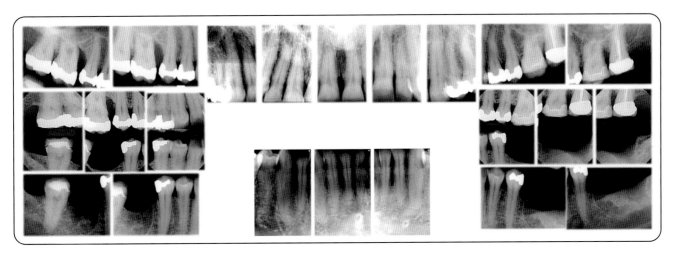

Figure 1.1.3 Complete series of intraoral radiographs.

Self-Study Questions

A. What is the significance of obtaining medical and dental history in treating a patient with periodontal conditions?

B. Aside from conventional parameters such as probing depth, recession, mobility and bleeding on probing, what are the additional parameters that should be obtained during a comprehensive periodontal evaluation?

C. How did we derive periodontal diagnosis for this case of interest?

D. What is the importance of conducting a comprehensive periodontal evaluation for a patient who needs a dental implant?

E. Aside from periodontal charting, are there any other clinical findings that clinicians should record during their routine comprehensive examinations?

Answers located at the end of the chapter.

References

1. Papapanou PN, Sanz M, Buduneli N, et al. Periodontitis: Consensus report of workgroup 2 of the 2017 World Workshop on the Classification of Periodontal and Peri-Implant Diseases and Conditions. *J Periodontol* 2018; 89(Suppl 1):S173–S182.

2. Kwon T, Levin L. Cause-related therapy: a review and suggested guidelines. *Quintessence Int* 2014;45(7):585–591.

3. Eke PI, Wei L, Thornton-Evans GO, et al. Risk indicators for periodontitis in US adults: NHANES 2009 to 2012. *J Periodontol* 2016;87(10):1174–1185.

4. Grossi SG, Zambon JJ, Ho AW, et al. Assessment of risk for periodontal disease. I. Risk indicators for attachment loss. *J Periodontol* 1994;65(3):260–267.

5. Grossi SG, Genco RJ, Machtei EE, et al. Assessment of risk for periodontal disease. II. Risk indicators for alveolar bone loss. *J Periodontol* 1995;66(1):23–29.

6. Loe H, Theilade E, Jensen SB. Experimental gingivitis in man. *J Periodontol* 1965;36:177–187.

7. Hirschfeld L, Wasserman B. A long-term survey of tooth loss in 600 treated periodontal patients. *J Periodontol* 1978;49(5):225–237.

8. McFall WT. Tooth loss in 100 treated patients with periodontal disease. A long-term study. *J Periodontol* 1982;53(9): 539–549.

9. McGuire MK, Nunn ME. Prognosis versus actual outcome. III. The effectiveness of clinical parameters in accurately predicting tooth survival. *J Periodontol* 1996;67(7):666–674.

10. Lang NP, Löe H. The relationship between the width of keratinized gingiva and gingival health. *J Periodontol* 1972;43(10):623–627.

11. Thakur AM, Baburaj MD. Analysis of spontaneous repositioning of pathologically migrated teeth: a clinical and radiographic study. *Quintessence Int* 2014;45(9):733–741.

12. Berglundh T, Armitage G, Araujo MG, et al. Peri-implant diseases and conditions: Consensus report of workgroup 4 of the 2017 World Workshop on the Classification of Periodontal and Peri-Implant Diseases and Conditions. *J Periodontol* 2018;89(Suppl 1):S313–S318.

13. Schwarz F, Derks J, Monje A, Wang H-L. Peri-implantitis. *J Clin Periodontol* 2018;45(Suppl 20):S246–S266.

14. Ferreira SD, Martins CC, Amaral SA, et al. Periodontitis as a risk factor for peri-implantitis: systematic review and meta-analysis of observational studies. *J Dent* 2018;79:1–10.

15. Swierkot K, Lottholz P, Flores-de-Jacoby L, Mengel R. Mucositis, peri-implantitis, implant success, and survival of implants in patients with treated generalized aggressive periodontitis: 3- to 16-year results of a prospective long-term cohort study. *J Periodontol* 2012;83(10):1213–1225.

16. Clark D, Levin L. Dental implant management and maintenance: how to improve long-term implant success? *Quintessence Int* 2016;47(5):417–423.

17. Jepsen S, Caton JG, Albandar JM, et al. Periodontal manifestations of systemic diseases and developmental and acquired conditions: Consensus report of workgroup 3 of the 2017 World Workshop on the Classification of Periodontal and Peri-Implant Diseases and Conditions. *J Periodontol* 2018;89(Suppl 1):S237–S248.

18. Fan J, Caton JG. Occlusal trauma and excessive occlusal forces: narrative review, case definitions, and diagnostic considerations. *J Periodontol* 2018;89(Suppl 1):S214–S222.

19. Cortellini P, Tonetti MS, Lang NP, et al. The simplified papilla preservation flap in the regenerative treatment of deep intrabony defects: clinical outcomes and postoperative morbidity. *J Periodontol* 2001;72(12):1702–1712.

20. Seibert JS. Reconstruction of deformed, partially edentulous ridges, using full thickness onlay grafts. Part II. Prosthetic/periodontal interrelationships. *Compend Contin Educ Dent* 1983;4(6):549–562.

21. Coslet JG, Vanarsdall R, Weisgold A. Diagnosis and classification of delayed passive eruption of the dentogingival junction in the adult. *Alpha Omegan* 1977;70(3):24–28.

22. Mele M, Felice P, Sharma P, et al. Esthetic treatment of altered passive eruption. *Periodontol 2000* 2018;77(1):65–83.

TAKE-HOME POINTS

A. The pathogenesis of periodontal diseases is multifactorial in nature, involving dental plaque, susceptible host, and environmental factors (Figure 1.1.4) [2]. Thus, during medical and dental history-taking, clinicians should obtain information related to these factors.

Susceptible Host

Patients with diabetes may be at greater risk for developing periodontal diseases compared to healthy counterparts, especially when the diabetic condition is not under control (HbA$_{1c}$ >7.0%) [1,3]. If necessary, medical consultation with the patient's physician should be considered. Furthermore, some patients may be susceptible to periodontal diseases genetically. Thus, under family history-taking, the patient should be asked about the periodontal conditions of his or her family members.

Environmental Factor

Cigarette smoking is a risk factor for developing periodontal diseases [1,4,5]. Under social history-

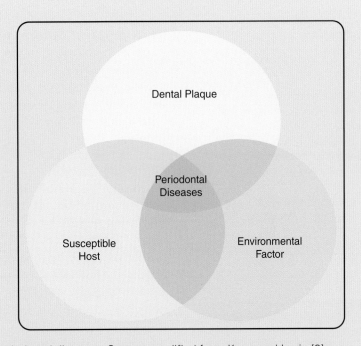

Figure 1.1.4 Pathogenesis of periodontal diseases. Source: modified from Kwon and Levin [2].

taking, the patient should be asked about their smoking habit (i.e. never smoked, past smoker, or active smoker). Smoking habit should be recorded as number of cigarettes consumed per day as well as number of years of active smoking.

Dental Plaque

Dental plaque is the etiologic factor for periodontal diseases [6]. Under dental history-taking, patients should be asked about their routine home oral care or dental plaque control. Their daily frequency of toothbrushing as well as interproximal cleaning (i.e. floss, interdental brush, interdental toothpick) should be recorded. During clinical evaluation, a plaque disclosing tablet may be used to objectively record the patient's plaque control as well. Furthermore, patients should be asked about their previous periodontal treatment as well as its outcome, all of which should be recorded. If necessary, a consultation with the patient's previous dental or periodontal provider may be considered.

B.

Furcation Involvement

According to previous studies, furcated molars have a significantly greater chance to be lost than nonfurcated molars [7–9]. Thus clinicians should proactively evaluate molars (or any other multirooted

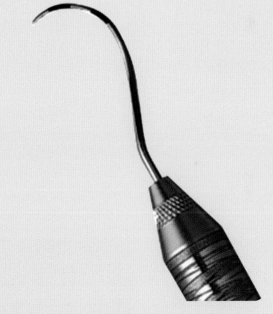

Figure 1.1.5 Nabers probe (Hu-Friedy, IL, USA).

teeth) for furcation involvement, which would ensure their treatment in a timely manner, improving their periodontal prognosis. For easier detection of furcation involvement, a Nabers probe (Figure 1.1.5) may be used instead of a regular periodontal probe.

Glickman's Furcation Classification

Grade I   Incipient suprabony lesion. Radiographic changes are rarely found.

Grade II   Furcation bone loss with a horizontal component. Radiographs may not show bone loss in the furcation.

Grade III A through-and-through lesion that is not clinically visible because it is filled. Radiographs show a radiolucency in the furcation.

Grade IV   A through-and-through lesion that is clinically visible. The soft tissue has receded apically. Radiolucency is clearly visible in the furcation area.

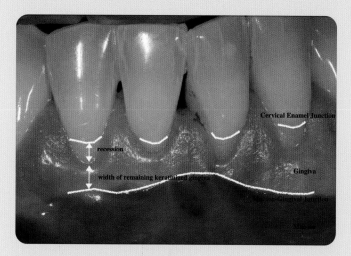

Figure 1.1.6 Mucogingival anatomy.

Mucogingival Deformity

In general, to maintain gingival health (Figure 1.1.6), the presence of at least 2 mm width of remaining keratinized gingiva is preferred [10]. Mucogingival deformity may be recorded as present for any tooth with less than 2 mm width of remaining keratinized gingiva.

Pathologic Migration

A tooth with a significant periodontal breakdown with severe bone loss may undergo pathologic migration (Figure 1.1.7) [11]. In the case presented above, tooth #3 showed evidence of pathologic migration resulting in supraeruption as well as acquired open interproximal contact between tooth #3 and tooth #4. Clinicians should also evaluate any possible acquired pre-mature occlusal contact in these teeth with pathologic migration, resulting in occlusal trauma or fremitus.

C. *Stage* [1] (Tables 1.1.1 and 1.1.2)
The greatest interdental clinical attachment loss of 14 mm (probing depth of 12 mm + gingival recession of 2 mm) was noted on tooth #3 mesiopalatal aspect, with bone loss extending beyond the apical third of the root. Tooth #3, as well as tooth #14 with interdental clinical attachment loss >5 mm, were assigned to stage III. Considering only two of 25 teeth were affected to the same severity, the extent and distribution descriptor "localized" was assigned. *Grade* [1]

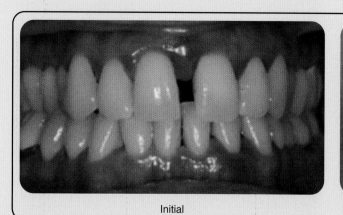
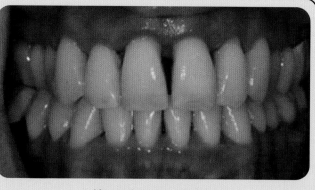

Initial   After periodontal treatment

Figure 1.1.7 Resolution of pathologic migration after successful periodontal treatment, resulting in reduction in acquired diastema between the maxillary central incisors.

Table 1.1.1 Classification of periodontitis based on stages defined by severity (according to the level of interdental clinical attachment loss [CAL], radiographic bone loss and tooth loss), complexity and extent and distribution.

Periodontal stage		Stage I	Stage II	Stage III	Stage IV
Severity	Interdental CAL at site of greatest loss	1–2 mm	3–4 mm	≥5 mm	≥5 mm
	Radiographic bone loss	Coronal third (<15%)	Coronal third (15–33%)	Extending to middle or apical third of root	Extending to middle or apical third of root
	Tooth loss	No tooth loss due to periodontitis		Tooth loss due to periodontitis of ≤4 teeth	Tooth loss due to periodontitis of ≤5 teeth
Complexity	Local	Max. probing depth ≤4 mm Mostly horizontal bone loss	Max. probing depth ≤5 mm Mostly horizontal bone loss	In addition to stage II complexity: • Probing depth ≥6 mm • Vertical bone loss ≥3 mm • Furcation involvement Class II or III • Moderate ridge defect	In addition to stage III complexity, need for complete rehabilitation due to: • Masticatory dysfunction • Secondary occlusal trauma (tooth mobility degree ≥2) • Severe ridge defect • Bite collapse, drifting, flaring • Less than 20 remaining teeth (10 opposing pairs)
Extent and distribution	Add to stage as descriptor	For each stage, describe extent as localized (<30% of teeth involved), generalized, or molar/incisor pattern			

Source: Papapanou et al. [1].

Table 1.1.2 Classification of periodontitis based on grades that reflect biologic features of the disease including evidence of, or risk for, rapid progression, and anticipated treatment response, and systemic health.

Periodontitis grade			Grade A: slow rate of progression	Grade B: moderate rate of progression	Grade C: rapid rate of progression
Primary criteria	Direct evidence of progression	Longitudinal data (radiographic bone loss or CAL)	Evidence of no loss over 5 years	<2 mm over 5 years	≥2 mm over 5 years
	Indirect evidence of progression	% bone loss/age	<0.25	0.25–1.0	≥1.0
		Case phenotype	Heavy biofilm deposits with low levels of destruction	Destruction commensurate with biofilm deposits	Destruction exceeds expectation given biofilm deposits; specific clinical patterns suggestive of periods of rapid progression and/or early-onset disease (e.g. molar/incisor pattern, lack of expected response to standard bacterial control therapies)
Grade modifiers	Risk factors	Smoking	Nonsmoker	Smoker <10 cigarettes/day	Smoker ≥10 cigarettes/day
		Diabetes	Normoglycemic/no diagnosis of diabetes	HbA_{1c} <7.0% in patients with diabetes	HbA_{1c} ≥7.0% in patients with diabetes

Source: Papapanou et al. [1].

As direct evidence of progression was not available, indirect evidence was used instead. The percentage bone loss/age was calculated as follows: 80% of alveolar bone loss on #3/44 years old = 1.82. Thus, grade C was assigned.

D. According to the latest 2017 World Workshop on the topic of peri-implantitis [12,13], there is strong evidence indicating a higher risk of peri-implantitis development in patients who have a history of periodontitis, poor oral plaque control, and lack of regular periodontal maintenance therapy after implant placement. Furthermore, patients with active periodontal diseases or deep periodontal pockets may be at greater risk of developing peri-implant diseases than periodontally healthy patients [14,15]. Thus, prior to proceeding with dental implant therapy, clinicians should carefully examine the periodontal conditions carefully and ensure that the patient does not have any active periodontal diseases. Oral hygiene habits need to be developed and meticulous home care abilities should be achieved prior to dental implant planning [16].

E. Clinical signs of occlusal trauma are often overlooked by clinicians; however, the following findings can provide valuable diagnostic information and help formulate the proper treatment plan for patients. According to the 2017 World Workshop on Classification of Periodontal and Peri-Implant Diseases and Conditions on the topic of occlusal trauma [17], the following list of clinical/radiographic indicators could help identify occlusal trauma: fremitus, progression of mobility, occlusal discrepancies, wear facets, tooth migration, fractured tooth, thermal sensitivity, discomfort/pain on chewing, widening PDL space, root resorption, and cemental tear (Figure 1.1.8). It is important to understand that occlusal trauma by itself does not initiate periodontitis; however, there is evidence suggesting that it alters progression of the disease when combined with dental plaque [18]. It is also important to perform proper occlusal analysis when performing

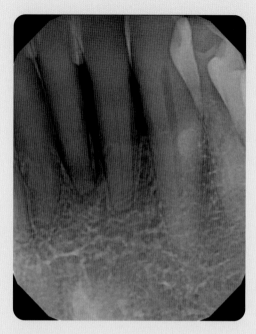

Figure 1.1.8 Cemental tear on tooth #24 resulting in localized alveolar bone loss and increase in mobility. Secondary occlusal trauma was noted during clinical evaluation.

regenerative periodontal surgery, as there evidence to support the view that tooth mobility plays a role in the regenerative outcome [19].

Edentulous alveolar ridge width/height should be recorded during the initial comprehensive examination [20]. This would ensure proper execution of dental implant therapy (implant size selection, depth/angulation of implant fixture, distance between adjacent tooth and implant, prosthetic emergence profile, screw vs. cement retained prosthesis and prosthetic occlusal form).

Esthetic plastic periodontal therapy is also a component of periodontal specialty; therefore, proper documentation of the patient's smile line (low, average, high) and gingival margin harmony plays a crucial role in treatment planning. When a patient presents with high smile line, it is important to determine the main causative reason (altered passive eruption, vertical maxillary excess, hypermobile lip or combination) [21,22].

Case 2

Dental Plaque-Induced Gingivitis

CASE STORY

A 27-year-old Caucasian male presented with the chief complaint of "My gums bleed when I brush my teeth." The patient noticed blood in the gingiva whenever he brushed or flossed (A). There had never been any swelling or pain associated with his gums, and the patient had never had an episode like this before. The patient claimed to brush his teeth once daily, and he flossed two to three times a wee k (B).

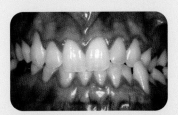

Figure 1.2.1 Preoperative presentation (frontal view).

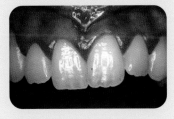

Figure 1.2.2 Preoperative frontal view of maxillary anteriors.

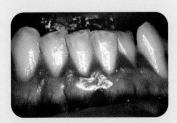

Figure 1.2.3 Preoperative frontal view of mandibular anteriors.

LEARNING GOALS AND OBJECTIVES

- To be able to diagnose gingivitis
- To identify the possible etiology for the same condition and to address them
- To understand the importance of oral hygiene in preventing gingivitis

Medical History

There were no significant medical problems. On questioning, the patient stated he was taking no medications and he had no allergies.

Review of Systems

- Vital signs
  - Blood pressure: 120/65 mmHg
  - Pulse rate: 72 beats/minute (regular)
  - Respiratory rate: 15 breaths/minute

Social History

The patient did not drink alcohol. He did smoke (started at age 23 and currently smoked half a pack of cigarettes daily).

Extraoral Examination

No significant findings. The patient had no masses or swelling, and the temporomandibular joint was within normal limits.

Intraoral Examination

- The soft tissues of the mouth (except gingiva) including the tongue appeared normal.
- A gingival examination revealed a mild marginal erythema, with rolled margins and swollen papillae (Figures 1.2.1–1.2.3).
- A hard tissue and soft tissue examination were completed (Figure 1.2.4) (F).

Occlusion

There were no occlusal discrepancies or interferences.

Radiographic Examination

A full-mouth set of radiographs was ordered (G). (See Figure 1.2.5 for the patient's bitewing radiographs.)

Diagnosis

After reviewing the history and both the clinical and radiographic examinations, a differential diagnosis was generated (H).

Treatment Plan

The treatment plan of the periodontal problems for this patient included an initial phase of scaling with polishing and a six-week reevaluation.

Treatment

The patient received a scaling and polishing. At the six-week reevaluation, the clinical signs and symptoms had not improved, even though the patient claimed to be practicing excellent oral hygiene as per the instructions (I).

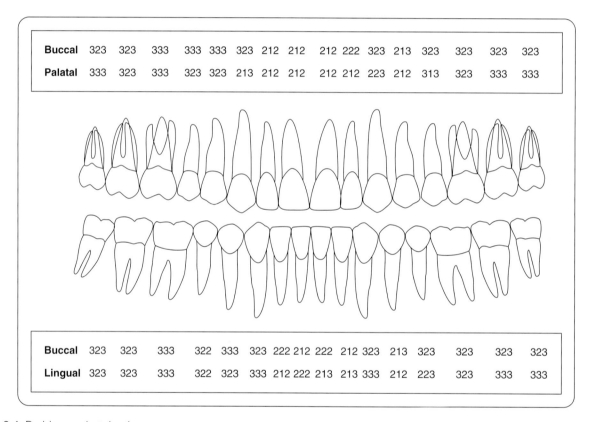

Buccal	323	323	333	333	333	323	212	212	212	222	323	213	323	323	323	323
Palatal	333	323	333	323	323	213	212	212	212	212	223	212	313	323	333	333

Buccal	323	323	333	322	333	323	222	212	222	212	323	213	323	323	323	323
Lingual	323	323	333	322	323	333	212	222	213	213	333	212	223	323	333	333

Figure 1.2.4 Probing pocket depth measurements.

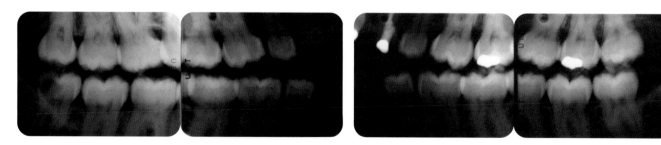

Figure 1.2.5 Bitewing radiographs depicting the interproximal bone levels.

Discussion

In dental plaque-induced gingivitis, the inflammation is confined to the gingiva without attachment or bone loss, making it a reversible condition (with treatment). Gingivitis can also occur on a reduced but healthy periodontium. Reduced but healthy periodontium is when there is attachment loss due to past non-periodontitis cause (e.g. gingival recession) or due to past history of periodontitis and/or its treatment but currently exhibiting shallow sulci (J). A thorough history and periodontal examination must be completed to arrive at a diagnosis. Other characteristic features associated with dental plaque-induced gingivitis include the presence of plaque at the gingival margin, increased gingival exudate, and bleeding on probing (K). With good plaque control, the condition should resolve [1]. If there is a medical concern, it is typically identified by obtaining a thorough medical history. Conditions such as diabetes and leukemia have a profound effect on gingival health, and therefore the patient must be evaluated accordingly. In women, hormonal changes, such as those that occur during the onset of puberty, pregnancy, or menstruation, have a transient effect on the gingival inflammatory status of these patients [2], which when combined with poor plaque control will lead to severe gingivitis [3,4]. After a diagnosis is reached, the treatment plan will include oral hygiene instructions, an initial phase of treatment (scaling or scaling and root planing) with a four- to six-week reevaluation. If the symptoms persist at this visit (despite an improvement in the patient's oral hygiene), the patient should be referred to a physician to rule out any potential systemic conditions that might cause bleeding.

Self-Study Questions

A. How are gingival diseases classified in the 2017 Periodontal Disease Classification?

B. What are the "ideal" brushing/flossing habits and techniques for a patient?

C. What effects can smoking have on the periodontium? On the oral cavity?

D. How would you perform an oral cancer screening?

E. What are the components of a periodontal examination?

F. What information should be recorded on a periodontal or soft tissue charting?

G. What kind of radiographs should be ordered for a periodontal examination?

H. What are the components that make one diagnose a case as gingivitis versus periodontitis?

I. What should a practitioner do in the case where gingival/periodontal symptoms have not resolved despite the prescribed dental care?

J. What are the different clinical situations gingivitis can manifest?

K. What are the common signs and symptoms of dental plaque-induced gingivitis?

Answers located at the end of the chapter.

References

1. Mariotti A. Dental plaque-induced gingival diseases. *Ann Periodontol* 1999;4:7–17.
2. Mariotti A. Sex steroid hormones and cell dynamics in the periodontium. *Crit Rev Oral Biol Med* 1994;5:27–53.
3. Hugoson A. Gingivitis in pregnant women. A longitudinal clinical study. *Odontologisk Revy* 1971;22:25–42.
4. Löe H. Periodontal changes in pregnancy. *J Periodontol* 1965;36:209–216.
5. Chapple ILC, Mealey BL, Van Dyke TE, et al. Periodontal health and gingival diseases and conditions on an intact and a reduced periodontium: Consensus report of workgroup 1 of the 2017 World Workshop on the Classification of Periodontal and Peri-Implant Diseases and Conditions. *J Periodontol* 2018;89(Suppl 1):S74–S84.
6. Moran JM, Addy M, Newcombe RG. A comparative study of stain removal with two electric toothbrushes and a manual brush. *J Clin Dent* 1995;6(4):188–193.
7. Tritten CB, Armitage GC. Comparison of a sonic and a manual toothbrush for efficacy in supragingival plaque removal and reduction of gingivitis. *J Clin Periodontol* 1996;23:641–648.
8. Grossi SG, Zambon JJ, Ho AW, et al. Assessment of risk for periodontal disease. I. Risk indicators for attachment loss. *J Periodontol* 1994;65:260–267.
9. Mullally B, Breen B, Linden GJ. Smoking and patterns of bone loss in early-onset periodontitis. *J Periodontol* 1999;70:394–401.
10. Rose LF, Mealy BL (eds). *Periodontics: Medicine, Surgery, and Implants.* St. Louis, MO: Mosby, 2004:871.
11. Blot WJ, McLaughlin JK, Winn DM, et al. Smoking and drinking in relation to oral and pharyngeal cancers. *Cancer Res* 1988;48:3282–3287.
12. Neville BW, Damm DD, Allen C, Bouquot J. *Oral and Maxillofacial Pathology*, 2nd edn. Philadelphia, PA: Lippincott, 2005:356–362.

TAKE-HOME POINTS

A. Based on the 2017 periodontal disease classification, gingival diseases are broadly classified into those that are dental plaque induced and those that are not [5].

Dental plaque-induced gingival diseases
A. Associated with plaque alone
B. Mediated by systemic or local risk factors
 • Systemic factors (e.g. smoking, diabetes, puberty, pregnancy, hematologic conditions)
 • Local factors (e.g. plaque-retentive restorative margins, dry mouth)
C. Medication-induced gingival enlargement

Non-plaque-induced gingival diseases
A. Genetic disorders (hereditary gingival fibromatosis)
B. Infections (e.g. herpes simplex, *Neisseria gonorrhoeae*, human papillomavirus, candidosis)
C. Inflammatory and immune conditions (contact allergy, pemphigus, lichen planus, sarcoidosis)
D. Reactive processes (epulis, peripheral giant cell granuloma)
E. Neoplasms: premalignant (leukoplakia) and malignant (squamous cell carcinoma) conditions
F. Endocrine, nutritional and metabolic diseases (vitamin C deficiency)
G. Traumatic lesions (chemical or thermal burns)

Questions to help develop a differential diagnosis include the following:
• How often do you brush or floss?
• Do you bruise easily?
• When you wake up do you notice any blood in your mouth?
• When you cut yourself, do you tend to clot within a normal amount of time?
• What medicines are you taking currently?
• Are you pregnant (for female patients)?
• Are you a mouth breather? Do you have difficulty breathing through your nose?

B. A patient should ideally brush twice daily and floss once daily. Evidence indicates that use of rotary brushes is better than manual brushes for interproximal plaque removal and stain removal [6,7]. A toothbrush with soft bristles is strongly recommended. The bristles should be positioned at a 45-degree angle to the junction of the tooth and marginal gingiva, and then the brushing should be initiated using short circular gentle motions (Bass method of brushing). The same technique should be repeated for the rest of the mouth. If a patient has gingival recession, coronal sweeping motion of bristles from the gingiva to the teeth is recommended to prevent the progression of recession (modified Stillman's technique).

C. Smoking has been identified as an important risk factor for periodontitis [8]. The number of cigarettes an individual smokes per day and the number of years an individual has been smoking are two important parameters strongly associated with the degree of attachment loss [9]. It is well established that smoking affects the host immune response, causes local tissue ischemia, and also alters the bacterial profile, shifting the plaque ecology and increasing the periodontal pathogens in the host [10]. This risk factor is "behavioral" and can be modified. Smoking causes an increased risk for oral and throat cancers [11]. Oral cancer is the sixth most common cancer in males and the twelfth most common cancer in women in the United States [12].

D. A thorough extraoral examination should be conducted. Visualization and palpation of the soft tissues of the head and neck should be completed including palpation of the muscles and lymph nodes. The intraoral examination should consist of visualization and palpation of the tongue. The tongue represents the most common site (50%) for oral cancer, and the ventral and lateral surfaces (20%) in particular have a higher predilection for cancer than the dorsal surface of the tongue (4%) [12]. The floor of the mouth is the second most common site for oral cancer, and therefore careful examination of this area of the mouth should be a part of cancer screening. Other areas that should be examined specifically for oral cancer include the soft palate, gingiva, and buccal and labial mucosa [12].

E. A periodontal examination includes visually assessing and recording the gingival color, contour, consistency, texture, presence or absence of exudates from sulcus, and bleeding on probing. Six probing depths (mesiobuccal, midbuccal, distobuccal, mesiolingual, midlingual, and distolingual) per tooth should be recorded. Areas of recession, mobility, and furcation involvement are also recorded and graded according to the established classifications for each of these parameters. In addition, the width of the keratinized gingiva for each tooth is recorded. Radiographs and study models are also important because they offer valuable information that is not obtained from the clinical oral examination.

F. The following are essential components of a periodontal chart:
- Name of the patient and the date of recording.
- Missing teeth should be recorded.
- Probing pocket depth: measured on six surfaces of each tooth in the mouth using a periodontal probe.
- Degree of recession: measured using a periodontal probe.
- Mobility: measured using two flat ends of dental instruments such as dental mirror and/or periodontal probe and pushing the teeth with one instrument against the second instrument.
- Fremitus: assessed by placing the inner pad of the fingers on the gingiva of the teeth in question and asking the patient to tap teeth three or four times. In traumatic occlusion, fremitus is usually felt by the examiner's fingers, which is then recorded.
- Degree of furcation involvement: examined using Naber's probe.
- Mucogingival complex: the width of the mucogingival complex (keratinized gingiva) should be measured from the gingival margin to the apical-most part of the attached gingiva in every tooth, using a periodontal probe, and recorded.

G. Radiographs form an essential component of a periodontal examination. Apart from providing information about the supporting hard tissue apparatus of the tooth in question, other valuable information such as root length, root form, periapical lesions, and root proximity can be ascertained. The American Dental Association recommends taking a full-mouth set of radiographs for a full diagnosis (typically every five years). A set of four bitewings should be exposed every two years. The diagnosis of periodontal disease can be made using clinical findings and radiographic findings provided by periapical radiographs and bitewing radiographs. Bitewing radiographs are the most diagnostic for reading bone height because the head of the X-ray tube is perpendicular to the film. Vertical bitewings are recommended for areas with extensive bone loss. In general, paralleling technique is recommended over bisecting angle technique because it reduces the errors associated with film angulations.

H. Clinical attachment loss (CAL) (distance from the cementoenamel junction to the base of a periodontal pocket) and bone loss as seen on a radiograph are the gold standards used to help distinguish a patient with periodontitis versus gingivitis. Patients with gingivitis do not exhibit CAL and bone loss (radiographically) making it a reversible condition (with treatment), whereas if the diseases progresses to periodontitis, CAL and bone loss are characteristically observed.

I. Referral to a physician should be made to rule out any systemic conditions.

J. Gingivitis can occur on an intact periodontium, a reduced periodontium due to non-periodontitis causes (mainly gingival recession induced) or a reduced periodontium induced by periodontitis (but successfully treated).

K. The clinical signs of gingivitis include bleeding on probing, swelling, redness and sensitivity to probing. The symptoms include bleeding gums, pain, halitosis, unesthetic appearance, and difficulty in consuming food.

Case 3

Non-Plaque-Induced Gingivitis

CASE STORY

A 41-year-old Latin American female presented with a chief complaint of "My gums and teeth are sensitive." She had been referred by her general dentist for periodontal treatment. She reported a five-year history of gingival sensitivity and progressive gingival recession. She experienced lingering pain after drinking hot and cold liquids and also noted sensitivity when brushing.

LEARNING GOALS AND OBJECTIVES

- To distinguish desquamative gingivitis from plaque-induced gingivitis
- To formulate a differential diagnosis for common causes of desquamative gingivitis
- To develop a definitive diagnosis and properly manage a patient with desquamative gingivitis

Medical History

The patient denied a significant medical history. The patient had been seeing a primary care physician annually for physical examination. She did not take any medications and she had no known drug allergies.

Review of Systems

- Vital signs
  - Blood pressure: 120/70 mmHg
  - Pulse rate: 78 beats/minute
  - Respiratory rate: 15 breaths/minute

Dental History

The patient had received sporadic general dental care and orthodontics in Brazil and was unsure if the city water she had consumed in her childhood was fluoridated. She had received dental care more regularly since moving to the United States 13 years ago. She had her teeth cleaned twice yearly. She reported that her teeth and gums were very sensitive and that local anesthesia was often needed during her cleanings.

Social History

The patient had been born and raised in Brazil and had moved to the United States when she was 28 years old. She was married and had two daughters. She worked as a housecleaner. The patient consumed one to three alcohol drinks per week and denied the use of tobacco products.

Family History

Both of the patient's parents resided in Brazil and were in good health. She had one brother who lived in the United States and was also in good health. The patient was unaware of any dental problems in the members of her immediate family.

Extraoral Examination

The patient had no detectable lesions, masses, or swelling. The temporomandibular joint was within normal limits.

Intraoral Examination

- The buccal mucosa adjacent to the mandibular third molars demonstrated diffuse white reticulation.
- Generalized gingival erythema was present with desquamation of the maxillary and mandibular anterior gingiva (Figure 1.3.1).

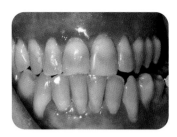

Figure 1.3.1 Frontal view.

Hard Tissue Examination

- The patient had several restorations in her posterior dentition. All of the restorations appeared clinically and radiographically sound.
- No carious lesions were detected.

Periodontal Examination

- The periodontal examination revealed probing depths of 1–4 mm with generalized bleeding on probing.
- There was diffuse gingival erythema with varying degrees of mucosal sloughing and erosion.
- There was generalized mild to moderate gingival recession on the facial and lingual/palatal surfaces of her teeth.
- The patient had mild plaque accumulations on her posterior teeth.

Occlusion

- The patient had class III occlusion with an open bite on the posterior left side.

Radiographic Examination

- A full-mouth set of radiographs was taken.
- No carious lesions were detected.

- There was generalized mild horizontal bone loss.
- There were no other pathologic findings noted.

Diagnosis

Following review of the history and clinical evaluation, a clinical diagnosis of *desquamative gingivitis* was rendered.

Treatment Plan

The patient received a dental scaling with oral hygiene instructions. The treatment of her desquamative gingivitis will be determined after a definitive diagnosis is established.

Discussion

Desquamative gingivitis is not a definitive diagnosis but a clinical term referring to the manifestation of a variety of underlying conditions. To arrive at a definitive diagnosis, a tissue biopsy is required. In this case, punch biopsies of the gingiva and buccal mucosa were performed and submitted for pathologic evaluation. One sample was placed in 10% formalin for hematoxylin and eosin staining and the second in Michel's medium for direct immunofluorescence studies. The pathology report was signed out as oral lichen planus (LP).

After the diagnosis was established, the patient was prescribed a topical corticosteroid (fluocinonide gel 0.05%) and instructed to apply it two to three times daily. The patient returned after two weeks of treatment with improvement of gingival erythema. The patient was informed that because there is no cure for her condition, the medication would need to be reapplied whenever she became symptomatic.

Self-Study Questions

A. How are non-plaque-induced gingival lesions classified?

B. What is desquamative gingivitis, and how does it differ from plaque-induced gingivitis?

C. What is the differential diagnosis for desquamative gingivitis?

D. How is desquamative diagnosis managed?

E. What is the presentation and prevalence of oral LP?

F. How is a diagnosis of oral LP rendered?

G. What is the etiology of oral LP?

H. What are the histopathologic features of oral LP?

I. How is oral LP managed?

J. What is the long-term prognosis for oral LP?

Answers located at the end of the chapter.

References

1. Holmstrup P, Plemons J, Meyle J. Non-plaque induced gingival diseases. *J Periodontol* 2018;89(Suppl 1):S9–S16.
2. American Academy of Periodontology Position Paper. Oral features of mucocutaneous disorders. *J Periodontol* 2003;74:1545–1556.
3. Lo Russo L, Fierro G, Guiglia R, et al. Epidemiology of desquamative gingivitis: evaluation of 125 patients and review of the literature. *Int J Dermatol* 2009;48:1049–1052.
4. Leao JC, Ingafou M, Khan A, et al. Desquamative gingivitis: retrospective analysis of disease associations of a large cohort. *Oral Dis* 2008;14(6):556–560.
5. Guiglia R, Di Liberto C, Pizzo G, et al. A combined treatment regimen for desquamative gingivitis in patients with oral lichen planus. *J Oral Pathol Med* 2007;36(2):110–116.
6. Chams-Davatchi D, Valikhani M, Daneshpazhooh M, et al. Pemphigus: analysis of 1209 cases. *Int J Dermatol* 2005;44:470–476.
7. Eisen D. The evaluation of cutaneous, genital, scalp, nail, esophageal, and ocular involvement in patients with oral lichen planus. *Oral Surg Oral Med Oral Pathol Oral Radiol Endod* 1999;88(4):431–436.
8. Scully C, Almeida OPD, Welbury R. Oral lichen planus in childhood. *Br J Dermatol* 1994;130:131–133.
9. Scully C, Beyli M, Ferreiro MC, et al. Update on oral lichen planus: etiopathogenesis and management. *Crit Rev Oral Biol Med* 1998;9:86–122.
10. Eisen D. The clinical manifestations and treatment of oral lichen planus. *Dermatol Clin* 2003;21(1):79–89.
11. Ingafou M, Leao JC, Porter SR, et al. Oral lichen planus: a retrospective study of 690 British patients. *Oral Dis* 2006;12:463–468.
12. Neville BW, Damm DD, Allen C, Chi A. *Oral and Maxillofacial Pathology*, 4th edn. St. Louis, MO: Elsevier, 2016:317–320.
13. Eversole LR. Immunopathology of oral mucosal ulcerative, desquamative and bullous diseases. *Oral Surg Oral Med Oral Pathol* 1994;77:555–571.
14. Holmstrup P, Schiøtz AW, Westergaard J. Effect of dental plaque control on gingival lichen planus. *Oral Surg Oral Med Oral Pathol* 1990;69:585–590.
15. Fitzpatrick SG, Hirsch SA, Gordon SC. The malignant transformation of oral lichen planus and oral lichenoid lesions. *J Am Dent Assoc* 2014;145(1):45–56.
16. Aghbari SMH, Abushouk AI, Attia A, et al. Malignant transformation of oral lichen planus and oral lichenoid lesions: a meta-analysis of 20095 patient data. *Oral Oncol* 2017;68:92–102.

TAKE-HOME POINTS

A. According to the 2017 World Workshop on the Classification of Periodontal and Peri-Implant Diseases and Conditions, the etiology of the non-plaque-induced gingival lesions can be divided into several categories [1]. It should be emphasized that even though the direct cause of the lesions in these cases is not plaque, the severity of the inflammation often depends on the interaction with the bacterial plaque present.

- Genetic/developmental disorders (e.g. hereditary gingival fibromatosis)
- Specific infections (e.g. bacterial, viral, fungal)
- Inflammatory and immune conditions and lesions (e.g. hypersensitivity reactions, autoimmune diseases of skin and mucous membranes, granulomatous inflammatory conditions)
- Reactive processes (e.g. epulides)
- Neoplasms (e.g. premalignant, malignant)
- Endocrine, nutritional, and metabolic diseases (e.g. vitamin deficiencies)
- Traumatic lesions (e.g. physical/mechanical insults, chemical [toxic] insults, thermal insults)
- Gingival pigmentation

Arriving at a specific diagnosis may be a complex process and requires taking a detailed history along with the specific clinical presentation of a particular patient.

B. Desquamative gingivitis (DG) is a clinical term used to describe a condition characterized by intense erythema, desquamation, and/or ulceration of the gingiva [2]. A variety of different conditions can manifest as DG, but it is most often associated with one of the vesiculoerosive diseases (see answer to Question C).

Plaque-induced gingivitis is a response to inadequate oral hygiene practices and generally presents with inflammation at the gingival margin. This inflammation often causes the tissue to become erythematous and edematous. There is commonly bleeding on probing and an increase in gingival crevicular fluid or exudate. The clinical signs and symptoms of plaque-induced gingivitis are usually reversed after removing the primary etiology of bacteria-laden plaque. Refer to Chapter 1, Case 2 for a detailed description of plaque-induced gingivitis.

C. DG may be a manifestation of multiple dermatologic conditions, most commonly LP, mucous membrane pemphigoid, or pemphigus vulgaris [3]. Other conditions that can present as DG include linear immunoglobulin A disease, dermatomyositis, or mixed connective tissue disease [4]. Once a clinical diagnosis of DG is rendered, a definitive diagnosis must be established.

D. Regardless of the underlying cause of DG, it has been shown that improved oral hygiene can decrease the severity of the lesions [5]. However, this will not bring about complete resolution and, more importantly, does not address the underlying cause. A biopsy of the lesion must be taken to establish a definitive diagnosis. The biopsy should include intact epithelium because the center of an ulcer histologically reveals only nonspecific granulation tissue. A second specimen submitted for immunofluorescence studies may aid in the diagnosis.

The symptoms of DG are managed based on the underlying cause of the condition. In most cases, the oral lesions themselves may be managed with topical corticosteroids. A common first line of treatment is 0.05% fluocinonide gel, which may be applied to the lesions four times daily. This may be delivered directly to the gingiva or, in the case of diffuse gingival involvement, placed in a custom-fabricated tray comparable to a bleaching tray typically used for tooth whitening. Alternatively, a dexamethasone elixir may be prescribed for patients to swish and expectorate three times daily. It is important to monitor the patients for signs of oral candidiasis that may develop in the setting of steroid use.

Patients diagnosed with mucous membrane pemphigoid should be referred to an ophthalmologist who is familiar with the ocular lesions of this condition to guard against vision loss. Although corticosteroid therapy has helped to reduce the mortality rate associated with pemphigus vulgaris to less than 10% [6], patients with this diagnosis should be evaluated by their primary care physicians or dermatologists for the evaluation of cutaneous lesions.

E. Oral LP is one of the most common mucocutaneous diseases manifesting on the gingiva. Oral involvement alone is common; concomitant skin lesions develop in patients with oral lesions in approximately 15% of cases [7]. Most patients who present with oral LP are middle aged. Children are rarely affected [8]. A predilection for women is shown in most series of cases by a ratio of 3 : 2 over men. The prevalence of oral LP in various populations has been found to be 0.1–4% [9].

Different classifications have been used for oral LP, and a recent classification groups lesions into three categories: reticular, atrophic, and ulcerated [10]. The reticular form is most common and often goes unnoticed by the patient. It generally involves the posterior buccal mucosa bilaterally, but any area of the oral mucosa may be affected. Reticular LP is named because of its characteristic pattern of interlacing white lines (Wickham striae). Erosive/erythematous and ulcerated LP are less common but more significant for the patient because the lesions are usually symptomatic. The periphery is usually bordered by the fine white radiating striae of reticular LP. Erythema with or without ulcers involving the gingiva are characteristic features of DG.

F. The most characteristic clinical manifestations of oral LP are white interlacing white striae appearing bilaterally on the posterior buccal mucosa [11]. A diagnosis of reticular LP can often be made based on simply the clinical presentation of the lesions. Erosive and ulcerated LP can be more challenging to diagnose based on clinical features alone. Unilateral lesions or presentations lacking typical radiating white striae may be difficult to distinguish from other ulcerative or erosive diseases. If the diagnosis is in question after clinical examination, a biopsy is necessary to confirm a diagnosis.

G. The etiology of most oral LP cases is idiopathic. Oral lichenoid lesions can also be associated with various types of medications including nonsteroidal anti-inflammatory drugs, antihypertensive agents, antimalarials, gold salts, and penicillamine [12]. Unilateral oral lichenoid lesions are rare and may be secondary to contact with amalgam dental restorations.

H. Oral LP presents histologically with varying degrees of orthokeratosis and/or parakeratosis. There is disruption of the basal cells and transmigration of T lymphocytes into the basal and parabasal cell layers of the epithelium. Degenerating keratinocytes termed *Civatte bodies* (colloid bodies) are often found at the junction of the epithelium and connective tissue. There is typically a subepithelial bandlike accumulation of T lymphocytes and macrophages characteristic of a type IV hypersensitivity reaction [13] (Figure 1.3.2). These features are characteristic but not specific to oral LP. Other interface processes including lupus erythematosus and chronic ulcerative stomatitis have similar histopathologic presentations.

I. Reticular LP often causes no symptoms and need not be treated. The first line of treatment for symptomatic erosive LP is topical corticosteroids. Fluocinonide gel applied to the most symptomatic areas or dexamethasone elixir used as a mouth rinse up to four times per day is often sufficient to induce healing within one to two weeks. Patients should be informed that the lesions will likely return and the corticosteroids should be reapplied. Patients should be monitored for their response and for the possibility of candidiasis induced by use of the steroids. Another important part of the therapeutic regimen in

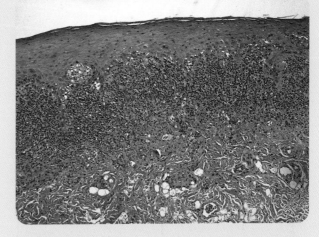

Figure 1.3.2 Characteristic histopathology of lichen planus demonstrates parakeratinized and/or orthokeratinized stratified squamous epithelium with sawtooth-shaped rete ridges, squamatization of basal cells, and a bandlike infiltrate of lymphocytes in the superficial connective tissue.

patients with DG is meticulous plaque control, which results in significant improvement in many patients [14].

J. LP is a chronic condition with lesions that wax and wane over time. The erosive form should be monitored and treated as necessary to improve patient comfort. There has long been controversy over the malignant potential of LP. Recent studies suggest malignant transformation appears to be more common in older females, often with erythematous LP, and the rate has been reported to range from 0.9 to 1.1% [15,16].

Case 4

Gingival Enlargement

Medical History
The patient was diagnosed with epilepsy 13 years ago. Since that time she has been taking Dilantin 500 mg daily, and currently in addition 2000 mg Depakote daily (1000 mg b.i.d.) and 10 mg Zyprexa at bedtime. There were no other significant medical problems and the patient had no known allergies.

Social History
The patient did not smoke or drink alcohol.

Extraoral and Intraoral Examinations
- There were no significant findings on extraoral examination. The patient had no masses or swelling and the temporomandibular joint was within normal limits.
- With the exception of the gingiva, the soft tissues of the mouth including the tongue appeared normal.
- Examination of the gingiva revealed generalized marginal erythema, edema, rolled margins, enlarged papillae, and bleeding on probing (Figures 1.4.1 and 1.4.2). Probing depths ranged from 2 to 5 mm (pseudo-pockets due to gingival enlargement; Figure 1.4.3).
- The hard tissue examination found multiple restorations.

Occlusion
Angle class II, division 2 occlusion with tooth #12 in crossbite due to arch incongruence.

Radiographic Examination
A full-mouth set of radiographs revealed normal levels of alveolar bone throughout the mouth including the maxillary and mandibular anterior where clinical gingival enlargement was present (Figure 1.4.4).

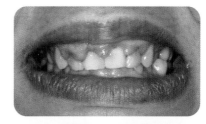

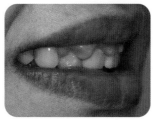
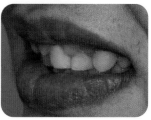

Figure 1.4.1 Initial presentation of a patient with phenytoin-induced gingival enlargement: smile frontal, right, and left views.

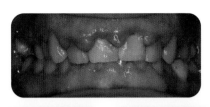

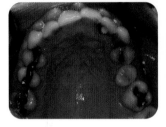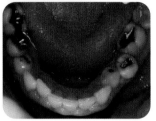

Figure 1.4.2 Initial presentation of a patient with phenytoin-induced gingival enlargement: buccal view in occlusion, maxilla and mandible occlusal views. Note that gingival enlargement is localized to anterior and facial segments on both maxilla and mandible.

Diagnosis

After reviewing the history and the clinical and radiographic examinations, the patient was diagnosed with phenytoin-associated drug-influenced gingival enlargement and a differential diagnosis was generated (A).

Treatment Plan

The treatment plan for the phenytoin-associated gingival enlargement includes interdisciplinary consultation (to include the primary care physician regarding alternative medication for treatment of epilepsy), oral hygiene instructions, initial phase therapy consisting of supragingival and subgingival scaling with polishing, reevaluation at six weeks, and surgical phase (gingivectomy) if gingival enlargement persists. Routine maintenance therapy should be performed every three months following resolution of the gingival enlargement (G).

Treatment

The patient received full-mouth scaling and polishing. The patient was referred to a restorative dentist for detailed hard tissue examination and treatment of active decay. At six-week reevaluation, the patient demonstrated excellent oral hygiene, but the clinical signs and symptoms had improved only slightly. Therefore, gingivectomy and gingivoplasty were performed to restore gingival contours (G; see also Chapter 3, Case 1). The patient is currently on three-month recall.

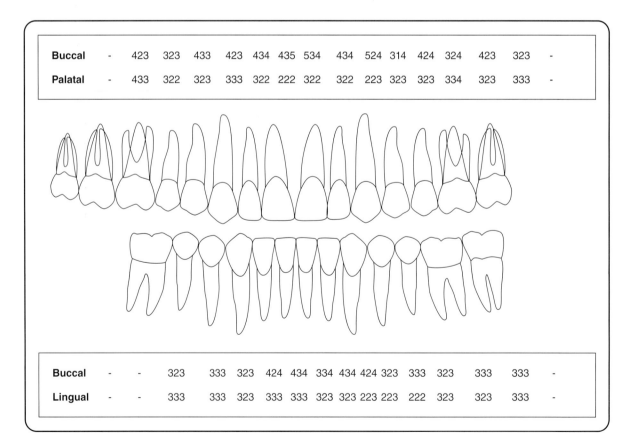

| Buccal | - | 423 | 323 | 433 | 423 | 434 | 435 | 534 | 434 | 524 | 314 | 424 | 324 | 423 | 323 | - |
| Palatal | - | 433 | 322 | 323 | 333 | 322 | 222 | 322 | 322 | 223 | 323 | 323 | 334 | 323 | 333 | - |

| Buccal | - | - | 323 | 333 | 323 | 424 | 434 | 334 | 434 | 424 | 323 | 333 | 323 | 333 | 333 | - |
| Lingual | - | - | 333 | 333 | 323 | 333 | 333 | 323 | 323 | 223 | 223 | 222 | 323 | 323 | 333 | - |

Figure 1.4.3 Probing pocket depth measurements.

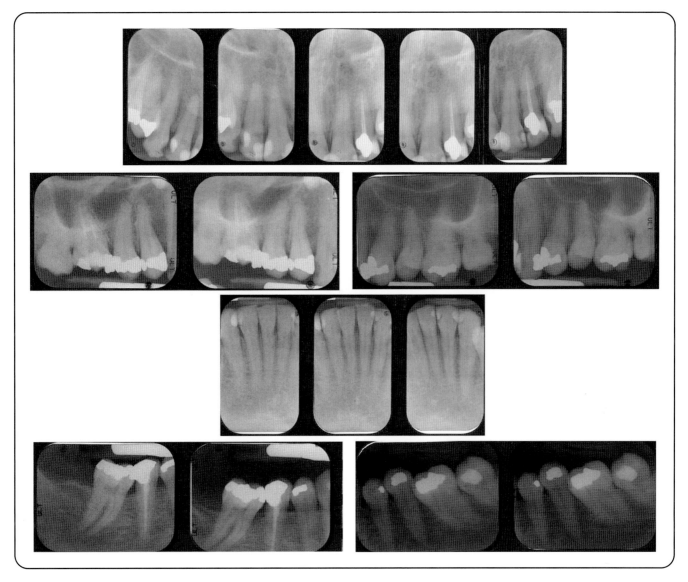

Figure 1.4.4 Periapical radiographs depicting the interproximal bone levels.

Discussion

Most patients who have gingival enlargement present with the chief complaint of an unesthetic smile. Comprehensive medical and dental histories (A) as well as a complete periodontal examination are needed to come to the appropriate diagnosis. Most commonly, gingival enlargement is a dental plaque-induced gingival condition modified by medications such as phenytoin, cyclosporine, or calcium channel blockers [1]. In some rare cases, a non-plaque-induced gingival enlargement called hereditary gingival fibromatosis (A) may be seen.

Once the diagnosis is determined, the treatment plan includes oral hygiene instructions, an initial phase of treatment (scaling and polishing), and communication with the primary care physician for potential alternative medication to address the systemic condition (G). Phase 1 therapy is followed by periodontal reevaluation at four to six weeks. If the gingival enlargement persists at this visit, surgical excision of excessive gingiva is recommended with subsequent reinforcement of home care oral hygiene and a periodontal maintenance every three months is instituted (G).

In a recent case report, Capodiferro et al. [2] showed that nonsurgical periodontal treatment by an Er:YAG laser also promoted regression of gingival overgrowth in patients taking cyclosporine.

Self-Study Questions

A. What is the etiology for gingival enlargement? What questions in a dental history might help you begin to form a differential diagnosis?

B. What are the characteristics of drug-induced gingival enlargement?

C. How would you differentiate between a "true" periodontal pocket and a "pseudo-pocket"?

D. What are the clinical characteristics that distinguish gingival enlargement versus periodontitis?

E. What is the pathogenesis of gingival enlargement?

F. What is another reason for a short clinical crown?

G. What is the current treatment for patients with drug-induced gingival enlargement? What is the long-term prognosis with treatment for these patients?

Answers located at the end of the chapter.

References

1. Murakami S, Mealey BL, Mariotti A, Chapple ILC. Dental plaque-induced gingival conditions. *J Periodontol* 2018;89 (Suppl 1):S17–S27.
2. Capodiferro S, Tempesta A, Limongelli L, et al. Nonsurgical periodontal treatment by erbium:YAG laser promotes regression of gingival overgrowth in patient taking cyclosporine A: a case report. *Photobiomodul Photomed Laser Surg* 2019;37:53–56.
3. Caton JG Jr, Rees T, Pack A, et al. Consensus report: Non-plaque-induced gingival lesions. *Ann Periodontol* 1999;4:30–31.
4. Hart TC, Pallos D, Bozzo L, et al. Evidence of genetic heterogeneity for hereditary gingival fibromatosis. *J Dent Res* 2000;79:1758–1764.
5. Hart TC, Zhang Y, Gorry MC, et al. A mutation in the SOS1 gene causes hereditary gingival fibromatosis type 1. *Am J Hum Genet* 2002;70:943–954.
6. Lynch MA, Ship II. Initial oral manifestations of leukemia. *J Am Dent Assoc* 1967;75:932–940.
7. Dreizen S, McCredie KB, Keating MJ. Chemotherapy-associated oral hemorrhages in adults with acute leukemia. *Oral Surg Oral Med Oral Pathol* 1984;57:494–498.
8. Mariotti A. Dental plaque-induced gingival diseases. *Ann Periodontol* 1999;4:7–19.
9. Listgarten MA. Periodontal probing: what does it mean? [review]. *J Clin Periodontol* 1980;7:165–176.
10. Trackman PC, Kantarci A. Connective tissue metabolism and gingival overgrowth. *Crit Rev Oral Biol Med* 2004; 15;165–175.
11. Black SA Jr, Palamakumbura AH, Stan M, Trackman PC. Tissue-specific mechanisms for CCN2/CTGF persistence in fibrotic gingiva: interactions between cAMP and MAPK signaling pathways, and prostaglandin E2-EP3 receptor mediated activation of the c-JUN N-terminal kinase. *J Biol Chem* 2007;282:15416–15429.
12. Kantarci A, Black SA, Xydas CE, et al. Epithelial and connective tissue cell CTGF/CCN2 expression in gingival fibrosis. *J Pathol* 2006;210:59–66.
13. Uzel MI, Kantarci A, Hong HH, et al. Connective tissue growth factor in drug-induced gingival overgrowth. *J Periodontol* 2001;72:921–931.
14. Kantarci A, Augustin P, Firatli E, et al. Apoptosis in gingival overgrowth tissues. *J Dent Res* 2007;86:888–892.
15. Volchansky A, Cleaton-Jones P. Delayed passive eruption: a predisposing factor to Vincent's infection. *J Dent Assoc S Africa* 1974;29:291–294.
16. Volchansky A, Cleaton-Jones P. The position of the gingival margin as expressed by clinical crown height in children ages 6–16 years. *J Dent* 1975;4:116–122.
17. Goldman HM, Cohen DW. *Periodontal Therapy*, 4th edn. St. Louis, MO: Mosby, 1968.
18. Marshall RI, Bartold PM. A clinical review of drug-induced gingival overgrowths. *Aust Dent J* 1999;44:219–232.
19. Hall EE. Prevention and treatment considerations in patients with drug-induced gingival enlargement. *Curr Opin Periodontol* 1997;4:59–63.
20. Ilgenli T, Atilla G, Baylas H. Effectiveness of periodontal therapy in patients with drug-induced gingival overgrowth. *Long-term results. J Periodontol* 1999;70:967–972.
21. Ciancio SG, Bartz NW Jr, Lauciello FR. Cyclosporine-induced gingival hyperplasia and chlorhexidine: a case report. *Int J Periodontics Restorative Dent* 1991;11:241–245.
22. Prasad VN, Chawla HS, Goyal A, et al. Folic acid and phenytoin induced gingival overgrowth: is there a preventive effect? *J Indian Soc Pedod Prev Dent* 2004;22:82–91.
23. Chand DH, Quattrocchi J, Poe SA, et al. Trial of metronidazole vs. azithromycin for treatment of cyclosporine-induced gingival overgrowth. *Pediatr Transplant* 2004;8:60–64.

TAKE-HOME POINTS

A. Gingival overgrowth or enlargement is a common side effect and unwanted outcome of certain systemic medications. Drug-influenced gingival enlargement refers to an abnormal growth of the gingiva secondary to use of systemic medication and is classified by the 2017 World Workshop as a form of dental plaque-induced gingival disease modified by medications [1]. Currently three pharmaceutical categories of medication (anticonvulsants, immunosuppressants, and calcium channel blockers) are associated with gingival enlargement. However, a strong association has been noted only with phenytoin (when used in a chronic regimen to control epileptic seizures), cyclosporine (powerful immunoregulator drug primarily used in the prevention of organ transplant rejection), and nifedipine (commonly prescribed as an antihypertensive, antiarrhythmic, and antianginal agent). The prevalence of gingival overgrowth varies widely: the prevalence related to use of phenytoin is approximately 50%, whereas cyclosporine and nifedipine produce significant gingival changes in about 25% of the patients treated.

Among the non-plaque-induced gingival lesions, gingival fibromatosis of genetic origin has been also described as associated with gingival overgrowth [3]. Hereditary gingival fibromatosis (HGF) is an uncommon disorder that can occur as an isolated finding or as part of a genetic syndrome. HGF is most frequently reported to be transmitted as an autosomal dominant trait, but autosomal recessive inheritance has also been reported [4]. The clinical presentation of HGF is variable, both in the distribution (number of teeth involved) and in the degree (severity) of expression [4]. Affected individuals have a benign, slowly progressive, nonhemorrhagic, fibrous enlargement of the oral masticatory mucosa [5]. A mutation in the *SOS1* (Son of Sevenless-1) gene was reported to cause HGF type 1 [5]. HGF usually develops before the person reaches 10 years of age, often at or about the time of eruption of the permanent incisors. However, cases have been reported to occur during the eruption of the deciduous dentition and even to appear at birth [4].

Gingival enlargement has been found to be one of the oral manifestations associated with acute leukemias [6], in addition to cervical adenopathy, petechiae, mucosal ulcers, and gingival inflammation. Gingival bleeding is a common and usually the initial oral sign and/or symptom in 17.7% and 4.4% of patients with acute and chronic leukemias, respectively [6]. Gingival inflammation in leukemic patients presents as swollen, glazed, and spongy tissues that are red to deep purple in appearance [7]. Gingival enlargement has been associated with leukemia beginning at the interdental papilla and extending to the marginal and attached gingiva [7].

Questions important in the development of a differential diagnosis include the following.
- When did your gingiva start to swell?
- Did anybody in your family describe a similar pattern of gingival enlargement?
- Are you taking any medication?
- How long have you been taking the specific medication?
- Do your gums bleed easily?

B. As detailed in Mariotti [8], the common clinical characteristics of drug-related gingival enlargement include variation in interpatient and intrapatient pattern (such as genetic predisposition), predilection for anterior and facial segments, higher prevalence in children (due to phenytoin most often used in young patients and having the highest prevalence of all medication-induced gingival enlargement), onset within one to three months of drug use, change in gingival contour leading to modification of gingival size, enlargement starting at the interdental papilla, change in gingival color, pronounced inflammatory response of gingiva in association with bacterial plaque and reduction in severity with decrease in dental plaque, bleeding upon provocation, increased gingival exudate, and found in gingiva with or without bone loss but is not associated with attachment loss. Patients with this diagnosis are usually taking one of the following: phenytoin, cyclosporine, or certain channel blocker drugs.

C. The probing depth is the distance from the gingival margin to the base of the gingival sulcus. The normal sulcus, measuring between 1 and 3 mm, is normally measured to the nearest millimeter by means of a graduated periodontal probe with a standardized tip diameter of approximately 0.4–0.5 mm. The measurements recorded clinically with the periodontal probe have generally been considered a reasonably accurate estimate of sulcus or pocket depth. A probing of the sulcus depth (PPD) of ≥4 mm suggests a diseased state and represents a true periodontal pocket. A "true" periodontal pocket is the measurement from the gingival margin to the bottom of the pocket, recording an increased value (PPD ≥4 mm) beyond that found in the normal gingival sulcus. This depth increase is the result of apical migration of the junctional epithelium subsequent to alveolar bone resorption in patients with periodontitis.

Pocket depths of more than 3–4 mm may also be caused by the swelling of the gingiva without concomitant apical migration of dentogingival epithelium from the cementoenamel junction (CEJ), as in the case of gingival enlargement. This increase in pocket depth is called a "pseudo-pocket" because it is not associated with bone loss or apical migration of the junctional epithelium.

Probing depth is, in fact, a histologic term expressing the distance from the gingival margin to the most coronal level of the junctional epithelium. Clinical probing depth measured from the gingival margin seldom corresponds to sulcus or pocket depth. The discrepancy is least in the absence of inflammation and increases with increasing degrees of inflammation [9]. In the presence of periodontitis the probe tip passes through the inflamed tissues to stop at the level of the most coronal intact dentogingival fibers, approximately 0.3–0.5 mm apical to the apical termination of the junctional epithelium. Decreased probing depth measurements following periodontal therapy may be in part due to decreased penetrability of the gingival tissues by the probe. Therefore, a distinction should be made between the histologic and the clinical PPD to differentiate between the actual depth of anatomic defect and the measurement recorded by the periodontal probe [9].

D. Gingival enlargement is usually associated with certain medications (i.e. phenytoin, nifedipine, cyclosporine), and the clinical presentation is typically characteristic: papillary and free marginal gingiva is enlarged, mostly localized in anterior facial segments, increased probing depth with normal bone levels generally; possibly there are signs of inflammation.

Periodontitis is characterized by plaque-induced inflammation localized at the marginal gingiva, with bleeding on probing, increased probing depth and loss of periodontal tissues (cementum, periodontal ligament and crestal bone resorption) – therefore displaying "true" periodontal pockets. Depending on the degree of clinical attachment loss, periodontitis can be mild, moderate, or severe.

Diagnosis of each disease type is critical due to the distinct treatment that is needed to restore form and function and/or stabilize the periodontal disease progression, as mainly in the case of periodontitis.

E. The biologic origins for gingival overgrowth are complex. Recent studies indicate that molecular markers and clinical features of gingival overgrowth differ in their response to medication and that multiple genetic loci are linked to the inherited forms of gingival overgrowth [10].

Multiple hypotheses have been suggested and tested to better understand the molecular mechanisms underlying the clinical features of drug-induced gingival overgrowth. One leading theory is that substances that cause gingival overgrowth may do so by altering the normal balance of cytokines in gingival tissues, because abnormally high levels of specific cytokines were found in enlarged gingival tissues. Among the cytokines and growth factors found to be at elevated levels in human drug-induced gingival overgrowth are interleukin (IL)-6, IL-1β, platelet-derived growth factor-B, fibroblast growth factor-2, transforming growth factor-β, and connective tissue growth factor [10].

Connective tissue growth factor (CTGF, or CCN2), is a 38-kDa secreted protein belonging to the CCN family of growth factors. It has been shown to promote the synthesis of various components of the extracellular matrix, and its overexpression is associated with the onset and progression of fibrosis in many organs including human gingiva [11]. Moreover, fibrotic human gingival tissues express CTGF/CCN2 in both epithelium [12] and connective tissues [13], suggesting that interactions between epithelial and connective tissues could contribute to gingival fibrosis.

It has also been suggested that variations in the balance between cell proliferation and apoptosis contribute to the etiology of gingival overgrowth. Increased fibroblast proliferation and a simultaneous decrease in apoptosis were found to contribute to gingival overgrowth [14].

F. Short clinical crowns associated with healthy-appearing gingiva can be due to gingival tissue located more incisally or occlusally on the anatomic crown. Volchansky and Cleaton-Jones described this condition as delayed passive eruption [15,16]. They reported an incidence of 12% of patients examined demonstrating delayed passive eruption. Goldman and Cohen [17] also described this condition where the gingival margin fails to recede to the CEJ during tooth eruption as altered (retarded) passive eruption.

G. The treatment of patients with drug-induced gingival enlargement consists of oral hygiene instructions, supragingival and subgingival scaling and polishing, and referral to the primary care physician for possible substitution of one medication for another (i.e. phenytoin can be replaced with carbamazepine or valproic acid, cyclosporine with tacrolimus, and nifedipine with one of many dihydropteridines) not as strongly associated with gingival overgrowth. If the previously described treatment does not result in significant resolution of gingival enlargement, surgical excision of the excessive gingiva is performed using a classic external bevel gingivectomy or an internal bevel gingivectomy approach [18] (see Chapter 3, Case 1).

The internal bevel approach provides primary closure and reduction of postoperative bleeding, discomfort, and infection. More recently, a carbon dioxide laser has been used for surgical excision and provides rapid hemostasis and compatibility with a host with underlying medical conditions. It also has been reported to reduce surgical time [18].

Having the patient in a rigorous home plaque control regimen as well as regular three-month periodontal maintenance are strongly recommended [19] and may considerably reduce the risk of recurrence. In a study of 38 individuals, 18 months after surgical therapy, the recurrence rate of gingival overgrowth in patients taking cyclosporine or nifedipine was 34%. Age, gingival inflammation, and attendance at periodontal maintenance visits were all significantly related to recurrence, and they suggest that regular remotivation and professional care at frequent recall appointments are of great importance in patients with a history of drug-induced gingival overgrowth [20]. To prevent postsurgical recurrence, a chlorhexidine rinse twice daily is recommended [21].

Several medications have been shown to ameliorate gingival enlargement, such as systemic or topical folic acid [22] or a short course of metronidazole or azithromycin. The latter drugs work particularly well for significant resolution of cyclosporine-induced gingival overgrowth [23]. The mechanism of action for these antibiotics is not clear, but it is suggested they may contribute to inhibition of collagen fiber proliferation in addition to their antimicrobial action.

Case 5

Aggressive Periodontitis

CASE STORY

A 23-year-old African American female patient presented with a chief complaint of "Bleeding gums on brushing and swollen gums in specific areas of the mouth." The patient's dentist observed 7–10 mm probing depths in several teeth in all four quadrants of the mouth and referred her to a periodontist for a periodontal consultation.

LEARNING GOALS AND OBJECTIVES

- To be able to understand the definition and diagnostic criteria of molar/incisor pattern periodontitis
- To understand the various treatment options available for this condition
- To understand the prognosis of periodontal and implant treatment in these patients

Medical History

There were no findings on medical history and the patient did not report any allergies to food or to drugs. The patient was not taking any medications.

Review of Systems

- Vital signs
  - Blood pressure: 120/80 mmHg
  - Pulse rate: 73 beats/minute (regular)
  - Respiratory rate: 15 breaths/minute

Social History

The patient was a nonsmoker and reported that she did not consume alcohol.

Extraoral Examination

There were no significant findings. The patient had no masses or swelling and the temporomandibular joint was within normal limits.

Intraoral Examination

- There were no abnormal findings with respect to the tongue, floor of the mouth, palate, and buccal mucosa.
- A gingival examination revealed mild marginal erythema with areas of rolled margins and swollen papillae in the areas of all first molars and mandibular incisors (Figures 1.5.1–1.5.5).
- A periodontal charting was completed (Figure 1.5.6). Teeth #3, #14, #19 and #30 exhibited probing depths of more than 7 mm especially in the interproximal

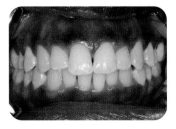

Figure 1.5.1 Preoperative frontal view.

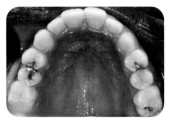

Figure 1.5.2 Preoperative maxillary dentition.

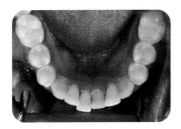

Figure 1.5.3 Preoperative mandibular dentition.

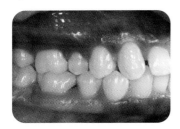

Figure 1.5.4 Preoperative left occlusal view.

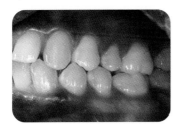

Figure 1.5.5 Preoperative right occlusal.

areas. The mandibular incisors also exhibited probing depths in the range of 6–7 mm (Figure 1.5.7).

- Grade 3 mobility was observed in mandibular lateral incisors.
- The teeth other than incisors and molars exhibited probing depths in the range of 2–4 mm.
- Grade II furcation involvements were recorded for all the affected molars.
- The patient's oral hygiene was good.

Occlusion

There were no occlusal discrepancies or interferences.

Radiographic Examination

A full-mouth set of radiographs was ordered. The periapical radiographs of the affected molars are shown in Figure 1.5.8. The radiographs show vertical bone defects around all first molars. The bone defects are confined to interproximal areas of the maxillary molars (involving the proximal furcations) and are circumferential in the mandibular molars involving the buccal or lingual furcation areas. Radiographs also revealed severe vertical bone loss in the maxillary and mandibular incisors (radiographs not shown).

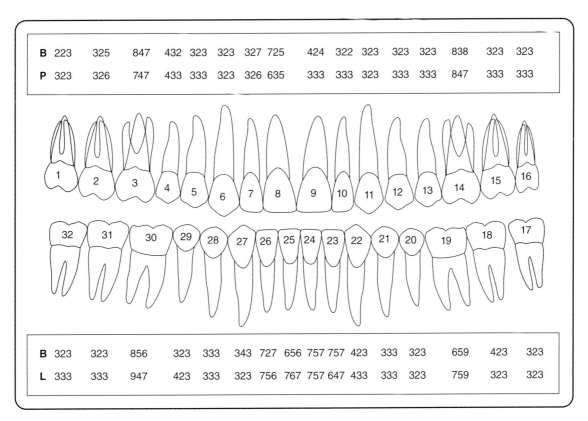

Figure 1.5.6 Probing pocket depth measurements during phase 1 reevaluation. B, buccal; P, palatal; L, lingual.

Maxillary:

	1	2	3	4	5	6	7	8	9	10	11	12	13	14	15	16
B	223	325	847	432	323	323	327	725	424	322	323	323	323	838	323	323
P	323	326	747	433	333	323	326	635	333	333	323	333	333	847	333	333

Mandibular:

	32	31	30	29	28	27	26	25	24	23	22	21	20	19	18	17
B	323	323	856	323	333	343	727	656	757	757	423	333	323	659	423	323
L	333	333	947	423	333	323	756	767	757	647	433	333	323	759	323	323

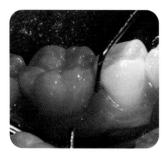
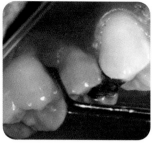

Figure 1.5.7 Intraoral clinical photographs depicting deeper probing depth associated with maxillary and mandibular molars.

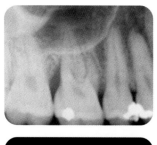
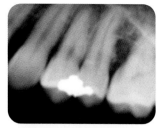
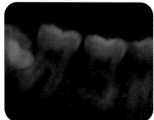
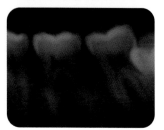

Figure 1.5.8 Periapical radiographs demonstrating the intrabony defects surrounding all four molars and the relatively normal premolars and second molars.

Diagnosis and Prognosis

The patient's age, ethnicity, history, and clinical and radiographic exams led to the diagnosis of molar/incisor pattern stage III grade C periodontitis. The molars were not mobile and the defects surrounding them were intrabony, which are highly amenable to regeneration by guided tissue regeneration or enamel matrix protein. Moreover, the patient also had very good oral hygiene and was highly compliant. Therefore these molars will have a fair prognosis. However, the long-term prognosis of mandibular incisors is questionable as the sites exhibited severe destruction of the periodontium with bone loss almost to the apex of the teeth.

Treatment Plan

The treatment plan for a typical case of molar/incisor pattern periodontitis consists of the following phases.
- The diagnostic phase consists of a comprehensive periodontal examination, radiographs and study models. In some cases, microbial testing and genetic testing can be performed.
- The disease control phase includes oral hygiene instruction, splinting of mandibular incisors and scaling/root planing of all the affected areas with adjunctive systemic antibiotics (amoxicillin and metronidazole combination). Extractions of all the third molars can be included in this phase.
- The reevaluation phase consists of revisiting her probing pocket depths and her overall periodontal condition plus treatment planning for sites that did not improve after the initial phase of therapy or those that warrant further treatment.
- The sites that need further treatment can be treated surgically.
- Guided tissue regeneration or bone grafts with enamel matrix protein is commonly employed to treat the intrabony defects associated with molars.
- After surgical phase, the sites will again be evaluated for improvement in the periodontal condition.
- Once the periodontal condition is stabilized, patient will be placed on a three- to six-month maintenance protocol.

Discussion

Following the 2017 World Workshop on the Classification of Periodontal and Peri-implant Diseases and Conditions, the previous classification of chronic periodontitis and aggressive periodontitis was amended so that now they are grouped under a single category – "periodontitis" [1]. With the new 2017 classification system, grading estimates the aggressiveness of the disease by focusing on the factors contributing to progression rather than previously focusing on the identification of a form of periodontitis. The characteristic clinical and radiographic features associated with molar/incisor pattern periodontitis allow the oral healthcare provider to diagnose the condition without much difficulty. The case that we present in this book chapter exhibited the classical clinical and radiographic features of molar/incisor pattern periodontitis, including age of onset of disease, the pattern of disease progression and aggressiveness in clinical attachment loss. Stage III was determined after considering both severity (including interdental attachment loss ≥5 mm and bone loss beyond more than middle third of root) and complexity (including probing depths ≥6 mm with vertical bone loss ≥3 mm). Grade C was due to the high risk of progression. Therefore a diagnosis of molar/incisor pattern stage III grade C periodontitis was made. In some cases, microbiological and immunological tests can be used as an adjunct to diagnose this disease. Increased levels of

Aggregatibacter actinomycetemcomitans (especially serotype b) microbes and a robust antibiotic response to the same microorganism are expected in such testing. After completing phase 1 therapy consisting of scaling and root planing with adjunctive use of systemic antibiotics, a drastic improvement in probing depth reduction and clinical attachment gain are expected in deeper pockets. Residual pockets (>6 mm) remaining after phase 1 therapy will be usually treated with surgical periodontal therapy. Adequate oral hygiene is critical in the successful outcome of any periodontal therapy. Usually patients with molar/incisor pattern periodontitis tend to exhibit

insignificant amounts of local factors such as plaque and calculus and tend to have good oral hygiene. In the case described in this chapter, the patient had insignificant amounts of local factors (Figures 1.5.1–1.5.5). With respect to outcomes of surgeries performed in patients with molar/incisor pattern periodontitis, long-term stability after regenerative therapy has been shown. The success rates of dental implants in patients with molar/incisor pattern periodontitis are inconclusive. Some studies have indicated that the success rates in these patients are slightly lower (<10%) than in patients with grade A or B periodontitis [2,3].

Self-Study Questions

A. How do you define molar/incisor pattern periodontitis and how do you classify it?

B. What are the other terms used to describe molar/incisor pattern periodontitis?

C. What are the characteristic presentations common to molar/incisor pattern grade C periodontitis and generalized grade C periodontitis?

D. What are the features that distinguish molar/incisor pattern grade C periodontitis from generalized grade C periodontitis?

E. How common is molar/incisor pattern periodontitis and which sector of the population is more susceptible to this disease?

F. What are the etiologic agents responsible for molar/incisor pattern periodontitis?

G. How do you treat patients with molar/incisor pattern periodontitis?

H. In molar/incisor pattern periodontitis patients, what will be the prognosis after treatment?

Answers located at the end of the chapter.

References

1. Caton JG, Armitage G, Berglundh T, et al. A new classification scheme for periodontal and peri-implant diseases and conditions. Introduction and key changes from the 1999 classification. *J Periodontol* 2018;89(Suppl 1):S1–S8.
2. De Boever AL, Quirynen M, Coucke W, et al. Clinical and radiographic study of implant treatment outcome in periodontally susceptible and non-susceptible patients: a prospective long-term study. *Clin Oral Implants Res* 2009;20:1341–1350.
3. Al-Zahrani MS. Implant therapy in aggressive periodontitis patients: a systematic review and clinical implications. *Quintessence Int* 2008;39:211–215.
4. Meng H, Xu L, Li Q, et al. Determinants of host susceptibility in aggressive periodontitis. *Periodontol 2000* 2007;43:133–159.
5. Armitage GC. Development of a classification system for periodontal diseases and conditions. *Ann Periodontol* 1999;4:1–6.
6. Brown LJ, Albandar JM, Brunelle JA, Loe H. Early-onset periodontitis: progression of attachment loss during 6 years. *J Periodontol* 1996;67:968–975.
7. Orban B. A diffuse atrophy of the alveolar bone (periodontosis). *J Periodontol* 1942;13:31.
8. Baer PN. The case for periodontosis as a clinical entity. *J Periodontol* 1971;42:516–520.

9. Lang N, Bartold PM, Cullinan M, et al. Consensus report: aggressive periodontitis. *Ann Periodontol* 1999;4:53.

10. Benjamin SD, Baer PN. Familial patterns of advanced alveolar bone loss in adolescence (periodontosis). *Periodontics* 1967;5:82–88.

11. Kantarci A, Oyaizu K, Van Dyke TE. Neutrophil-mediated tissue injury in periodontal disease pathogenesis: findings from localized aggressive periodontitis. *J Periodontol* 2003;74:66–75.

12. Fredman G, Oh SF, Ayilavarapu S, et al. Impaired phagocytosis in localized aggressive periodontitis: rescue by Resolvin E1. *PLoS One* 2011;6:e24422.

13. Shaddox L, Wiedey J, Bimstein E, et al. Hyper-responsive phenotype in localized aggressive periodontitis. *J Dent Res* 2010;89:143–148.

14. Fine DH, Armitage GC, Genco RJ, et al. Unique etiologic, demographic, and pathologic characteristics of localized aggressive periodontitis support classification as a distinct subcategory of periodontitis. *J Am Dent Assoc* 2019;150:922–931.

15. Loe H, Brown LJ. Early onset periodontitis in the United States of America. *J Periodontol* 1991;62:608–616.

16. Albandar JM, Muranga MB, Rams TE. Prevalence of aggressive periodontitis in school attendees in Uganda. *J Clin Periodontol* 2002;29:823–831.

17. Miller K, Treloar T, Guelmann M, et al. Clinical characteristics of localized aggressive periodontitis in primary dentition. *J Clin Pediatr Dent* 2018;42:95–102.

18. Merchant SN, Vovk A, Kalash D, et al. Localized aggressive periodontitis treatment response in primary and permanent dentitions. *J Periodontol* 2014;85:1722–1729.

19. Marazita ML, Burmeister JA, Gunsolley JC, et al. Evidence for autosomal dominant inheritance and race-specific heterogeneity in early-onset periodontitis. *J Periodontol* 1994;65:623–630.

20. Hart TC, Marazita ML, Schenkein HA, Diehl SR. Re-interpretation of the evidence for X-linked dominant inheritance of juvenile periodontitis. *J Periodontol* 1992;63:169–173.

21. Fine DH, Markowitz K, Furgang D, et al. *Aggregatibacter actinomycetemcomitans* and its relationship to initiation of localized aggressive periodontitis: longitudinal cohort study of initially healthy adolescents. *J Clin Microbiol* 2007;45:3859–3869.

22. Haraszthy VI, Hariharan G, Tinoco EM, et al. Evidence for the role of highly leukotoxic *Actinobacillus actinomycetemcomitans* in the pathogenesis of localized juvenile and other forms of early-onset periodontitis. *J Periodontol* 2000;71:912–922.

23. Fine DH, Markowitz K, Fairlie K, et al. A consortium of *Aggregatibacter actinomycetemcomitans*, *Streptococcus parasanguinis*, and *Filifactor alocis* is present in sites prior to bone loss in a longitudinal study of localized aggressive periodontitis. *J Clin Microbiol* 2013;51:2850–2861.

24. Fine DH, Markowitz K, Fairlie K, et al. Macrophage inflammatory protein-1α shows predictive value as a risk marker for subjects and sites vulnerable to bone loss in a longitudinal model of aggressive periodontitis. *PLoS One* 2014;9:e98541.

25. Faveri M, Figueiredo LC, Duarte PM, et al. Microbiological profile of untreated subjects with localized aggressive periodontitis. *J Clin Periodontol* 2009;36:739–749.

26. Zambon JJ, Christersson LA, Slots J. *Actinobacillus actinomycetemcomitans* in human periodontal disease. Prevalence in patient groups and distribution of biotypes and serotypes within families. *J Periodontol* 1983;54:707–711.

27. Ebersole JL, Cappelli D, Steffen MJ. Antigenic specificity of gingival crevicular fluid antibody to *Actinobacillus actinomycetemcomitans*. *J Dent Res* 2000;79:1362–1370.

28. Teughels W, Dhondt R, Dekeyser C, Quirynen M. Treatment of aggressive periodontitis. *Periodontol 2000* 2014;65:107–133.

29. Miller KA, Branco-de-Almeida LS, Wolf S, et al. Long-term clinical response to treatment and maintenance of localized aggressive periodontitis: a cohort study. *J Clin Periodontol* 2017;44:158–168.

30. Gorski B, Jalowski S, Gorska R, Zaremba M. Treatment of intrabony defects with modified perforated membranes in aggressive periodontitis: a 12-month randomized controlled trial. *Clin Oral Investig* 2018;22:2819–2828.

31. Artzi Z, Sudri S, Platner O, Kozlovsky A. Regeneration of the periodontal apparatus in aggressive periodontitis patients. *Dent J (Basel)* 2019;7(1):29.

32. Momen-Heravi F, Kang P. Treatment of localized aggressive periodontitis with guided tissue regeneration technique and enamel matrix derivative. *Clin Adv Periodontics* 2017;7:182–189.

33. Pavicic MJ, van Winkelhoff AJ, Douque NH, et al. Microbiological and clinical effects of metronidazole and amoxicillin in *Actinobacillus actinomycetemcomitans*-associated periodontitis. A 2-year evaluation. *J Clin Periodontol* 1994;21:107–112.

34. Winkel EG, van Winkelhoff AJ, van der Velden U. Additional clinical and microbiological effects of amoxicillin and metronidazole after initial periodontal therapy. *J Clin Periodontol* 1998;25:857–864.

35. Buchmann R, Nunn ME, Van Dyke TE, Lange DE. Aggressive periodontitis: 5-year follow-up of treatment. *J Periodontol* 2002;73:675–683.

36. Kamma JJ, Baehni PC. Five-year maintenance follow-up of early-onset periodontitis patients. *J Clin Periodontol* 2003;30:562–572.

37. Baumer A, Weber D, Staufer S, et al. Tooth loss in aggressive periodontitis: results 25 years after active periodontal therapy in a private practice. *J Clin Periodontol* 2020;47(2):223–232.

38. Petit C, Huck O, Amar S, Tenenbaum H. Management of localized aggressive periodontitis: a 30-year follow-up. *Quintessence Int* 2018;49:615–624.

39. Mros ST, Berglundh T. Aggressive periodontitis in children: a 14–19-year follow-up. *J Clin Periodontol* 2010;37:283–287.

40. Dopico J, Nibali L, Donos N. Disease progression in aggressive periodontitis patients. A retrospective study. *J Clin Periodontol* 2016;43:531–537.

41. Goh V, Nihalani D, Yeung KWS, et al. Moderate- to long-term therapeutic outcomes of treated aggressive periodontitis patients without regular supportive care. *J Periodontal Res* 2018;53:324–333.

42. Kaner D, Bernimoulin JP, Kleber BM, Friedmann A. Minimally invasive flap surgery and enamel matrix derivative in the treatment of localized aggressive periodontitis: case report. *Int J Periodontics Restorative Dent* 2009;29:89–97.

TAKE-HOME POINTS

A. Molar/incisor pattern periodontitis was designated as a separate disease – localized aggressive periodontitis – in the 1999 AAP classification because of the location of lesions and its aggressive nature, characterized by early onset and familial aggregation; affected individuals are otherwise systemically healthy [4,5].

Molar/incisor pattern is defined as interproximal loss of attachment localized to at least two permanent first molars/incisors, one of which is a first molar, and involving no more than two teeth other than first molars and incisors. When the interproximal loss of attachment extends to at least three permanent teeth other than first incisors and molars, then the condition is classified as generalized periodontitis. If left untreated, 35% of originally classified molar/incisor pattern periodontitis may progress to generalized periodontitis [6].

B. Molar/incisor pattern periodontitis was formerly called "periodontosis" [7,8] and later called "early-onset periodontitis" and "localized prepubertal/juvenile periodontitis" in the 1989 AAP classification because the disease generally affects young patients. Molar/incisor pattern periodontitis was later called "localized aggressive periodontitis" in the 1999 AAP classification, based on clinical, radiographic, historical and/or laboratory findings, rather than the age of the patient.

The current classification grouped "chronic" and "aggressive" under a single category "periodontitis" because the specific etiologic or pathologic elements that account for early onset and molar/incisor pattern clinical presentation are insufficiently defined. Current evident does not support the distinction between chronic and aggressive periodontitis as two separate diseases.

C. The following are primary features [9].
• Rapid attachment loss accompanied with severe bone destruction. The progression rate of molar/incisor pattern periodontitis is about three to four times faster than that of periodontitis with grade A or B. The rapidly progressive vertical bone loss is often half-moon shaped and symmetric to the contralateral tooth [10].

• Patients will usually be medically healthy children or adolescents.
• Strong familial aggregation.
   Secondary features that are frequently but not always present include the following.
• Inconsistency in the relationship between the amount of microbial deposits (i.e. supragingival plaque) and the severity of periodontal destruction.
• Elevated levels of *Aggregatibacter actinomycetemcomitans* and/or *Porphyromonas gingivalis*.
• Patients usually exhibit hyperactive polymorphonuclear neutrophils (PMNs) in chemotaxis and superoxide (O_2^-) production with hyperresponsive macrophages [11,12].
• Elevated levels of inflammatory cytokines (e.g. PGE_2, IL-1α, IL-1β) from primed macrophages.
• Progression of attachment loss and bone loss may be self-arresting and remain stationary for years.

D.

Table 1.5.1 Features distinguishing molar/incisor pattern grade C periodontitis from generalized grade C periodontitis.

Features	Molar/incisor pattern grade C periodontitis	Generalized grade C periodontitis
Age of onset	Circumpubertal	<30 years but may be older
Clinical manifestation	Involves no more than two teeth other than incisors and first molars	Involves at least three teeth other than incisors and first molars
Serum antibody response to infecting agents [13]	Robust response	Poor response

E. The prevalence of molar/incisor pattern periodontitis varies among racial and geographic groups. Molar/incisor pattern periodontitis has a 10-fold higher prevalence in African Americans, Middle Easterners, and Hispanics [14]. The prevalence is ~0.2% in Caucasian populations and ~2% in those of African descent [15,16]. Molar/incisor pattern periodontitis may also start in the primary dentition [17,18]. The proportion of affected males and females is similar [19,20].

F. Nonmotile Gram-negative anaerobic rods such as *A. actinomycetemcomitans, P. gingivalis* [21–24], and red and some orange complex species [25] are the most numerous and prevalent periodontal pathogens in molar/incisor pattern periodontitis and are present in most of the diseased sites compared to healthy sites. The microbiomes of molar/incisor pattern periodontitis may vary among different ethnic groups, but *A. actinomycetemcomitans* (especially serotype b) was found in higher numbers and frequency, at least in the early stage, when compared with other pathogens [21,26]. *Aggregatibacter actinomycetemcomitans* produces a leukotoxin that affects the antibacterial function of neutrophils. The heightened antibody responses to *A. actinomycetemcomitans* may also be responsible for the localized periodontal destruction [27].

The exact reason why the disease is localized to first molars and incisors with such early onset in young adults is still debatable. However, those young patients' hormonal changes and the fact that the first molars and incisors are the first permanent teeth to erupt may alter the microbial environment in some unique way that causes the periodontal destruction [14].

G. The general treatment methods should be similar to those used for periodontitis, including oral hygiene instruction/reinforcement, plaque control, scaling and root planing, and occlusal adjustment (if necessary).

Additional treatments that may be required in certain patients include the following.
• General medical evaluation to determine the presence of any systemic diseases. Consultation with the physician may be indicated.
• Counseling of family members.
• Adjunctive use of amoxicillin combined with metronidazole [28]. Tetracycline is contraindicated in young patients due to the problem of tooth staining. Systemic administration of amoxicillin 500 mg plus metronidazole 250 mg three times daily for seven days with maintenance every three months resulted in significant clinical improvement and reduced

levels of key periodontal pathogens in the long term [29].
• Periodontal maintenance with short interval may be needed.

Teeth with poor prognosis are usually extracted mostly in phase 1 or sometimes phase 2 of periodontal therapy. Most of the intrabony defects that result from molar/incisor pattern periodontitis and that are amenable to regeneration are surgically treated using either guided tissue regeneration (GTR) [30] or enamel matrix derivative (EMD) with xenografts/allografts [31,32] (Figure 1.5.9). See the appropriate chapters in this textbook for more details on these surgical techniques. Limited studies have shown that the adjunctive use of local subgingival antimicrobials does not result in additional improvement of clinical parameters.

H. Scaling and root planing in combination with amoxicillin 375 mg and metronidazole 250 mg (t.i.d. for seven days) in patients with *A. actinomycetemcomitans*-associated periodontitis improved clinical parameters and suppressed A. actinomycetemcomitans below cultivable levels in most of the patients for up to two years with supportive periodontal therapy once every three to six

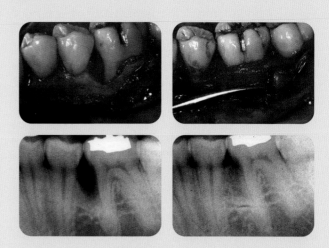

Figure 1.5.9 Classical intrabony defect affecting a mandibular first molar in another patient with localized aggressive periodontitis (top left). Guided tissue regeneration (GTR) was performed to regenerate the periodontal defect using bone grating and membrane (top right). Periapical radiographs depict the vertical bony defect before (lower left) and after (lower right) GTR therapy. Significant radiographic bone fill was obtained after GTR therapy.

months [33,34]. Patients showing compliance with the antibiotic regimen also have better treatment outcome. Long-term stabilization of periodontal health after amoxicillin 500 mg and metronidazole 250 mg plus periodontal surgeries has been reported, with a small percentage (5–10%) showing recurrence in five years [35,36].

Most patients have a relatively good prognosis if kept in a maintenance protocol. It has been shown that 73% of patients undergoing supportive periodontal therapy (SPT) at least every six months would not need further retreatment in over 20 years [37]. Long-term follow-up case reports have also shown a low recurrence rate with SPT every three to six months for 30 years [38] or in the absence of consistent maintenance for 15 years [39]. However, 8–30% of patients may progress to a generalized pattern of disease [40,41]. Successful regenerative treatment outcomes have also been shown following GTR [30] or using EMD with xenografts [31,32,42].

The success rate of tooth implants in patients with molar/incisor pattern periodontitis is not conclusive. Overall, molar/incisor pattern stage C periodontitis shows less progression and tooth loss than generalized stage C periodontitis. Considering the defect in host response in these patients, it is reasonable to expect lower survival rates of the teeth and implants in these patients, compared to grade A or B periodontitis patients. Clinicians should be aware that these patients are generally younger than those with grade A or B periodontitis. The implant prosthesis would need to remain esthetic and functional for a longer period of time in these patients. Consultation with other specialists to evaluate the alterative restorative options, such as orthodontic treatment, might also help to determine whether or not to extract.

Case 6

Chronic Periodontitis

CASE STORY

The patient had been referred by his general dentist for periodontal treatment. Although he had a long history of dental treatment, he had never been diagnosed with periodontal disease. At the time of his first visit he had no chief complaint. He did report occasional gingival bleeding during toothbrushing.

LEARNING GOALS AND OBJECTIVES

■ To be able to identify the clinical features and overall characteristics of periodontitis
■ To be able to list difficulties in the proper diagnosis of early presentations of periodontitis
■ To understand possible aggressiveness patterns on the progression of periodontitis
■ To know what clinical changes can be anticipated in the response of periodontitis to anti-infective therapy

Medical History

There were no significant medical problems, and the patient had no known allergies. He had been previously hospitalized for a day surgery to remove polyps from his vocal cords. At the time of his first appointment he was not taking any medication.

Review of Systems

• Vital signs
  ○ Blood pressure: 120/75 mmHg
  ○ Pulse rate: 70 beats/minute (regular)

Social History

The patient was a 43-year-old white man, originally from Texas, but had been living in Massachusetts for the past 10 years. He drank alcohol socially, quit smoking 10 years ago, and reported not consuming recreational drugs. He was a musician, divorced, and had no children. His mother had heart disease, and his father died of lung cancer.

Extraoral Examination

His extraoral examination was unremarkable: skin, head, neck, temporomandibular joint, and muscles were all within normal limits.

Intraoral Examination

The oral cancer screen was negative. His gingiva was pink, firm, with pointed papillae on the buccal aspect (Figure 1.6.1). However, the lingual and palatal aspects presented with signs of inflammation, with erythematous and edematous gingival margins. Adequate amounts of attached tissue were present around most teeth. Gingival recession was present at several sites (see periodontal chart for details). Supragingival and subgingival calculus could be detected on several tooth surfaces, particularly on the buccal surface of upper molars and lingual surfaces of lower incisors. There was generalized plaque accumulation. Saliva was of normal flow and consistency.

The periodontal chart presented in Figure 1.6.2 includes the following periodontal parameters: (i) probing pocket depth (PD) in millimeters; (ii) measurement from the cementoenamel junction (CEJ) to the free gingival margin (FGM) in millimeters (gingival recession was recorded as a positive value); (iii) clinical attachment level (CAL), which was calculated by adding the CEJ–FGM distance to the PD; and (iv) presence (1) or absence (blank) of bleeding on probing (BOP). Each clinical parameter was measured at six sites per tooth excluding third molars. Probing values were colored in black and red to highlight shallow (<4 mm), and intermediate to deep (≥4 mm) pockets. BOP was detected

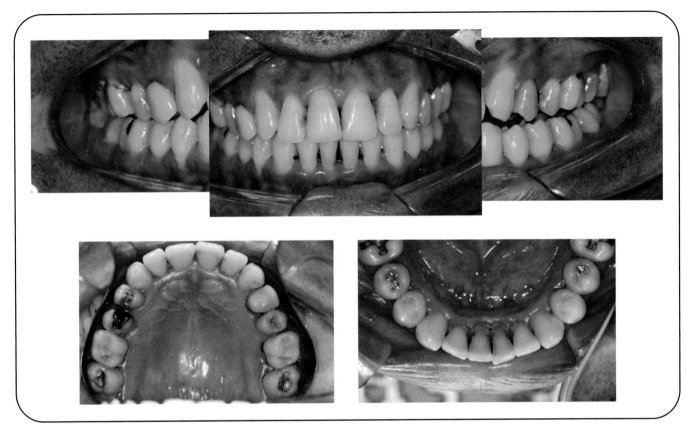

Figure 1.6.1 Clinical presentation of the case at initial visit. Source: courtesy of Dr. Eduardo Sampaio and Dr. Marcelo Faveri.

Initial Exam

Facial	1	2	3	4	5	6	7	8	9	10	11	12	13	14	15	16
PD		8 3 4	5 3 4	7 2 5	4 2 4	4 2 3	5 1 3	3 1 4	4 1 2	3 1 3	4 1 4	4 1 6	5 2 6	6 2 6	6 2 7	
FGM		-2 2 1	1 2 1	-1 1 -1	-1 1 -1	-2 0 0	-1 0 0	0 0 -1	-2 1 1	0 0 0	-1 0 -2	-2 1 -2	-1 1 -2	-2 2 -1	-1 1 -2	
AL		6 5 5	6 5 5	6 3 4	3 3 3	2 2 3	4 1 3	3 1 3	2 2 3	3 1 3	3 1 2	2 2 4	4 3 4	4 4 5	5 3 5	
Bleed		1 1 1	1 1 1	1	1	1	1	1	1		1	1	1 1 1	1 1 1	1 1 1	

Lingual	1	2	3	4	5	6	7	8	9	10	11	12	13	14	15	16
PD		8 2 7	7 2 6	7 2 5	5 2 5	4 3 4	5 4 4	3 2 3	3 3 3	4 3 4	3 3 3	3 2 4	4 2 7	6 3 7	7 3 8	
FGM		-2 0 -2	-2 1 -2	-2 0 -2	-2 0 -2	-2 -1 -1	-1 -1 -1	-1 0 -1	-1 0 0	0 0 -1	-1 0 -1	-1 -1 -1	-1 0 -2	-2 0 -2	-2 -1 -2	
AL		6 2 5	5 3 4	5 2 3	3 2 3	2 2 3	4 3 3	2 2 2	2 3 3	4 3 3	2 3 2	2 1 3	3 2 5	4 3 5	5 2 6	
Bleed		1 1 1	1 1 1	1 1 1	1 1 1		1 1 1	1 1 1	1 1 1	1 1 1		1 1 1	1 1 1	1 1 1	1 1 1	

Lingual	32	31	30	29	28	27	26	25	24	23	22	21	20	19	18	17
Bleed		1 1 1	1 1 1	1 1 1	1 1 1		1	1 1 1	1 1 1	1 1 1	1 1 1	1	1 1 1	1 1 1	1 1 1	1 1 1
AL		0 0 4	4 3 3	3 2 2	2 1 0	1 1 2	2 3 4	4 4 4	5 6 6	6 4 3	2 0 1	3 2 3	4 1 3	2 0 4	4 1 0	
FGM		-4 -2 -2	-2 -1 -2	-2 -2 -2	-2 0 -2	-2 0 -1	-1 1 2	2 3 3	3 3 2	2 1 0	-2 -1 -2	-1 0 -2	-2 -2 -2	-2 -2 -2	-2 -2 -2	
PD		4 2 6	6 4 5	5 4 4	4 1 2	3 1 3	3 2 2	2 1 1	2 3 4	4 3 3	4 1 3	4 2 5	6 3 5	4 2 6	6 3 2	

Facial	32	31	30	29	28	27	26	25	24	23	22	21	20	19	18	17
Bleed		1	1 1	1									1	1 1	1 1	1
AL		0 2 1	3 2 3	2 1 2	1 3 1	2 1 2	2 1 3	3 1 4	4 1 4	2 1 1	0 1 1	1 2 0	1 2 1	1 1 2	2 2 1	
FGM		-3 0 -2	-2 1 0	-1 0 -1	0 2 -1	0 0 1	1 0 2	2 0 2	2 0 2	1 0 0	-1 0 0	0 1 -1	-1 1 -1	-1 0 -1	-1 1 -2	
PD		3 2 3	5 1 3	3 1 3	1 1 2	2 1 1	1 1 1	1 1 2	2 1 2	1 1 1	1 1 1	1 1 1	2 1 2	2 1 3	3 1 3	

Figure 1.6.2 Periodontal chart at initial visit. Source: courtesy of Dr. Eduardo Sampaio and Dr. Marcelo Faveri.

in 68% of sites, and the mean values for full-mouth PD and CAL were 3.2 mm and 2.7 mm, respectively.

Occlusion

There were no signs of trauma from occlusion, no major occlusal discrepancies and interferences, and no significant mobility.

Radiographic Examination

A full-mouth set of radiographs (Figure 1.6.3) was exposed. There was generalized moderate to severe horizontal bone loss, consisting of more than 50% loss of the original bony support. There was furcation involvement seen in teeth #1, #2, #3, #14, #15, #16, #18, #19 and #30. There was a periapical radiolucency noted on tooth #5. There were root canal treatments seen on teeth #5 and #12. There were several amalgam restorations and recurrent decay noted on tooth #13.

Diagnosis

Periodontitis stage III, localized, grade C.

Treatment Plan

The treatment plan for this case consisted primarily of four to six sessions of scaling and root planing (SRP) accompanied by oral hygiene instructions for the complete dentition. A reassessment of the case was planned for three months after the completion of this initial phase when the need for additional therapy would be decided.

Treatment

After the patient's initial examination, radiographs, and charting (Figures 1.6.1–1.6.3), a comprehensive treatment plan was presented and agreed upon. The first session involved full-mouth gross scaling and oral hygiene instructions on the proper toothbrushing technique and use of dental floss. Due to the presence of large amounts of subgingival calculus, the patient required six sessions of subgingival SRP under local anesthesia (one sextant of the mouth was instrumented per session). During this active phase of anti-infective therapy, previously instrumented sextants were constantly reexamined for residual supragingival and subgingival calculus, and whenever detected, residual calculus was removed. Every SRP session was accompanied by reinforcement of the oral hygiene instructions.

Three months after the last SRP session, the patient was reexamined (Figures 1.6.4 and 1.6.5), residual pockets ≥4 mm received additional SRP, a full-mouth plaque removal was performed, and oral hygiene instructions reinforced. Mean full-mouth PD and CAL were reduced to 2.3 and 2.4 mm, respectively, and there was a reduction in BOP to 13%. At that time no additional periodontal therapy was deemed necessary. The patient was placed in a recall system for supportive periodontal therapy every three months. Figures 1.6.6 and 1.6.7 illustrate the clinical presentation and the periodontal parameters one year after completion of SRP.

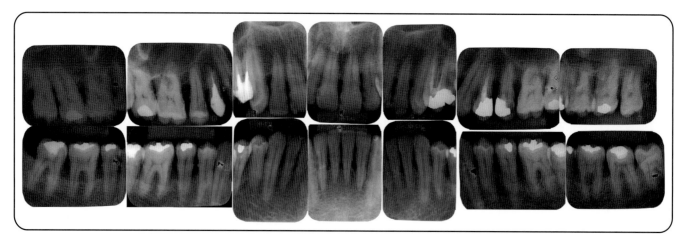

Figure 1.6.3 Full-mouth periapical radiographs of the case at initial visit. Source: courtesy of Dr. Eduardo Sampaio and Dr. Marcelo Faveri.

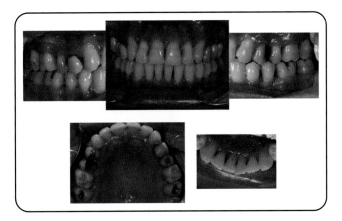

Figure 1.6.4 Clinical presentation of the case three months after therapy. Source: courtesy of Dr. Eduardo Sampaio and Dr. Marcelo Faveri.

Discussion

Periodontitis is a debilitating disease that is very prevalent and which can significantly impair quality of life, with the potential to negatively affect multiple systemic conditions. Early diagnosis and treatment has been shown to improve considerably the oral health of patients, and also biomarkers associated with their overall well-being. This disease is diagnosed based on the clinical signs of inflammation and clinical evidence of periodontal tissue destruction. Radiographs also help to determine the extent of bone loss. According to the 2017 World Workshop on the Classification of Periodontal and Peri-Implant Diseases and Conditions (https://www.perio.org/2017wwdc) [1], periodontitis has been identified in three distinct forms: periodontitis; periodontitis as a direct manifestation of systemic diseases; and necrotizing periodontitis. This case has focused on periodontitis, since this is the most prevalent form of this disease, and corresponds to what has been previously classified as either chronic or aggressive periodontitis.

Periodontitis is distinguished from gingivitis primarily on the basis of the presence of loss of attachment and resorption of alveolar bone. Therefore, in addition to common signs found in gingivitis, such as redness, swelling, bleeding tendency, and possibly suppuration, the diagnosis of periodontitis requires the presence of periodontal pockets associated with clinical loss of attachment. Alveolar bone loss is also a hallmark of the pathology and can be detected radiographically. It is not uncommon to detect extensive accumulation of dental plaque and calculus, although this can also be found in gingivitis [2]. According to the 2017 World Workshop, the severity and complexity of periodontitis can be categorized into a staging system that ranges from stage I to IV, from the least to the most complex conditions. The distinctions between these stages are clearly provided in the published proceeding of the 2017 World Workshop, and consider parameters such as interdental CAL, bone loss, tooth loss due to periodontitis, PD, furcation involvement, ridge defects, and masticatory dysfunctions. The stage can also be described in terms of its extent and distribution as localized (<30% of teeth involved) or generalized

3 months post-therapy

Teeth 1–16:

	1	2	3	4	5	6	7	8	9	10	11	12	13	14	15	16
Facial																
PD		6 2 3	4 3 3	4 1 3	2 2 2	2 2 3	3 1 2	2 1 2	2 1 2	2 1 2	2 1 2	2 1 3	3 2 4	4 2 4	4 2 4	
FGM		0 3 3	2 2 1	1 2 1	1 1 1	-1 0 0	1 1 2	1 1 0	1 1 1	1 1 1	0 0 0	0 1 2	1 1 1	0 2 1	2 2 0	
AL		6 5 6	6 5 4	5 3 4	3 3 3	1 2 3	4 2 4	3 2 2	3 2 3	3 2 3	2 1 2	2 2 5	4 3 5	4 4 5	6 4 4	
Bleed		1		1										1	1 1	1
Lingual																
PD		5 2 4	3 2 4	4 2 4	3 2 3	2 3 2	3 2 2	3 2 3	2 2 3	3 2 3	3 2 3	3 2 3	4 2 4	4 2 4	4 2 5	
FGM		-1 0 -1	-2 1 -1	-1 0 -1	-2 0 -2	-1 -1 -1	-1 -1 -1	-1 0 -1	-1 0 0	0 0 -1	-1 0 -1	-1 -1 -1	-1 0 -1	-1 0 -1	-2 -1 -1	
AL		4 2 3	1 3 3	3 2 3	1 2 1	1 2 1	2 1 1	2 2 2	1 2 3	3 2 2	2 2 2	2 1 2	3 2 3	3 2 3	2 1 4	
Bleed		1		1										1	1	

Teeth 32–17:

	32	31	30	29	28	27	26	25	24	23	22	21	20	19	18	17
Lingual																
Bleed		1		1										1	1	
AL	0 0 3	3 3 3	1 0 1	1 1 0	1 1 3	3 4 4	4 4 5	5 4 4	4 3 2	2 1 1	1 2 2	3 1 2	1 0 2	3 0 0		
FGM	-3 -2 -1	-1 0 -1	-2 -2 -2	-2 0 -2	-2 0 0	1 2 2	2 3 3	3 3 2	2 2 0	0 0 -1	-1 0 -1	-1 -1 -1	-2 -2 -2	-1 -2 -2		
PD	3 2 4	4 3 4	3 2 3	3 1 2	3 1 3	2 2 2	2 1 2	2 1 2	2 1 2	2 1 2	2 1 2	2 2 3	4 2 3	3 2 4	4 2 2	
Facial																
Bleed	1	1	1											1	1	
AL	1 2 2	4 2 2	3 2 2	1 3 1	2 1 2	2 1 3	3 1 4		4 1 4	2 1 1	1 1 1	1 2 1	2 3 2	2 1 2	2 2 2	
FGM	-2 0 -1	0 1 0	1 1 0	0 2 -1	0 0 1	1 0 2	2 0 2		2 0 2	1 0 0	0 0 0	0 1 0	1 2 1	0 0 0	0 1 0	
PD	3 2 3	4 1 2	2 1 2	1 1 2	2 1 1	1 1 1	1 1 2		2 1 2	1 1 1	1 1 1	1 1 1	1 1 1	2 1 2	2 1 2	

Figure 1.6.5 Periodontal chart three months after therapy. Source: courtesy of Dr. Eduardo Sampaio and Dr. Marcelo Faveri.

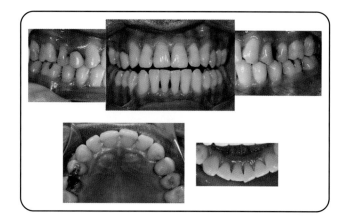

Figure 1.6.6 Clinical presentation of the case one year after therapy. Source: courtesy of Dr. Eduardo Sampaio and Dr. Marcelo Faveri.

(≥30%), and/or molar/incisor pattern [3]. The extension should be assessed after the stage has been determined, and it should refer to the stage that captures the overall severity and complexity of the case [4]. This classification system also categorizes the case in a grade system based on historical disease progression and risk for potential continuation, including the factors that modify progression of the disease such as diabetes and smoking burden (grade modifiers). In this way the provider and the patient can have a clearer idea of the aggressiveness of the manifestation of periodontal disease, the likelihood of successful outcomes with most modalities of treatment, and the impact of the disease on systemic health. Other than the grade

modifiers (smoking and diabetes), the primary factors considered in establishing the grade include direct and indirect evidence of progression, such as longitudinal bone loss or CAL, percentage bone loss/age, and case phenotype (level of destruction proportional to magnitude of local factors, such as biofilm and calculus). The grades are described as A, B or C, in which grade A represents the lowest risk of progression and grade C the highest risk.

Based on the criteria established by this current classification, the present case would be diagnosed as periodontitis stage III, localized, grade C. A brief discussion of this diagnosis follows.

- *Periodontitis case*: periodontitis was defined based on the presence of two or more nonadjacent teeth with CAL >2 mm, associated with bone loss and periodontal pockets. The case is not associated with necrosis of gingival tissues or with rare forms of systemic disease that severely affect periodontal tissues.
- *Stage III*: most of the teeth present with bone loss extending to the middle of the root, CAL is more than 5 mm for multiple teeth, and more than one site presents with PD >6 mm. However, there is no tooth loss due to periodontitis, neither is any tooth expected to be extracted because of it, and apparently there is no significant need of complex rehabilitation.
- *Localized extension*: less than 30% of teeth were affected at the stage III level, as the chart and radiographs show. Of the 28 teeth present, eight (28.5%) had CAL >5 mm.

1 year post-therapy

Facial	1	2	3	4	5	6	7	8	9	10	11	12	13	14	15	16
PD		6 2 3	4 3 3	5 1 3	2 2 2	2 2 3	3 1 2	2 1 2	2 1 2	2 1 2	2 1 3	3 2 4	4 2 5	5 3 4		
FGM		0 3 3	2 2 1	0 2 1	1 1 1	-1 0 0	1 1 2	1 1 0	1 1 1	1 1 1	0 0 0	0 1 2	1 1 1	0 2 0	1 1 0	
AL		6 5 6	6 5 4	5 3 4	3 3 3	1 2 3	4 2 4	3 2 2	3 2 3	3 2 3	2 1 2	2 2 5	4 3 5	4 4 5	6 4 4	
Bleed			1		1									1	1 1	1

Lingual	1	2	3	4	5	6	7	8	9	10	11	12	13	14	15	16
PD		5 2 5	4 2 4	4 2 4	3 2 3	2 3 2	3 2 2	3 2 3	2 2 3	3 2 3	3 2 3	3 2 3	4 2 4	4 2 5	5 2 5	
FGM		-1 0 -2	-2 1 -1	-1 0 -1	-2 0 -2	-1 -1 -1	-1 -1 -1	-1 0 -1	-1 0 0	0 0 -1	-1 0 -1	-1 -1 -1	-1 0 -1	-1 0 -1	-2 -1 -1	
AL		4 2 3	2 3 3	3 2 3	1 2 1	1 2 1	2 1 1	2 2 2	1 2 3	3 2 2	2 2 2	2 1 2	3 2 3	3 2 4	3 1 4	
Bleed	1		1											1	1 1	

Lingual	32	31	30	29	28	27	26	25	24	23	22	21	20	19	18	17
Bleed	1	1	1		1	1						1	1 1	1 1	1 1	
AL		0 0 3	4 3 3	1 0 1	1 1 0	1 1 3	3 4 4	4 4 5	5 4 4	4 3 2	2 1 1	1 2 2	3 1 2	1 0 2	3 0 0	
FGM		-3 -2 -2	-1 0 -1	-2 -2 -2	-2 0 -2	-2 0 0	1 2 2	2 3 3	3 3 2	2 2 0	0 0 -1	-1 0 -1	-1 -1 -1	-2 -2 -2	-1 -2 -2	
PD		3 2 5	5 3 4	3 2 3	3 1 2	3 1 3	2 2 2	2 1 2	2 1 2	2 1 2	2 1 2	2 2 3	4 2 3	3 2 4	4 2 2	

Facial	32	31	30	29	28	27	26	25	24	23	22	21	20	19	18	17
Bleed	1	1												1	1	
AL		1 2 2	4 2 2	3 2 2	1 3 1	2 1 2	2 1 3	3 1 4	4 1 4	2 1 1	1 1 1	1 2 1	2 3 2	2 1 2	2 2 2	
FGM		-2 0 -1	0 1 0	1 1 0	0 2 -1	0 0 1	1 0 2	2 0 2	2 0 2	1 0 0	0 0 0	0 1 0	1 2 1	0 0 0	0 1 0	
PD		3 2 3	4 1 2	2 1 2	1 1 2	2 1 1	1 1 1	1 1 2	2 1 2	1 1 1	1 1 1	1 1 1	1 1 1	2 1 2	2 1 2	

Figure 1.6.7 Periodontal chart one year after periodontal therapy. Source: courtesy of Dr. Eduardo Sampaio and Dr. Marcelo Faveri.

- *Grade C (rapid rate of progression)*: percentage bone loss/age was more than 1.0 (50%/43 years).

Although the diagnosis of periodontitis for cases such as the one presented here is straightforward, the determination of cases at the beginning of the disease process and the distinction between severe generalized cases and more aggressive forms of periodontitis is not always easy. The new classification system presents numerous tools to help clarify such distinctions. Such understanding is very valuable in determining prognosis and establishing a treatment plan and guiding the follow-up on these cases. Although this classification is fairly new, some recent longitudinal data has validated its staging and grading parameters for long-term prognosis and outcomes following treatment of periodontal patients [5,6]. However, clinical technical issues still exist, especially in the distinction between early signs of periodontitis and more advanced forms of gingivitis, complicated by difficulties in determining initial clinical attachment loss in the absence of clear radiographic evidence of alveolar bone loss, mainly in areas where severe gingival inflammation causes hyperplasia of the gingival margin.

Clinicians should also be careful while distinguishing between patients with periodontitis and those presenting with areas of incidental attachment loss not caused by the bacterial-induced inflammation characteristic of periodontitis – what is currently described as "reduced periodontium in non-periodontitis patient" [7]. For instance, isolated sites of gingival recession caused by toothbrush trauma should not be confused as a sign of periodontitis. These lesions are easily distinguishable from recession of the gingival margin as a consequence of periodontitis on the basis of their clinical features. They involve primarily the buccal surface of teeth, with no loss of adjacent interproximal tissue, and are primarily associated with teeth with thin buccal soft tissues such as maxillary canines and premolars – what is described as "periodontal phenotype." The presence of these isolated lesions is not sufficient for the diagnosis of periodontitis, even though they are associated with attachment and alveolar bone loss. However, if lesions such as these present with CAL ≥3 mm and PD >3 mm in two or more teeth, especially in the context of plaque and gingival inflammation, then the diagnosis of periodontitis would be more likely and therefore recommended [8].

Other common examples of incidental attachment loss lesions include the bone loss associated with restorations invading the biologic width and defects on the distal aspect of second molars caused by the malposition of unerupted or partially erupted third molars. The mesial tipping of teeth can also lead to a clinically deepened sulcus and a radiographic image suggestive of a vertical bone loss. This appearance is the consequence of the apical displacement of the mesial CEJ and should not lead to the erroneous diagnosis of periodontitis. It should be noted, however, that a condition such as this may predispose the site to greater accumulation of plaque, and therefore greater risk of development of any form of periodontal disease. As one can see, there are several circumstances where the early diagnosis of periodontitis can be complicated.

The distinction among more aggressive manifestations of periodontitis, what previously was differentiated as chronic and aggressive periodontitis, can also be difficult. These two conditions have since been understood as one single disease – periodontitis – as no significant evidence could corroborate a distinct etiologic or pathologic process for each of the former [3,9,10]. Such distinctions now are helped by the use of the grading system and among other features aim to find aggressive manifestations, i.e. those that show a faster rate of tissue loss and a greater risk for further progression. However, clinicians rarely have the opportunity to measure rates of disease progression, and therefore indirect measures may assist in this understanding, especially using the percentage bone loss/age formula incorporated in the grading. Although periodontitis can affect individuals of any age, chronological age remains an essential component of the natural progression of periodontitis if left untreated. If a younger individual presents with advanced attachment and bone loss, it is concluded that these subjects are presenting a faster rate of progression.

Although the description of a specific disease called "aggressive periodontitis" is no longer adopted, the classical presentation of several clinical features that made it easily distinguishable, such as age of onset, primarily incisors and firsts molars affected by the disease (including a tendency to manifest infrabony angular defects around these molars), and an overall lack of clinical signs of inflammation and minimal amounts of gross plaque and calculus accumulation despite severe bone loss around the affected teeth is accounted for by the new grading system, especially the grade C pattern.

The treatment of periodontitis as discussed in later chapters depends on the ability of the clinician to remove plaque and calculus from the root surfaces, allowing for proper healing of the gingival tissues, and on the capacity of the patient to perform proper plaque control. These are the cornerstones of periodontal therapy. Although the focus of this case is the diagnosis, but not treatment, of periodontitis, it is important to emphasize that the results obtained with anti-infective periodontal therapy will determine the long-term prognosis of the case and the need for additional treatment. Therefore, it is essential that clinicians examine the outcome of the initial therapy before any additional decisions regarding the case can be made, and this reevaluation could be considered part of the diagnostic process.

Studies examining the prognostic ability of periodontal clinical parameters have demonstrated that the presence of plaque, BOP, and suppuration have very low positive predictive values but very high negative predictive values [11,12]. This indicates that sites without clinical signs of inflammation are at very low risk for disease progression and might not require additional therapy. In addition, the accumulation of information regarding the clinical parameters for a given site over time increases the prognostic value of these parameters. Sites with constant BOP have a much higher chance of progression than sites that bleed sporadically [12]. These findings support the notion that any site cleared of periodontitis, but still presenting with PD ≥4 mm and BOP should be carefully monitored during the maintenance phase [7]. It is also well established that the prognosis of periodontitis directly depends on the patient's ability to control plaque accumulation. A longer follow-up will afford the clinician a better assessment of the patient's oral hygiene skills.

The presence of residual pockets after initial therapy, rather than the presence of deep pockets at the initial examination, is associated with an increased risk of future attachment loss [13]. This information is readily available to periodontists and can add great insights into the long-term prognosis of the case. When clinicians are trying to assess the outcome of their initial periodontal therapy, another key piece of information is how much improvement one can anticipate. In other words, what should be the realistic expectation of a therapist regarding the treatment outcome? This clearly will depend on the severity and extent of the periodontal condition at the beginning of treatment, also understood by the given staging and grading of the case. A few clinical end points for the active phase of periodontal treatment have been recently suggested, such as the presence of at most four sites with PD ≥5 mm [14], absence of sites with PD ≥4 mm and bleeding on probing and <10% of sites with BOP in the mouth [7], and absence of sites with PD ≥5 mm with BOP and no sites with PD ≥6 mm [15]. All these authors have suggested that successful anti-infective treatment should lead to a minimal number of deep pockets and of sites with BOP in the mouth after treatment.

In addition, several longitudinal studies have been conducted, and guidelines regarding the amount of pocket depth reduction and clinical attachment gains for each initial pocket depth are available and should be used to keep the outcome of treatment in perspective [16,17]. It is unrealistic, for instance, to expect a 9-mm pocket to convert to a 3-mm sulcus after SRP. The staging of the case may therefore allow a better understanding of what to expect of the case and what course of action a clinician should take. For example, a case described as periodontitis stage I/II will need anti-infective therapies, but likely will not need any further treatment if this initial phase is successful. A periodontitis stage III is one where the patient may expect some teeth loss following long-term care, but is likely to maintain most of the dentition, if not all, if proper anti-infective treatment and good home care are maintained. However, because of the multiple complexities of such cases, they may benefit from a consultation with a periodontist, and may need adjunctive antimicrobials and periodontal surgery, especially those with a generalized extent. A periodontitis stage IV is one where the patient may expect complete loss of the dentition if appropriate treatment is not timely rendered, or if successful outcomes are not established. These cases would significantly benefit from multidisciplinary treatment, especially a team of professionals with advanced restorative/prosthodontic and periodontal skills. If part of the dentition remains, these cases may also benefit from adjunctive antimicrobials and periodontal surgery. The grading of the case may also help establish expectations and course of action. Especially in cases that have modifiers affecting the grade, such as diabetes and smoking, an integrative approach involving the medical care team in the management of the case would be of benefit to the outcomes of periodontal treatment and the overall health of the patient. Cases without known systemic conditions, but presenting with grade C features, may also benefit from a more careful analysis by such an integrated healthcare team, or at least may need more attention and special care from the dental providers.

Self-Study Questions

A. What are the clinical features that differentiate incidental loss of attachment resulting from mechanical trauma from periodontitis-induced loss of attachment?

B. If a clinician is unsure about the diagnosis of the case based on the presence of some aggressive characteristics (i.e. periodontitis as a manifestation of systemic disease or generalized periodontitis), how should he or she proceed?

C. What are the possible therapeutic consequences of a differential diagnosis between periodontitis of

different gradings or of other potentially aggressive manifestations?

D. If the initial outcome of a periodontal anti-infective therapy is below the standards indicated by the literature, what should the therapist suspect and how should he or she proceed?

E. How should the periodontist proceed if, by the reexamination, the case has several residual pockets?

Answers located at the end of the chapter.

References

1. Caton JG, Armitage G, Berglundh T, et al. A new classification scheme for periodontal and peri-implant diseases and conditions: introduction and key changes from the 1999 classification. *J Clin Periodontol* 2018;45(Suppl 20):S1–S8.
2. Page RC, Eke PI. Case definitions for use in population-based surveillance of periodontitis. *J Periodontol* 2007;78:1387–1399.
3. Papapanou PN, Sanz M, Buduneli N, et al. Periodontitis: consensus report on workgroup 2 of the 2017 World Workshop on the Classification of Periodontal and Peri-Implant Diseases and Conditions. *J Clin Periodontol* 2018;45(Suppl 20):S162–S170.
4. Sanz M, Papapanou PN, Tonetti MS, et al. Guest Editorial: clarifications on the use of the new classification of periodontitis. *J Clin Periodontol* 2020;47(6):658–659.
5. Ravidà A, Troiano G, Qazi M, et al. Development of a nomogram for the prediction of periodontal tooth loss using the staging and grading system: a long-term cohort study. *J Clin Periodontol* 2020;47(11):1362–1370.
6. Ravidà A, Qazi M, Troiano G, et al. Using periodontal staging and grading system as a prognostic factor for future tooth loss: a long-term retrospective study. *J Periodontol* 2020;91(4):454–461.
7. Chapple ILC, Mealey BL, Van Dyke TE, et al. Periodontal health and gingival diseases and conditions on an intact and a reduced periodontium: consensus report of workgroup 1 of the 2017 World Workshop on the Classification of Periodontal and Peri-implant Diseases and Conditions. *J Clin Periodontolol* 2018;45(Suppl 20):S68–S77.
8. Tonetti MS, Greenwell H, Kornman KS. Staging and grading of periodontitis: framework and proposal of a new classification and case definition. *J Periodontol* 2018;89(Suppl 1):S159–S172.
9. Duarte PM, Bastos MF, Fermiano D, et al. Do subjects with aggressive and chronic periodontitis exhibit a different cytokine/chemokine profile in the gingival crevicular fluid? A systematic review. *J Periodontal Res* 2015;50(1):18–27.
10. Montenegro SCL, Retamal-Valdes B, Bueno-Silva B, et al. Do patients with aggressive and chronic periodontitis exhibit specific differences in the subgingival microbial composition? A systematic review. *J Periodontol* 2020; 91(11):1503–1520.
11. Claffey N, Nylund K, Kiger R, et al. Diagnostic predictability of scores of plaque, bleeding, suppuration and probing depth for probing attachment loss: 3½ years of observation following initial periodontal therapy. *J Clin Periodontol* 1990;17:108–114.
12. Lang NP, Adler R, Joss A, Nyman S. Absence of bleeding on probing. An indicator of periodontal stability. *J Clin Periodontol* 1990;17:714–721.
13. Matuliene G, Pjetursson BE, Salvi GE, et al. Influence of residual pockets on progression of periodontitis and tooth loss: results after 11 years of maintenance. *J Clin Periodontol* 2008;35(8):685–695.
14. Feres M, Retamal-Valdes B, Faveri M, et al. Proposal of a clinical endpoint for periodontal trials: the treat-to-target approach. *J Int Acad Periodontol* 2020;22(2):41–53.
15. Loos BG, Needleman I. Endpoints of active periodontal therapy. *J Clin Periodontol* 2020;47(Suppl 22):61–71.
16. Hung HC, Douglass CW. Meta-analysis of the effect of scaling and root planing, surgical treatment and antibiotic therapies on periodontal probing depth and attachment loss. *J Clin Periodontol* 2002;29:975–986.
17. Heitz-Mayfield LJ, Trombelli L, Heitz F, et al. A systematic review of the effect of surgical debridement vs non-surgical debridement for the treatment of chronic periodontitis. *J Clin Periodontol* 2002;29(Suppl 3):92–102; discussion 160–162.

18. Jepsen S, Caton JG, Albandar JM, et al. Periodontal manifestations of systemic diseases and developmental and acquired conditions: consensus report of workgroup 3 of the 2018 World Workshop on the Classification of Periodontal and Peri-Implant Diseases and Conditions. *J Clin Periodontol* 2018;45(Suppl 20):S219–S229.

19. Mongardini C, van Steenberghe D, Dekeyser C, Quirynen M. One stage full-versus partial-mouth disinfection in the treatment of chronic adult or generalized early-onset periodontitis. I. Long-term clinical observations. *J Periodontol* 1999;70:632–645.

20. Claffey N, Egelberg J. Clinical indicators of probing attachment loss following initial periodontal treatment in advanced periodontitis patients. *J Clin Periodontol* 1995; 22:690–696.

21. Nyman S, Rosling B, Lindhe J. Effect of professional tooth cleaning on healing after periodontal surgery. *J Clin Periodontol* 1975;2:80–86.

TAKE-HOME POINTS

A. Incidental loss of attachment associated with mechanical trauma has distinct clinical features that make it clearly distinguishable from infection/inflammation-induced attachment loss. It tends to be circumscribed to buccal surfaces, particularly in areas of a very thin soft tissue, and the neighboring papilla present normal height. The tissue surrounding the recession has a very healthy appearance, and it is not uncommon to have toothbrush abrasion associated with the gingival recession. The collapse of gingival tissues on buccal surfaces can also be associated with marginal gingival inflammation, but in this case the presence of plaque and calculus is not an uncommon finding and the tissues surrounding the gingival recession tend to show clinical signs of inflammation.

B. The distinction between the two diagnoses can be difficult at times. The differences are typically determined by the age of onset, rate of progression, and the patterns of bone loss. In general, periodontitis starts at age 30–35 years and progresses in random bursts in different sites throughout life. If the disease presents in younger patients or can be documented to have occurred in a short period, it tends to be classified as of more aggressive nature, increasing the grading of the case for periodontitis, or considering the possibility of a systemic disease that may have major impact on periodontal tissues. Both forms of periodontitis can occur in a localized or generalized pattern. Familial aggregation is one of the features of many forms of aggressive patterns of periodontitis; therefore, if this is suspected, the clinician should inquire about the periodontal status of close relatives or suggest they receive an oral examination. Many common chronic diseases, such as diabetes, may affect the course of periodontitis, or at least are intrinsically associated with it, but do not necessarily have a distinguishable phenotype, and thus the diagnosis still is of periodontitis. However, a careful review of the medical history is imperative, including referral for further evaluations or consultations for any systemic comorbidities, including rare medical disorders that may have major impact on the periodontal tissues. Those medical evaluations should confirm the periodontal diagnosis and direct the treatment plan. Because of the much higher prevalence of periodontitis compared with other aggressive forms associated with rare systemic diseases, this will be the most prevalent diagnosis, but the potential for the latter should not be dismissed [18].

C. Although it is not the intent here to address therapy, which is discussed extensively in other chapters of the book, the relevance of the distinction between different aggressive forms of periodontitis, especially considering the grading system of the new classification, depends on the assumption that these clinical forms of the disease would require specific types of treatment. Classical literature has indicated that subjects with different aggressive forms of periodontitis (aggressive forms compared to "chronic periodontitis" in previous classifications) with comparable extent and severity of the conditions tend to respond similarly to periodontal therapy [19]. This would imply that the prognosis of the case would depend more on the extent and severity (staging) of the periodontal disease, and also the progression and risk factors associated with it (grading).

Therefore, the new classification system could be helpful in establishing different treatment protocols according to the combination of the findings already discussed. A general dentist should be especially mindful in consulting a periodontist whenever the diagnosis reaches stage III or grade B, and potentially other dental and healthcare providers the diagnosis reaches stage IV or grade C, or if the case presents with other signs of potential aggressiveness or major complexity.

D. In these circumstances, the clinician should confirm the grading of the case, ruling out any systemic causes for the disease (risk factors such as smoking or uncontrolled diabetes, immunocompromise, endocrine disorders, or syndromes). The next thing to check is the efficiency of the patient's plaque control. This can be easily ascertained by the gingival and plaque indices. In the presence of large amounts of plaque, reinfection of pockets occurs fast and healing is compromised. Once the level of oral hygiene of the patient has been assessed, provided it was not the problem, the next steps will depend greatly on the level of periodontal training of the therapist. If the clinician is an experienced periodontist, the chances are that therapy was properly executed and there is very little room for improvement. The clinician might be dealing with a rare case of refractory periodontitis, where the subject does not respond to conventional therapy. The next step would be to consider adjunctive or complementary approaches such as systemic antibiotics and/or periodontal surgery. If a less experienced clinician is involved, the fair assumption is there was failure in calculus removal to a level compatible with resolution of the periodontal

condition. Particularly for severe generalized forms (higher staging) of the disease this should not be a surprise because subgingival debridement of deep pockets is not an easy task and requires highly skilled and well-trained individuals. Residual pockets should be carefully reinstrumented, and this step should involve as many sessions as needed. A new period of three months of healing should be given before an assessment of the outcome of this new cycle of SRP is conducted. Clinicians should keep in mind that there is very little risk to the patient in delaying a possible surgical phase of treatment to make every effort to guarantee an optimal outcome of the anti-infective therapy.

E. Although the presence of residual pockets has been demonstrated as a good predictor of future attachment loss [20], clinicians should interpret this information with caution. Several other clinical aspects will impact the prognosis of the case. such as the level of plaque control by the subject, the presence of BOP, and the presence of furcation defects. Further, one must keep in mind that periodontal surgical procedures involve nonaffected periodontally diseased sites adjacent to residual pockets. If residual pockets are isolated nonbleeding lesions, they present a very low risk of progression and can be easily addressed with SRP during supportive periodontal therapy. Conversely, if residual pockets cluster around a few adjacent teeth and BOP is a recurrent finding over several sessions of maintenance, a surgical approach seems adequate. Periodontal surgery in the absence of proper plaque control exposes the periodontal patient to the risk of accelerated attachment loss [21] and should be avoided at all costs.

Case 7

Local Anatomic Factors Contributing to Periodontal Disease

CASE STORY

A 63-year-old woman was referred for evaluation of periodontal condition on tooth #19. The patient reported tenderness around tooth #19 from time to time when she applied pressure on the buccal gingiva (Figures 1.7.1 and 1.7.2).

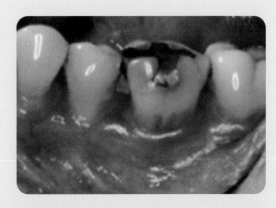

Figure 1.7.1 Clinical presentation of tooth #19.

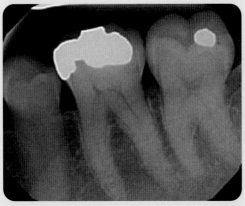
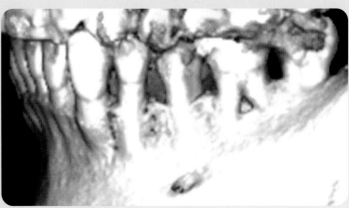

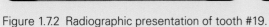

Figure 1.7.2 Radiographic presentation of tooth #19.

LEARNING GOALS AND OBJECTIVES

■ To be able to identify local anatomic factors that may contribute to periodontal disease
■ To understand the anatomy of the furcation and root
■ To be able to diagnose a furcation invasion using a furcation classification system

Medical History

The patient's medical history was not significant. The patient reported no allergies to any medication, latex, metal, or food.

Review of Systems

• Vital signs
  ○ Blood pressure: 119/71 mmHg

○ Pulse rate: 56 beats/minute
○ Respiratory rate: 15 breaths/minute

Social History

The patient denied smoking, occasionally drank alcohol during social events, and denied the use of recreational drugs. The patient was a yoga instructor and claimed that she had a very healthy lifestyle.

Oral Hygiene Status

The patient brushed twice a day with electric toothbrush and flossed every day.

Extraoral Examination

No significant findings were present.

Intraoral Examination

- Soft tissues including buccal mucosa, hard and soft palate, floor of the mouth, and tongue were all within normal limits.
- There was generalized gingival recession, although most teeth still had adequate amounts of attached keratinized gingiva.

- Refer to Figure 1.7.3 for the periodontal charting.
- Tooth #19 exhibited a probing depth of 8 mm on the midbuccal aspect and clinically had grade II furcation invasion. No significant mobility was detected.
- A cervical enamel projection (CEP) was detected at the buccal furcation area below the gingival margin on #19.

Occlusion

No occlusal interferences were detected.

Radiographic Examination

Periapical radiograph of tooth #19 did not show a significant amount of bone loss around the furcation area. Cone beam computed tomography (CT) was used to further examine the periodontal condition of tooth #19 and showed evidence of bone loss over the buccal furcation area (Figure 1.7.2).

Diagnosis

A diagnosis of stage III grade B periodontitis was made based on the clinical and radiographic examinations with respective to the severity of furcation involvement (grade II) and the rate of progression of bone loss (<2 mm over

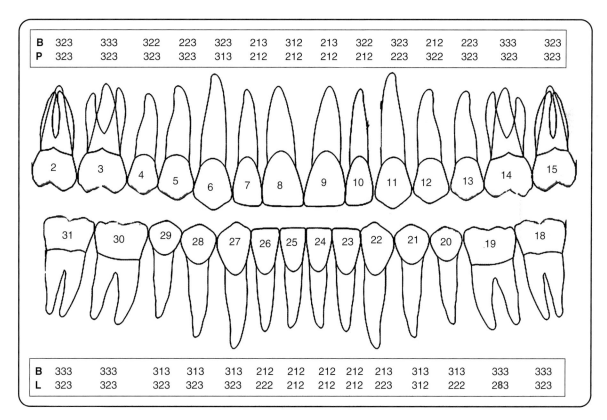

Figure 1.7.3 Periodontal probing depth measurements during initial visit.

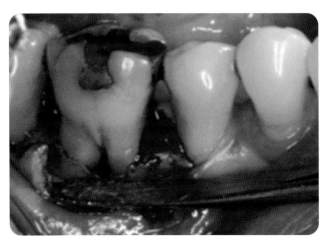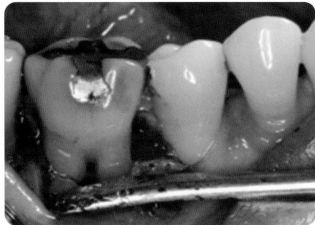

Figure 1.7.4 Cervical enamel projection (CEP) on buccal of tooth #19 (left); CEP removed (right).

five years). The attachment loss and grade II furcation invasion on tooth #19 required definitive periodontal treatment. The prognosis of #19 was questionable because the grade II furcation made the patient's daily oral hygiene maintenance in this area very difficult [1].

Treatment Plan

The treatment plan and sequence were as follows.
- Diagnostic phase: comprehensive dental and peri-odontal examination, radiographic examination.
- Disease control phase: oral hygiene instruction, adult prophylaxis, localized scaling, and root planing of the buccal furcation of tooth #19.
- Reevaluation phase: periodontal reevaluation of tooth #19, oral hygiene evaluation and reinforcement.
- Surgical phase: open flap debridement and removal of the CEP on the buccal aspect of tooth #19.
- Maintenance phase: regular three-month periodontal maintenance visits.

Treatment

Localized scaling and root planing of tooth #19 was performed using a Cavitron and hand instruments. After a healing period of six weeks, periodontal reevaluation revealed a probing depth of 8 mm with bleeding on probing on the midbuccal of #19. The treatment plan at this point included surgical treatment to remove the CEP. An intrasulcular incision was made from the distal line angle of tooth #18 to mesial line angle of tooth #20 using a 15C blade. Full-thickness buccal and lingual flaps were raised to expose the furcation area of tooth #19 and allow adequate visualization of, and access to, the

CEP. Figure 1.7.4 shows that the CEP extended apically almost to the level of bone crest. A diamond burr was then used to remove the CEP completely (Figure 1.7.4) and the furca was debrided using a Cavitron and hand instruments. The flap was eventually sutured back into its original position. Postoperative instructions were given and the patient was seen two weeks later for a follow-up. Six months later, localized probing at tooth #19 showed a probing depth of 4 mm without bleeding on probing.

Discussion

The patient presented with a probing depth of 8 mm on the buccal furcation area of tooth #19, possibly due to the presence of a CEP that extended deep into the furcation. The presence of the CEP prevented proper soft tissue attachment at the furcal area, leading to the formation of a deep periodontal pocket. Bone loss at the furcal area was most likely due to prolonged plaque accumulation in this periodontal pocket that subsequently led to chronic inflammation and hence attachment loss. By removing the CEP, enamel at the furcation was eliminated to expose the underlying dentin, thereby allowing soft tissue attachment to occur over this area. In so doing, a periodontal pocket was eliminated. Note that a grade II furcation can also be treated with guided tissue regeneration or a bone graft.

It is critical to identify all local etiologic factors because they may accelerate periodontal disease progression and affect the diagnosis, prognosis, and treatment of the disease.

Self-Study Questions

A. What are some anatomic factors that may contribute to periodontal disease?

B. Describe the anatomy of a furcation and define furcation invasion.

C. Name different classification systems of furcation invasion.

D. How should you diagnose a furcation invasion?

Answers located at the end of the chapter.

ACKNOWLEDGMENT
We would like to thank Dr. David Yu for providing Figure 1.7.8.

References

1. McGuire MK, Nunn ME. Prognosis versus actual outcome. II. The effectiveness of clinical parameters in developing an accurate prognosis. *J Periodontol* 1996;67:658–665.
2. Masters DH, Hoskins SW. Projection of cervical enamel into molar furcations. *J Periodontol* 1964;35:49–53.
3. Bissada NF, Abdelmalek RG. Incidence of cervical enamel projections and its relationship to furcation involvement in Egyptian skulls. *J Periodontol* 1973;44:583–585.
4. Swan RH, Hurt WC. Cervical enamel projections as an etiologic factor in furcation involvement. *J Am Dent Assoc* 1976;93:342–345.
5. Moskow BS, Canut PM. Studies on root enamel (2). Enamel pearls. A review of their morphology, localization, nomenclature, occurrence, classification, histogenesis and incidence. *J Clin Periodontol* 1990;17:275–281.
6. Bower RC. Furcation morphology relative to periodontal treatment. Furcation root surface anatomy. *J Periodontol* 1979;50:366–374.
7. Haskova JE, Gill DS, Figueiredo JAP, et al. Taurodontism: a review. *Dent Update* 2009;36:235–236.
8. Everett FG, Jump EB, Holder TD, Williams GC. The intermediate bifurcational ridge: a study of the morphology of the bifurcation of the lower first molar. *J Dent Res* 1958;37:162–169.
9. Burch JG, Hulen S. A study of the presence of accessory foramina and the topography of molar furcations. *Oral Surg Oral Med Oral Pathol* 1974;38:451–455.
10. Ben-Bassat Y, Brin I. The labiogingival notch: an anatomical variation of clinical importance. *J Am Dent Assoc* 2001;132:919–921.
11. Schwartz SA, Koch MA, Deas DE, Powell CA. Combined endodontic–periodontic treatment of a palatal groove: a case report. *J Endod* 2006;32:573–578.
12. Vertucci FJ, Williams RG. Furcation canals in the human mandibular first molar. *Oral Surg Oral Med Oral Pathol* 1974;38:308–314.
13. Dunlap RM, Gher ME. Root surface measurements of the mandibular first molar. *J Periodontol* 1985;56:234–238.
14. Tal H. Relationship between the depths of furcal defects and alveolar bone loss. *J Periodontol* 1982;53:631–634.
15. Bower RC. Furcation morphology relative to periodontal treatment. Furcation entrance architecture. *J Periodontol* 1979;50:23–27.
16. Hermann DW, Gher ME Jr, Dunlap RM, Pelleu GB Jr. The potential attachment area of the maxillary first molar. *J Periodontol* 1983;54:431–434.
17. Gher MW Jr, Dunlap RW. Linear variation of the root surface area of the maxillary first molar. *J Periodontol* 1985;56:39–43.
18. Booker BW 3rd, Loughlin DM. A morphologic study of the mesial root surface of the adolescent maxillary first bicuspid. *J Periodontol* 1985;56:666–670.
19. Gher ME, Vernino AR. Root morphology: clinical significance in pathogenesis and treatment of periodontal disease. *J Am Dent Assoc* 1980;101:627–633.
20. Glickman I. *Clinical Periodontology*, 2nd edn. Philadelphia, PA: Saunders, 1958:694–696.
21. Hamp SE, Nyman S, Lindhe J. Periodontal treatment of multirooted teeth. Results after 5 years. *J Clin Periodontol* 1975;2:126–135.
22. Tarnow D, Fletcher P. Classification of the vertical component of furcation involvement. *J Periodontol* 1984;55:283–284.
23. Hardekopf JD, Dunlap RM, Ahl DR, Pelleu GB Jr. The "furcation arrow." A reliable radiographic image? *J Periodontol* 1987;58:258–261.
24. Ross IF, Thompson RH Jr. Furcation involvement in maxillary and mandibular molars. *J Periodontol* 1980;51:450–454.

TAKE-HOME POINTS

A.

Proximal Contact Relation

Open interproximal contacts or uneven marginal ridge relations may encourage food impaction between the teeth. If proper oral hygiene is absent, food impaction can lead to inflammation, thereby potentially resulting in attachment loss in the interproximal area (Figure 1.7.5).

Root Proximity

Close root proximity between the two adjacent teeth will render oral hygiene difficult to maintain for both the patient and the dental professionals. Hence without good oral hygiene there can be loss of attachment between the two teeth (Figure 1.7.6).

Cervical Enamel Projections and Enamel Pearls

CEPs are extensions of enamel to the furcal area of the root surface. CEPs may potentially predispose a furcation to attachment loss because they pre-vent connective tissue attachment at furcation. As such, a periodontal pocket may form, leading to plaque accumulation and possibly furcation invasion.

Most clinicians agree there is a correlation between CEPs and the incidence of furcation invasion. Masters and Hoskins reported that 90% of mandibular furcation

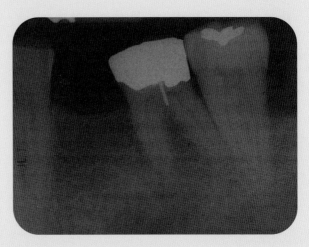

Figure 1.7.6 Close root proximity between teeth #18 and #19.

invasions have CEPs [2]. Bissada and Abdelmalek reported a 50% correlation between CEPs and furcation invasion [3]. Swan and Hurt observed a statistically significant association between CEPs and furcation invasion [4].

In descending order of occurrence, CEPs are most commonly seen in mandibular second molars, maxillary second molars, mandibular first molars, and maxillary first molars. When CEPs are observed, they are usually seen on buccal aspects of molars [2] (Figure 1.7.7).

Enamel pearls are ectopic globules of enamel and sometimes pulpal tissue that often adhere to the cementoenamel junction (CEJ). They are present in roughly 2.7% of the molars and are mostly found on maxillary third and second molars [5]. Moskow and Canut suggested that enamel pearls may also predis-pose a furcation to attachment loss [5] (Figure 1.7.8).

Root Concavity

The furcal aspects of the roots frequently have concavities with a certain amount of depth (see Question B for details) that will encourage plaque accumulation and prevent proper instrumentation of furcation. Hence a root concavity may predispose the furcation to attachment loss (Figure 1.7.9).

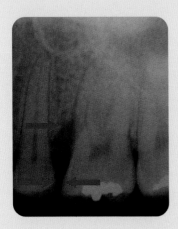

Figure 1.7.5 Interproximal open contact between teeth #13 and #14 (indicated by the red arrows) and vertical bone loss on #14 mesial.

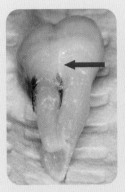
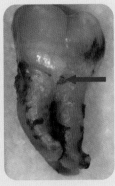

Figure 1.7.7 Cervical enamel projection (indicated by the red arrow).

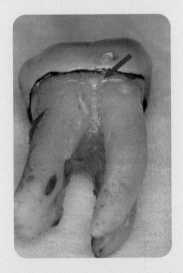

Figure 1.7.8 Enamel pearl (indicated by the red arrow).

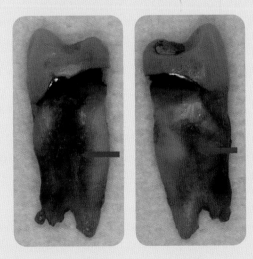

Figure 1.7.9 Mesial and distal root concavities of maxillary first premolar.

Size of Furcation Entrance

Approximately 80% of all furcation entrances are less than 1.0 mm in diameter, with about 60% less than 0.75 mm [6]. Because frequently used curettes and scalers have a face width of 0.75–1.10 mm, it is unlikely that effective removal of accretions at furcation can be achieved by using these instruments alone. Hence a small furcation entrance may predispose a furcation to attachment loss (Figure 1.7.10).

Root Divergence and Root Fusion

The degree of root divergence in a multirooted tooth will influence the ability of the patient and dental professionals to control plaque level. Diverging roots allow easier instrumentation to the furcation area, whereas converging roots (e.g. root fusion) render access to the furcation area very difficult, resulting in poor plaque control and possible attachment loss (Figure 1.7.11).

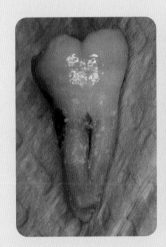
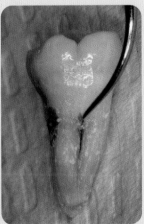

Figure 1.7.10 The size of the Cavitron tip is too big to enter the furcated area, rendering scaling and root planing in this area very difficult.

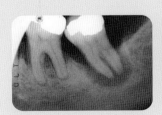
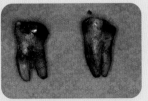

Figure 1.7.11 The root divergence of #19 is more prominent than that of #17.

Root Trunk Length

The length of root trunk affects attachment loss. The longer a given root trunk, the less likely a furcation will be predisposed to attachment loss. Teeth with taurodontism usually have apically displaced furcation and longer root trunk length [7] (Figure 1.7.12).

Intermediate Bifurcation Ridge

Intermediate bifurcation ridges are ridges spanning the bifurcation of mandibular molars in the mesio-distal direction. These ridges are present in 70–77% of the mandibular molars [8,9]. Just like other anatomic structures, the presence of an intermediate bifurcation ridge may hinder effective plaque control and root preparation by both the patient and dentist.

Buccal Radicular Groove and Palato-gingival Groove

Buccal radicular grooves and palato-gingival grooves are developmental phenomena that affect mainly the maxillary anterior teeth [10,11]. These grooves run on the roots in the coronal-apical direction. Due to their anatomy, the grooves frequently provide a plaque-retentive area that is very difficult to instrument, making teeth with these developmental grooves more prone to attachment loss (Figure 1.7.13).

Accessory Pulpal Canals

Accessory pulpal canals are small endodontic canals branching off from the main root canal that may furnish a communication between the pulpal chamber and the periodontal ligament. These accessory canals are usually located near the root apex; however, they can also be found anywhere along the root, including the furcation area. There is a theory that some periodontal infections can originate from endodontic sources, traveling through accessory/lateral canals located in the furcation areas. In these cases there is periodontal involvement in the furcation, but the infec-

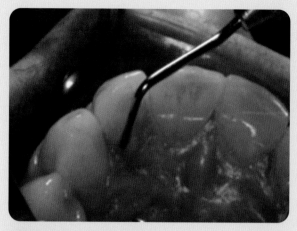

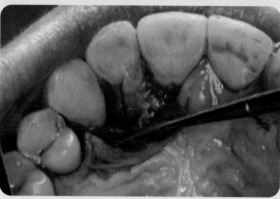

Figure 1.7.13 Palato-gingival groove present on tooth #10 as indicated by the probe tip.

tion originated in the pulp. Although still controversial, it has been proposed that periodontal disease can result from pulpal infection. An endodontic infection may be present at the furcation area when the infection travels through accessory canals that end at the furca. Vertucci and Williams reported that accessory canals at furcations are present in 46% of human lower first molars [12]. Burch and Hulen observed accessory canals in 76% of maxillary and mandibular molars [9].

Restorative Considerations

Dental restorations with overhangs or open margins are plaque-retentive areas that may result in gingival inflammation and attachment loss. Restorative margins are most compatible with the periodontium when located either supragingivally or at the level of the gingival margin. Should the restorative margin violate the biologic width, the resulting inflammatory process may lead to gingival recession, bone loss, and

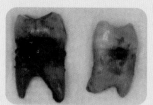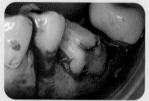

Figure 1.7.12 Long root trunk length (left) and short root trunk at #19 (right).

exposure of the restorative margin. The restorative contour (e.g. crown contour) should follow the root surface contour rather than accentuating the cervical bulge to support periodontal health. In the case of bridges, the design of the pontic can affect its ability to be cleaned and hence the periodontal health of the teeth (Figure 1.7.14).

B. A furcation is an anatomic area where the roots of a multirooted tooth start to diverge. Mandibular molars and maxillary first premolars are bifurcated because they each have two roots. Maxillary molars are trifurcated because they each have three roots.

A furcation consists of two parts: (i) root separation area, where alveolar bone begins to separate the roots, and (ii) fluting area, the part of the root that is directly coronal to the root separation area.

There are often concavities in the furcal side of the roots. In mandibular molars, all the mesial roots have concavities on the furcal side, with each concavity averaging 0.7 mm in depth [13]. Likewise, 99% of the distal roots of mandibular molars have concavities on the furcal side, with an average depth of 0.5 mm [13]. The root trunk, which is the distance from the CEJ to the level of root separation, is about 4.0 ± 0.7 mm in mandibular first molars [13,14].

In maxillary molars, 94% of the mesiobuccal roots have concavities on the furcal side, with each concavity averaging 0.3 mm in depth [15]. Roughly one-third (31%) of the mesiodistal roots and one-quarter (17%) of the palatal roots have concavities, and each concavity is about 0.1 mm in depth [15]. The lengths of root trunks of maxillary molars are

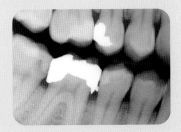

Figure 1.7.14 Overhangs on the mesial and distal of tooth #30 that may eventually lead to bone loss on the mesial and distal of #30.

3.6, 4.2, and 4.8 mm on the mesial, buccal, and distal surfaces, respectively [16,17].

All bifurcated maxillary first premolars have a mesial and distal root trunk of about 8 mm. In addition, almost all the buccal roots have "developmental depressions" also known as "buccal furcation groove" present at the 9.4-mm level on the furcal side [18,19].

Furcation invasion is defined as a loss of attachment within a furcation. When there is a loss of clinical attachment, the presence of concavities on these roots at furcation will hinder effective plaque control at these areas.

C. There are a number of different classification systems of furcation invasion. The three most commonly used systems are as follows.

Glickman Classification

The Glickman classification [20] describes both the vertical and horizontal components of the furcation invasion.

Grade I	Pocket formation into the fluting area but with intact interradicular bone.
Grade II	Pocket formation into the root separation area with interradicular bone loss that is not completely through to the opposite side of the furcation.
Grade III	Same as grade II but with through-and-through interradicular bone loss (the soft tissue still covers part of the entrance of the furcation).
Grade IV	Same as grade III but with gingival recession making furcation clinically visible.

Hamp Classification

The Hamp et al. classification [21] describes the horizontal component of the furcation invasion.

Degree I	Horizontal bone loss going into the furcation <3 mm.
Degree II	Horizontal bone loss going into the furcation >3 mm but not to the opposite side.
Degree III	A through-and-through horizontal bone loss in the furcation.

Tarnow and Fletcher Classification

The Tarnow and Fletcher classification [22] describes the vertical component of the furcation invasion.

Subclass A	Vertical attachment loss 0–3 mm in furcation.
Subclass B	Vertical attachment loss of 4–6 mm in furcation.
Subclass C	Vertical attachment loss of >7 mm.

D. The most effective way to diagnose a furcation invasion is to use a combination of clinical examination and radiographic evaluation. The clinical examination involves using periodontal and furcation probes to detect the furcation invasion.

Radiographs must be taken with a paralleling technique to minimize distortion of the images. Note that radiographically the palatal root of maxillary molars may leave a grade III furcation invasion undetected due to the overlapping of the palatal root with mesiobuccal and distobuccal roots. In addition, the presence of a furcation arrow (a triangular shadow seen at either the mesial or distal roots in the interproximal area on maxillary molars) may possibly suggest the presence of grade II–III furcation invasion on maxillary molars [23] (Figure 1.7.15). The more extensive a given furcation invasion, the higher the likelihood of observing the furcation arrow. However, it must be noted that the absence of furcation arrow does not necessarily suggest the absence of a furcation invasion.

Generally, interproximal surfaces of the maxillary molars are more prone to furcation invasion than buccal surfaces [24].

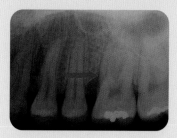

Figure 1.7.15 Furcation arrow (red arrow) is showing furcal involvement on the mesial of #14 radiographically.

Case 8

Oral–Systemic Links

CASE STORY

A 64-year-old Hispanic female presented as a referral to a periodontist from a general dental practice because of her severe periodontal condition. Her chief concern was I need to have my gums treated. She stated that her last professional prophylaxis was seven years before, and reported brushing with a manual and electric toothbrush once daily. The patient denied flossing and reported use of mouthwash once a day in the morning. On observation at her initial examination, her techniques of both brushing and flossing were inadequate to remove subgingival cervical and interproximal plaque. She reported loss of teeth due to periodontal disease and decay.

LEARNING GOALS AND OBJECTIVES

■ To evaluate the effects that diabetes may cause on oral health
■ To show the role of periodontal treatment on diabetic patients

Medical History

The patient reported that she suffered from hypertension, hyperlipidemia, type 2 diabetes mellitus, and gastroesophageal reflux disease, for which she was taking, respectively, losartan/hydrochlorothiazide 100/25 mg daily, simvastatin 20 mg daily, metformin 500 mg q.i.d., and omeprazole 20 mg daily. No specific information could be collected regarding HbA_{1c}, but the patient reported levels higher than 7%.

Review of Systems

- Vital signs
  - Blood pressure: 150/70 mmHg
  - Pulse rate: 88 beats/minute
  - Respiratory rate: 16 breaths/minute
- Height 1.55 m, weight 74.4 kg so BMI = 31.0, which classifies her as obese

Social History

The patient had never smoked and did not drink alcohol.

Extraoral Examination

The extraoral examination revealed no significant findings. The patient presented with no suspicious masses or swellings. Her face was symmetric, and there were no swollen lymph nodes noted on palpation and direct observation. Her eyes were of normal dimension, with the interpupillary line parallel to the occlusal plane. An assessment of the temporomandibular joints showed no alteration of the anatomic structures and her mandibular excursions and function. The patient's skin was of normal color. Her smile line was high.

Intraoral Examination

- Oral cancer screening was negative.
- The soft tissues including tongue, floor of the mouth, and the throat appeared to be normal in color, shape, and dimension.
- The gingival tissue exhibited a thick morphotype. The color was pale pink with localized erythematous dark-red areas and pigmentation. The gingiva was enlarged on the margins and papillae. The shape was bulbous with flat papillae. The consistency appeared edematous and soft, with localized areas of firm gingiva. The gingival surface texture was smooth and shiny with localized stippling. The gingival margins were asymmetric with generalized recession.

- The patient was missing natural teeth #2, #16, #19, and #30. No caries was detected but defective restorations on #3, #7, and #10 were detected. The patient presented with multiple open contacts, with her maxillary and mandibular teeth presenting noticeable wear facets. No crowding was detected but tilting rotation and extrusion were noted on #1, #3, #7, #9, #10, #14, #18, and #31. All maxillary teeth presented fremitus, in particular #5, #7 and #10. Pathologic migration was noted on #9 and #10. On cold testing, tooth #10 was not responsive.

Clinical Investigations

- Intraoral and extraoral photographs were taken (Figure 1.8.1).
- A complete series of periapical, bitewing and panoramic radiographs were ordered (Figure 1.8.2).
- Study casts were made.
- Periodontal charting was performed, including probing depth, bleeding on probing, clinical attachment loss, mobility, suppuration, furcation, mucogingival defects, and recessions (Figure 1.8.3). This revealed the following.
  - Periodontal probing:
    - 4–6 mm: #3, 8, 13, 17, 20, 21, 22, 27, 28, 29, 32
    - 7–9 mm: #1, 4, 5, 7, 11, 15, 31
    - ≥10 mm: #6, 9, 10, 12, 14, 18
  - Furcations:
    - Class I: #31
    - Class II: #3, 18
    - Class III: #14
  - The patient presented with plaque index class 2 [1], plaque score [2] of 85%, and gingival bleeding index [3] of 80% with no evidence of suppuration.
  - Localized presence of subgingival plaque and slight subgingival calculus accumulation was noted on teeth #4, #5, #7, #18 and #31.
  - The patient exhibited generalized and reduced keratinized tissue levels on #17, #18, #20, #21, #31, and #32.
  - Mobility grade 3 for #10 and #18.

Occlusion

The patient exhibited canine class III on the right and class I on the left. Right side guidance was performed by #6 and #26 with interference #14 and #18. Left side showed group function with interference #3 and #31. Protrusion was guided by #7, #8 on #26 with interferences #14 on #18 and #3 on #31.

Radiographic Examination

The radiographic examination (Figure 1.8.2) revealed the presence of generalized horizontal bone loss with localized vertical defects (#1, #4, #5, #6, #14, #18, #31) and generalized absence of crestal lamina dura. Furcae entrances were noted on #3, #14, #15, #18, and #31. Radiographic calculus appeared on #4, #5, #7, and #9. Funneling and periodontal ligament (PDL) widening was shown on #4, #5, #7, #9, #11, #12, #14, #15, and #18.

Diagnosis

- Partial edentulism
- Generalized stage 3 grade C periodontitis [4]
- Periodontal manifestation of systemic diseases and developmental and acquired conditions
  - Other periodontal conditions: endodontic–periodontal lesions #10
  - Mucogingival deformities and conditions around teeth: localized tooth-related factors that modify or predispose to plaque-induced periodontitis
  - Mucogingival deformities and conditions around teeth:
    - Gingival/soft tissue recession
    - Lack of gingiva
  - Traumatic occlusal forces: secondary occlusal trauma
  - Prosthesis- and tooth-related factors that modify or predispose to plaque-induced gingival diseases/periodontitis
    - Localized tooth-related factors
    - Localized dental prostheses-related factors

Prognosis

The teeth prognosis followed the classification proposed by McGuire et al. [5].
- Good: #23, 24, 25, 26, 27
- Fair: #13, 20, 21, 22, 28, 29
- Poor: #3, 4, 5, 6, 8, 9, 11, 23, 17, 31, 32
- Questionable: #1, 7, 14, 15
- Hopeless: #18, 10

Treatment Plan

The treatment plan for this patient consisted of phase 1 therapy or inflammation control as follows.
- Patient motivation.
- Oral hygiene technique instructions.
- Medical consult for diabetes control.
- Interdisciplinary consultation: prosthetic/endodontic for #10, caries control and extraction of hopeless teeth #10 and #18.

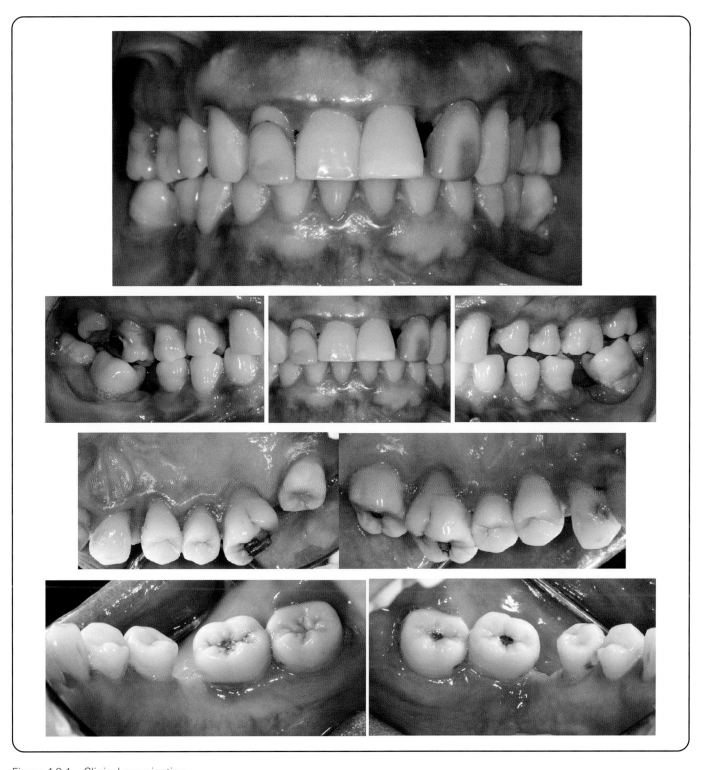

Figure 1.8.1   Clinical examination.

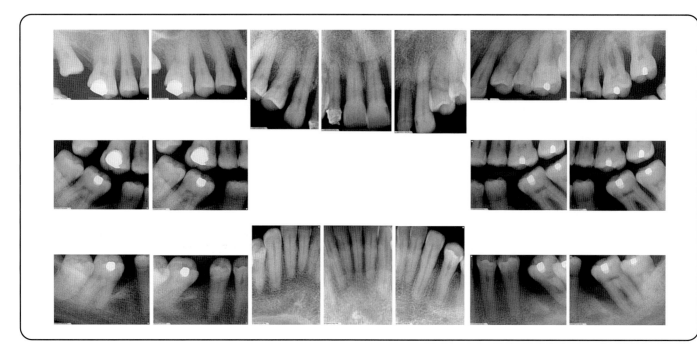

Figure 1.8.2   Full-mouth radiographs.

- Complete mouth debridement: prophylaxis and scaling and root planing of dentition.
- Reevaluation of initial phase (four to six weeks) and occlusal adjustment.

Treatment

Before initiating mechanical periodontal treatment, a clinician needs to identify potential systemic and local factors that may pose risks of disease progression. A thorough and comprehensive medical history interview is of paramount importance. After collecting all data regarding past and present systemic conditions as well as medications, the patient's primary care physician (PCP) was contacted in order to identify a strategy to bring diabetes under control. Clinically, patient motivation was assessed by observing the patient's plaque removal techniques, and these were modified in order to achieve better control of the biofilm. As an important part of this first phase, the patient demonstrated the recommended plaque control techniques for the clinician in front of a mirror. It is critical to observe the patient perform the suggested methods in order to ensure its effectiveness and to help correct improper and ineffective techniques. She was instructed in the use of all recommended plaque removal aids that were compatible with her manual capabilities. A tailored protocol was selected to suit her profile.

Following her plaque control technique instruction, her teeth were scaled and root planed, as per treatment plan recommendation, in two sessions one week apart utilizing local anesthesia. The oral hygiene techniques were again reviewed during the second session of root planing and debridement, in order to assess the patient's technical abilities. Following the assessment, the remaining half of the mouth was debrided.

Six weeks after the initial phase 1 therapy, a comprehensive periodontal reevaluation was performed to evaluate efficacy of treatment (Figures 1.8.4 and 1.8.5). A note from the physician was received confirming improvement in glucose levels, but not sufficient to consider the blood values under control and below the HbA_{1c} threshold of <7%.

Discussion

Many systemic diseases are associated with a profound loss of periodontal attachment and alveolar bone, and for some of these disorders the periodontal manifestations may be among the first signs of the disease. Systemic disorders may affect periodontal inflammation by altering the host immune response to periodontal infections; others cause defects in the connective tissue, trigger metabolic shifts in the host, or operate by other mechanisms. For some more common systemic disorders, their contribution to the loss of periodontal

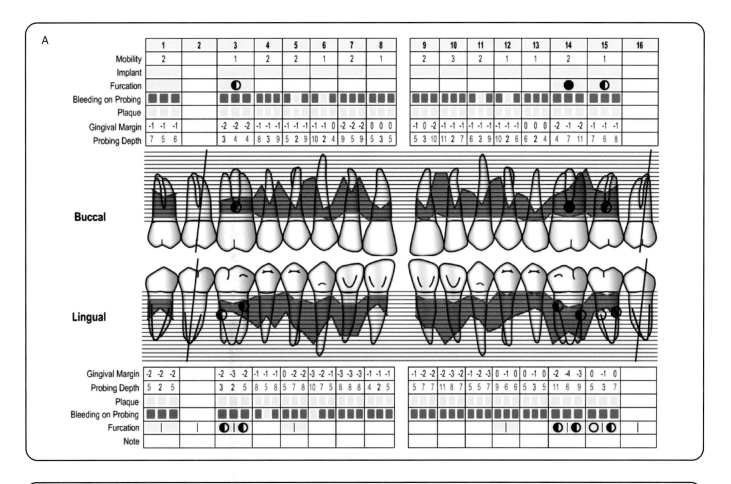

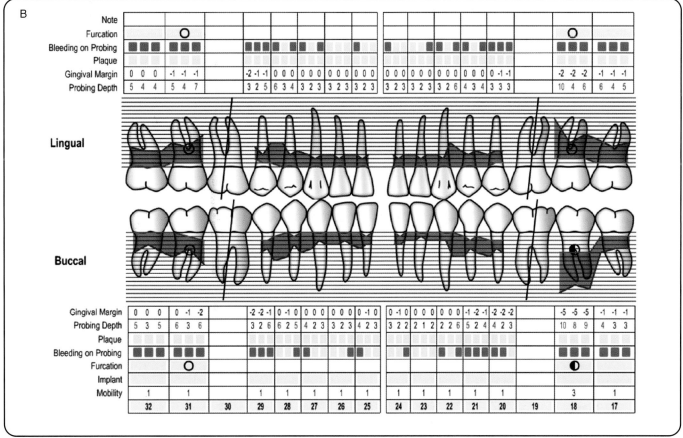

Figure 1.8.3 Periodontal charting: (A) maxilla; (B) mandible.

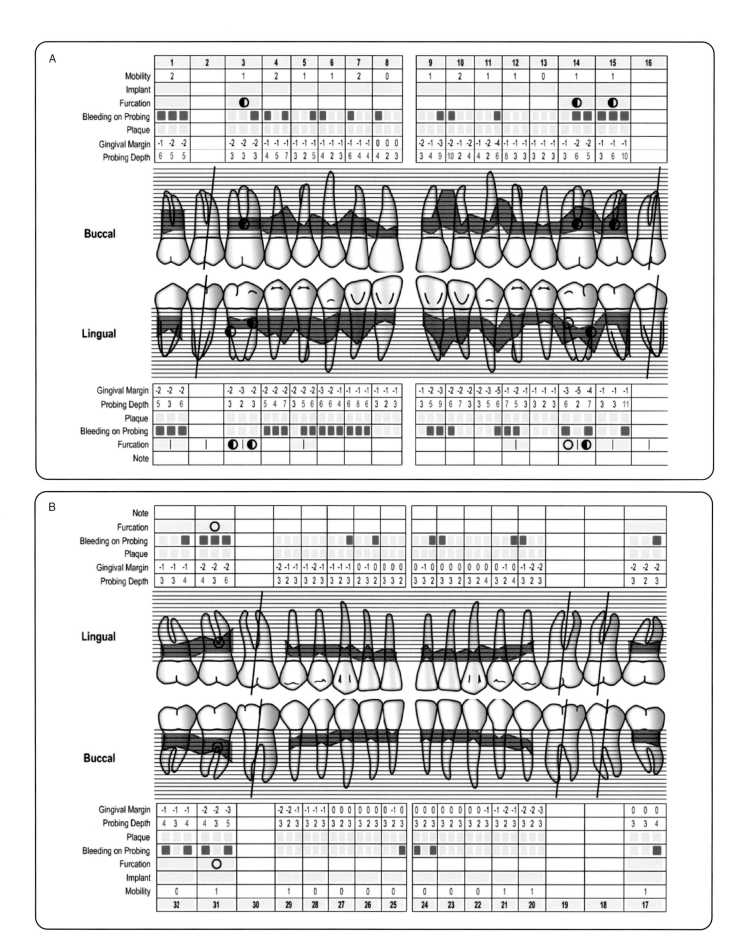

Figure 1.8.4   Follow-up periodontal charting six weeks post treatment: (A) maxilla; (B) mandible.

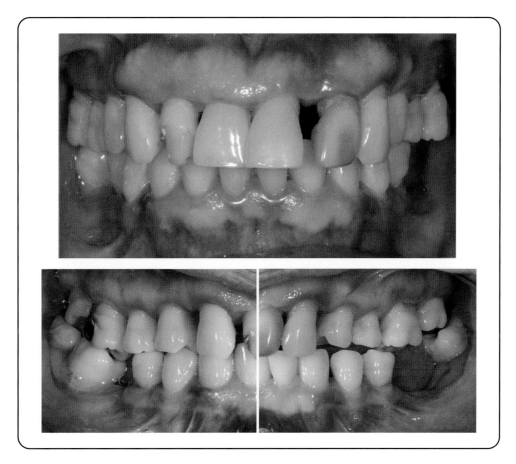

Figure 1.8.5 Follow-up views six weeks post treatment.

tissue is modest, while for others the contribution is not supported by clear evidence [6].

Although there is moderate evidence showing a reduction of hyperglycemia in uncontrolled type 2 diabetes following periodontal treatment, there is insufficient evidence to support the converse view [7–9]. However, there is evidence that periodontitis can negatively affect glycemic control in diabetes mellitus, supporting the bidirectional relationship between the two diseases [10].

Patients with diabetes should be informed that they are at increased risk of periodontitis. If they are affected by periodontal disease, their glycemic control may be more difficult and they are at higher risk for other complications like cardiovascular and kidney disease. Of all the clinical features of diabetes mellitus, chronic hyperglycemia has attracted the most attention because of its direct and indirect influences on the development of periodontal disease [6]. The pronounced inflammation and elevated production of inflammation-related end products in patients with hyperglycemia has been linked with a variety of systemic inflammatory diseases, including periodontitis [11–13]. The hyperinflammation

elevates the release of proinflammatory cytokines, giving rise to changes in the host response to bacterial invasion and wound healing impairment in the oral cavity [13]. The accumulation of advanced glycation end products (AGEs) and of their binding receptor (RAGE) have been highlighted for their potential role in hyperglycemia-related complications [14]. Patients with periodontal disease manifest higher levels of circulating AGEs and expression of RAGE, leading to triggered production of interleukin (IL)-1, IL-6, and tumor necrosis factor (TNF)-α [15]. However, all these findings should be interpreted with caution because of other confounding systemic diseases, including obesity and hypertension [12].

The most important step is to diagnose both systemic diseases and treat them concurrently. Uncontrolled diabetes is associated with increased progression of periodontitis [16]. Early diagnosis of diabetes can reduce the risk of complications. A good relationship with the patient's PCP or endocrinologist needs to be established to monitor the patient from both the dental and medical point of view. The patient needs to be motivated with oral hygiene maneuvers as well as diet counseling and habit control. From a dental point of view, the first goal should be patient education to assist understanding of why proficient plaque removal is necessary. The decreased immune response to infections should lead the patient to increase their efforts in plaque control procedures. If the patient understands the benefits of self-plaque removal, they will likely be motivated to be consistent and thorough in performing the necessary techniques for plaque removal. The second task is to assist the patient with the techniques for plaque removal which best address the specific needs.

The role of adjunctive antibiotic therapy seems to be of secondary importance. A recent systematic

review [17] disproved the benefit of adjunctive use of systemic antibiotic in terms of HbA_{1c} improvement in periodontal treatment of patients with diabetes. The use of systemic antibiotics does not offer additional benefits in terms of HbA_{1c} values in diabetic patients. The consensus report of the Joint EFP/AAP Workshop on Periodontitis and Systemic Diseases reported that adjunctive antibiotic therapy does not appear to confer additional benefits. There is insufficient evidence to suggest a specific periodontal treatment regimen. Patients with type 2 diabetes benefit from standard mechanical debridement along with effective personal oral hygiene [10].

Self-Study Questions

A. What are the risk factors for periodontal disease?

B. What are the systemic diseases that place patients at risk for periodontal conditions?

C. What are the links between oral health (periodontitis) and systemic diseases?

D. Can the treatment of periodontal disease have an impact on general health?

References

1. Silness J, Löe H. Periodontal disease in pregnancy. II. Correlation between oral hygiene and periodontal condition. *Acta Odontol Scand* 1964;22:121–135.
2. O'Leary TJ, Drake RB, Naylor JE. The plaque control record. *J Periodontol* 1972;43:38.
3. Ainamo J, Bay I. Problems and proposals for recording gingivitis and plaque. *Int Dent J* 1975;25:229–235.
4. Tonetti MS, Greenwell H, Kornman KS. Staging and grading of periodontitis: framework and proposal of a new classification and case definition. *J Periodontol* 2018;89(Suppl 1):S159–S172.
5. McGuire MK. Prognosis versus actual outcome: a long-term survey of 100 treated periodontal patients under maintenance care. *J Periodontol* 1991;62:51–58.
6. Albandar JM, Susin C, Hughes FJ. Manifestations of systemic diseases and conditions that affect the periodontal attachment apparatus: case definitions and diagnostic considerations. *J Periodontol* 2018;89(Suppl 1):S183–S203.
7. Sanz M, Ceriello A, Buysschaert M, et al. Scientific evidence on the links between periodontal diseases and diabetes: consensus report and guidelines of the joint workshop on periodontal diseases and diabetes by the International Diabetes Federation and the European Federation of Periodontology. *J Clin Periodontol* 2018;45:138–149.
8. Engebretson SP, Hyman LG, Michalowicz BS, et al. The effect of nonsurgical periodontal therapy on hemoglobin A1c levels in persons with type 2 diabetes and chronic periodontitis: a randomized clinical trial. *JAMA* 2013;310:2523–2532.
9. Madianos PN, Koromantzos PA. An update of the evidence on the potential impact of periodontal therapy on diabetes outcomes. *J Clin Periodontol* 2018;45:188–195.
10. Chapple ILC, Genco R; Working Group 2 of the Joint EFP/AAP Workshop. Diabetes and periodontal diseases: consensus report of the Joint EFP/AAP Workshop on Periodontitis and Systemic Diseases. *J Periodontol* 2013; 84(4 Suppl):S106–S112.
11. Mealey BL, Ocampo GL. Diabetes mellitus and periodontal disease. *Periodontol 2000* 2007;44:127–153.
12. Polak D, Shapira L. An update on the evidence for pathogenic mechanisms that may link periodontitis and diabetes. *J Clin Periodontol* 2018;45:150–166.
13. Taylor JJ, Preshaw PM, Lalla E. A review of the evidence for pathogenic mechanisms that may link periodontitis and diabetes. *J Clin Periodontol* 2013;40(Suppl 14):S113–S134.
14. Del Turco S, Basta G. An update on advanced glycation end-products and atherosclerosis. *Biofactors* 2012;38:266–274.
15. Lalla E, Papapanou PN. Diabetes mellitus and periodontitis: a tale of two common interrelated diseases. *Nat Rev Endocrinol* 2011;7:738–748.

16. Genco RJ, Sanz M. Clinical and public health implications of periodontal and systemic diseases: an overview. *Periodontol 2000* 2020;83(1):7–13.

17. Lira Junior R, Santos CMM, Oliveira BH, et al. Effects on HbA$_{1c}$ in diabetic patients of adjunctive use of systemic antibiotics in nonsurgical periodontal treatment: a systematic review. *J Dent* 2017;66:1–7.

18. Papapanou PN. Periodontal diseases: epidemiology. *Ann Periodontol* 1996;1:1–36.

19. Löe H. Periodontal disease. The sixth complication of diabetes mellitus. *Diabetes Care* 1993;16:329–334.

20. Tsai C, Hayes C, Taylor GW. Glycemic control of type 2 diabetes and severe periodontal disease in the US adult population. *Community Dent Oral Epidemiol* 2002;30:182–192.

21. Taylor GW, Burt BA, Becker MP, et al. Non-insulin dependent diabetes mellitus and alveolar bone loss progression over 2 years. *J Periodontol* 1998;69:76–83.

22. Winning L, Patterson CC, Neville CE, et al. Periodontitis and incident type 2 diabetes: a prospective cohort study. *J Clin Periodontol* 2017;44:266–274.

23. Falcao A, Bullón P. A review of the influence of periodontal treatment in systemic diseases. *Periodontol 2000* 2019;79:117–128.

24. Lockhart PB, Bolger AF, Papapanou PN, et al. Periodontal disease and atherosclerotic vascular disease: does the evidence support an independent association?: a scientific statement from the American Heart Association. *Circulation* 2012;125:2520–2544.

25. Friedewald VE, Kornman KS, Beck JD, et al. The American Journal of Cardiology and Journal of Periodontology editors' consensus: periodontitis and atherosclerotic cardiovascular disease. *J Periodontol* 2009;80:1021–1032.

26. Blaizot A, Vergnes JN, Nuwwareh S, et al. Periodontal diseases and cardiovascular events: meta-analysis of observational studies. *Int Dent J* 2009;59:197–209.

27. Humphrey LL, Fu R, Buckley DI, et al. Periodontal disease and coronary heart disease incidence: a systematic review and meta-analysis. *J Gen Intern Med* 2008;23:2079–2086.

28. Janket SJ, Baird AE, Chuang SK, Jones JA. Meta-analysis of periodontal disease and risk of coronary heart disease and stroke. *Oral Surg Oral Med Oral Pathol Oral Radiol Endod* 2003;95:559–569.

29. Reyes L, Herrera D, Kozarov E, et al. Periodontal bacterial invasion and infection: contribution to atherosclerotic pathology. *J Clin Periodontol* 2013;40(Suppl 14):S30–S50.

30. Bahrani-Mougeot FK, Paster BJ, Coleman S, et al. Diverse and novel oral bacterial species in blood following dental procedures. *J Clin Microbiol* 2008;46:2129–2132.

31. Roth GA, Moser B, Huang SJ, et al. Infection with a periodontal pathogen induces procoagulant effects in human aortic endothelial cells. *J Thromb Haemost* 2006;4:2256–2261.

32. D'Aiuto F, Orlandi M, Gunsolley JC. Evidence that periodontal treatment improves biomarkers and CVD outcomes. *J Clin Periodontol* 2013;40(Suppl 14):S85–S105.

33. Teeuw WJ, Slot DE, Susanto H, et al. Treatment of periodontitis improves the atherosclerotic profile: a systematic review and meta-analysis. *J Clin Periodontol* 2014; 41:70–79.

34. Sanz M, Kornman K, Working group 3 of the joint EFP/AAP workshop. Periodontitis and adverse pregnancy outcomes: consensus report of the Joint EFP/AAP Workshop on Periodontitis and Systemic Diseases. *J Clin Periodontol* 2013;40(Suppl 14):S164–S169.

35. Ide M, Papapanou PN. Epidemiology of association between maternal periodontal disease and adverse pregnancy outcomes: systematic review. *J Periodontol* 2013;84(4 Suppl):S181–S194.

36. Madianos PN, Bobetsis YA, Offenbacher S. Adverse pregnancy outcomes (APOs) and periodontal disease: pathogenic mechanisms. *J Clin Periodontol* 2013;40(Suppl 14):S170–S180.

37. de Molon RS, Rossa C Jr, Thurlings RM, et al. Linkage of periodontitis and rheumatoid arthritis: current evidence and potential biological interactions. *Int J Mol Sci* 2019;20(18):4541.

38. McInnes IB, Schett G. The pathogenesis of rheumatoid arthritis. *N Engl J Med* 2011;365:2205–2219.

39. Gabriel SE, Michaud K. Epidemiological studies in incidence, prevalence, mortality, and comorbidity of the rheumatic diseases. *Arthritis Res Ther* 2009;11(3):229.

40. Linos A, Worthington JW, O'Fallon WM, Kurland LT. The epidemiology of rheumatoid arthritis in Rochester, Minnesota: a study of incidence, prevalence, and mortality. *Am J Epidemiol* 1980;111:87–98.

41. van Vollenhoven RF. Sex differences in rheumatoid arthritis: more than meets the eye. *BMC Med* 2009;7:12.

42. Bodkhe R, Balakrishnan B, Taneja V. The role of microbiome in rheumatoid arthritis treatment. *Ther Adv Musculoskelet Dis* 2019;11:1759720X19844632.

43. Chang K, Yang SM, Kim SH, et al. Smoking and rheumatoid arthritis. *Int J Mol Sci* 2014;15:22279–22295.

44. Edwards CJ, Cooper C. Early environmental factors and rheumatoid arthritis. *Clin Exp Immunol* 2006;143:1–5.

45. Kallberg H, Padyukov L, Plenge RM, et al. Gene–gene and gene–environment interactions involving HLA-DRB1, PTPN22, and smoking in two subsets of rheumatoid arthritis. *Am J Hum Genet* 2007;80:867–875.

46. Abdollahi-Roodsaz S, Abramson SB, Scher JU. The metabolic role of the gut microbiota in health and rheumatic disease: mechanisms and interventions. *Nat Rev Rheumatol* 2016;12:446–455.

47. Evans-Marin H, Rogier R, Koralov SB, et al. Microbiota-dependent involvement of Th17 cells in murine models of inflammatory arthritis. *Arthritis Rheumatol* 2018;70: 1971–1983.

48. de Smit M, Westra J, Vissink A, et al. Periodontitis in established rheumatoid arthritis patients: a cross-sectional clinical, microbiological and serological study. *Arthritis Res Ther* 2012;14:R222.

49. Laugisch O, Wong A, Sroka A, et al. Citrullination in the periodontium: a possible link between periodontitis and rheumatoid arthritis. *Clin Oral Investig* 2016;20: 675–683.

50. Ogrendik M. Rheumatoid arthritis is linked to oral bacteria: etiological association. *Mod Rheumatol* 2009;19:453–456.

51. McGraw WT, Potempa J, Farley D, Travis J. Purification, characterization, and sequence analysis of a potential

virulence factor from *Porphyromonas gingivalis*, peptidylarginine deiminase. *Infect Immun* 1999;67:3248–3256.

52. Wegner N, Wait R, Sroka A, et al. Peptidylarginine deiminase from *Porphyromonas gingivalis* citrullinates human fibrinogen and α-enolase: implications for autoimmunity in rheumatoid arthritis. *Arthritis Rheum* 2010;62:2662–2672.

53. Avouac J, Gossec L, Dougados M. Diagnostic and predictive value of anti-cyclic citrullinated protein antibodies in rheumatoid arthritis: a systematic literature review. *Ann Rheum Dis* 2006;65:845–851.

54. Bingham CO 3rd, Moni M. Periodontal disease and rheumatoid arthritis: the evidence accumulates for complex pathobiologic interactions. *Curr Opin Rheumatol* 2013;25:345–353.

55. Mikuls TR, Payne JB, Yu F, et al. Periodontitis and *Porphyromonas gingivalis* in patients with rheumatoid arthritis. *Arthritis Rheumatol* 2014;66:1090–1100.

56. Nielen MM, van Schaardenburg D, Reesink HW, et al. Specific autoantibodies precede the symptoms of rheumatoid arthritis: a study of serial measurements in blood donors. *Arthritis Rheum* 2004;50:380–386.

57. Nishimura K, Sugiyama D, Kogata Y, et al. Meta-analysis: diagnostic accuracy of anti-cyclic citrullinated peptide antibody and rheumatoid factor for rheumatoid arthritis. *Ann Intern Med* 2007;146:797–808.

58. Äyräväinen L, Leirisalo-Repo M, Kuuliala A, et al. Periodontitis in early and chronic rheumatoid arthritis: a prospective follow-up study in Finnish population. *BMJ Open* 2017;7:e011916.

59. Unriza-Puin S, Bautista-Molano W, Lafaurie GI, et al. Are obesity, ACPAs and periodontitis conditions that influence the risk of developing rheumatoid arthritis in first-degree relatives? *Clin Rheumatol* 2017;36:799–806.

60. Araujo VM, Melo IM, Lima V. Relationship between periodontitis and rheumatoid arthritis: review of the literature. *Mediators Inflamm* 2015;2015:259074.

61. Bartold PM, Marshall RI, Haynes DR. Periodontitis and rheumatoid arthritis: a review. *J Periodontol* 2005;76(11 Suppl):2066–2074.

62. Obesity: preventing and managing the global epidemic. Report of a WHO consultation. *World Health Organ Tech Rep Ser* 2000;894:1–253.

63. Clinical guidelines on the identification, evaluation, and treatment of overweight and obesity in adults: executive summary. Expert Panel on the Identification, Evaluation, and Treatment of Overweight in Adults. *Am J Clin Nutr* 1998;68:899–917.

64. Hales CM, Carroll MD, Fryar CD, Ogden CL. Prevalence of obesity among adults and youth: United States, 2015–2016. *NCHS Data Brief* 2017;(288):1–8.

65. Ahima RS, Flier JS. Adipose tissue as an endocrine organ. *Trends Endocrinol Metab* 2000;11:327–332.

66. Lyon CJ, Law RE, Hsueh WA. Minireview: adiposity, inflammation, and atherogenesis. *Endocrinology* 2003;144:2195–2200.

67. Suvan JE, Finer N, D'Aiuto F. Periodontal complications with obesity. *Periodontol 2000* 2018;78:98–128.

68. Al-Zahrani MS, Bissada NF, Borawskit EA. Obesity and periodontal disease in young, middle-aged, and older adults. *J Periodontol* 2003;74:610–615.

69. Dalla Vecchia CF, Susin C, Rosing CK, et al. Overweight and obesity as risk indicators for periodontitis in adults. *J Periodontol* 2005;76:1721–1728.

70. Keller A, Rohde JF, Raymond K, Heitmann BL. Association between periodontal disease and overweight and obesity: a systematic review. *J Periodontol* 2015;86:766–776.

71. Martinez-Herrera M, Silvestre-Rangil J, Silvestre FJ. Association between obesity and periodontal disease. A systematic review of epidemiological studies and controlled clinical trials. *Med Oral Patol Oral Cir Bucal* 2017;22:e708–e715.

72. Nascimento GG, Leite FRM, Do LG, et al. Is weight gain associated with the incidence of periodontitis? A systematic review and meta-analysis. *J Clin Periodontol* 2015;42:495–505.

73. Suvan J, D'Aiuto F, Moles DR, et al. Association between overweight/obesity and periodontitis in adults. A systematic review. *Obes Rev* 2011;12:e381–404.

74. Miller WD. The human mouth as a focus of infection. *Lancet* 1891;138(3546):340–342.

75. Scannapieco FA. Systemic effects of periodontal diseases. *Dent Clin North Am* 2005;49:533–550.

76. Seymour RA. Is gum disease killing your patient? *Br Dent J* 2009;206:551–552.

77. Wade WG. The oral microbiome in health and disease. *Pharmacol Res* 2013;69:137–143.

78. Van Dyke TE, van Winkelhoff AJ. Infection and inflammatory mechanisms. *J Clin Periodontol* 2013;40(Suppl 14):S1–S7.

79. Rock KL, Kono H. The inflammatory response to cell death. *Annu Rev Pathol* 2008;3:99–126.

80. Bullon P, Newman HN, Battino M. Obesity, diabetes mellitus, atherosclerosis and chronic periodontitis: a shared pathology via oxidative stress and mitochondrial dysfunction? *Periodontol 2000* 2014;64:139–153.

81. Jeffcoat MK, Jeffcoat RL, Gladowski PA, et al. Impact of periodontal therapy on general health: evidence from insurance data for five systemic conditions. *Am J Prev Med* 2014;47:166–174.

82. Stratton IM, Adler AI, Neil HA, et al. Association of glycaemia with macrovascular and microvascular complications of type 2 diabetes (UKPDS 35): prospective observational study. *BMJ* 2000;321(7258):405–412.

83. Engebretson S, Kocher T. Evidence that periodontal treatment improves diabetes outcomes: a systematic review and meta-analysis. *J Clin Periodontol* 2013;40(Suppl 14):S153–S163.

84. Saffi MAL, Furtado MV, Polanczyk CA, et al. Relationship between vascular endothelium and periodontal disease in atherosclerotic lesions: review article. *World J Cardiol* 2015;7:26–30.

85. Beeraka SS, Natarajan K, Patil R, et al. Clinical and radiological assessment of effects of long-term corticosteroid therapy on oral health. *Dent Res J (Isfahan)* 2013;10:666–673.

86. Savioli C, Ribeiro ACM, Fabri GMC, et al. Persistent periodontal disease hampers anti-tumor necrosis factor treatment response in rheumatoid arthritis. *J Clin Rheumatol* 2012;18:180–184.

87. Han JY, Reynolds MA. Effect of anti-rheumatic agents on periodontal parameters and biomarkers of inflammation: a

systematic review and meta-analysis. *J Periodontal Implant Sci* 2012;42:3–12.

88. Kobayashi T, Yokoyama T, Ito S, et al. Periodontal and serum protein profiles in patients with rheumatoid arthritis treated with tumor necrosis factor inhibitor adalimumab. *J Periodontol* 2014;85:1480–1488.

89. Coat J, Demoersman J, Beuzit S, et al. Anti-B lymphocyte immunotherapy is associated with improvement of periodontal status in subjects with rheumatoid arthritis. *J Clin Periodontol* 2015;42:817–823.

90. Kobayashi T, Okada M, Ito S, et al. Assessment of interleukin-6 receptor inhibition therapy on periodontal condition in patients with rheumatoid arthritis and chronic periodontitis. *J Periodontol* 2014;85:57–67.

91. Silvestre FJ, Silvestre-Rangil J, Bagan L, Bagan JV. Effect of nonsurgical periodontal treatment in patients with periodontitis and rheumatoid arthritis: a systematic review. *Med Oral Patol Oral Cir Bucal* 2016;21:e349–354.

92. Kurgan S, Fentoğlu Ö, Önder C, et al. The effects of periodontal therapy on gingival crevicular fluid matrix metalloproteinase-8, interleukin-6 and prostaglandin E2 levels in patients with rheumatoid arthritis. *J Periodontal Res* 2016;51:586–595.

93. Kurgan S, Önder C, Balcı N, et al. Gingival crevicular fluid tissue/blood vessel-type plasminogen activator and plasminogen activator inhibitor-2 levels in patients with rheumatoid arthritis: effects of nonsurgical periodontal therapy. *J Periodontal Res* 2017;52:574–581.

94. Kaur S, Bright R, Proudman SM, Bartold PM. Does periodontal treatment influence clinical and biochemical measures for rheumatoid arthritis? A systematic review and meta-analysis. *Semin Arthritis Rheum* 2014;44:113–122.

95. Papageorgiou SN, Reichert C, Jager A, Deschner J. Effect of overweight/obesity on response to periodontal treatment: systematic review and a meta-analysis. *J Clin Periodontol* 2015;42:247–261.

96. Akram Z, Safii SH, Vaithilingam RD, et al. Efficacy of nonsurgical periodontal therapy in the management of chronic periodontitis among obese and non-obese patients: a systematic review and meta-analysis. *Clin Oral Investig* 2016;20:903–914.

TAKE-HOME POINTS

A. Periodontitis is a host-mediated inflammatory disease associated with pathologic microorganisms that leads to loss of periodontal attachment. Its pathogenesis features an interaction between different host and environmental factors, immune response, and local anatomic factors. The complexity of these mechanisms represents a combination of the host's genetic profile influenced by environmental and host behavioral factors. For instance, smoking and the presence of certain strains of pathologic microorganisms (*Aggregatibacter actinomycetemcomitans, Porphyromonas gingivalis, Tannerella forsythia*, among others) have been proven to be true risk factors. The 2017 classification of periodontal disease indicated that there is no evidence to suggest that different forms of periodontitis have a unique pathophysiology (i.e. aggressive compared to chronic periodontitis). Instead the above-mentioned complex combination of risk factors in a multifactorial disease model may explain the different disease phenotypes. One of the features of the 2017 classification system is the grading of a patient with periodontitis, which provides tools to identify risks or evidence of periodontal disease progression. Individuals presenting with different severity and extent of disease and resulting complexity of management may possess different rates of progression and/or risk factors. As stated in the Consensus statement on the new classification structure [4], the goals of grading a periodontal patient are to estimate the future risk of disease progression and responsiveness to basic therapeutic principles as well as to provide guidance on frequency and intensity of therapy and follow-up. The second aim is to estimate the potential impact of periodontitis on systemic disease and, conversely, to monitor and coordinate systemic therapy with medical colleagues.

B. Many systemic diseases are associated with a profound loss of periodontal attachment and alveolar bone, and for some of these disorders the periodontal manifestations may be among the first signs of the disease. Systemic disorders may affect periodontal inflammation by altering the host immune response to periodontal infections; others cause defects in the connective tissue, trigger metabolic shifts in the host, or operate by other mechanisms. For some systemic disorders that are more common, their contribution to the loss of periodontal tissue is modest, while for others the contribution is not supported by clear evidence [6]. There is an abundance of evidence that periodontitis correlates with certain systemic diseases such as cardiovascular disease (CVD), preterm labor and low birthweight infants, diabetes mellitus, and obesity.

Diabetes and Periodontal Disease

Diabetes mellitus (DM) represents a risk for periodontal disease that is independent of the effect of other significant factors [18]. Diabetes and periodontal disease have a two-way relationship. Research suggests that diabetic patients are more likely to develop periodontal disease which, in return, can increase blood sugar levels and diabetic complications. The most plausible reason is the fact that diabetics are more susceptible to infections, especially the uncontrolled conditions. The importance of this combination was described in an early paper by Löe [19] that defined periodontal disease as the "sixth complication of diabetes mellitus."

For decades, DM has been observed to be associated with the initiation and progression of periodontal disease by representative periodontal parameters in epidemiologic studies. The accumulating evidence has mainly focused on the effects of type 2 DM on periodontal disease development since it accounts for most DM patients. The association was previously recognized in epidemiologic studies [20] and further investigated in longitudinal studies [19,21] in which diabetes increased the risks and rates of periodontal bone loss and attachment loss over time compared with subjects without diabetes. According to the new classification system from the 2017 World Workshop, diabetes is listed as a risk factor for periodontal disease progression. Currently, there is a lack of evidence to consider periodontitis in poorly controlled diabetes a different entity with unique pathophysiology that requires specific periodontal treatment other than control of both comorbidities [7]. Periodontitis observed in patients affected by systemic diseases that severely impair host response should be considered a periodontal manifestation of the systemic disease itself and that should be the main diagnosis [6].

Recently, longitudinal studies have proved that the persistence of periodontal inflammation contributes to the onset or progression of hyperglycemia [22], leading to the hypothesis that the relationship between DM and periodontal disease is bidirectional. While DM increases the risk of periodontal complications, the inflammatory mechanisms that result from periodontal disease are also adversely associated with metabolic control of DM and its complications [23]. The third National Health and Nutrition Examination Survey (NHANES III) in the United States reported a difference in prevalence of DM between patients with and without periodontal disease (12.5% vs. 6.3%, respectively), while the same survey also reported a difference in prevalence of periodontal disease between patients with and without DM (17.3% vs. 9%, respectively).

Cardiovascular Disease and Periodontal Disease

Cardiovascular diseases involve a variety of clinical disorders of the heart and blood vessels, including cardiomyopathy, hypertension, myocardial infarction, and atherosclerotic vascular disease (ASVD). ASVD draws the most attention because it is the main cause of death, accounting for 30% of all deaths globally [24]. The association between periodontal disease and atherosclerosis has been subject to different levels of evidence, ultimately leading to a consensus by the editors of the *American Journal of Cardiology* and *Journal of Periodontology* in 2009 [25] and a statement by the American Heart Association in 2012 [24]. Several prevalent risk indicators are shared by periodontal disease and ASVD, which initially made clinicians interested in investigating the possible relationship between the two diseases, but which also confounded the relationship. The documented impacting risk indicators for both diseases include increasing age, smoking, alcohol abuse, ethnicity, DM, and stress [24].

Epidemiologic studies of periodontal disease using different periodontal parameters (clinical/radiographic measurements, tooth loss, and serologic assessments) to investigate ASVD-associated outcomes have proved that there is a positive association between periodontal disease and ASVD with sufficient level of evidence [23,24].

Supporting data from different meta-analyses have shown that the risk ratio of having ASVD in patients with periodontal disease ranges from 1.19 to 1.34 [26–28].

Several pathogenic mechanisms linking periodontal disease and ASVD have been proposed and categorized into two groups: indirect and direct mechanisms. Generally, indirect mechanisms describe the systemic inflammatory responses triggered by local periodontal diseases, leading to higher levels of several ASVD-associated cytokines, including IL-1β, IL-6, IL-8 and TNF-α. The proposed indirect mechanisms also involve the periodontal disease-promoted synthesis of some intravascular plasma proteins, including C-reactive protein (CRP) and fibrinogen [28]. The proposed direct mechanisms are derived from the fact that transient bacteremia from the oral cavity is often seen in patients with periodontal disease, resulting in possible atherosclerotic processes [29,30]. Specifically, attention has been focused on some periodontal pathogens with the ability to adhere to and invade host cells and influence host response. For instance, *P. gingivalis* can infect endothelial cells and induce a procoagulant response [31].

In recent years, several clinical studies have been conducted to investigate whether treatments for periodontitis reduce the risk of ASVD, by monitoring associated biomarkers. According to the most recent systematic reviews and meta-analyses, the progressive improvement in cardiovascular disease, in terms of improved endothelial function and reduced biomarkers, can last for up to six months postoperatively [32,33]. However, these results need to be interpreted with caution because of the limitations of the studies, including heterogeneity of study sample size, types of periodontal disease, and types of periodontal interventions.

Adverse Pregnancy Outcomes and Periodontal Disease

Adverse pregnancy outcomes include low birthweight (<2500 g), preterm birth (<37 weeks), growth restriction, preeclampsia, miscarriage, and stillbirth [34]. These outcomes have been statistically associated with exposure to maternal periodontal disease in epidemiologic studies [35].

The proposed mechanisms for the association can be divided into direct and indirect pathways [34]. The direct mechanism involves the dissemination of periodontal pathogens from the oral cavity to the fetal–placental unit, leading to several complications [36]. The indirect mechanism involves a systemic inflammatory response triggered by local periodontal disease, with the fetal–placental unit being influenced by increased inflammatory mediators such as TNF-α, prostaglandin (PG)E$_2$, matrix metalloproteinases (MMPs), fibronectin, IL-1, IL-6, and IL-8 [34]. The severity of adverse outcomes is dependent on the severity and duration of exposure.

Rheumatoid Arthritis and Periodontal Disease

Rheumatoid arthritis (RA) is a chronic autoimmune disease characterized by synovial inflammation and hyperplasia leading to irreversible damage of the bone and cartilage in the joints. It is associated with significant systemic comorbidities (cardiovascular, pulmonary, psychological, and skeletal disorders), leading to loss of function, chronic pain, and progressive disability (swelling, stiffness, and deformation of the joints) [37,38]. It is estimated to affect 0.5–1% of the population worldwide [39] and is more common in women, with a reported male to female ratio of 1 : 3 [40,41]. Although the etiology of RA is not completely understood, it appears to be multifactorial. There is evidence that several environmental, genetic, hormonal, and infectious risk factors [37,42–45] result in the formation of autoantibodies and therefore in the development of RA.

Recently, the gut microbiome has been suggested as an environmental factor related to the development of RA [42,46,47]. In this context, it is plausible that there is a relationship between the microorganisms found in the gut and in the periodontal tissues, and the pathogenesis of RA. In fact, it appears that periodontal disease and RA share some common etiologic and pathophysiologic characteristics.

An association between RA and periodontal disease has been reported. Indeed, high levels of oral anaerobic bacterial antibodies have been found in the serum and synovial fluid of RA patients [48–50]. Specifically, antibodies against *P. gingivalis* have been identified in RA patients. It has been shown that *P. gingivalis* expresses peptidylarginine deiminase (PAD), an enzyme capable of citrullinating both host and bacterial peptides [51,52], which may be related to the onset of RA [53–57]. Moreover, epidemiologic and case–control studies have shown that patients with active RA exhibit a significantly increased prevalence of periodontal disease compared with non-RA patients [55,58,59]. Additionally, the prevalence of RA in periodontitis patients is higher in comparison to matched periodontally healthy controls [37,60,61].

Obesity and Periodontal Disease

Obesity is defined as a condition of abnormal or excessive fat accumulation in the adipose tissue, to the extent that health may be impaired [62]. According to World Health Organization (WHO) criteria [62], individuals with a body mass index (BMI) ≥ 30.0 kg/m^2 are classified as obese. Both the WHO and the National Institutes of Health (NIH) have reported that obesity is a complex multifactorial disease which develops from an interaction between genotype and the environment [62,63]. According to the results from the National Center for Health Statistics, between 2016 and 2017 the prevalence of obesity among US adults was 39.8% and among US youth (2–19 years) 18.5% [64].

Adipose tissue is both a dynamic endocrine organ and a highly active metabolic tissue that may secrete hormones, cytokines, and other proinflammatory mediators, contributing to inflammation [65,66]. Therefore, obesity-related systemic inflammation triggered by these mediators may act as the link to many of the comorbidities associated with obesity, such as metabolic syndrome, hypertension, dyslipidemia, type 2 diabetes, coronary heart disease, stroke, gallbladder disease, osteoarthritis, sleep apnea and respiratory problems, and endometrial, breast, prostate, and colon cancers [63,67].

Evidence suggests that obese individuals are two to three times more likely to suffer from periodontitis independently of traditional risk factors (age, gender, and cigarette smoking) [67–73].

C. Periodontitis and some systemic diseases and conditions are activated by similar genetic and/or environmental etiologic factors, and in certain instances patients can be affected by both diseases. Their diagnosis and recognition could lead to important therapeutic advances to prevent progression to the most severe manifestations. The effort to understand this complex relationship has evolved over the years and the impact on treatment protocols has changed accordingly. Initially, some authors hypothesized that oral infections (also referred to as oral sepsis) were the origin of a wide range of systemic symptoms and conditions [74]. The result was a routine practice of complete tooth extraction or prophylaxis for almost all patients. Fortunately, the realization of the ineffectiveness of these procedures switched the therapeutic focus to the maintenance of teeth.

In the last few decades, the hypothesis that the oral microbiota might play an important role in systemic health has regained popularity. In particular, the presence of periodontal disease might be a causative or precipitating factor of some systemic conditions [75–77]. The focused question of several publications is whether the simultaneous occurrence of periodontal disease and systemic diseases is a coincidence (i.e. they share similar risk factors) or there is a causal association. Some authors [78] have hypothesized that the link between periodontal disease and systemic conditions can be explained by two main pathways – infectious and inflammatory – that mostly occur simultaneously and are therefore not independent.

The *infectious pathway* identifies the oral cavity as a reservoir of microorganisms that may include potential systemic pathogens. Ulceration of periodontal pockets may aggravate this pathogen collection so that they and their products can access the bloodstream or respiratory tract, resulting in a diffused bacteremia that can trigger complications in susceptible and immunocompromised individuals. On the other hand, the *inflammatory pathway* refers to the role of inflammatory molecules released by bacteria and the diseased periodontium that have the potential to promote systemic inflammation via several pathways. In some susceptible subjects, these factors can exacerbate inflammatory-associated systemic diseases or act as risk factors. Inflammation represents a complex system of defense of the organism. A cascade of molecular reactions and cellular processes act to identify, control, and eliminate the invader. The system is in a state of constant alert for immediate response; sometimes this response may lead to collateral damage, the main objective being to preserve the organism [79]. Dysfunction of these immune responses can lead to pathologic processes that can trigger or worsen a systemic disease or condition [80]. The focus of periodontal therapy is to decrease local oral inflammation, and this may reduce the overall burden of inflammation on the organism.

D. There is little evidence to support the view that direct treatment of periodontitis will benefit overall health. Current but limited evidence that effective treatment of certain cases of periodontitis can favorably influence systemic diseases or their surrogates may lead to further developments.

The analysis of health-related epidemiologic studies has allowed collection of vast amounts of data on the possible relationships between different systemic diseases, their epidemiology, and the outcome of treatments. Jeffcoat et al. [81] were the first to analyze the possible beneficial relationship between periodontal treatment and certain systemic diseases: type 2 DM, coronary artery disease, cerebrovascular disease, RA, and pregnancy. The main limitations of those findings were the inconsistent criteria of inclusion in the periodontally treated group, the definition of the control group, the lack of information on periodontal status and treatment, and the overall very small, treated group.

Diabetes

There is moderate evidence showing reduction of hyperglycemia in uncontrolled type 2 diabetes following periodontal treatment, although this was not supported in larger studies where the periodontal treatment outcomes were less clear. Stratton et al. reported that a 1% reduction in glycated hemoglobin leads to a 37% reduction of risk of diabetes-associated microvascular complications [82]. Moreover, a reduction in glycated hemoglobin by 0.4% following periodontal therapy has a

similar clinical effect, equivalent to adding a second drug to a pharmacologic regimen for DM management [10].

However, whether periodontal treatment can benefit diabetes control still remains controversial. A systematic review including nine randomized clinical trials reported a 0.36% reduction in glycated hemoglobin after periodontal treatment at three- to four-months follow-up [83]. However, another multicenter clinical trial reported that there was no significant improvement in glycated hemoglobin resulting from periodontal treatment for type 2 DM patients at three-months follow-up [8]. Researchers have concluded that the mixed results were due to the difficulty of adjusting all the possible confounders, including different medications patients were taking, initial DM management, and different periodontal treatment regimens. Despite the controversy, the Joint EFP/AAP Workshop determined that the existing evidence is sufficient to conclude that periodontal disease has dose-dependent negative effect on diabetes control in DM patients [10].

Pregnancy

Although it is considered safe to receive periodontal treatments during pregnancy, there is controversy about the benefit of periodontal treatments to reduce adverse pregnancy outcomes. The current evidence is insufficient to demonstrate the beneficial effects of periodontal treatments in decreasing adverse pregnancy outcomes [23,34].

Cardiovascular Disease

The current data suggest that periodontal treatment could reduce the risk of cardiovascular disease by improving the plasma levels of inflammatory biomarkers associated with cardiovascular events [84]. Yet there is still a need for further long-term interventional studies, with less heterogeneous methodologies.

Rheumatoid Arthritis

What Are the Effects of Treating RA on Periodontal Patients?

The treatment of RA involves several pharmacologic approaches. Nonsteroidal anti-inflammatory drugs, glucocorticoids, and synthetic and biologic disease-modifying antirheumatic drugs (DMARDs, e.g. methotrexate, sulfasalazine, leflunomide, TNF-α inhibitors, IL-1β monoclonal antibody, anti-B cell agents) are currently the most prescribed drugs for the treatment of RA. Since these medications act in different ways, there is great variability in the literature. Most of the medications will inhibit an inflammatory component of the host response, which could potentially act as a double-edged sword. Specifically, Beeraka et al. [85] found that patients treated long term with corticosteroids had higher levels of attachment loss and deepened probing pocket depth. In contrast, several prospective cohort studies treating RA patients with DMARDs found no worsening of their periodontal status [58,86]. In fact, the beneficial effects of pharmacologic treatment with anti-TNF-α agents [87,88], anti-human IL-6 receptor antibody [89,90] or anti-B lymphocyte therapy [89] on periodontal parameters have also been reported.

What Are the Effects of Treating Periodontal Disease on RA Patients?

A recent systematic review by Silvestre et al. [91] found that nonsurgical periodontal treatment had beneficial effects on laboratory test parameters such as erythrocyte sedimentation rate (ESR) and on clinical parameters assessed by the DAS28 (Disease Activity Score in 28 joints). Additionally, in two observational clinical cohort studies, Kurgan et al. [92,93] assessed the outcomes of nonsurgical periodontal treatment on RA biomarkers. The results of these studies demonstrated that periodontal treatment significantly reduced the levels of PGE_2, MMP-8, tissue/blood vessel-type plasminogen activator, and IL-6 in the gingival crevicular fluid of RA patients. Nevertheless, several systemic biomarkers of RA such as ESR, CRP, and rheumatoid factor were not improved. A systematic review and meta-analysis of periodontal treatment and its clinical and biochemical influence on RA concluded that nonsurgical treatment in individuals with periodontitis and RA could lead to improvements in markers of disease activity [94].

In conclusion, DMARDs and other medications used to treat RA have a host modulatory and anti-inflammatory effect which may affect the outcomes of periodontal tissue destruction in a protective way. On the other hand, nonsurgical periodontal therapy may also have some effect on inflammatory cytokines/markers related to RA, as well as in improving RA clinical scores, although its effect may be limited. However, these results should be interpreted with caution, since all studies were observational and had small sample sizes and different criteria for definition of RA and periodontal disease, lacked control of confounding/environmental factors, and had a follow-up post intervention no longer than six months.

Obesity

Studies on the association between overweight/obesity and response to periodontal therapy are heterogeneous. In a recent systematic review, Papageorgiou et al. [95] found that overweight/obese patients responded similarly to normal-weight patients following periodontal treatment. Akram et al. [96] assessed the effect of nonsurgical periodontal therapy (NSPT) in obese patients compared to nonobese patients and concluded that it was unclear whether NSPT had a significantly higher impact on clinical periodontal outcomes in obese than in nonobese patients with chronic periodontitis.

Case 9

Developments in Diagnostics

CASE STORY
A 53-year-old male presented for consultation regarding missing tooth #3. The patient was interested in a dental implant for edentulous site #3. He was being treated for high blood pressure and Crohn's disease. Tooth #3 was extracted a year ago and the patient had been informed of the potential need for a sinus augmentation before placement of the dental implant.

LEARNING GOALS AND OBJECTIVES
■ Recognize that different radiographic imaging techniques are available in dentistry: full-mouth series, individual periapical radiographs/bitewings, panoramic radiographs, and CBCT
■ Understand when it is appropriate to prescribe each of these modalities in clinical practice
■ Describe the ideal radiographic images that should be prescribed to diagnose periodontal disease
■ Describe the ideal radiographic images that should be prescribed to distinguish between periodontal and endodontic diagnoses
■ Understand the differences in exposure to radiation

Medical History
The patient was diagnosed with Crohn's disease and benign prostatic hyperplasia. The patient reported no food or drug allergies. His blood pressure was 145/87 mmHg and pulse 97 beats/minute. The patient was taking a number of medications for management of Crohn's disease and benign prostatic hyperplasia:

- Mesalamine (Pentasa) 500 mg (eight capsules) per day
- Adalimumab (Humira) 40 mg (0.8 ml) subcutaneous administration once every two weeks
- Tamsulosin 0.4 mg once a day for enlarged prostate.

Social History
The patient indicated that he smoked a cigarette per day and drank one glass of alcohol per day.

Extraoral Examination
The extraoral examination was unremarkable: eyes, skin, lips, temporomandibular joint, lymph nodes, and soft tissue profile were all within normal limits. Smile line was within the average.

Intraoral Examination
- Oral cancer screening was negative. Grade 1 mobility was noted in teeth #4, #7, #14, #18, #21, #23, #24, #25, #26, #29, #30.
- Plaque control was very poor with generalized plaque and localized calculus deposits.
- In general the gingival examination (Figure 1.9.1) revealed color and texture to be within normal limits, with rolled margins and blunted interdental papilla. There was localized moderate gingival inflammation and bleeding on probing with suppuration associated with tooth #30 in the mid-buccal region. Localized recession (1 –5 mm) was noted on teeth #19, #20, #21, #28, and #29. See Figure 1.9.2 for details of the initial periodontal evaluation.

Occlusion
- Generalized wear facets were noted.
- Static analysis of conclusion: canine and molar class I.
- Overjet: 3 mm.
- Overbite: 3 mm.
- No interferences were noted during protrusion and lateral extrusion.

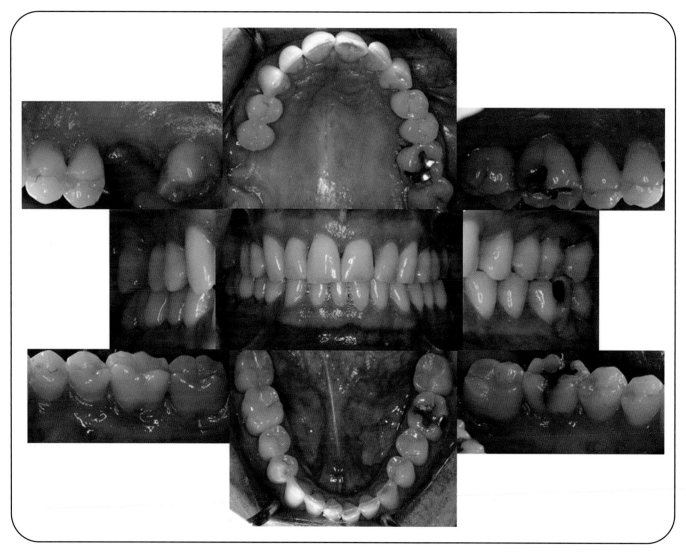

Figure 1.9.1 Intraoral images at the initial consultation.

Radiographic Examination

A panoramic radiograph was taken for initial evaluation (Figure 1.9.3). The imaging findings were compared with findings from a full-mouth set of radiographs (Figure 1.9.4) dated a year ago and a panoramic radiograph from six years previously (Figure 1.9.5). Generalized mild to moderate horizontal bone loss was noted in the radiographs. Angular bone loss and furcation involvement associated with teeth #18, #19, #30 and #31 were more severe compared to the previous images. There was widening of the apical periodontal ligament space associated with the distal root of tooth #19 and sclerotic bone surrounding the distal root.

Diagnosis and Prognosis

Review of clinical and radiographic evaluations resulted in the following diagnoses.

- Localized stage IV (teeth #12, #14, #15, #18, #19, #30 and #31).
- Generalized stage II, grade B.
- Partial edentulism (tooth #3).

Factors contributing to this condition were determined to be the patient's poor oral hygiene, parafunctional habits and smoking.

Overall prognosis was determined to be fair, with poor prognosis for teeth #12, #14, and #15, and questionable prognosis for teeth #18, #19, #30, and #31 due to the angular bone loss detected in the intraoral and panoramic radiographs.

Treatment

The patient received full-mouth scaling using ultrasonics to remove as much of the supragingival and subgingival calculus as possible. All clinically detectable supragingival

Maxillary arch (teeth 1–16)

	1	2	3	4	5	6	7	8	9	10	11	12	13	14	15	16	
	323			324	323	323	323	222	223	323	323	723	423	466	827		P.D.
	001			320	000	001	101	110	000	100	000	021	011	121	120		FGM
	324			644	323	324	424	332	223	423	323	744	434	587	947		ATTACH
														3	2		FURCA
	P P			P . .	. . P	P . .	P . .	. . . .	P . P	P . P	F . P	P . P	P . P	P . P	P . P		PLAQUE
	. B			B . .	. . .	. . .			. . .	. . .	. . .	. . .	. . .	. . B	B B B		BL/SUP
	. .			. . .	. . .	. . .			. . .	. . .	. . .	. . .	. . .	. . C	. . .		Calculus
				.		.		.		.		.		.	.		MGDEF

1	2	3	4	5	6	7	8	9	10	11	12	13	14	15	16	
335			324	423	322	222	323	323	323	322	542	223	027	734		P.D.
000			210	000	000	000	000	000	000	000	000	011	221	100		FGM
335			534	423	322	222	323	323	323	322	542	234	248	834		ATTACH
P P			P . P	P . P	P . P	P . P	P . P	P . P	P . P	F . P	P . P	P . P	P . P	P . P		PLAQUE
1													1 1	1 2		FURCA
. B			. . .	. . 3					. . B				. . B	B . B		BL/SUP
N			1	N	N	1	N	N	N	N	N	N	1	N		MOBILITY
													C . C			Calculus

Mandibular arch (teeth 32–17)

32	31	30	29	28	27	26	25	24	23	22	21	20	19	18	17	
. . .	. . .	. . .	. . .	. . .	. . C	C C C	C C C	C C C	C	. . .	. . .	. . .	. . C	. . .		Calculus
	N	1	1	N	N	1	1	1	1	N	1	N	N	1		MOBILITY
	. . .	. . .	. . .	B . .	. . .	. . B	. . .	. . .	. . .	. . .	. . .	. . .	. . B	. . B		BL/SUP
	3	3											4	4		FURCA
	P . P	P . P	P . P	P . P	P . P	P . P	P . P	P . P	P	P . P	P . P	P . .	P . P	P . P		PLAQUE
	153	263	132	101	100	120	030	030	030	000	101	100	381	376		ATTACH
	+22 +1	+13 +1	+21 +2	+2+2+2	+2+2+2	+20 +2	+21 +2	+21 +2	+2? +2	+2+2+3	+2+2+2	+2+2+3	+13 +2	+23 2		FGM
	334	334	324	323	322	322	222	222	222	223	323	323	453	544		P.D.

32	31	30	29	28	27	26	25	24	23	22	21	20	19	18	17	
	.	.	MG	MG	.	.	.	.	.	.	MG	MG	MG	.		MGDEF
	. C .	. C .	. . .	. . .	. . .	. . .	. . .	. . .	. . .	. . .	. . .	. . .	. . C	. . .		Calculus
		S											R	R R		BL/SUP
	P . P	. . P	P . P	P . P	P . P	P . P	P . P	P . P	P	P . P	P . P	P . P	. . P	P . P		PLAQUE
	3	3											4	4		FURCA
	060	0 120	030	030	321	120	020	020	020	122	131	233	464	465		ATTACH
	+31 +3	+32 +3	+31 +3	+31 +3	+20 +2	+20 +2	+20 +2	+20 +2	+20 +2	+10 +1	+21 +2	+11 0	020	032		FGM
	353	3 103	323	323	523	322	222	222	222	223	323	323	444	433		P.D.

Figure 1.9.2 Periodontal chart during initial evaluation.

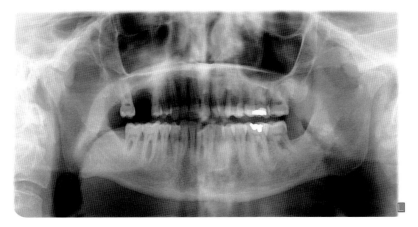

Figure 1.9.3 Panoramic radiograph taken during initial evaluation.

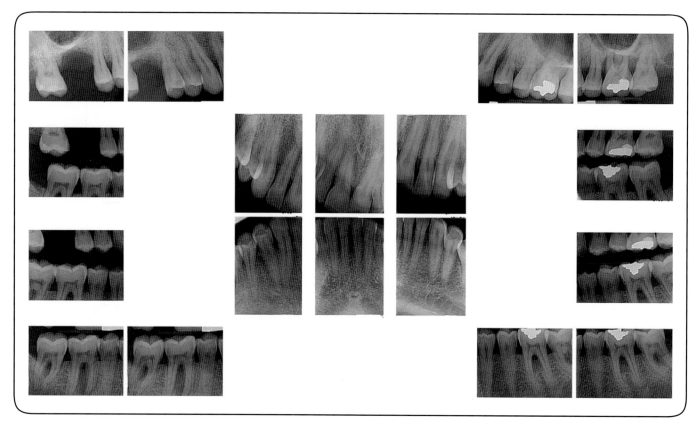

Figure 1.9.4 Full-mouth series taken a year prior to initial evaluation.

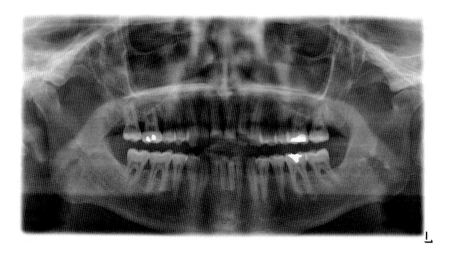

Figure 1.9.5 Panoramic radiograph taken six years previously.

and subgingival calculus was removed using hand scalers and curettes. All exposed tooth surfaces were polished. Home care was reviewed and reinforced with the patient, along with a demonstration of appropriate brushing and flossing techniques.

At two-month reevaluation, a gingival flap was raised in the lower right quadrant to provide open access and

debridement of subgingival calculus for the purpose of pocket reduction, followed by the same procedure in the lower left quadrant at four-month reevaluation. Both quadrants healed without incident.

Currently the patient is wearing an occlusal guard to control his parafunctional habit (bruxism). Extraction of tooth #2 was recommended due to severe distal bone loss. Sinus augmentation for implant treatment planning for site #3 was recommended.

Cone-beam computed tomography (CBCT) scan of the maxilla (Figures 1.9.6–1.9.9) was used to evaluate the edentulous site #3. Findings from the CBCT data included generalized mild to moderate periodontal bone loss with localized severe periodontal bone loss associated with teeth #2, #12, #14 and #15; severe disuse atrophy of edentulous site was noted in the scan.

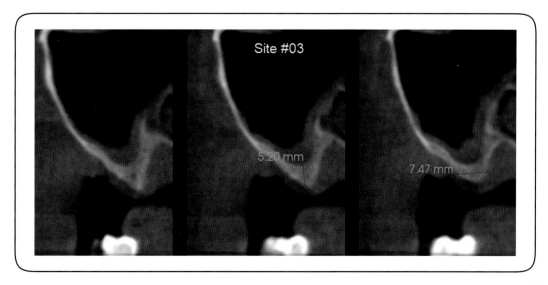

Figure 1.9.6 Cross-sections of severe disuse atrophy (Siebert Class III defect) of edentulous site #3.

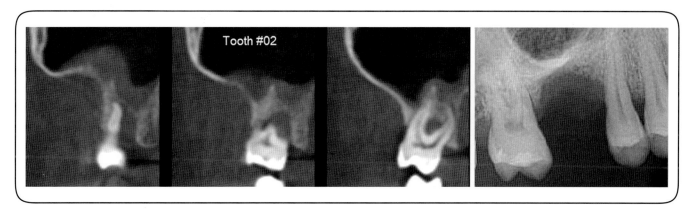

Figure 1.9.7 Comparison of cross-sections from CBCT and periapical radiographs: angular bone loss of tooth #2.

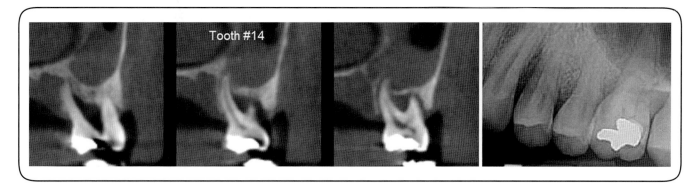

Figure 1.9.8 Comparison of cross-sections from CBCT and periapical radiographs: angular bone loss of tooth #14.

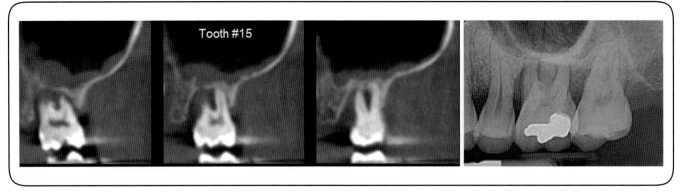

Figure 1.9.9 Comparison of cross-sections from CBCT and periapical radiographs: angular bone loss of tooth #15.

Discussion

This patient presented with a chief complaint of edentulous site #3 and requested the area be restored with a dental implant. A diagnosis of generalized slight with localized severe chronic periodontitis based on the clinical and radiographic findings was made. Clinical and radiographic evaluation play an important role in the diagnosis and for planning comprehensive treatment options. Different radiographic imaging techniques are available in dentistry: full-mouth series, individual periapical radiographs/bitewings, panoramic radiographs, and CBCT. It is important to understand when it is appropriate to prescribe each of these modalities in clinical practice.

Self-Study Questions

A. What is the recommended imaging technique for evaluating patients with periodontal disease?

B. How often are radiographic images recommended in patients with periodontal disease?

C. What are the advantages and disadvantages of two-dimensional imaging (full-mouth series and panoramic radiographs)?

D. When is CBCT recommended in periodontal management?

E. How would you identify a vertical fracture in a radiograph?

F. What imaging technique is recommended for evaluating an endodontic–periodontal lesion?

G. What are the differences in exposure to radiation for the recommended imaging techniques in periodontics?

Answers located at the end of the chapter.

References

1. Cobert EF, Ho DKL, Lai SML. Radiographs in periodontal disease diagnosis and management. *Aust Dent J* 2009;54(1 Suppl):S27–S43.
2. American Dental Association. *Dental Radiographic Examinations: Recommendations for Patient Selection and Limiting Radiation Exposure.* Chicago: ADA, 2012.
3. Mol A. Imaging methods in periodontology. *Periodontol 2000* 2004;34:34–48.
4. White S, Pharoah M. *Oral Radiology: Principles and Interpretation*, 7th edn. St. Louis, MO: Mosby Elsiever, 2014:299–313.
5. Research, Science and Therapy Committee. Position paper: Diagnosis of periodontal diseases. *J Periodontol* 2003;74(8):1237–1247.
6. Misch K, Yi E, Sarment D. Accuracy of cone beam computed tomography for periodontal defect measurements. *J Periodontol* 2006;77(7):1261–1266.

7. Grimard B, Hoidal M, Mills M, et al. Comparison of clinical, periapical radiograph and cone beam volume tomography measurement techniques for assessing bone level changes following regenerative periodontal therapy. *J Periodontol* 2009;8(1):48–55.

8. Åkesson L, Håkansson J, Rohlin M. Comparison of panoramic and intraoral radiography and pocket probing for the measurement of the marginal bone level. *J Clin Periodontol* 1992;19:326–332.

9. Flint D, Paunovich E, Moore W, et al. A diagnostic comparison of panoramic and intraoral radiograph. *Oral Surg Oral Med Oral Pathol Oral Radiol Endod* 1998;85(6): 731–735.

10. Bean LR, Ackerman WY Jr. Intraoral or panoramic radiography? *Dent Clin North Am* 1984;28(1):47–55.

11. Goodarzi Pour D, Romoozi E, Soleimani Shayesteh Y. Accuracy of cone beam computed tomography for detection of bone loss. *J Dent Tehran* 2015; 12(7):513–523.

12. Nikolic-Jakoba N, Spin-Neto R, Wenzel A. Cone beam computed tomography for detection of intrabony and furcation defects: a systematic review based on a hierarchical model for diagnostic efficacy. *J Periodontol* 2016;87(6): 630–644.

13. Mandelaris G, Scheyer T, Evans M, et al. American Academy of Periodontology Best Evidence consensus statement on

14. Queiroz PM, Nascimento HAR, Jacome da Paz TD, et al. Accuracy of digital subtraction radiography in the detection of vertical root fractures. *J Endod* 2016;42(6): 896–899.

15. Chang E, Lam E, Shah P, Azarpazhooh A. Cone-beam computed tomography for detecting vertical root fractures in endodontically treated teeth: a systematic review. *J Endod* 2016;42(2):177–185.

16. Edlund M, Nair MK, Nair UP. Detection of vertical root fractures by using cone-beam computed tomography: a clinical study. *J Endod* 2011;37(6):768–772.

17. Wanderley VA, Freitas DQ, Haiter-Neto F, Oliveira ML. Influence of tooth orientation on the detection of vertical root fracture in cone-beam computed tomography. *J Endod* 2018;44(7):1168–1172.

18. Al-Fouzan KS. A new classification of endodontic–periodontal lesions. *Int J Dent* 2014;2014:919173.

19. Rotstein I. Interaction between endodontics and periodontics. *Periodontol 2000* 2017;74(1):11–39.

20. Singh P. Endo-perio dilemma: a brief review. *Dent Res J (Isfahan)* 2011;8(1):39–47.

21. Shenoy N, Shenoy A. Endo-perio lesions: diagnosis and clinical considerations. *Indian J Dent Res* 2010;21(4):579–585.

selected oral applications for cone bean computed tomography. *J Periodontol* 2017;88(10):939–945.

TAKE-HOME POINTS

A. Radiographic images play an important role in the assessment of periodontal disease; however, this must be considered as an adjunct and not a substitute for clinical evaluation. The American Dental Association (ADA) has established that radiographic screening to detect possible disease should not be performed. A clinical evaluation, medical history, and review of previous exams and previous radiographic images should precede any radiographic prescription. Any radiograph needs to be justified, with adherence to the principle of ALARA (as low as reasonably achievable), offering the best diagnostic option for the patient with the lowest radiation dose [1,2].

There are different techniques to be considered: panoramic radiographs and intraoral radiographs including periapical radiographs and bitewings, which offer important diagnostic information but which present two-dimensional information derived from three-dimensional anatomy. Newer imaging techniques that could overcome this challenge in the diagnosis of periodontal disease include digital subtraction, optical coherence tomography, computed tomography (CT), and cone beam computed tomography [3,4]. In any of these techniques, the reference for periodontal evaluation is the distance from the cementoenamel junction (CEJ) to the crestal bone or the base of the osseous defects.

Periapical Radiographs

This technique is recommended when evaluation of the entire tooth, including alveolar bone, periodontal ligament space and lamina dura, is needed. A paralleling technique is recommended to obtain relatively accurate measurements. With the paralleling technique, the receptor is positioned parallel to the long axis of the teeth to be imaged and the X-ray beam oriented perpendicular to the surface of the receptor and long axis of the tooth.

Bitewing Radiographs

There are two types of bitewing radiographs used in dentistry, horizontal and vertical. Horizontal bitewings are the most used routinely to evaluate the level of the crestal bone; however, in cases of advanced periodontal bone loss, vertical bitewings are recommended. This technique includes the crowns of maxillary and mandibular teeth with alveolar crestal levels in a single image.

Panoramic Radiographs

A panoramic radiograph is one of the most used imaging modalities in dentistry, consisting of a single image that includes all dentoalveolar structures with good resolution and relatively low dose compared with an intraoral full-mouth series [3]. A panoramic radiograph may be sufficient as an adjunct to the clinical evaluation of periodontal disease; however, supplementary intraoral images such as periapical or bitewing radiographs may be needed to obtain more detail in a specific region [1].

Digital Subtraction

This technique consists of the superimposition of two digital intraoral images with matched density and projection geometry, where the information on one radiograph is subtracted from the other. The biggest limitation of this technique is the challenge of reproducible projection geometry of the images. However, digital subtraction allows detection of minimal changes in bone density as low as 5% that are undetectable with other techniques [5].

Computed Tomography

This advanced imaging technique allows the dentist to evaluate the alveolar bone height in three dimensions, with no superimposition. The area of interest can be visualized in three planes, sagittal, axial and coronal, allowing comparison of each view. Despite the advantages, CT presents limited spatial resolution, making small changes in bone level (1–2 mm) undetectable. Another limitation is the high radiation dose compared with other imaging techniques [6].

Cone Beam Computed Tomography

This is an advanced imaging technique that allows evaluation of the level of the crestal bone in three planes without any superposition of other structures. Compared to CT, CBCT has a cone-shaped X-ray beam that captures the region of interest in a single rotation around the patient, contributing to a significant reduction in radiation dose. Additionally, optimization of the voxel size is possible, with options to select a 75-µm voxel size to improve the spatial resolution, making small osseous changes (1–2 mm) detectable [3,5–7]. It is important to understand that because CBCT imparts an effective dose higher than that of panoramic and intraoral radiography, it is not recommended as a routine radiographic technique, but is specifically prescribed when the diagnostic task justifies it.

B. There is no predetermined frequency or type of imaging established for reevaluation of a patient with periodontal disease, and the need for imaging should be based on the diagnosis and prognosis. Imaging techniques recommended for reevaluation include panoramic radiographs with or without bitewings and/or selected intraoral radiographs [1–3]. In cases of severe periodontal bone loss where treatment planning involves combined implants, CBCT is recommended. Radiographs should aid in visualization of the level of supporting alveolar bone, interproximal crestal bone, furcation areas, patterns of bone loss, calculus, and length of the roots. These images need to be compared with previous images to determine the evolution of the periodontal disease.

The ADA has established guidelines recommending selection, frequency, and radiation exposure for radiographic examinations in dentistry. According to these guidelines, clinical evaluation and medical history will determine the type of radiographic images and their frequency of use. In cases of caries the ADA does recommend the frequency of radiographic examination based on the incidence of disease. However, the frequency of radiographic examination for periodontal evaluation should be based on the clinical judgment of the dentist, applying the principle of ALARA to any recommended procedure to reduce the patient's exposure [2].

C.
Intraoral Radiographs: Full-mouth Series/Bitewing Radiographs (with Paralleling Technique)

Advantages
- More detail than panoramic radiograph
- Less distortion
- Measurements are more accurate
- No need to take the full series, only the regions of interest

Disadvantages
- Sensor can be uncomfortable for patients
- Challenge in patients with gag reflex
- Variations of anatomy: mandibular tori and torus palatinus can interfere with the positioning of the receptor

Panoramic Radiographs
Advantages
- Rapid and single technique, requiring minimal time
- Good method for visualization of the crestal bone level
- Broad anatomic coverage
- Less radiation dose
- Recommended for patients with gag reflex
- Useful technique for patient education

Disadvantages
- Uneven magnification, linear measurements not completely accurate
- Distortion of the image due to positioning of the patient
- Lower resolution than intraoral images
- Presence of double images and ghost images
- Difficult to obtain accurate image when there is maxillomandibular discrepancy

Both imaging techniques are useful as an adjunct to clinical evaluation, but there are some limitations relating to the evaluation of periodontal disease:
- Provide two-dimensional images of three-dimensional structures.
- Size of bone lesions are bigger than visualized in radiographic images.
- Soft tissue is not visible [4,8–11].

D. One of the biggest limitations with intraoral and panoramic radiographs in the evaluation of periodontal bone loss is that these imaging techniques present a two-dimensional projection of the oral maxillofacial structures. CBCT allows visualization in multiplanar reconstructions (sagittal, coronal and axial views) as well as cross-sections and panoramic views, without superimposition or magnification.

One of the most common uses of CBCT in periodontology is related to the evaluation of edentulous sites or prospective sites for dental implant treatment. CBCT allows the evaluation of tooth morphology, implant sites, osseous morphology, trabecular pattern and density of edentulous sites, and proximity and relationship to anatomic structures (e.g. floor of the maxillary sinus and inferior alveolar nerve canal), and facilitates fabrication of surgical guides.

One of the most important limitations of CBCT is the presence of artifacts due to multiple metallic restorations, endodontic treatment, or any other metal adjacent to the region of interest. These artifacts may interfere with the visualization of edentulous or prospective sites for implant treatment planning.

CBCT is not considered a standard diagnostic tool for diagnosis of periodontal disease, although it is an excellent diagnostic adjunct when it is necessary to assess alveolar bone defects, advanced periodontal bone loss, and endodontic–periodontal lesions, and for the diagnosis and management of peri-implantitis or the localization of osseous defects [6,11–13].

E. Vertical root fracture is a fracture oriented parallel to the long axis of the root of the tooth. Vertical root fractures are commonly associated with endodontically treated teeth, attributed to excessive root canal instrumentation, pressure during gutta-percha filling, or inappropriate placement of an intraradicular post.

Radiography is a useful diagnostic test for vertical root fracture, which is visible as a vertical radiolucent line in the region of the root. Vertical root fracture is visible only if the X-ray beam is aligned perpendicular to the fracture plane and there is some separation of the fragments, making a confirmatory radiographic diagnosis possible only in one-third of cases.

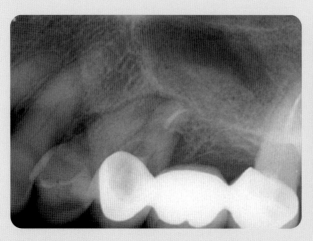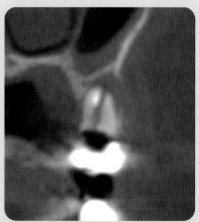

Figure 1.9.10 Vertical fracture of tooth #13. This vertical root fracture is not visible in the periapical radiograph. In the CBCT cross-sectional view, the vertical fracture and disruption of the buccal plate are clearly visualized.

CBCT is recommended for the evaluation of teeth with root fractures because of the lack of superposition of structures and the capacity to evaluate the tooth in different views (Figure 1.9.10). CBCT analysis with limited-area field of view (FOV) with voxel size between 80 and 125 μm is recommended for evaluation of vertical root fractures.

When vertical fractures are not radiographically visible with any modality, indirect features such as focal widening of the periodontal ligament space can be considered a sign of root fracture when clinical symptoms are present [4,14–17].

F. Endodontic–periodontal lesions are defined as lesions that are due to both endodontic and periodontal etiology. It is important to understand the interaction between endodontic and periodontal disease to achieve the correct diagnosis of the endodontic–periodontal lesion and this will guide successful treatment.

Endodontic–periodontal lesions are classified according to the location of the primary lesion: primary endodontic disease, primary periodontal disease, or combined diseases. The factors that may contribute to the development of endodontic–periodontal lesions include poor endodontic treatment, poor restorations, trauma, root resorption, and root fractures and perforations during endodontic preparation.

Radiographic evaluation plays an important role in the detection of the factors that may contribute to the development of endodontic–periodontal lesions.

Table 1.9.1 Median effective dose for various radiographic techniques.

Radiographic technique	Median effective dose	Equivalent background exposure
Intraoral		
Rectangular collimation		
Posterior bitewings: PSP or F-speed film	5 μSv	0.6 day
Full-mouths series: PSP or F-speed film	40 μSv	5 days
Full-mouth series: CCD sensor	20 μSv	2.5 days
Extraoral		
Panoramic	20 μSv	2.5 days
CBCT small field of view	50 μSv	6 days
CBCT medium field of view	100 μSv	12 days
CBCT large field of view	120 μSv	15 days
Computed tomography maxillofacial	650 μSv	2 months
Computed tomography head	2 mSv	8 months

One of the most common radiographic findings in endodontic–periodontal lesions is bone loss extending from the level of the crestal bone to, or near, the apical region of the teeth and widening of the periodontal ligament space [18–21].

Periapical radiographs are commonly used in the evaluation of endodontic–periodontal lesions; however, a limited FOV CBCT scan is recommended to assess for associated fractures, accessory root canals, root perforation, or other features not visualized in a periapical radiograph.

G. Dentists need to consider the type of radiographic image recommended to evaluate periodontal disease based on the clinical evaluation and medical history; additionally, they need to evaluate the effective dose patients will receive for this radiographic evaluation.

Effective dose is used to estimate the risk in humans by comparing different exposure types. This takes into account volume, radiosensitivity of the tissue irradiated, and the biologic effectiveness of radiation. The SI unit of effective dose is the sievert (Sv); however, for the purposes of patient education it is recommended that the clinician knows the equivalence of the effective dose to background exposure. Equivalent background radiation is calculated based on a background radiation of 3.1 mSv per year.

Because of the availability of multiple types of radiographic unit, median effective dose from the dentomaxillofacial region with typical exposure protocols is calculated based on multiple published studies.

2

Nonsurgical Periodontal Therapy

Case 1: Hand and Automated Instrumentation 86
Helen Livson, DMD, MMSc

Case 2: Local Drug Delivery 92
Emilio I. Arguello, DDS, MSc and Naciye G. Uzel, DMD, DMSc

Case 3: Systemic Antibiotics 101
Flavia Teles, DDS, MS, DMSc, Ricardo Teles[†], DDS, DMSc, Magda Feres, DDS, MSc, PhD,
Belen Retamal-Valdes, DDS, MSc, PhD, and Vinicius Souza Rodrigues, DDS, SDD, DMSc

Case 4: Use of Lasers in Periodontology 114
Abiar Alwael, DDS, MS, Irina F. Dragan, DDS, DMD, MS, and Charles Hawley, DDS, PhD

[†] Deceased

Case 1

Hand and Automated Instrumentation

CASE STORY

A 25-year-old Caucasian male presented with a chief complaint of "I need a cleaning." The patient had noticed significant staining as well as plaque and calculus buildup, particularly in the mandibular anterior region (Figures 2.1.1–2.1.3).

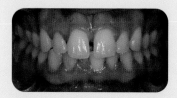

Figure 2.1.1 Frontal view.

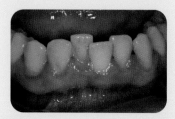

Figure 2.1.2 Buccal view, mandibular anterior.

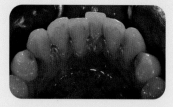

Figure 2.1.3 Lingual view, mandibular anterior.

LEARNING GOALS AND OBJECTIVES

■ To identify appropriate instruments that may be used for scaling and/or scaling and root planing
■ To learn the importance of primary phase nonsurgical therapy
■ To learn the advantages and disadvantages of hand versus power instrumentation
■ To understand the limitations of these instruments in the nonsurgical management of periodontal disease

Medical History

The patient reported a history of asthma and used an albuterol inhaler once per day. Otherwise, there were no significant medical problems, and the patient had no known allergies.

Review of Systems

- Vital signs
  - Blood pressure: 120/65 mmHg
  - Pulse rate: 72 beats/minute (regular)
  - Respiratory rate: 15 breaths/minute

Social History

The patient does not drink alcohol. He reported smoking one time per week.

Extraoral Examination

No significant findings. The patient had no masses or swelling, and the temporomandibular joint was within normal limits.

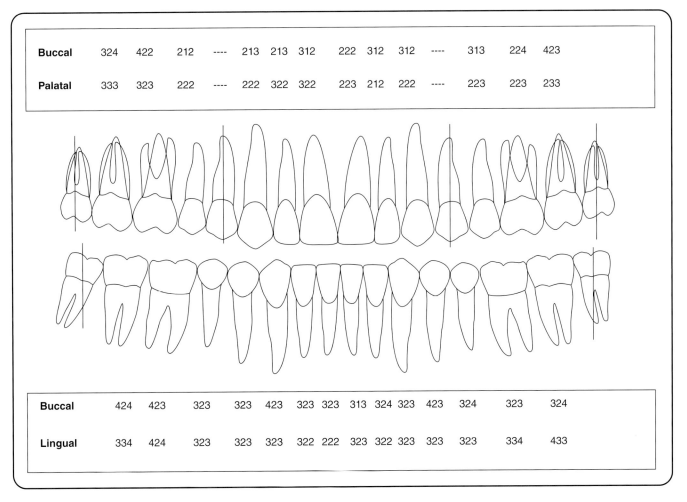

Buccal	324	422	212	----	213	213	312	222	312	312	----	313	224	423
Palatal	333	323	222	----	222	322	322	223	212	222	----	223	223	233

Buccal	424	423	323	323	423	323	323	313	324	323	423	324	323	324
Lingual	334	424	323	323	323	322	222	323	322	323	323	323	334	433

Figure 2.1.4 Probing pocket depth measurements.

Intraoral Examination
- The soft tissues of the mouth, including the tongue and buccal mucosa, appeared normal.
- A gingival examination revealed localized marginal erythema, with rolled margins and inflamed papillae (Figures 2.1.1–2.1.3).
- A complete periodontal examination and charting were completed (Figure 2.1.4).

Radiographic Examination
Given the patient's young age and lack of caries history, only bitewing radiographs were taken (Figure 2.1.5).

Occlusion
There were no occlusal discrepancies or interferences.

Diagnosis
After reviewing the patient's history as well as the clinical and radiographic examination, a differential diagnosis of dental biofilm-induced gingivitis was made.

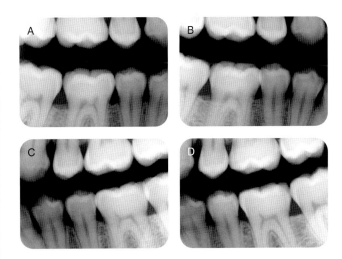

Figure 2.1.5 Bite-wing radiographs.

Treatment Plan
The treatment plan for this patient includes oral hygiene instructions, followed by scaling and polishing using hand instruments and powered mechanical instruments.

Treatment

After thorough oral hygiene instructions were reviewed, the patient received a scaling and polishing. The procedure began with an ultrasonic-powered mechanical instrument to loosen any tenacious supragingival deposits as well as initial stain removal. Hand scalers were then employed, including a sickle scaler for removal of supragingival calculus and stain in the mandibular anterior areas, Gracey curettes were utilized in the interproximal areas posteriorly, and universal curettes for the buccal and lingual aspects of the teeth. The ultrasonic was then used again for a final lavage, and the teeth were ultimately polished for any additional stain elimination using prophylaxis paste and a rubber cup (Figures 2.1.6–2.1.8).

Discussion

The patient presented with heavy supragingival plaque and calculus, gingival inflammation, and generalized bleeding on probing with no concurrent bone loss around the teeth. After a detailed medical history was completed, a diagnosis of dental biofilm-induced gingivitis was assigned. To restore the patient to periodontal health, comprehensive oral hygiene instructions were provided, and a professional scaling was arranged.

A combination of hand instruments and power-driven instruments were used for removal of plaque, calculus, and stain from the teeth. Hand instruments are available in various lengths, shapes, and designs to effectively

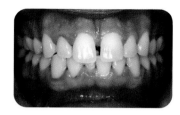

Figure 2.1.6 Frontal view.

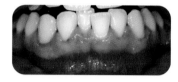

Figure 2.1.7 Buccal view, mandibular anterior.

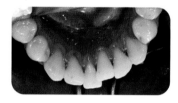

Figure 2.1.8 Lingual view, mandibular anterior.

reach and treat all areas of the teeth. An ultrasonic instrument (Cavitron) was used as an adjunct for stain removal, mechanical debridement, lavage, and cavitation. Regularly scheduled reevaluations and prophylaxis in addition to routine home care are recommended for maintaining optimal oral hygiene and periodontal health in this patient.

Self-Study Questions

A. What are the chief instruments available in our armamentarium for scaling and root planing?

B. What are some examples of hand instruments?

C. What is the mechanism of action of powered mechanical instruments?

D. Are there any contraindications to using powered mechanical instruments?

E. Are there differences in efficacy of treatment between hand scalers and automated scalers?

F. What are some advantages and disadvantages of hand instruments versus powered mechanical instruments?

G. What are the limitations to prophylaxis and scaling and root planing?

Answers located at the end of the chapter.

References

1. Ewen SJ, Glickstein BA. *Ultrasonic Therapy in Periodontics.* Springfield, IL: Charles C. Thomas, 1968:12–34.
2. Clarke PR, Hill CR. Physical and chemical aspects of ultrasonic disruption of cells. *J Acoust Soc Am* 1970;47: 649–653.
3. Gantes BG, Nilveus R. The effects of different hygiene instruments on titanium surfaces: SEM observations. *Int J Periodontics Restorative Dent* 1991;11:225–239.
4. Miller CS, Leonelli FM, Latham E. Selective interference with pacemaker activity by electrical dental devices. *Oral Surg Oral Med Oral Pathol Oral Radiol Endod* 1998;85: 33–36.
5. Breininger D, O'Leary T, Blumenshine RV. Comparative effectiveness of ultrasonic and hand scaling on removal of subgingival plaque and calculus. *J Periodontol* 1987;58: 9–18.
6. Thornton S, Garnick J. Comparison of ultrasonic to hand instruments in the removal of subgingival plaque. *J Periodontol* 1982;53:35–37.
7. Baeni P, Thilo B, Chapuis B, Pernet D. Effects of ultrasonic and sonic scalers on dental plaque microflora in vitro and in vivo. *J Clin Periodontol* 1992;19:455–459.
8. Nishimine D, O'Leary TJ. Hand instrumentation versus ultrasonics in the removal of endotoxins from root surface. *J Periodontol* 1979;50:345–349.
9. Hunter R, P'Leary T, Kafrawy AH. The effectiveness of hand versus instrumentation in open-flap root planing. *J Periodontol* 1984;55:697–703.
10. Matia J, Bissada N, Maybury JE, Ricchetti P. Efficiency of scaling the molar furcation area with and without surgical access. *Int J Periodontics Restorative Dent* 1986;6:24–35.
11. Gellin R. The effectiveness of the Titan-S sonic scaler versus curettes in the removal of subgingival calculus. A human evaluation. *J Periodontol* 1986;57:672–680.
12. Bower RC. Furcation morphology relative to periodontal treatment: furcation entrance architecture. *J Periodontol* 1979;50:23–27.
13. Dragoo M. A clinical evaluation of hand and ultrasonic instruments on subgingival debridement. Part I. With unmodified and modified ultrasonic inserts. *Int J Periodontics Restorative Dent* 1992;12:311–313.
14. Leon L, Vogel R. A comparison of the effectiveness of hand scaling and ultrasonic debridement in furcations as evaluated with dark-field microscopy. *J Periodontol* 1987;58:86–94.
15. Ritz L, Hefti A, Rateitschak KH. An in vitro investigation on the loss of root substance in scaling with various instruments. *J Clin Periodontol* 1991;18:643–647.
16. Larato DC, Ruskin PF, Martin A. Effect of an ultrasonic scaler on bacterial counts in air. *J Periodontol* 1967;38:550–554.
17. Waerhaug J. Healing of the dento-epithelial junction following subgingival plaque control II: as observed on extracted teeth. *J Periodontol* 1978;49:119–134.
18. Caffesse RG, Sweeney PL, Smith BA. Scaling and root planing with and without periodontal flap surgery. *J Clin Periodontol* 1986;13:205–210.
19. Lindhe J, Socransky S, Nyman S, et al. "Critical probing depths" in periodontal therapy. *J Clin Periodontol* 1982;9:323–336.
20. Philstrom BL, McHugh RB, Oliphant TH, Ortiz-Campos C. Comparison of surgical and nonsurgical treatment of periodontal disease. A review of current studies and additional results after 6½ years. *J Clin Periodontol* 1983;10:524–541.
21. Isidor F, Karring T. Long-term effect of surgical and nonsurgical periodontal treatment. A 5-year clinical study. *J Periodontal Res* 1986;21:462–472.

TAKE-HOME POINTS

The most fundamental objective of primary phase nonsurgical therapy is to reestablish periodontal health in a patient by reduction of putative periodontal pathogens from the periodontium. Literature has demonstrated that instrumentation can effectively decrease these periodontal pathogens and help restore a healthier bacterial flora in the mouth.

A. In our armamentarium, the chief instruments available for scaling and root planing include:
- Scalers and curettes: manual mechanical instrumentation.
- Ultrasonic devices (magnetorestrictive, piezoelectric): powered mechanical instrumentation.
- Air abrasives/rubber cups (for stain removal).

B. Manual instrumentation is an essential skill necessary to optimize results from initial nonsurgical therapy; it is paramount that the practitioner has a thorough understanding of these instruments.
- Scalers are designed for removal of supragingival calculus. They include two straight cutting edges and a pointed toe (e.g. sickle scalers; Figure 2.1.9A,B).
- Curettes are designed for subgingival instrumentation but can be used for supragingival scaling as well.
  o Universal curettes have two cutting edges (Figure 2.1.9C).

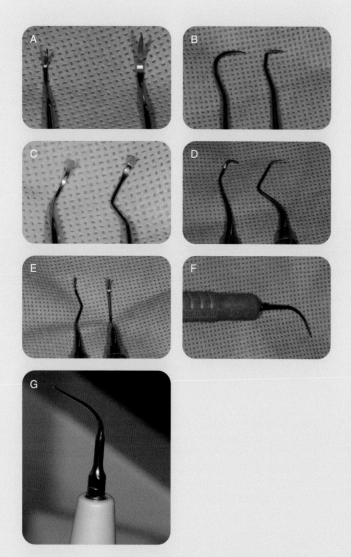

Figure 2.1.9   (A, B) Sickle scalers; (C) universal curettes; (D, E) Gracey curettes; (F) magnetorestrictive ultrasonic scalers; (G) piezoelectric ultrasonic scalers.

o Area-specific curettes have only one cutting edge (i.e. Gracey curettes; Figure 2.1.9D,E).

C. Powered mechanical instruments such as sonic and ultrasonic scalers have been used by practitioners to remove plaque, calculus, and stain from tooth and root surfaces. These automated scalers work by way of vibration; as the tip oscillates, it helps break apart adherent deposits that may be present on the teeth. While operating, the tip sprays a jet of water that flushes away debris and helps dissipate heat produced by the instrument. Additionally, when the

water passes over the vibrations of the oscillating tip of an ultrasonic instrument, cavitation is observed. Cavitation is a process by which formation and destruction of small air cavities releases energy that may disrupt bacterial cell membranes [1,2].

Powered mechanical instruments are classified based on their frequencies, and are very effective for nonsurgical debridement of teeth.
- Sonic scalers operate at a frequency of 3000–8000 cycles per second and are driven by compressed air from the dental unit. A rotor system is then activated and the sonic tip oscillates in an elliptical to circular pattern.
- Ultrasonic scalers can be further classified as follows.
  o Magnetorestrictive ultrasonic scalers: operate inaudibly; the tip oscillates at 18–42 kHz (thousand cycles per second). The motion of the tip is elliptical to circular, and all surfaces of the tip are useful in debridement (Figure 2.1.9F).
  o Piezoelectric ultrasonic scalers: operate inaudibly; the tip oscillates at 24–45 kHz. The motion of the tip is linear, so unlike the magnetorestrictive ultrasonics, only its lateral surfaces are useful in debridement (Figure 2.1.9G).

D. Concerns that the practitioner should be aware of if using powered mechanical instruments are both dental and medical in nature.

Dental

As with manual instrumentation, mechanical instruments may remove excessive tooth structure causing subsequent dental hypersensitivity. It is not recommended that sonic and ultrasonic instruments be used directly on dental implants as the metal tips may scratch the softer titanium. Ideally, hand periodontal scalers made of plastic, Teflon, wood, or titanium, or gold-plated scalers should be used for cleaning dental implants [3]. If used too vigorously, these instruments may also damage certain restorative margins.

Medical

Cardiac pacemakers, particularly those placed before the mid-1980s, may suffer electromagnetic interference from *magnetorestrictive* ultrasonics (piezoelectric scalers are a safe alternative) [4]. Patients with significant respiratory problems may be intolerant to the aerosols produced during power instrumentation. Powered mechanical instruments should be avoided in patients with infectious diseases that could be transmitted via aerosol production.

E. Several studies have evaluated the efficacy of plaque and calculus removal using manual versus automated instrumentation. These studies have demonstrated that both hand instrumentation and ultrasonic instrumentation are very effective at plaque removal [5]. There were no significant differences observed between the use of manual instruments and ultrasonic instruments [6] or between sonic and ultrasonic instrumentation in terms of the ability to remove plaque [7]. Some studies have demonstrated that manual instrumentation is more effective than ultrasonic instrumentation in calculus removal [8,9]. However, powered instruments have been shown to access concavities and furcations of roots better than manual instruments [10]. According to Gellin, using these methods concurrently is more effective than using either method alone [11].

F. See Table 2.1.1

G. Although hand and powered instruments are effective in treating periodontal and gingival disease as part of the initial phase of therapy, we should be mindful of their limitations. Literature has established that even with all currently available instrumentation, there is a certain pocket depth up to which we can effectively eliminate subgingival plaque and calculus [17]. Caffesse and associates found that the extent of residual calculus is directly related to pocket depth; as pocket depth increased, the percentage of the tooth surfaces completely free of calculus gradually decreased [18]. This probing depth, referred to as the "critical probing depth," is 2.9 mm for scaling and

root planing. Any probing depth beyond 4.2 mm benefits from surgical periodontal therapy rather than nonsurgical treatment due to the limits of the effectiveness of hand and/or powered instruments [19]. Nonsurgical treatments are usually attempted first; if appropriate results are not achieved at reevaluation, surgical treatment should be pursued. Whether nonsurgical or surgical periodontal treatment modalities are used, longitudinal studies show that if treated appropriately and followed closely, patients with periodontal disease can be maintained in the long term [20,21].

Table 2.1.1 Advantages and disadvantages of using hand instruments versus powered mechanical instruments.

	Advantages	Disadvantages
Hand instruments	• Not as damaging to porcelain and composite restorations • More effective at removing endotoxin from periodontally involved root surfaces [8]	• Larger tip than furcation width [12] • Fatigue [13] • Longer scaling times [13]
Powered mechanical instruments	• Lavage effect of irrigation • Cavitation [1,2] • Slightly shorter scaling times [13] • Less skill required to be competent [13] • More effective in class II and III furcations [14] • Less removal of tooth structure [15] • Require no sharpening	• May be contraindicated for patients with older cardiac pacemakers [4] • Production of aerosols (30-fold increase of airborne microorganisms in the treatment room) [16]

Case 2

Local Drug Delivery

CASE STORY

A 35-year-old Caucasian male presented with a chief complaint of "My dentist told me I have gum disease." The patient had not experienced pain, discomfort, or swelling associated with his gums; however, he had noticed slight bleeding upon brushing and flossing. The patient claimed to brush his teeth at least once daily and he flossed once a week (Figures 2.2.1–2.2.3).

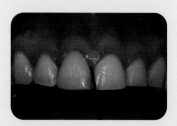

Figure 2.2.1 Preoperative view of maxillary anterior teeth and a 15-mm periodontal probe demonstrating a 5-mm probing on mesial of tooth #8 with bleeding on probing.

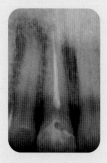

Figure 2.2.2 Preoperative periapical radiograph of tooth #8 demonstrating localized mild vertical bone loss.

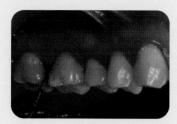

Figure 2.2.3 Preoperative view of maxillary posterior teeth and a 15-mm periodontal probe demonstrating a 4-mm probing on the distal of tooth #3 with bleeding on probing.

LEARNING GOALS AND OBJECTIVES

- To be able to diagnose periodontitis
- To identify the possible etiologic and contributing factors and to address them
- To be able to elaborate an initial treatment plan with a comprehensive phase 1 therapy to achieve initial periodontal stability
- To be able to identify the different local chemo-therapeutic agents and how, when, and why to use them

Medical History

There were no significant medical problems and the patient had no known allergies. He had no known medical illnesses. On questioning the patient stated he was not taking any medications and he had no allergies.

Review of Systems

- Vital signs
  - Blood pressure: 128/83 mmHg
  - Pulse rate: 69 beats/minute (regular)
  - Respiratory rate: 16 breaths/minute

Social History

The patient did not smoke and drank alcohol twice a month in social gatherings.

Extraoral Examination

There were no significant findings. The patient had no masses or swelling, and the temporomandibular joint was within normal limits.

Intraoral Examination

- The soft tissues of the mouth (except gingiva) including the tongue appeared normal.
- A gingival examination revealed a mild marginal erythema and swollen papillae (Figures 2.2.1 and 2.2.3).
- The patient exhibited localized areas with bleeding on probing as well as localized areas with probing depths of 4 and 5 mm (Figures 2.2.1 and 2.2.3).
- A periodontal chart was completed. Note that the clinical attachment levels (CALs) are not displayed because all gingival margins are at the level of the cementoenamel junction, and thus the CAL equals probing depth (Figure 2.2.4).

BUCCAL																
PD Pre-op	423	324	423	323	313	323	212	425	323	322	323	413	324	424	323	323
PD Re-eval	323	313	322	213	323	213	312	212	212	312	323	223	323	323	223	323
BOP Pre-op	1--1	1--1	1--1	1--1	1--1	111	---1	111	1--1	1--1	---1	---1	---1	1--1	1--1	1---
LINGUAL																
PD Pre-op	323	324	433	313	323	323	212	424	212	212	323	213	323	324	423	323
PD Re-eval	322	223	312	312	313	223	212	212	213	312	223	212	223	322	323	323
BOP Pre-op	---1	1--1	1--1	1--	---1	1--1	---1	1--1	1--1	1---	---1	1--1	----	---1	1--1	1---
Tooth #	1	2	3	4	5	6	7	8	9	10	11	12	13	14	15	16

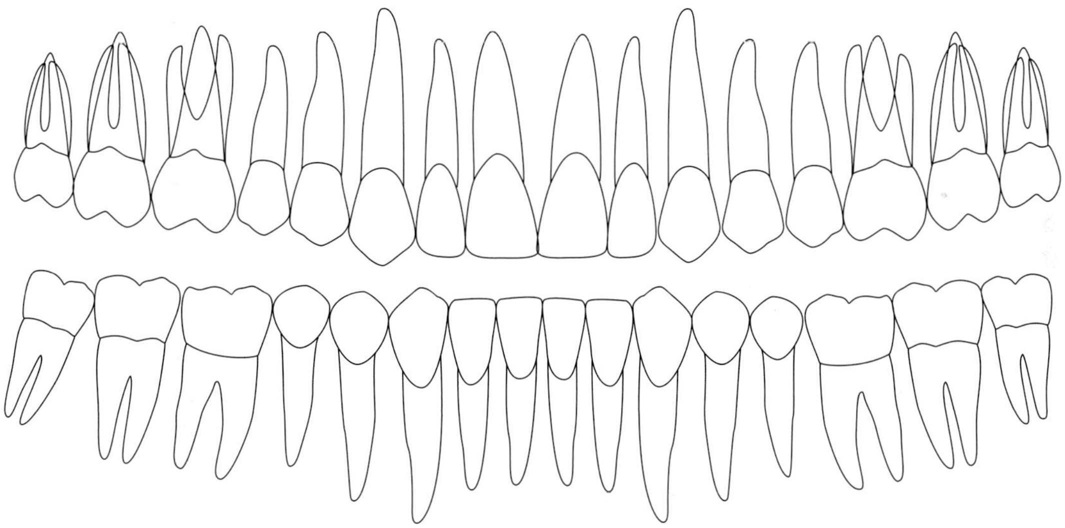

Tooth #	32	31	30	29	28	27	26	25	24	23	22	21	20	19	18	17
LINGUAL																
PD Pre-op	324	324	423	313	323	323	312	212	212	222	313	213	324	424	424	423
PD Re-eval	323	322	222	213	222	322	212	211	112	212	213	212	322	323	323	323
BOP	---1	1--1	1---	---1	1--1	----	----	----	1---	---1	----	---1	---1	1--1	1--	1---
BUCCAL																
PD Pre-op	323	314	423	423	313	322	222	222	212	212	222	214	224	324	324	323
PD Re-eval	323	323	223	313	312	222	212	212	212	222	212	213	222	223	322	323
BOP	---1	1--1	1--1	1--1	1--1	---1	----	----	1--1	---1	---1	---1	---1	1--1	1--1	1---

Figure 2.2.4 Probing pocket depth measurements.

Occlusion

There were no occlusal discrepancies or interferences.

Radiographic Examination

A full-mouth set of radiographs was ordered; there were localized areas of mild vertical bone loss on the mesial and distal surfaces of tooth #8 (Figure 2.2.2).

Diagnosis

After reviewing the history and the clinical and radiographic examinations, the periodontal diagnosis was localized stage I grade A periodontitis. The American Dental Association diagnosis is type II.

Treatment Plan

The treatment plan consisted of addressing the primary etiology that causes the periodontal disease for this patient (phase 1) in the following order: oral hygiene instruction; subgingival scaling and root planing (SRP) of all sites with initial probing depths >3 mm, and supragingival scaling and polishing of all other surfaces; concomitant administration of a local antibiotic immediately after scaling (Figures 2.2.5 and 2.2.6) and only for sites with probing depths >3 mm followed by a minimum of four- to six-week reevaluation to assess the need for further periodontal therapy (phase 2).

Reevaluation of Post-initial Treatment

At the six-week reevaluation, the clinical parameters had improved, and certain probing depths that were initially >3 mm were reduced (Figures 2.2.7 and 2.2.8). Thus no further periodontal treatment was needed; only periodontal maintenance therapy every three months is required.

Discussion

Elements that will lead to a successful outcome include an accurate diagnosis based on a thorough history and a periodontal examination, as well as the knowledge of the etiologic factors that lead to disease. Next, a variety of treatment choices must be selected with the understanding that the primary goal will be to provide initial stability of the disease or condition, in this particular case periodontitis. Once the initial stability has been achieved, either one can proceed to further treatment such as restorative procedures or have the patient on a three-month periodontal maintenance protocol. However, initial therapy or phase 1 with or without the concomitant use of local chemotherapeutics may not achieve the optimal periodontal stability desired, and thus it is the responsibility of the treating clinician to identify what areas will need to proceed to the second phase of therapy that could involve periodontal surgery.

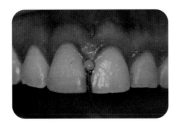

Figure 2.2.5 Application of local delivery Atridox on a 5-mm pocket mesial of tooth #8 immediately after scaling and root planing.

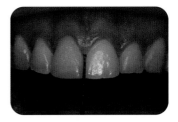

Figure 2.2.7 A six-week postoperative image of maxillary anterior teeth demonstrating a 2-mm probing on mesial of tooth #8.

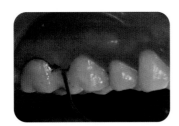

Figure 2.2.6 Application of local delivery Atridox on a 4-mm pocket distal of tooth #3 immediately after scaling and root planing.

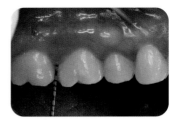

Figure 2.2.8 A six-week postoperative image of maxillary posterior teeth demonstrating a 3-mm probing on distal of tooth #3.

Self-Study Questions

A. What is the rationale for using local antibiotics and other agents for the treatment of periodontal disease?

B. Which local drug delivery agents are available?

C. What type of patients will benefit from the use of a local antibiotic?

D. What is the existing research that justifies the use of local drug delivery?

E. What are the techniques and devices used to deliver local antibiotics?

F. What are the considerations for patients to observe after receiving the local antibiotic?

G. What are the determinants of success in local drug delivery therapy?

H. What does rescue therapy mean, and how can local antibiotics help patients with periodontal disease that recurs over time?

Answers located at the end of the chapter.

ACKNOWLEDGMENTS

Thanks to Dr. Campo Elias Perez for his contribution to this chapter.

References

1. Haffajee AD, Arguello EI, Ximenez-Fyvie LA, Socransky SS. Controlling the plaque biofilm. *Int Dent J* 2003;53(Suppl 3):191–199.
2. Haffajee AD, Socransky SS. Introduction to microbial aspects of periodontal biofilm communities, development and treatment. *Periodontol 2000* 2006;42:7–12.
3. Hanes P, Purvis J. Local anti-infective therapy: pharmacological agents. A systematic review. *Ann Periodontol* 2003;8:79–98.
4. Golub LM, Goodson JM, Lee HM, et al. Tetracyclines inhibit tissue collagenases. *J Periodontol* 1985;56(11 Suppl):93–97.
5. Magnusson I. The use of locally-delivered metronidazole in the treatment of periodontitis. Clinical results. *J Clin Periodontol* 1998;25:959–963.
6. Slot DE, Kranendonk AA, Paraskevas S, Van der Weijden F. The effect of a pulsed Nd:YAG laser in non-surgical periodontal therapy. *J Periodontol* 2009;80:1041–1056.
7. Sanz M, Teughels W; Group A of European Workshop on Periodontology. Innovations in non-surgical periodontal therapy: Consensus Report of the Sixth European Workshop on Periodontology. *J Clin Periodontol* 2008;35(8 Suppl):3–7.
8. Armitage GC. Development of a classification system for periodontal diseases and conditions. *Ann Periodontol* 1999;4:1–6.
9. Caffesse RG, Sweeney PL, Smith BA. Scaling and root planing with and without periodontal flap surgery. *J Clin Periodontol* 1986;13:205–210.
10. Cobb CM. Non-surgical pocket therapy: mechanical. *Ann Periodontol* 1996;1:443–490.
11. Goodson IM, Holborow D, Dunn RL, et al. Monolithic tetracycline-containing fibres for controlled delivery to periodontal pockets. *J Periodontol* 1983;54:575–579.
12. Bonito A, Lux L, Lohr KN. Impact of local adjuncts to scaling and root planing in periodontal disease therapy: a systematic review. *J Periodontol* 2005;76:1227–1236.
13. Tanner ACR, Goodson JM. Sampling of microorganisms associated with periodontal disease. *Oral Microbiol Immunol* 1986;1:15–20.
14. Haffajee AD, Uzel NG, Arguello EI, et al. Clinical and microbiological changes associated with use of combined antimicrobial therapies to treat "refractory" periodontitis. *J Clin Periodontol* 2004;31:869–877.

TAKE-HOME POINTS

A. To understand the use of local antibiotics and other agents in the treatment of periodontal disease, one should understand the etiology of this disease, the bacterial colonization as well as the biofilm development. Bacterial colonization reaches a saturation gradient from the supragingival plaque, and it migrates vertically to colonize the subgingival sulcus or periodontal pocket. Bacteria in the supragingival plaque are composed mainly of Gram-positive aerobes, while bacteria in the subgingival plaque are made up mainly of Gram-negative anaerobes. These diverse bacterial communities that interact and exist with each other are called biofilms. Although bacterial biofilms exist in very diverse settings, it is well known that biofilm infections in the medical field are challenging to treat because of the complexity of the bacterial organization [1]. Periodontal disease is caused by a biofilm infection, and although some of the main causative bacteria have been isolated, such as the so-called red complex (*Porphyromonas gingivalis*, *Treponema denticola*, and *Tannerella forsythia*) as described by Haffajee and Socransky, periodontal disease has multiple variables. These variables include the host immune response and risk factors such as genetic predisposition and environmental factors such as smoking [2].

The use of antibiotics as well as other agents for the treatment of periodontal diseases has been widely studied, and the aim of these therapies is to minimize the bacterial colonization within the biofilm, allowing a positive host response. The concomitant use of local antibiotics delivered into the sulcus, when combined with mechanical debridement of the supragingival and subgingival plaque, reduce this bacterial burden, increase the attachment level, and reduce the pocket depth in patients with periodontal disease [3]. However, it should be noted that the use of local antibiotics and other agents should be considered as an adjunct therapeutic approach and that this approach is just one of many that can help in slowing down the progression of this complex disease.

B. The most common local drug delivery agents used in dental practice today are antibiotics such as tetracyclines and tetracycline derivatives such as doxycycline and minocycline. These are broad-spectrum antibiotics that are effective against both Gram-positive and Gram-negative bacteria; however, the concentration of the local drug is usually higher than those used systemically. In addition, tetracyclines inhibit matrix metalloproteinases (MMPs), enzymes that degrade the extracellular matrix like collagen [4] and are produced by the bacteria associated with periodontal disease. These commercially available antimicrobials include Arestin (minocycline microspheres), Atridox (10% doxycycline hyclate in a gel), and Actisite (tetracycline 12.7 mg in an ethylene/vinyl acetate copolymer fiber).

In addition to the category just described, another antibiotic that has been widely studied is metronidazole, which targets anaerobic bacteria by affecting their DNA but not the aerobic microorganisms. The brand name of the local delivery form is Elyzol, which consists of a gel containing metronidazole benzoate in a mixture of monoglycerides and triglycerides [5]. It should be noted that not all the local antibiotics mentioned here are still available in all markets.

Some other agents that are not antibiotics have proven effective in the management of the disease by affecting the host response, inflammation, and, to a certain extent, the bacterial burden. An example of this is PerioChip (chlorhexidine gluconate 2.5 mg in a biodegradable matrix of hydrolyzed gelatin cross-linked with glutaraldehyde). This product is also indicated as an adjunct to SRP procedures in patients with periodontitis or during a periodontal maintenance program. Chlorhexidine is active against broad-spectrum microorganisms that due to its positive charge reacts with the microbial cell surface and destroys the integrity of the cell membrane and precipitates the cytoplasm, causing cell death.

Other nondrug delivery devices that have been used as adjuncts to periodontal therapy are lasers and photodynamic light therapy. The word *laser* is an acronym for "light amplification by stimulated emission of radiation"; lasers are categorized according to the medium used to provide atoms to the emitting system. Although existing research has shown that lasers at specific wavelengths can kill bacteria, the conclusions of current systematic reviews and consensus reports have stated that there is insufficient evidence to support the clinical application of CO_2, Nd:YAG, Nd:YAP, or other diode lasers to treat periodontal disease. This is because the available clinical studies that used these laser applications as adjuncts to mechanical debridement did not demonstrate significant added clinical value [6,7]. The use of these devices is not discussed in this chapter.

C. The successful treatment of periodontal disease depends on the control and management of multiple variables as previously discussed. However, the appropriate diagnosis constitutes the primary step in selecting the treatment modality that is most appropriate for each case. The current reference to help the clinician formulate the proper diagnosis is based on the 1999 International Workshop for a Classification of Periodontal Diseases and Conditions [8]. However, it is well recognized among the scientific and clinical community that the deeper the periodontal probing or pocket, the greater the concentration of bacterial burden and the less effective the SRP. Mechanical debridement or scaling of subgingival pockets with probing >3 mm is the most commonly used anti-infective therapy in the treatment of periodontal diseases [9,10]. Cobb [10] calculated the mean probing depth reduction and gain of clinical attachment that can be achieved with subgingival SRP, and concluded that probing depth reduction usually was greater at sites with larger initial probing depths. However, with an initial pocket depth ≥5 mm, clinicians have been shown to inadequately debride roots 65% of the time [9].

Most studies have concluded that the optimum time of administration of the local agent is immediately after SRP. Because there might be an optimum access for close instrumentation determined by the probing depth, these agents should be used for sites with probing depth >3 mm and with at least a moderate form of periodontitis and should be used as adjuncts to SRP because the use of a local drug delivery system alone without the mechanical debridement is not sufficient to provide an optimum outcome.

D. An extensive amount of data has been generated in the last decade justifying the use of local delivery adjunctive chemotherapeutics for the treatment of periodontitis. A prototype fiber-like device to deliver drugs to the periodontal pocket was first introduced by Goodson and coworkers in 1983 [11]. Systematic reviews report on the efficacy of most available agents. In a review by Hanes and Purvis [3] that comprised a meta-analysis of 19 prospective studies that included SRP and local sustained-release agents compared with SRP alone, a significant adjunctive probing depth reduction or attachment level gain was observed for minocycline, chlorhexidine chip, doxycycline gel, and tetracycline fibers when compared with SRP alone.

However, findings from the meta-analysis indicate that the average amount of pocket depth (PD) reduction achieved by the addition of sustained-release antimicrobials to SRP is quite small, although highly statistically significant. With this amount of additional PD reduction, it is necessary to consider clinically if is worth the extra time and expense required to insert the antimicrobial system. Although irrigants or rinses are not discussed in this case, this systematic review found no evidence for adjunctive effect on reduction of probing depth and bleeding on probing of therapist-delivered chlorhexidine irrigation during SRP compared with SRP alone [3]. A separate review performed by Bonito et al. [12] found that among the locally administered adjunctive antimicrobials, the most positive results occurred for tetracycline, minocycline, metronidazole, and chlorhexidine. Adjunctive local therapy generally reduced PD levels. Differences between treatment and SRP-only groups in the baseline to follow-up period typically favored treatment groups but usually only modestly (e.g. from about 0.1 mm to nearly 0.5 mm) even when the differences were statistically significant. These authors evaluated a total of 50 published studies that were appropriate for analysis from 599 algorithm-identified articles [12].

It should be noted that these systematic reviews produce an average that is a summary statistic that combines negative, neutral, and positive effects into one number; this average could potentially mask individually significant results that may be clinically important to the patient [3].

E. The primary goal is to remove soft and hardened microbial deposits from the pathologically exposed root surfaces. The immediate effect of SRP is an enormous disruption of the subgingival biofilm, and curettes and ultrasonics can remove up to 90% of the subgingival plaque [13]. Thus SRP is strongly recommended prior to the time of insertion of any of the local agents to obtain the maximum benefit.

The following techniques correspond to the ones suggested by the manufacturers based on the clinical research presented and approved for the specific use by the Food and Drug Administration.

Actisite

Each Actisite fiber is 23 cm (9 inches) long and individually packaged. Remove the fiber from package and insert it into the periodontal pocket until the pocket is filled. An instrument such as a cord packer should be used to condense the fiber into the pocket. The length of fiber used will vary with pocket depth and contour. The fiber should be placed to closely approximate the pocket anatomy and should be in contact with the base of the pocket. An appropriate cyanoacrylate adhesive should be used to help secure the fiber in the pocket.

When placed within a periodontal pocket, Actisite fibers provide continuous release of tetracycline for 10 days. At the end of 10 days of treatment, all fibers must be removed. Fibers lost before seven days should be replaced. Fibers should not be used in an acutely abscessed periodontal pocket (Figure 2.2.9).

Atridox

Atridox® is removed from the refrigerator 15 minutes before use. Assemble "syringe A" that contains liquid polymer (red stripe) with "syringe B" that contains doxycycline hyclate powder. Mix

the contents of both syringes, pushing the contents back and forth about 100 times, about 1.5 minutes. The final contents must be in syringe A (indicated by red stripe) when finished. Attach a blunt cannula and bend it to resemble a periodontal probe. Insert the cannula tip into the periodontal pocket near the base. Express product into pocket until gel reaches the top of the gingival margin. Slowly withdraw the cannula coronally as the pocket begins to fill. Consider using a moistened dental hand instrument to hold product in place and to pack it lightly.

Considerations: Atridox is most retentive in posterior interproximal sites, deeper sites, and furcations. It is least retentive in shallow pockets and single-rooted teeth, in which case you should overflow Atridox, pack it into the embrasure, and cover with periodontal dressing. For least retentive sites, overflow Atridox and pack it into the embrasure and cover with periodontal dressing. It is not necessary to remove Atridox from the pocket because it will absorb completely (Figure 2.2.10).

Arestin

Arestin is packaged in a specially designed unit-dose cartridge that is inserted into a cartridge handle for product administration. Each cartridge contains enough for one periodontal pocket. It does not require preparation before administration because it is already premixed and premeasured, and does not require refrigeration.

Insert the cartridge into the handle while exerting slight pressure and twist it until you feel and hear the cartridge "lock" into place. If you need to reach difficult-to-access areas, gently bend the tip, leaving the blue cap on. Bending the tip after removal of the blue cap may cause the integral plunger to rupture the cartridge wall. Place the cartridge tip into the periodontal pocket, parallel to the long axis of the tooth. Be sure not to force the tip into the base of the pocket. Gently

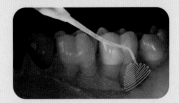

Figure 2.2.9   Placement of Actisite.

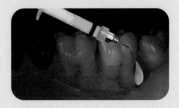

Figure 2.2.10   Placement of Atridox.

press the thumb ring to express the Arestin powder while withdrawing the cartridge tip away from the base of the pocket. If you feel any resistance during delivery, withdraw the device further. Once delivery is complete, retract the thumb ring and remove the cartridge with your free hand. Discard the cartridge appropriately and sterilize the handle before reuse. Arestin does not need to be removed because it is completely bioresorbable (Figure 2.2.11).

Elyzol

Elyzol comes packed in a carton containing a single-use applicator and a blunt needle. The applicator is preloaded with a cartridge containing the gel. Remove the protective cover at the base of the needle. Attach the needle to the applicator. Remove the upper protective cover from the needle and bend to the preferred angle.

Slowly pump up the pressure in the applicator by depressing the blue lever until flowing gel is visible at the tip of the needle. Release the lever and carefully move the needle down to the bottom of the pocket. Now press the lever down to its lowest position and keep it depressed until gel is visible at the gingival margin. Release the lever and repeat this procedure for all teeth to be treated.

When application is completed, dispose of the needle and the applicator including any remaining gel. Repeat the treatment with Elyzol 25% Dental Gel one week later (Figure 2.2.12).

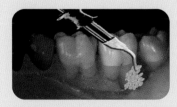

Figure 2.2.11   Placement of Arestin.

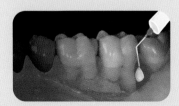

Figure 2.2.12   Placement of Elyzol.

F. The following patient recommendations correspond to the ones suggested by the product manufacturers.

Actisite

The most frequently reported adverse reactions in the pivotal clinical trials were discomfort on fiber placement (10%) and local erythema following removal. When Actisite fiber is in place, patients should avoid actions that may dislodge the fiber.

Instruct them not to chew hard, crusty, or sticky foods; not to brush or floss near any treated areas (continue to clean other teeth); not to engage in any other hygienic practices that could potentially dislodge the fibers; and not to probe at the treated area with tongue or fingers. Patients should notify the dentist promptly if the fiber is dislodged or falls out before the scheduled recall visit, or if pain or swelling or other problems occur.

Atridox

The most common side effects may include headache; common cold; gum discomfort, pain, or soreness. Instruct the patient to contact a dental professional about any unusual discomfort. Patients should not brush or floss the treated area for seven days. Dentists may prescribe or recommend an oral rinse to use during the seven days following Atridox application, which is the length time that patients cannot brush or floss.

Patients should not be alarmed if small amounts of Atridox are dislodged as it is harmless if swallowed.

As the gums heal and swelling begins to subside they may recede a bit, and the patient may notice some "white material" at the gum line; this is the Atridox and most of it will dissolve and be absorbed within 28 days.

After seven days, patients should brush and floss as recommended by the dental professional.

Arestin

The most frequent dental treatment-emergent adverse experience is inflammation of the gums.

After treatment, the patient should avoid touching areas of the gums that the dental professional has treated. Arestin does not require bandages and will not leak or fall out. The patient should also wait 12 hours after treatment before brushing their teeth in the affected area, and should avoid eating hard, crunchy, or sticky foods for one week.

The patient should also postpone the use of dental floss, dental tape, toothpicks, or any other devices that clean between the teeth and the affected area for at least 10 days.

Some mild to moderate sensitivity is expected during the first week after SRP and administration of Arestin.

Patients should notify their dental professional promptly if pain, swelling, or other problems occur.

Elyzol

The most frequent side effects are local and occur directly in connection with the application, such as bitter taste and temporary local tenderness. Headache has been reported.

The patient may eat and drink normally. Normal dental hygiene can be observed, but dental floss, interdental brushes, and toothpicks should not be used on the day following the application.

G. The most recognized clinical parameters for measuring the success of a periodontal treatment reported in the literature are periodontal probing depth, CAL, and bleeding on probing. In a systematic review of the literature, Hanes and Purvis [3] concluded that SRP and sustained-release agents compared with SRP alone indicated significant adjunctive PD reduction or CAL gain for all the antibiotics discussed in this chapter. However,

improvement could vary from patient to patient and from site to site in the same mouth. Thus it is strongly recommended that a full periodontal evaluation is performed between one and three months after treatment. Most studies in the literature agree that if the periodontal probing is 5 mm or more, further periodontal therapy might be needed.

Success in the treatment of periodontal disease is relative because although a periodontal site could have been reduced below the 5-mm threshold, close monitoring through a full periodontal evaluation every three months is strongly recommended.

H. Rescue therapy refers to an intervention treatment that is usually performed after optimal periodontal therapy has been carried out on a specific patient with poor short- or long-term success or recurrence. In a long-term follow-up study conducted by Haffajee et al. [14], it was found that the combination of local and systemic antibiotic therapy in conjunction with SRP in "refractory" periodontitis patients produced statistically significant reductions of already low levels of highly pathogenic microbial species as well as improvements in probing depth reductions and CAL gain. Thus it is suggested that clinicians consider a combination therapy approach for the treatment of recurrent lesions >5 mm that include local and systemic antibiotics among other treatments.

All the recommendations made in this chapter should be considered cautiously and with the understanding that results will vary from patient to patient and from site to site.

Case 3

Systemic Antibiotics

CASE STORY

A 42-year-old Hispanic white male presented with a chief complaint of pain and bleeding associated with his gums. At the time of his first examination he had not received any periodontal treatment and reported having his lower first molars extracted over five years before. The patient claimed that the reason the teeth were extracted was due to "pain," but he could not describe whether the cause for the pain was due to caries, periodontal problems, endodontic infections or any other reason.

LEARNING GOALS AND OBJECTIVES

- To be able to list the theoretical advantages for the use of systemic antibiotics in the treatment of periodontal infections
- To be able to identify periodontal cases that could benefit from the adjunctive use of systemic antibiotics
- To be able to list the antibiotics most commonly used in the treatment of periodontal diseases, the criteria used in their selection, and which ones are currently the drugs of choice for these infections
- To know what clinical benefits can be anticipated with the adjunctive use of systemic antibiotics in comparison to mechanical therapy
- To understand the main risks associated with the use of systemic antibiotics
- To know at which stage of the periodontal treatment antibiotics should be prescribed

Medical History

The patient reported a history of high blood pressure, which he managed with diet and exercise; otherwise his medical history was unremarkable. At the time of his first appointment he was not taking any medication besides an occasional aspirin for headaches.

Review of Systems

- Vital signs
  - Blood pressure: 140/80 mmHg
  - Pulse rate: 75 beats/minute (regular)

Social History

The patient was married with two children. He drank alcohol socially, had never smoked, and had not used recreational drugs. His father was diabetic and his mother died of breast cancer 10 years ago. His attitude was very positive and he considered his treatment a priority.

Extraoral Examination

His extraoral examination was unremarkable: skin, head, neck, temporomandibular joint, and muscles were all within normal limits.

Intraoral Examination

The oral cancer screening was negative. There was no dental caries present at the time of examination. The gingival examination revealed generalized severe erythema, with rolled margins and swollen papillae with an edematous consistency and absent stippling (Figure 2.3.1). Spontaneous bleeding and exudation upon pressure was present in a few teeth. There was an adequate amount of attached tissue around most teeth. Gingival recession was present at several sites (see periodontal chart in Figure 2.3.2 for details).

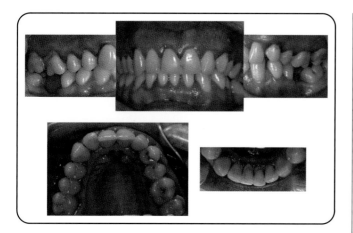

Figure 2.3.1 Clinical presentation of the case at initial visit. Source: courtesy of Dr. Eduardo Sampaio and Dr. Marcelo Faveri.

Supragingival and subgingival calculus could be detected on several teeth, particularly on the buccal surface of upper molars and lingual surfaces of lower incisors. Teeth #11, #19 and #30 were missing. Due to the absence of the lower first molars, teeth #3 and #14 had supererupted and the lower second molars had tipped mesially. The absence of #11 resulted in the mesialization of the upper left posterior teeth. There was generalized plaque accumulation. A few amalgam restorations of adequate quality were present in the posterior teeth. Saliva was of normal flow and consistency.

The periodontal chart presented in Figure 2.3.2 includes the following periodontal parameters:

(i) probing pocket depth (PD) in millimeters (mm); (ii) measurement from the cementoenamel junction (CEJ) to the gingival margin (GM) in mm (gingival recession was recorded as a negative value); (iii) clinical attachment level (CAL), which was calculated by subtracting the CEJ–GM distance from the PD; and (iv) presence (1) or absence (0) of bleeding on probing (BOP). Each clinical parameter was measured at six sites per tooth excluding third molars. Probing values were colored in blue, green or red to highlight shallow (<4 mm), intermediate (4–6 mm), and deep (>6 mm) pockets, respectively. BOP was detected in 81% of sites and the mean values for PD and CAL were 4.4 mm and 4.3 mm, respectively.

Occlusion

There were no signs of trauma from occlusion, no interferences, and no significant mobility. Despite the migration of certain teeth due to the absence of teeth #11, #19 and #30, there were no major occlusal discrepancies. The patient denied any sign or symptoms associated with his temporomandibular joint like crepitus, clicking or pain.

Radiographic Examination

A full-mouth set of radiographs (Figure 2.3.3) was obtained. There was generalized moderate to severe horizontal bone loss. There were images compatible with subgingival calculus on several teeth. Several amalgam restorations were noted on teeth #1, #2,

Visit: Initial Exam

Surface	Buccal																																										
Tooth	2			3			4			5			6			7			8			9			10			11			12			13			14			15		
PD	3	4	5	5	4	6	5	3	5	4	6	5	6	3	6	7	2	6	6	3	6	4	2	7	7	2	7	-	-	-	8	4	8	7	3	6	6	3	5	6	3	6
CEJ-GM	0	-2	-1	-1	-2	1	1	-1	1	1	-1	1	1	0	1	1	0	1	1	0	1	1	0	1	1	0	1	-	-	-	1	-1	1	1	0	0	0	-1	-1	0	-1	0
CAL	3	6	6	6	6	5	4	4	4	3	7	4	5	3	5	6	2	5	5	3	5	3	2	6	6	2	6	-	-	-	7	5	7	6	3	6	6	4	6	6	4	6
BOP	1	1	1	1	1	1	1	1	0	0	1	1	1	1	1	1	1	1	1	1	1	1	1	1	1	1	1	-	-	-	1	1	1	1	1	0	1	1	0	1	1	1
Surface	Palatal																																										
Tooth	2			3			4			5			6			7			8			9			10			11			12			13			14			15		
PD	8	3	6	6	3	5	5	3	6	5	2	7	6	3	7	6	4	5	5	3	5	4	4	5	5	5	7	-	-	-	7	3	7	7	3	5	6	3	6	6	3	6
CEJ-GM	0	1	1	1	-1	1	1	1	1	1	0	1	1	0	1	1	1	1	1	1	1	1	1	1	1	1	1	-	-	-	1	1	1	1	1	1	1	1	1	1	1	0
CAL	8	2	5	5	4	4	4	2	5	4	2	6	5	3	6	5	3	4	4	2	4	3	3	4	4	4	6	-	-	-	6	2	6	6	2	4	5	2	5	5	2	6
BOP	1	1	1	1	1	1	1	1	1	1	1	1	1	1	1	1	1	1	1	1	1	1	1	1	1	1	1	-	-	-	1	1	1	1	1	1	1	0	1	1	0	1
Surface	Buccal																																										
Tooth	31			30			29			28			27			26			25			24			23			22			21			20			19			18		
PD	5	3	4	-	-	-	3	2	3	3	2	4	4	3	5	5	3	5	5	2	4	2	2	6	6	2	5	6	2	6	4	3	3	3	3	3	-	-	-	8	2	3
CEJ-GM	0	0	0	-	-	-	0	0	0	0	0	1	1	0	1	1	0	0	0	-1	0	0	0	0	0	0	0	0	0	0	0	0	0	0	0	-1	-	-	-	0	0	0
CAL	5	3	4	-	-	-	3	2	3	3	2	3	3	3	4	4	3	5	5	3	4	4	2	6	6	2	5	6	2	6	4	3	3	3	3	4	-	-	-	8	2	3
BOP	1	1	1	-	-	-	0	0	0	0	0	1	1	1	1	1	1	1	1	1	0	1	1	0	1	1	0	1	1	0	1	0	0	0	0	0	-	-	-	1	0	0
Surface	Lingual																																										
Tooth	31			30			29			28			27			26			25			24			23			22			21			20			19			18		
PD	6	4	4	-	-	-	3	3	4	4	3	4	3	2	4	3	3	3	3	3	5	5	3	5	5	2	3	3	3	6	4	4	5	3	3	3	-	-	-	10	3	4
CEJ-GM	1	0	0	-	-	-	0	0	0	0	0	0	0	0	0	0	0	-1	-1	-1	-2	-2	-2	-2	-2	-2	-2	-2	0	1	1	0	0	0	0	-1	-	-	-	0	0	0
CAL	5	4	4	-	-	-	3	3	4	4	3	4	3	2	4	3	3	3	4	4	7	7	5	7	7	4	5	5	3	5	3	4	5	3	3	4	-	-	-	10	3	4
BOP	1	1	1	-	-	-	1	0	1	1	0	1	0	0	1	1	1	1	1	1	1	1	1	1	1	1	1	1	1	1	1	1	1	1	1	1	-	-	-	1	0	1

Figure 2.3.2 Periodontal chart, initial visit.

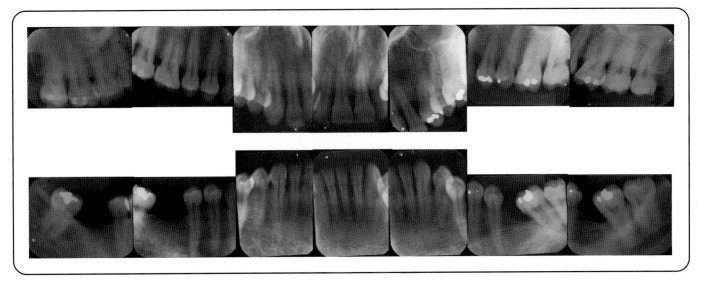

Figure 2.3.3 Full-mouth periapical radiographs of the case at initial visit. Source: courtesy of Dr. Eduardo Sampaio and Dr. Marcelo Faveri.

#12, #13, #14, #18, #21, and #31. There were images compatible with composite restorations on teeth #7, #8, and #9.

Diagnosis

According to the classification established by the 2017 World Workshop on the Classification of Periodontal and Peri Implant Diseases and Conditions [1], the case is of periodontitis stage III, generalized, grade C.

Treatment Plan

The treatment plan for this case consisted primarily of four to six sessions of scaling and root planing (SRP) accompanied by oral hygiene instructions with the concomitant use of adjunctive systemic antibiotics: amoxicillin (AMX) 500 mg three times a day (t.i.d.) plus metronidazole (MTZ) 250 mg t.i.d. for seven days. The antibiotic combination was prescribed immediately after the completion of the SRP sessions. A reassessment of the case was planned for three months after the completion of this initial active phase, when the need for additional therapy would be decided.

Treatment

After the patient's initial exam, radiographs and charting (Figures 2.3.1–2.3.3), a comprehensive treatment plan was presented and agreed upon. The first session involved full-mouth gross scaling and oral hygiene instructions on the proper toothbrushing technique and use of dental floss. Due to the presence of large amounts of subgingival calculus, the patient required six sessions of subgingival SRP under local anesthesia (one sextant of the mouth was instrumented per session). During this active phase of anti-infective therapy, previously instrumented sextants were constantly reexamined for the detection of residual supragingival and subgingival calculus, and whenever detected, residual calculus was removed. Every SRP session was accompanied by reinforcement of the oral hygiene instructions. At the end of his last SRP session, AMX 500 mg t.i.d. plus MTZ 250 mg t.i.d. were prescribed for seven days. The patients reported completing the antibiotic regimen without any adverse event.

Three months after the last SRP session, the subject was reexamined (Figures 2.3.4 and 2.3.5), residual

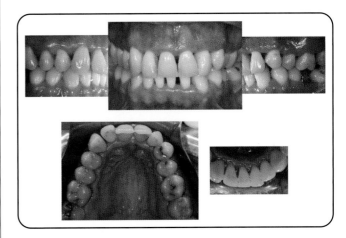

Figure 2.3.4 Clinical presentation of the case three months post therapy. Source: courtesy of Dr. Eduardo Sampaio and Dr. Marcelo Faveri.

Visit: 3 months post-therapy

Surface	Buccal													
Tooth	2	3	4	5	6	7	8	9	10	11	12	13	14	15
PD	3 3 4	4 2 3	3 2 3	2 3 2	3 2 3	3 3 3	3 3 3	3 3 3	3 2 3	- - -	3 2 3	3 2 3	3 3 3	3 3 4
CEJ-GM	0 -2 -1	-1 -2 0	0 -1 0	-1 -1 -1	0 0 -2	-1 -1 -2	-2 -1 0	-1 0 -2	-3 0 -2	- - -	0 -2 -1	0 0 0	0 -1 -2	-1 -1 0
CAL	3 5 5	5 4 3	3 3 3	3 4 3	3 2 5	4 4 5	5 4 3	4 3 5	6 2 5	- - -	3 4 4	3 2 3	3 4 5	4 4 4
BOP	1 0 0	0 0 0	0 0 0	0 0 0	0 0 0	0 0 0	0 0 0	0 0 0	0 0 0	- - -	0 0 0	0 0 0	0 0 0	0 0 0

Surface	Palatal													
Tooth	2	3	4	5	6	7	8	9	10	11	12	13	14	15
PD	4 3 4	3 3 3	3 3 3	3 2 2	3 2 3	3 2 3	3 3 4	3 3 3	3 3 3	- - -	4 3 3	4 3 3	4 3 3	4 3 4
CEJ-GM	0 0 0	0 -1 0	0 0 0	0 0 -1	-1 0 -2	-3 -1 -3	-1 0 0	0 0 -2	-3 0 -2	- - -	0 0 0	0 0 0	0 -1 -1	0 0 0
CAL	4 3 4	3 4 3	3 3 3	3 2 3	4 2 5	6 3 6	4 3 4	3 3 5	6 3 5	- - -	4 3 3	4 3 3	4 3 4	5 3 4
BOP	1 0 0	1 0 0	0 0 1	0 0 0	0 0 0	0 0 0	0 0 1	1 0 0	0 0 0	- - -	0 0 0	0 0 0	1 0 0	1 0 0

Surface	Buccal													
Tooth	31	30	29	28	27	26	25	24	23	22	21	20	19	18
PD	4 3 3	- - -	3 2 2	3 2 3	3 2 3	3 2 3	2 2 2	2 2 3	3 3 3	3 2 3	2 2 3	2 2 2	- - -	5 3 3
CEJ-GM	1 0 0	- - -	-1 0 0	0 0 0	0 0 0	0 -1 -2	-1 -1 -1	0 -2 -2	-1 -1 -2	0 0 0	-1 0 0	0 0 -1	- - -	-2 0 0
CAL	3 3 3	- - -	4 2 2	3 2 3	3 2 3	3 2 4	4 3 3	3 2 5	5 4 4	5 2 3	2 3 3	2 2 3	- - -	7 3 3
BOP	0 0 0	- - -	0 0 0	0 0 0	0 0 0	0 0 0	0 0 0	0 0 0	0 0 0	0 0 0	0 0 0	0 0 0	- - -	0 0 0

Surface	Lingual													
Tooth	31	30	29	28	27	26	25	24	23	22	21	20	19	18
PD	4 3 3	- - -	3 2 3	3 2 3	3 2 3	2 1 2	2 2 3	3 2 3	2 2 3	3 2 3	3 3 3	3 3 2	- - -	5 3 4
CEJ-GM	0 0 0	- - -	0 -1 0	0 0 0	0 0 0	-1 -1 -1	-1 -2 -2	-2 -2 -2	-2 -2 -1	-1 -1 0	0 0 -1	-1 -1 0	- - -	1 0 0
CAL	4 3 3	- - -	3 3 3	3 2 3	3 2 3	2 2 3	3 3 5	5 4 5	4 4 5	5 3 4	3 3 3	3 4 3	- - -	4 3 4
BOP	0 0 1	- - -	0 0 1	1 0 0	0 0 0	0 0 0	0 0 0	0 0 0	0 0 0	0 0 0	0 0 0	0 0 0	- - -	1 0 1

Figure 2.3.5 Periodontal chart, three months after therapy.

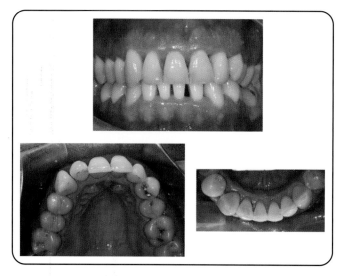

Figure 2.3.6 Clinical presentation of the case one year post therapy. Source: courtesy of Dr. Eduardo Sampaio and Dr. Marcelo Faveri.

pockets ≥4 mm received additional SRP, a full-mouth plaque removal was performed on the remaining dentition, and oral hygiene instructions reinforced. Mean PD and CAL were reduced from 4.4 to 2.8 mm and from 4.3 to 3.5 mm, respectively; there was also a reduction in percentage BOP from 81% to 9%. At this time no additional periodontal therapy was deemed necessary. The patient was placed in a recall system for supportive periodontal therapy every three months. Figures 2.3.6 and 2.3.7 illustrate the clinical presentation and the periodontal parameters one year after completion of periodontal therapy. The case remained stable with a mean PD of 2.9 mm, mean CAL of 3.5 mm and only 5% of sites with BOP.

Discussion

Since periodontal diseases are mixed infections, they should benefit from the use of systemic antibiotics. In fact, adjunct systemic antibiotic therapy offers several theoretical advantages over SRP alone.

1. Antibiotics achieve local levels that are distributed throughout the oral cavity, reaching all potential reservoirs for periodontal pathogens, including periodontal pockets of all depths and other intraoral surfaces.
2. Systemic antibiotics can achieve local concentrations at difficult-to-reach areas such as in the depth of infrabony defects and furcations.
3. Antibiotics enter the periodontal pocket through its epithelial lining, where bacteria actively involved in tissue destruction are more likely to be located.
4. Antibiotics may reach microorganisms inside the connective tissues and epithelial cells.

However, despite their potential benefits, the use of systemic antibiotics can be hazardous and common risks associated with their use include (i) toxicity; (ii) superinfection; (iii) allergic reactions; (iv) drug interactions; (v) disruption of gastrointestinal microflora; and (vi) bacterial resistance. In addition, their efficacy is dependent on the compliance of the patient with the prescribed regimen [2]. Therefore, when considering the

Visit: 1 year post-therapy

Surface	Buccal													
Tooth	2	3	4	5	6	7	8	9	10	11	12	13	14	15
PD	3 3 4	4 3 3	3 2 3	2 3 3	3 2 3	3 2 4	3 3 3	3 3 3	3 3 4	- - -	4 2 3	4 2 3	3 3 3	3 3 4
CEJ-GM	-1 -1 -1	-1 -1 -1	0 -1 0	-1 -1 -1	0 0 -1	-1 0 -1	-1 0 0	0 0 -1	-2 -1 0	- - -	-1 -2 0	0 0 0	0 -1 -2	-1 -1 0
CAL	4 4 5	5 4 4	3 3 3	3 4 4	3 2 4	4 2 5	4 3 3	3 3 4	5 4 4	- - -	5 4 3	4 2 3	3 4 5	4 4 4
BOP	0 0 1	0 0 1	0 0 0	0 0 0	0 0 0	0 0 0	0 0 0	0 0 0	0 0 0	- - -	0 0 0	0 0 0	0 0 0	0 0 0

Surface	Palatal													
Tooth	2	3	4	5	6	7	8	9	10	11	12	13	14	15
PD	3 3 4	3 3 3	3 3 3	3 2 3	3 2 3	3 2 3	3 3 3	3 3 3	3 3 3	- - -	3 3 3	3 3 3	3 3 3	4 3 4
CEJ-GM	0 0 0	0 -1 0	0 0 0	0 0 -1	-1 0 -1	-3 -1 -2	-1 0 0	0 0 -2	-3 0 -2	- - -	0 0 0	0 0 0	0 0 -1	-1 0 0
CAL	3 3 4	3 4 3	3 3 3	3 2 4	4 2 4	6 3 5	4 3 3	3 3 5	6 3 5	- - -	3 3 3	3 3 3	3 3 4	5 3 4
BOP	0 0 1	0 0 0	0 0 0	0 0 1	0 0 0	0 0 0	0 0 0	0 0 0	0 0 0	- - -	0 0 0	0 0 0	0 0 1	0 0 0

Surface	Buccal													
Tooth	31	30	29	28	27	26	25	24	23	22	21	20	19	18
PD	3 3 3	- - -	3 2 3	3 2 3	3 2 3	3 2 3	3 2 3	3 3 3	3 3 3	3 2 3	2 2 2	2 2 2	- - -	5 3 3
CEJ-GM	0 0 0	- - -	0 0 0	0 0 0	-1 0 0	0 -1 0	-1 0 -1	0 0 -1	-1 -1 0	0 0 0	-1 0 0	0 0 0	- - -	-2 0 0
CAL	3 3 3	- - -	3 2 3	3 2 3	3 3 3	3 2 4	4 2 4	3 3 4	4 4 3	3 2 3	2 3 2	2 2 2	- - -	7 3 3
BOP	0 0 0	- - -	0 0 0	1 0 0	0 0 0	0 0 0	0 0 0	0 0 0	0 0 0	0 0 0	0 0 0	0 0 0	- - -	0 0 0

Surface	Lingual													
Tooth	31	30	29	28	27	26	25	24	23	22	21	20	19	18
PD	3 3 3	- - -	3 2 3	3 2 3	3 3 3	3 2 3	3 2 3	3 2 3	3 2 3	3 3 4	3 3 3	4 3 2	- - -	5 2 4
CEJ-GM	0 0 0	- - -	0 -1 0	0 0 0	0 0 0	-1 -1 -1	-1 -1 -2	-2 -2 -2	-2 -2 -2	-2 -1 -1	-1 0 0	0 -1 -1	- - -	0 0 0
CAL	3 3 3	- - -	3 3 3	3 2 3	3 3 3	3 3 4	4 3 5	5 4 5	5 4 5	5 4 5	4 3 3	4 4 3	- - -	5 2 4
BOP	0 0 1	- - -	0 0 0	0 0 0	0 0 0	0 0 0	0 0 0	0 0 0	0 0 0	0 0 0	0 0 0	0 0 0	- - -	0 0 1

Figure 2.3.7 Periodontal chart, one year after periodontal therapy.

use of systemic antibiotics in periodontal therapy, the first question the clinician must ask is if they can offer any additional benefit to what can be obtained with traditional mechanical therapy. That implies that the decision for employing these agents has to be based on solid evidence from randomized clinical trials (RCTs) ideally double-blinded, placebo-controlled ones, that demonstrate a clinical outcome superior to the one obtained with SRP alone.

Evidence is accumulating that the use of systemic antibiotics as an adjunct to mechanical therapy can result in significant additional clinical benefits beyond what can be accomplished solely with SRP [3–5]. Particularly for severe cases, such as periodontitis stages III and IV generalized, and periodontitis with a molar/incisor pattern [5–8], the use of systemic antibiotics as an adjunct to mechanical therapy can result in statistically significant greater changes in periodontal clinical parameters compared to SRP only, for example greater mean PD reduction; increased gains in mean CAL; and higher reduction in the percentage of sites with BOP, of pocket closure and in frequency of pockets of ≥4 mm, ≥5 mm, ≥6 mm and ≥7 mm [5]. Although early reports suggested that the clinical benefits obtained with systemic antibiotics in cases previously classified as chronic periodontitis were somewhat inferior to the ones obtained in aggressive forms of the disease [3], a recent systematic review showed no indications that the benefits of systemic antimicrobials is different between aggressive and chronic periodontitis [5]. Several clinical trials have reported clinically

relevant improvements with the adjunctive use of antibiotics in severe forms of periodontitis in adults (especially for stages III and/or IV), particularly in generalized cases [9–17]. However, at times, the clinical relevance of these differences has been questioned due to their small magnitude. For instance, a meta-analysis using mean changes post treatment as primary outcomes indicated that adjunctive systemic antibiotics resulted in greater mean full-mouth attachment level (AL) gain of 0.3–0.4 mm or PD reduction of 0.5–0.6 mm from six months to one year after therapy [3]. These figures might seem clinically irrelevant. Nevertheless, if one considers data reported by Rosling et al. [18] describing a mean full-mouth attachment loss in subjects in supportive periodontal therapy of 0.042–0.067 mm, an AL gain of 0.3 mm would be equivalent to reversing four to seven years of disease progression. Even when the data from RCTs were analyzed taking into account information relevant to treatment planning decisions, such as the number of residual deep sites (i.e. PD ≥5 mm), the use of adjunctive systemic antibiotics still demonstrated clinical superiority to SRP alone. Feres et al. [19] have recently suggested that the presence of at most four sites with PD ≥5 mm is an effective clinical end point for periodontal treatment. RCTs reporting on this parameter [10,12,16,20–22] have shown that 53–72% of the patients taking adjunctive MTZ and AMX achieved this clinical outcome (four or less sites with PD ≥5 mm) at one or two years post therapy, as opposed to 6.6–36.5% of the patients receiving mechanical treatment only. The use of adjunctive systemic antibiotics has also been associated with a lower rate of disease progression [23,24]. For instance, in the Guerrero et al. study [24], disease progression occurred in 1.5% and 3.3% of the sites in the antibiotics and control groups, respectively. Further, there are data suggesting that the gains obtained with a single regimen of systemic antibiotics associated with mechanical therapy might last for up to one or two years even in the absence of subgingival SRP during maintenance [23,25].

It has been well recognized by clinicians and periodontal researchers that certain patients do not respond well to the traditional periodontal therapy and continue to show disease progression despite adequate treatment and proper plaque control [26]. These "refractory cases" form a heterogeneous population and the condition is rare, making the conduct of properly powered RCTs difficult. Regardless, reports of case series or small-scale clinical trials seem to indicate that these cases can also be controlled with the adjunctive use of systemic antibiotics [27–33]. However, since these subjects often have a history of several attempts to control their disease with systemic antibiotics, the choice of antibiotics to be used in these cases is complicated by the possibility of previous selection for resistant species. Therefore, it has been recommended that in refractory cases antimicrobial susceptibility testing be performed before the appropriate antibiotic is selected [34,35]. Systemic antibiotics have been recommended to treat necrotizing gingivitis [36,37] due to the presence of large numbers of bacteria, mainly strict anaerobes, within the tissues in such conditions [38]. However, systemic antibiotics for necrotizing gingivitis should be reserved for cases where there are signs of systemic dissemination of the infection [35,39]. When necrotizing gingivitis progresses to include attachment loss it is referred to as necrotizing periodontitis. Necrotizing periodontal diseases are commonly associated with HIV/AIDS and other pathologies where the immune system is compromised. In the presence of immunosuppression, systemic antibiotics should be used to control these infections, and a short course of three days of MTZ has been recommended [40]. Periodontal abscesses are treated primarily with local drainage and the use of systemic antibiotics is conditional on signs of systemic spreading of the infection [35,41].

In summary, data from RCTs support the use of systemic antibiotics in the treatment of severe periodontitis, independently of the phenotype previously categorized as "aggressive." According to the most recent literature, patients who benefit the most from

adjunctive systemic antibiotics are those with generalized stages III and IV periodontitis, and patients presenting periodontitis with a molar/incisor pattern. In addition, acute forms of periodontal diseases resulting in systemic symptoms such as fever and/or malaise or associated with immunosuppression might also require the use of systemic antibiotics. In addition, there is emerging literature suggesting that smokers and diabetic patients might also benefit from the use of these agents in the treatment of their periodontal condition [13,16,42].

Once the clinician has opted for the adjunctive use of systemic antibiotics to treat a case, he or she is still faced with several questions: (i) choice of antibiotic(s) to be used; (ii) dose and dosage of the antibiotic(s); and (iii) timing of drug administration in reference to mechanical therapy. When deciding which antibiotic(s) to select, the clinician is often advised to consider information regarding (i) in vitro activity against periodontopathogens, i.e. minimum inhibitory concentration (MIC); (ii) whether a concentration greater than the MIC is reached within the subgingival environment (i.e. gingival crevicular fluid levels); (iii) how long the dose should be maintained to affect the microbiota; and (iv) local and systemic adverse effects associated with the drug [43]. Parameters such as these have been used for the selection of agents in the treatment of periodontal infections. Although these considerations were essential in guiding the choice of antibiotics to be used in the treatment of periodontal infections, they were not particularly helpful in predicting the clinical outcome of their use. In fact, due to pharmacologic considerations [43] and the biofilm effect [44] it is almost impossible to predict based on in vitro data the clinical effects of systemic antibiotics. Therefore, clinicians should base their decision primarily on the results from RCTs.

The main antibiotics used so far in the treatment of periodontitis have been tetracycline, minocycline, doxycycline, clindamycin, clarithromycin, azithromycin, MTZ, AMX with clavulanic acid, and the combination of AMX and MTZ [5,45]. The reader should refer to the appropriate literature to become familiarized with the properties of these agents and the risks associated with their use, and the studies by Roberts [46] and Walker et al. [47] are suggested. Unfortunately, there are very few RCTs that have compared multiple antibiotics side by side and one cannot make definitive statements regarding the clinical superiority of an agent or combination of agents. However, there is some evidence indicating that the use of a combination of AMX and MTZ is superior to either antibiotic alone and to other antibiotics in the treatment of severe periodontitis in adults and young patients [10,12,13,15,16,22,24,48–54]. In fact, every published study comparing the adjunctive use of systemic AMX and MTZ with mechanical therapy alone has reported a significant clinical benefit associated with the use of this combination [9,11,13–15,17,23,24,54–64]. In addition, a recent systematic review showed that MTZ plus AMX adjunctive to SRP was the antibiotic protocol that presented the most consistent and relevant benefits for patients with periodontitis, independently of the chronic or aggressive diagnostic. This benefit was observed for PD, CAL, BOP, frequency of pocket closure, and of residual pockets [5]. Therefore, this combination of antibiotics should be the first protocol of choice in the treatment of periodontal infections. Clinicians should refrain from using last-generation antibiotics until clinical trials testing these drugs have demonstrated superiority not only to mechanical therapy alone, but also to drugs currently in use that have already demonstrated efficacy. This is important not only because the clinician needs evidence of the clinical effectiveness of the new drug but also due to the phenomenon of cross-resistance. If a microorganism develops resistance to a last-generation antibiotic, it might become resistant to the entire class of antibiotics that the new-generation drug belongs to [65].

The literature shows no consistency regarding the dose (the quantity of antibiotic to be administered at one time), dosage (the frequency and quantity of antibiotic administered to a patient), and duration of the course of antibiotics. The different regimens were somewhat arbitrarily defined and no scientific basis for their choice was presented in the reports, making a final decision on which one to choose difficult. In addition, most clinical trials did not report on the incidence of adverse events associated with the use of antibiotics, making it difficult to estimate if longer courses resulted in a higher incidence of adverse events. The only way of finding the best regimen for this combination of antibiotics would be through RCTs assessing not only the impact of different regimens on periodontal parameters but also on the incidence of adverse effects. Two studies have tested MTZ plus AMX for three or seven days [20,66]. Cosgarea et al. [20] showed similar benefits with both protocols, while Boia et al. [66] observed that seven days of antibiotic intake was more effective than three days in improving clinical and microbiological parameters. Evidence from another RCT reinforces the concept that this antibiotic regimen may exert greater benefit if given in long course (14 days) for patients with very severe disease [10]. These authors observed that approximately 60% of the patients achieved the clinical end point of "≤4 sites with PD ≥5 mm" [19] at one year post treatment, as opposed to approximately 30% in the group taking the antibiotics for seven days. However, it is important to note that in another study, Harks et al. [21] observed this same pattern of clinical response (i.e. approximately 60% of the patients achieving the clinical end point for treatment) using seven days intake of MTZ plus AMX, in a population with less severe disease.

In terms of dose, while there is good consensus that the ideal dose of AMX is 500 mg, there is some controversy regarding MTZ. The dose of MTZ was also tested by Borges et al. [10] and no critical differences were observed between 250 and 400 mg. These studies also did not detect important differences in terms of adverse events among all the protocols tested. Thus, there is some evidence suggesting that severity of disease should be considered while opting between 7 or 14 days of antibiotic intake. In addition, AMX should be prescribed at the dose of 500 mg and MTZ of 400 mg, or 250 mg when 400 mg is not available, three times daily. It should be noted that antibiotics used at low doses may contribute to the worldwide increase in microbial tolerance to these agents [67,68]. Furthermore, clinical trials that used lower dosages of MTZ (250 mg) and AMX (375 mg) t.i.d. for seven days did not observe important clinical and microbiological benefits over those achieved with mechanical treatment alone [14,69].

The timing of antibiotic administration is also an important consideration. Based on the biofilm effect of increased resistance to antimicrobials, clinicians have been instructed to initiate systemic antibiotic therapy concomitant or immediately once the mechanical therapy has been completed. The mechanical disruption of the biofilm would favor the antimicrobial effects of the antibiotics by decreasing the bacterial load and disrupting the glycocalyx, which increases antibiotic diffusion into the biofilm structure [44]. Although this recommendation makes biologic sense, data from studies using systemic antibiotics as a single therapy (i.e. without concomitant or prior mechanical treatment) have suggested that the subgingival biofilm can be significantly altered by systemic antibiotic administration even in the absence of mechanical therapy, resulting in beneficial clinical changes on the periodontium [60]. In fact, a few clinical trials demonstrating a superior clinical outcome with the adjunctive use of systemic AMX and MTZ have started the drug regimen concomitantly with the first SRP session, which included a full-mouth disruption of all subgingival biofilm followed by quadrant SRP sessions [10,12,13,22,42,52,70].

The American Academy of Periodontology (AAP) recommended in a position paper that systemic antibiotic therapy should be reserved for patients with unresolved and/or progressing sites after conventional mechanical periodontal treatment [35]. This implies that a reexamination of the outcome of mechanical therapy should be obtained prior to any decision on the use of systemic antibiotics. This would delay the use of antibiotics up to three months after initial therapy. A recent study has demonstrated that adjunctive systemic antibiotics result in improved clinical outcomes when administered immediately after mechanical therapy rather than three months post therapy [71]. Two cohorts of generalized "aggressive" periodontitis subjects (n = 17 for each group) were analyzed retrospectively; the group that received systemic AMX and MTZ immediately after SRP had greater improvements in mean PD and CAL compared to the late antibiotic therapy in deep sites (PD >6 mm). Similarly, Griffiths et al. [57] reported that when systemic AMX and MTZ were administered to a placebo group from a previous RCT six months after therapy, 67% of the pockets ≥5 mm converted to ≤4 mm, while in the original test group that received antibiotics at initial therapy, 83% of pockets showed this level of improvement. It is possible that delaying the beginning of antibiotic therapy might result in a return of the subgingival biofilm to its original complexity, diminishing the benefits offered by recent mechanical disruption of its structure. In addition, these three months of healing might decrease the amount of antibiotics being delivered to the site due to a decrease in gingival crevicular fluid flow and enhanced epithelial barrier. Therefore, systemic antibiotic therapy should start during the initial therapy either after the first session of SRP or immediately after completion of the final SRP and, ideally, not be delayed until after reexamination of the case as an alternative retreatment.

As discussed above, the use of systemic antibiotics is not without risks. Bacterial resistance is probably the single most important reason clinicians should refrain from the indiscriminate use of systemic antibiotics to treat periodontal infections [72]. However, concerns regarding antibiotic resistance should not preclude clinicians from using systemic antibiotics to treat periodontal diseases when indicated. Guidelines in the medical literature regarding the prudent use of antibiotics

in order to minimize the risk of antibiotic resistance include the following: (i) use antibiotics only when patient outcome can be improved; (ii) use narrow-spectrum antibiotics whenever possible; (iii) save last-generation antibiotics for serious life-threatening infections; and (iv) stop antibiotic therapy as soon as possible [65]. Clinicians can easily abide by these guidelines while still offering their patients the clinical benefits of the adjunctive use of systemic antibiotics.

Another important tenet of antibiotic use is that it should be used only to either treat an existing infection (therapeutic use) or to prevent the establishment of infection when a sterile body part is to be exposed to microorganisms (prophylactic use, e.g. surgical procedure) [65]. When used for prophylaxis a short course of antibiotics should be prescribed, typically only enough to last the duration of the surgical procedure, and administration should begin prior to surgery (two hours prior to the procedure), so that adequate systemic levels of the antibiotic (two to eight times above MIC) are present at the time of surgical incision [73]. The practice of prescribing antibiotics immediately after a surgical procedure should be avoided at all costs since it is neither therapeutic (there should be no infection at this time) nor prophylactic since the surgical wound is already closed. Most importantly this would bring no benefit to the patient, infringing on the guidelines regarding prudent use of antibiotics. The prophylactic use of antibiotics during periodontal surgeries is not recommended due to the extremely low incidence of postsurgical infections [74,75]. This is mainly a consequence of drainage at the gingival margin. In essence, during healing, the periodontal tissues can be considered an "open wound." The same degree of drainage and therefore protection against postsurgical infections is not present in closed procedures such as sinus-lifts or bone augmentations prior to implant placement. In these circumstances, prophylactic systemic antibiotics might be recommended. The insertion of endosseous dental implants also fits the recommendations for antibiotic prophylaxis in the medical literature [76] and there are a few studies suggesting that preoperative antibiotics might decrease the number of early implant failures [77]. However, an RCT conducted by Tan and co-workers [78] reported that systemic antibiotics, either prophylactic or after single implant placement, do not improve patient-reported outcomes or prevalence of postsurgical complications. Thus, there is no evidence in the literature to support the use of systemic antibiotics after single implant placement.

In summary, despite the lack of data on important issues regarding the use of systemic antibiotics as adjuncts in periodontal therapy, there is enough documentation of their additional clinical benefits, including oral health-related quality of life (OHRQoL) measures for patients with severe periodontitis [79], to warrant their use in clinical practice. The following general guidelines to the use of adjunctive systemic antibiotics to treat periodontal infections are recommended.

1. It should be restricted to generalized severe cases (stage III/IV) and periodontitis with a molar/incisor pattern, while mild to moderate (stage I/II) and localized forms of periodontitis are probably better addressed with local mechanical therapy.
2. AMX (500 mg t.i.d.) and MTZ (400 mg, or 250 mg when 400 mg is not available, t.i.d.) in combination is the protocol of choice unless the subject has a history of allergy or intolerance to either drug.
3. In the presence of refractory disease, an in vitro susceptibility test is recommended prior to deciding which antibiotic(s) to prescribe, particularly if the subject has a history of previous administrations of systemic antibiotics to treat the periodontal disease.
4. Smokers and diabetics might also benefit from the adjunctive use of systemic antibiotics.

Self-Study Questions

A. In which cases should the clinician consider the use of adjunctive systemic antibiotics?

B. What should be the antibiotic regimen of choice to treat periodontal infections and what are the alternatives in case of a history of allergy or intolerance to the antibiotic(s) of choice?

C. When during the periodontal treatment should you prescribe systemic antibiotics to obtain the greatest clinical benefit?

D. What are the general recommendations to be followed when using systemic antibiotics in order to minimize the risk of bacterial resistance?

E. What are the additional clinical benefits that one can expect from the adjunctive use of systemic antibiotics?

Answers located at the end of the chapter.

References

1. Papapanou PN, Sanz M, Buduneli N, et al. Periodontitis: Consensus report of workgroup 2 of the 2017 World Workshop on the Classification of Periodontal and Peri-Implant Diseases and Conditions. *J Periodontol* 2018;89(Suppl 1):S173–S182.
2. Guerrero A, Echeverria JJ, Tonetti MS. Incomplete adherence to an adjunctive systemic antibiotic regimen decreases clinical outcomes in generalized aggressive periodontitis patients: a pilot retrospective study. *J Clin Periodontol* 2007;34(10):897–902.
3. Haffajee AD, Socransky SS, Gunsolley JC. Systemic anti-infective periodontal therapy. A systematic review. *Ann Periodontol* 2003;8(1):115–181.
4. Herrera D, Sanz M, Jepsen S, et al. A systematic review on the effect of systemic antimicrobials as an adjunct to scaling and root planing in periodontitis patients. *J Clin Periodontol* 2002;29(Suppl 3):136–159.
5. Teughels W, Feres M, Oud V, et al. Adjunctive effect of systemic antimicrobials in periodontitis therapy: a systematic review and meta-analysis. *J Clin Periodontol* 2020;47(Suppl 22):257–281.
6. Allin N, Cruz-Almeida Y, Velsko I, et al. Inflammatory response influences treatment of localized aggressive periodontitis. *J Dent Res* 2016;95(6):635–641.
7. Beliveau D, Magnusson I, Bidwell JA, et al. Benefits of early systemic antibiotics in localized aggressive periodontitis: a retrospective study. *J Clin Periodontol* 2012;39(11):1075–1081.
8. Miller KA, Branco-de-Almeida LS, Wolf S, et al. Long-term clinical response to treatment and maintenance of localized aggressive periodontitis: a cohort study. *J Clin Periodontol* 2017;44(2):158–168.
9. Berglundh T, Krok L, Liljenberg B, et al. The use of metronidazole and amoxicillin in the treatment of advanced periodontal disease. A prospective, controlled clinical trial. *J Clin Periodontol* 1998;25(5):354–362.
10. Borges I, Faveri M, Figueiredo LC, et al. Different antibiotic protocols in the treatment of severe chronic periodontitis: a 1-year randomized trial. *J Clin Periodontol* 2017;44(8):822–832.
11. Cionca N, Giannopoulou C, Ugolotti G, Mombelli A. Amoxicillin and metronidazole as an adjunct to full-mouth scaling and root planing of chronic periodontitis. *J Periodontol* 2009;80(3):364–371.

12. Feres M, Soares GM, Mendes JA, et al. Metronidazole alone or with amoxicillin as adjuncts to non-surgical treatment of chronic periodontitis: a 1-year double-blinded, placebo-controlled, randomized clinical trial. *J Clin Periodontol* 2012;39(12):1149–1158.

13. Matarazzo F, Figueiredo LC, Cruz SE, et al. Clinical and microbiological benefits of systemic metronidazole and amoxicillin in the treatment of smokers with chronic periodontitis: a randomized placebo-controlled study. *J Clin Periodontol* 2008;35(10):885–896.

14. Ribeiro Edel P, Bittencourt S, Zanin IC, et al. Full-mouth ultrasonic debridement associated with amoxicillin and metronidazole in the treatment of severe chronic periodontitis. *J Periodontol* 2009;80(8):1254–1264.

15. Rooney J, Wade WG, Sprague SV, et al. Adjunctive effects to non-surgical periodontal therapy of systemic metronidazole and amoxycillin alone and combined. A placebo controlled study. *J Clin Periodontol* 2002;29(4):342–350.

16. Tamashiro NS, Duarte PM, Miranda TS, et al. Amoxicillin plus metronidazole therapy for patients with periodontitis and type 2 diabetes: a 2-year randomized controlled trial. *J Dent Res* 2016;95(7):829–836.

17. Winkel EG, Van Winkelhoff AJ, Timmerman MF, et al. Amoxicillin plus metronidazole in the treatment of adult periodontitis patients. A double-blind placebo-controlled study. *J Clin Periodontol* 2001;28(4):296–305.

18. Rosling B, Serino G, Hellstrom MK, et al. Longitudinal periodontal tissue alterations during supportive therapy. Findings from subjects with normal and high susceptibility to periodontal disease. *J Clin Periodontol* 2001;28(3):241–249.

19. Feres M, Retamal-Valdes B, Faveri M, et al. Proposal of a clinical endpoint for periodontal trials: the treat-to-target approach. *J Int Acad Periodontol* 2020;22(2):41–53.

20. Cosgarea R, Heumann C, Juncar R, et al. One year results of a randomized controlled clinical study evaluating the effects of non-surgical periodontal therapy of chronic periodontitis in conjunction with three or seven days systemic administration of amoxicillin/metronidazole. *PLoS One* 2017;12(6):e0179592.

21. Harks I, Koch R, Eickholz P, et al. Is progression of periodontitis relevantly influenced by systemic antibiotics? A clinical randomized trial. *J Clin Periodontol* 2015;42(9):832–842.

22. Mestnik MJ, Feres M, Figueiredo LC, et al. The effects of adjunctive metronidazole plus amoxicillin in the treatment of generalized aggressive periodontitis: a 1-year double-blinded, placebo-controlled, randomized clinical trial. *J Clin Periodontol* 2012;39(10):955–961.

23. Ehmke B, Moter A, Beikler T, et al. Adjunctive antimicrobial therapy of periodontitis: long-term effects on disease progression and oral colonization. *J Periodontol* 2005;76(5):749–759.

24. Guerrero A, Griffiths GS, Nibali L, et al. Adjunctive benefits of systemic amoxicillin and metronidazole in non-surgical treatment of generalized aggressive periodontitis: a randomized placebo-controlled clinical trial. *J Clin Periodontol* 2005;32(10):1096–1107.

25. Haffajee AD, Teles RP, Socransky SS. The effect of periodontal therapy on the composition of the subgingival microbiota. *Periodontol 2000* 2006;42:219–258.

26. Kornman KS. Refractory periodontitis: critical questions in clinical management. *J Clin Periodontol* 1996;23(3 Pt 2):293–298.

27. Collins JG, Offenbacher S, Arnold RR. Effects of a combination therapy to eliminate *Porphyromonas gingivalis* in refractory periodontitis. *J Periodontol* 1993;64(10):998–1007.

28. Gordon J, Walker C, Hovliaras C, Socransky S. Efficacy of clindamycin hydrochloride in refractory periodontitis: 24-month results. *J Periodontol* 1990;61(11):686–691.

29. Gordon J, Walker C, Lamster I, et al. Efficacy of clindamycin hydrochloride in refractory periodontitis. 12-month results. *J Periodontol* 1985;56(11 Suppl):75–80.

30. Haffajee AD, Uzel NG, Arguello EI, et al. Clinical and microbiological changes associated with the use of combined antimicrobial therapies to treat "refractory" periodontitis. *J Clin Periodontol* 2004;31(10):869–877.

31. Magnusson I, Clark WB, Low SB, et al. Effect of non-surgical periodontal therapy combined with adjunctive antibiotics in subjects with "refractory" periodontal disease. (I). Clinical results. *J Clin Periodontol* 1989;16(10):647–653.

32. Walker C, Gordon J. The effect of clindamycin on the microbiota associated with refractory periodontitis. *J Periodontol* 1990;61(11):692–698.

33. Winkel EG, Van Winkelhoff AJ, Timmerman MF, et al. Effects of metronidazole in patients with "refractory" periodontitis associated with *Bacteroides forsythus*. *J Clin Periodontol* 1997;24(8):573–579.

34. Shaddox LM, Walker C. Microbial testing in periodontics: value, limitations and future directions. *Periodontol 2000* 2009;50:25–38.

35. Slots J. Systemic antibiotics in periodontics. *J Periodontol* 2004;75(11):1553–1565.

36. Duckworth R, Waterhouse JP, Britton DE, et al. Acute ulcerative gingivitis. A double-blind controlled clinical trial of metronidazole. *Br Dent J* 1966;120(12):599–602.

37. Emslie RD. Treatment of acute ulcerative gingivitis. A clinical trial using chewing gums containing metronidazole or penicillin. *Br Dent J* 1967;122(7):307–308.

38. Loesche WJ, Syed SA, Laughon BE, Stoll J. The bacteriology of acute necrotizing ulcerative gingivitis. *J Periodontol* 1982;53(4):223–230.

39. Holroyd SV. Antibiotics in the practice of periodontics. *J Periodontol* 1971;42(9):584–589.

40. Ryder MI. An update on HIV and periodontal disease. *J Periodontol* 2002;73(9):1071–1078.

41. Dahlen G. Microbiology and treatment of dental abscesses and periodontal–endodontic lesions. *Periodontol 2000* 2002;28:206–239.

42. Miranda TS, Feres M, Perez-Chaparro PJ, et al. Metronidazole and amoxicillin as adjuncts to scaling and root planing for the treatment of type 2 diabetic subjects with periodontitis: 1-year outcomes of a randomized placebo-controlled clinical trial. *J Clin Periodontol* 2014;41(9):890–899.

43. van Winkelhoff AJ, Rams TE, Slots J. Systemic antibiotic therapy in periodontics. *Periodontol 2000* 1996;10:45–78.

44. Socransky SS, Haffajee AD. Dental biofilms: difficult therapeutic targets. *Periodontol 2000* 2002;28:12–55.

45. Slots J, Ting M. Systemic antibiotics in the treatment of periodontal disease. *Periodontol 2000* 2002;28:106–176.

46. Roberts MC. Antibiotic toxicity, interactions and resistance development. *Periodontol 2000* 2002;28:280–297.

47. Walker CB, Karpinia K, Baehni P. Chemotherapeutics: antibiotics and other antimicrobials. *Periodontol 2000* 2004; 36:146–165.

48. Araujo CF, Andere NMRB, Castro Dos Santos NC, et al. Two different antibiotic protocols as adjuncts to one-stage full-mouth ultrasonic debridement to treat generalized aggressive periodontitis: a pilot randomized controlled clinical trial. *J Periodontol* 2019;90(12):1431–1440.

49. Carvalho LH, D'Avila GB, Leão A, et al. Scaling and root planing, systemic metronidazole and professional plaque removal in the treatment of chronic periodontitis in a Brazilian population. I. Clinical results. *J Clin Periodontol* 2004;31(12):1070–1076.

50. Feres M, Haffajee AD, Allard K, et al. Change in subgingival microbial profiles in adult periodontitis subjects receiving either systemically-administered amoxicillin or metronidazole. *J Clin Periodontol* 2001;28(7):597–609.

51. Jentsch HF, Buchmann A, Friedrich A, Eick S. Nonsurgical therapy of chronic periodontitis with adjunctive systemic azithromycin or amoxicillin/metronidazole. *Clin Oral Investig* 2016;20(7):1765–1773.

52. Silva MP, Feres M, Sirotto TA, et al. Clinical and microbiological benefits of metronidazole alone or with amoxicillin as adjuncts in the treatment of chronic periodontitis: a randomized placebo-controlled clinical trial. *J Clin Periodontol* 2011;38(9):828–837.

53. Soares GM, Mendes JA, Silva MP, et al. Metronidazole alone or with amoxicillin as adjuncts to non-surgical treatment of chronic periodontitis: a secondary analysis of microbiological results from a randomized clinical trial. *J Clin Periodontol* 2014;41(4):366–376.

54. Xajigeorgiou C, Sakellari D, Slini T, et al. Clinical and microbiological effects of different antimicrobials on generalized aggressive periodontitis. *J Clin Periodontol* 2006;33(4): 254–264.

55. Flemmig TF, Milian E, Karch H, Klaiber B. Differential clinical treatment outcome after systemic metronidazole and amoxicillin in patients harboring *Actinobacillus actinomycetemcomitans* and/or *Porphyromonas gingivalis*. *J Clin Periodontol* 1998;25(5):380–387.

56. Flemmig TF, Milian E, Kopp C, et al. Differential effects of systemic metronidazole and amoxicillin on *Actinobacillus actinomycetemcomitans* and *Porphyromonas gingivalis* in intraoral habitats. *J Clin Periodontol* 1998;25(1):1–10.

57. Griffiths GS, Ayob R, Guerrero A, et al. Amoxicillin and metronidazole as an adjunctive treatment in generalized aggressive periodontitis at initial therapy or re-treatment: a randomized controlled clinical trial. *J Clin Periodontol* 2011;38(1):43–49.

58. Lopez NJ, Gamonal JA. Effects of metronidazole plus amoxicillin in progressive untreated adult periodontitis: results of a single 1-week course after 2 and 4 months. *J Periodontol* 1998;69(11):1291–1298.

59. Lopez NJ, Gamonal JA, Martinez B. Repeated metronidazole and amoxicillin treatment of periodontitis. A follow-up study. *J Periodontol* 2000;71(1):79–89.

60. Lopez NJ, Socransky SS, Da Silva I, et al. Effects of metronidazole plus amoxicillin as the only therapy on the microbiological and clinical parameters of untreated chronic periodontitis. *J Clin Periodontol* 2006;33(9):648–660.

61. Mestnik MJ, Feres M, Figueiredo LC, et al. Short-term benefits of the adjunctive use of metronidazole plus amoxicillin in the microbial profile and in the clinical parameters of subjects with generalized aggressive periodontitis. *J Clin Periodontol* 2010;37(4):353–365.

62. Moeintaghavi A, Talebi-ardakani MR, Haerian-ardakani A, et al. Adjunctive effects of systemic amoxicillin and metronidazole with scaling and root planing: a randomized, placebo controlled clinical trial. *J Contemp Dent Pract* 2007;8(5):51–59.

63. Winkel EG, van Winkelhoff AJ, van der Velden U. Additional clinical and microbiological effects of amoxicillin and metronidazole after initial periodontal therapy. *J Clin Periodontol* 1998;25(11 Pt 1):857–864.

64. Yek EC, Cintan S, Topcuoglu N, et al. Efficacy of amoxicillin and metronidazole combination for the management of generalized aggressive periodontitis. *J Periodontol* 2010;81(7):964–974.

65. Collignon PJ. 11: Antibiotic resistance. *Med J Aust* 2002;177(6):325–329.

66. Boia S, Boariu M, Baderca F, et al. Clinical, microbiological and oxidative stress evaluation of periodontitis patients treated with two regimens of systemic antibiotics, adjunctive to non-surgical therapy: a placebo-controlled randomized clinical trial. *Exp Ther Med* 2019;18(6):5001–5015.

67. Leekha S, Terrell CL, Edson RS. General principles of antimicrobial therapy. *Mayo Clin Proc* 2011;86(2):156–167.

68. Yap MNF. The double life of antibiotics. *Mo Med* 2013;110(4):320–324.

69. Casarin RC, Peloso Ribeiro ED, Sallum EA, et al. The combination of amoxicillin and metronidazole improves clinical and microbiologic results of one-stage, full-mouth, ultrasonic debridement in aggressive periodontitis treatment. *J Periodontol* 2012;83(8):988–998.

70. Goodson JM, Haffajee AD, Socransky SS, et al. Control of periodontal infections: a randomized controlled trial I. The primary outcome attachment gain and pocket depth reduction at treated sites. *J Clin Periodontol* 2012;39(6): 526–536.

71. Kaner D, Christan C, Dietrich T, et al. Timing affects the clinical outcome of adjunctive systemic antibiotic therapy for generalized aggressive periodontitis. *J Periodontol* 2007;78(7):1201–1208.

72. Pallasch TJ. Antibiotic resistance. *Dent Clin North Am* 2003;47(4):623–639.

73. Classen DC, Evans RS, Pestotnik SL, et al. The timing of prophylactic administration of antibiotics and the risk of surgical-wound infection. *N Engl J Med* 1992;326(5):281–286.

74. Callis S, Lemmer J, Touyz LZ. Antibiotic prophylaxis in periodontal surgery. A retrospective study. *J Dent Assoc S Afr* 1996;51(12):806–809.

75. Powell CA, Mealey BL, Deas DE, et al. Post-surgical infections: prevalence associated with various periodontal surgical procedures. *J Periodontol* 2005;76(3):329–333.

76. Paluzzi RG. Antimicrobial prophylaxis for surgery. *Med Clin North Am* 1993;77(2):427–441.

77. Esposito M, Grusovin MG, Coulthard P, et al. The efficacy of antibiotic prophylaxis at placement of dental implants: a

Cochrane systematic review of randomised clinical trials. *Eur J Oral Implantol* 2008;1(2):95–103.

78. Tan WC, Ong M, Han J, et al. Effect of systemic antibiotics on clinical and patient-reported outcomes of implant therapy: a multicenter randomized controlled clinical trial. *Clin Oral Implants Res* 2014;25(2):185–193.

79. Peikert SA, Spurzem W, Vach K, et al. Association of non-surgical periodontal therapy on patients' oral health-related quality of life: a multi-centre cohort study. *J Clin Periodontol* 2019;46(5):529–538.

80. Nibali L, Koidou VP, Hamborg T, Donos N. Empirical or microbiologically guided systemic antimicrobials as adjuncts to non-surgical periodontal therapy? A systematic review. *J Clin Periodontol* 2019;46(10):999–1012.

81. Fritoli A, Gonçalves C, Faveri M, et al. The effect of systemic antibiotics administered during the active phase of non-surgical periodontal therapy or after the healing phase: a systematic review. *J Appl Oral Sci* 2015;23(3):249–254.

TAKE-HOME POINTS

A. The use of systemic antibiotics is formally recommended by the AAP for "aggressive" periodontitis cases, refractory cases, and acute forms of periodontal diseases with systemic symptoms [35]. Several authors have discouraged the use of systemic antibiotics to treat chronic periodontitis on the grounds that this form of periodontal infection responds well to mechanical therapy. It has been suggested that systemic antibiotics should be reserved for cases of chronic periodontitis with a poor response to SRP as a retreatment option. However, papers reviewed in the discussion section have clearly demonstrated that severe cases of chronic periodontitis also benefit from the use of adjunctive antibiotics. In addition, a recent systematic review concluded that there are no indications that the effect of systemic antimicrobials is different between patients with aggressive and chronic periodontitis [5]. Finally, a few studies demonstrated that the clinical improvements were greater if the antibiotics were administered during the initial therapy rather than after reevaluation of the results obtained with the mechanical treatment.

B. Ideally, one would like to match the antibiotic therapy to clinical and microbiological characteristics of the patient that would indicate which subject would respond better to antibiotic, and to which one. Unfortunately, this is not the state of the art of systemic antibiotic use in periodontal therapy. The most reliable evidence available comes from randomized clinical trials. Based on some analysis, specific profiles of bacterial contamination associated with aggressive patterns could benefit the most

by antibiotics, but a systematic review on this subject failed to corroborate that finding [80]. And, based on the collective body of randomized clinical studies, a combination of AMX and MTZ is, hitherto, the first choice to treat periodontal infections. Several regimens have been employed in different studies, but while there may be only limited evidence of superiority of one over the other, the prudent use of these drugs would be to opt for the lowest doses and the shortest duration that have resulted in additional clinical benefits over SRP alone. Based on this criterion, the following regimen is suggested: AMX 500 mg t.i.d. and MTZ 400 mg t.i.d. for seven days, or for 14 days in very severe cases. MTZ 250 mg may also be used when 400 mg is not available. In case of a history of allergy to penicillins, the recommendation would be to use only MTZ, which has also demonstrated beneficial results in several clinical trials. In case of intolerance to MTZ and allergy to penicillin, an alternative would be the use of azithromycin, which also has shown positive results in a few clinical studies [5]. Patients should be told about the risk of allergies, and any other potential side effects (e.g. patients cannot drink any alcohol when taking MTZ).

C. Most available studies in the literature have used antibiotics during the active phase of periodontal treatment. There is some evidence [57,71,81] suggesting that we should not postpone this decision to the maintenance phase. Delaying the administration of antibiotics to a retreatment phase of the therapy might mitigate their clinical benefit. Therefore, they should be administered during the active phase of the mechanical therapy. To completely avoid interference by the biofilm structure, clinicians should start the antibiotic treatment immediately after the last SRP session or after an initial SRP session that includes an overall disruption of the full-mouth subgingival biofilm.

D. The prudent use of systemic antibiotics to minimize the risk of bacterial resistance should involve (i) using antibiotics only when patient outcome can be improved; (ii) using narrow-spectrum antibiotics whenever possible; (iii) saving last-generation antibiotics for serious life-threatening infections; and (iv) stopping antibiotic therapy as soon as possible. When used prophylactically a short course of antibiotics should

be prescribed, typically only enough to last the duration of the surgical procedure, and the administration should begin prior to surgery (two hours prior to the procedure), so that adequate systemic levels of the antibiotic (two to eight times above MIC) are present at the time of surgical incision.

E. Additional clinical benefits associated with the use of systemic antibiotics as adjuncts to mechanical therapy reported in the literature include (i) greater reduction in mean PD and gains in mean CAL; (ii) fewer residual deep pockets (≥5 mm); (iii) slower rate of disease progression during follow-up; and (iv) clinical gains can be maintained for at least two years after a single course of systemic antibiotics.

Case 4

Use of Lasers in Periodontology

Medical History

The patient reported that he took multivitamin supplements. Otherwise, there were no significant medical problems and no known allergies reported.

Review of Systems

• Height: 1.68 m
• Weight: 87 kg
• Body mass index (BMI): 31 kg/m²
• Vital signs
  o Blood pressure: 108/70 mmHg
  o Pulse rate: 67 beats/minute

Family History

The patient reported no significant family history of any particular periodontal conditions.

Social History

The patient had smoked 20–30 cigarettes per day for 15 years, but was interested in quitting. He had tried to quit twice but failed due to stress. He did not drink alcohol. He was self-employed and was expecting a child.

Extraoral Examination

Extraoral examination revealed no pathologic findings.

Intraoral Examination

The soft tissues of the mouth and the tongue appeared normal. There was generalized gingival erythema, bleeding on probing, and supragingival and subgingival calculus deposits (Figure 2.4.1). There were no occlusal interferences in lateral and protrusive movements.

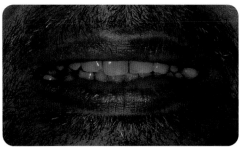
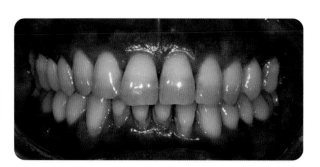

Figure 2.4.1 Appearance at initial presentation.

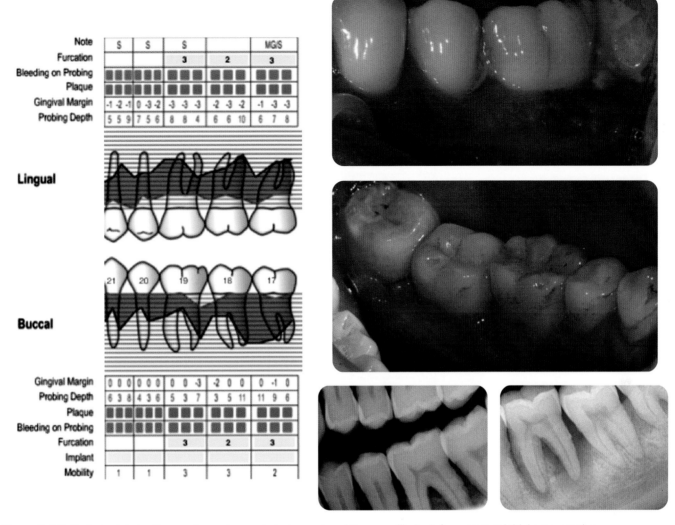

Figure 2.4.2 Periodontal charting, radiographs, and photographs of the mandibular left sextant at initial presentation.

The periodontal charting, radiographs, and photographs of the mandibular left sextant shown in Figure 2.4.2 are representative of the complete dentition.

Preoperative microbial testing was performed and the results are presented in Figure 2.4.3.

Diagnosis

According to the most recent EFP/AAP classification [1] this case can be diagnosed as periodontitis stage III, grade C.

Treatment Plan

The treatment plan for this patient included oral hygiene instructions, followed by scaling, root planing, and polishing using hand instruments as well as powered mechanical instruments.

Treatment

After thorough oral hygiene instructions were reviewed, the patient received scaling and polishing in all four quadrants (Figure 2.4.4). The procedure was started with an ultrasonic-powered mechanical instrument to loosen any tenacious supragingival deposits and for initial stain removal. Hand scalers were then used, including a sickle scaler for removal of supragingival calculus and stain in the mandibular anterior areas, Gracey curettes were used in the interproximal areas posteriorly, and universal curettes were used for the buccal and lingual aspects of the teeth. The Er:YAG laser was used in the lower left sextant to remove any subgingival calculus residuals and the teeth were finally polished to eliminate any additional stain using prophylaxis paste and a rubber cup.

Oral Microbiology Testing Service Laboratory
Temple University Kornberg School of Dentistry
3223 North Broad Street, Philadelphia, PA 19140
Telephone (215) 707-4237; Toll Free (800) 788-OMTS

Putative Periodontal Pathogens Presumptive Identification (critical % threshold level)		% Cultivable Microbiota	ANTIBIOTIC RESISTANCE TESTING S = 100% in vitro inhibition at threshold value, R = resistant			
			Doxycycline 4 µg/ml	Amoxicillin 8 µg/ml	Metronidazole 16 µg/ml	Clindamycin 4 µg/ml
A. actinomycetemcomitans	(0.01%)	0.0				
Red Complex Species:						
Porphyromonas gingivalis	(0.1%)	0.0				
Tannerella forsythia	(1%)	2.7	S	S	S	S
Orange Complex Species:						
Prevotella intermedia group	(2.5%)	7.3	R	R	S	S
Fusobacterium nucleatum	(10%)	16.4	S	S	S	S
Parvimonas micra (P. micros)	(3%)	10.9	S	S	S	R
Campylobacter rectus	(2%)	0.0				
Streptococcus constellatus	(2.5%)	0.0				
Other/Opportunistic Species:						
Streptococcus intermedius	(5%)	0.0				
Enteric gram negative rods	(5%)	0.0				
Enterococcus faecalis		0.0				
Staphylococcus aureus		0.0				
Candida species (yeast)		0.0				

% Microscopic Morphotypes: Spirochetes   Motile rods   Non-motile rods   Cocci

Pennsylvania Department of Health Clinical Laboratory Permit No. 021872 (Authorized for Bacteriology)
US Department of Health & Human Services CLIA Laboratory Certificate of Compliance No. 39007075B5

Figure 2.4.3 Preoperative microbial testing.

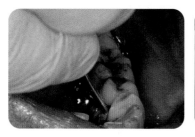
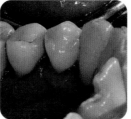

Figure 2.4.4 Scaling and polishing in all four quadrants.

Discussion

The patient presented with heavy supragingival and subgingival plaque and calculus, gingival inflammation and generalized bleeding on probing, with generalized moderate to severe bone loss around the teeth. After a detailed medical history was completed, a diagnosis of generalized severe chronic periodontitis was given. To restore the patient to periodontal health, comprehensive oral hygiene instructions were provided, and a professional scaling and root planing was arranged. A combination of hand and power-driven instruments were used for removal of plaque, calculus, and stain from the teeth. Hand instruments are available in various lengths, shapes, and designs to effectively reach and treat all areas of the teeth. An ultrasonic instrument (Cavitron) was used as an adjunct for stain removal, mechanical debridement, lavage, and cavitation. Er:YAG laser was used to remove subgingival calculus according to the manufacturer's settings and recommended tips root debridement. Regularly scheduled reevaluations and prophylaxis in addition to routine home care were recommended for maintaining optimal oral hygiene and periodontal health in this patient (Figure 2.4.5).

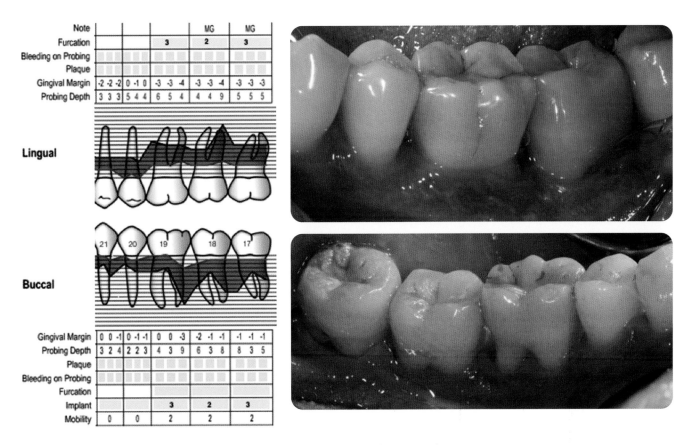

Figure 2.4.5 Periodontal charting and photographs of the mandibular left sextant after treatment.

Self-Study Questions

A. What types of lasers are used in periodontal therapy?

B. Why are lasers used/preferred in periodontal therapy?

C. What is the evidence for the use of lasers in nonsurgical periodontal therapy?

D. What is the evidence for the use of lasers in surgical periodontal therapy?

E. What are some potential risks of using laser therapy?

Answers located at the end of the chapter.

References

1. Caton JG, Armitage G, Berglundh T, et al. A new classification scheme for periodontal and peri-implant diseases and conditions: introduction and key changes from the 1999 classification. *J Clin Periodontol* 2018;45(Suppl 20):S1–S8.

2. Mills MP, Rosen PS, Chambrone L, et al. American Academy of Periodontology best evidence consensus statement on the efficacy of laser therapy used alone or as an adjunct to non-surgical and surgical treatment of periodontitis and peri-implant diseases. *J Periodontol* 2018;89:737–742.

TAKE-HOME POINTS [2]

A. The word "laser" stands for light amplification by stimulated emission of radiation. There are multiple types of lasers: argon, CO_2, diode, erbium (Er:YAG, Er,Cr:YSGG), and Nd:YAG. Some are penetrating (pigment lasers), such as Nd:YAG, diode, and argon; others are nonpenetrating (water lasers), such as erbium and CO_2. The most commonly known lasers that are commercially available include laser-assisted new attachment procedure or LANAP (Nd:YAG), Biolase (Er,Cr:YSGG) and Lares (Er:YAG).

B. There are multiple reasons why lasers have become popular for both patients and clinicians. They are used by clinicians because it is a new technology (improved marketing) and may produce positive clinical results. Patients have reported that they prefer the use of lasers because of minimal anesthesia, reduced pain, and minimal swelling/postoperative discomfort.

C. The American Academy of Periodontology Consensus reported in 2018 that laser therapy used as an adjunct to conventional periodontal therapy may provide some benefit (up to 1 mm improved probing depths and CAL). However, there is limited evidence that laser therapy alone is similar or superior to conventional periodontal therapy for patients with residual probing depths up to 5 mm.

D. Some studies report that lasers can be used as an alternative to conventional surgical therapy as it might provide some benefits: less patient bleeding, assistance in disease site disinfection, or facilitation of treatment for patients who are medically compromised (those on anticoagulation therapies) or the elderly, where a traditional approach may impose some risks.

E. There is evidence suggesting that the use of lasers in healthy individuals has more risks than benefits. The authors caution clinicians to review carefully the recommendations from the manufacturers (American National Standards Institute) prior to the use of this technology as overheating or improper use of the protocol can be damaging for the teeth or surrounding tissues.

3

Resective Periodontal Therapy

Case 1: Gingivectomy...120
  T. Howard Howell, DDS, Maria Dona, DMD, MSD, DMSc, and Thomas T. Nguyen, DMD, MSc, FRCD(C)

Case 2: Preprosthetic Hard Tissue and Soft Tissue Crown Lengthening 128
  Guillaume Campard, DDS, MMSc, Emilio I. Arguello, DDS, MSc, and Naciye G. Uzel, DMD, DMSc

Case 3: Flap Osseous Surgery 138
  Kevin Guze, DMD, DMSc, MSc, FRCD(C), FICOI

Case 4: Root Resection 145
  Philip Walton, DDS, MMSc and Paul A. Levi, Jr., DMD

Clinical Cases in Periodontics, Second Edition. Edited by Nadeem Karimbux.
© 2022 John Wiley & Sons, Inc. Published 2022 by John Wiley & Sons, Inc.
Companion website: www.wiley.com/go/karimbux/periodontics

Case 1

Gingivectomy

CASE STORY

A 16-year-old Caucasian male presented with a chief complaint of "My gums are puffy and bleed on flossing." After two years of orthodontic therapy, treatment had been discontinued two months before due to nonresolvable gingival enlargement (Figure 3.1.1). The patient had been informed of his gingival enlargement, and oral hygiene instructions had been reinforced. The patient had no significant gingival inflammation and/or enlargement before the start of orthodontic treatment. He stated that the gingival enlargement developed gradually during orthodontic treatment (Figures 3.1.2 and 3.1.3).

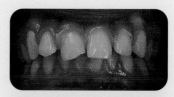
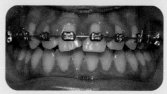

Figure 3.1.2 Clinical example of plaque-induced gingivitis with gingival enlargement: frontal occlusal views before orthodontic presentation (top) and during the orthodontic treatment (bottom).

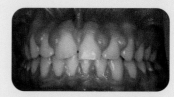

Figure 3.1.3 Clinical presentation two months after removal of orthodontic appliances: intraoral frontal view in occlusion.

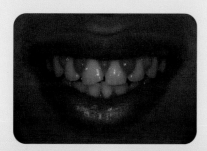
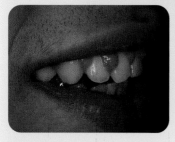
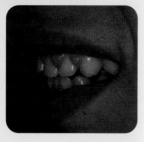

Figure 3.1.1 Clinical presentation after removal of orthodontic appliances: smile frontal and side views.

LEARNING GOALS AND OBJECTIVES

- To learn the indications for gingivectomy
- To understand the surgical technique for gingivectomy

Medical History

The patient reported no significant medical problems and no known allergies. He did not have a family history of gingival enlargement or a history of chronic or current medication.

Dental History

The patient reported that orthodontic treatment began two years ago to align his teeth. Slowly during this time, his gums became "puffy," and despite his best efforts at oral hygiene no improvement had been achieved. Therefore, two months ago, the orthodontic brackets were removed and the patient was referred to the Department of Periodontology for consultation and appropriate treatment. The patient was currently wearing a retainer. He denied a history of tooth extraction, restorations, or endodontic treatment. The anatomic crown of tooth #8 was previously chipped due to trauma.

Social History

The patient was a sophomore in high school and denied smoking and drinking alcohol.

Oral Hygiene

The patient used a manual toothbrush that was replaced every three months and reported toothbrushing and flossing in the morning only. He also used Listerine mouth rinse once a day.

Extraoral and Intraoral Examinations

- There were no significant findings on extraoral examination. The patient had no masses or swelling, and the temporomandibular joint was within normal limits.
- With the exception of the gingiva, the soft tissues of the mouth appeared normal.
- A periodontal examination revealed localized mild marginal erythema, localized rolled margins, swollen papillae, bleeding on probing, no recession or mobility, probing depths ranging from 2 to 5 mm, and keratinized gingiva ranging from 3 to 8 mm (Figures 3.1.3 and 3.1.4).
- The hard tissue examination found no active decay and no dental restorations. Tooth #8 was reported as fractured.

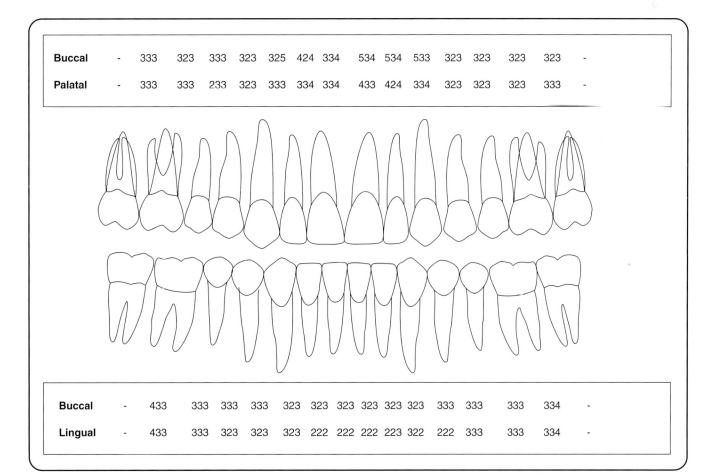

| Buccal | - | 333 | 323 | 333 | 323 | 325 | 424 | 334 | 534 | 534 | 533 | 323 | 323 | 323 | 323 | - |
| Palatal | - | 333 | 333 | 233 | 323 | 333 | 334 | 334 | 433 | 424 | 334 | 323 | 323 | 323 | 333 | - |

| Buccal | - | 433 | 333 | 333 | 333 | 323 | 323 | 323 | 323 | 323 | 323 | 333 | 333 | 333 | 334 | - |
| Lingual | - | 433 | 333 | 323 | 323 | 323 | 222 | 222 | 222 | 223 | 322 | 222 | 333 | 333 | 334 | - |

Figure 3.1.4 Probing pocket depth measurements.

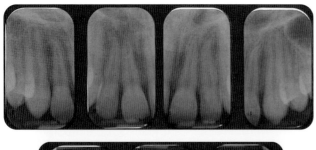

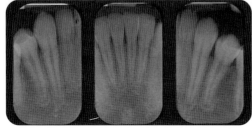

Figure 3.1.5 Periapical radiographs depicting interproximal bone levels.

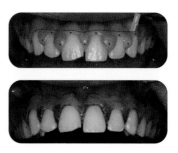

Figure 3.1.6 External bevel gingivectomy in anterior maxillary region: gingival marking for the external bevel incision (top) and immediately after gingivectomy (bottom).

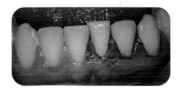

Figure 3.1.7 External bevel gingivectomy in anterior mandibular region: immediate post gingivectomy.

Occlusion

Class I angle occlusion was present after orthodontic treatment.

Radiographic Examination

The full-mouth set of radiographs demonstrated crestal bone levels to be within normal limits (Figure 3.1.5 shows the patient's anterior periapical X-rays).

Diagnosis

After reviewing the history and clinical and radiographic examinations, the patient was diagnosed with plaque-induced gingivitis resulting in gingival enlargement.

Treatment Plan

The treatment plan for this patient included prophylaxis, improved oral hygiene, and surgical correction (with gingivectomy/gingivoplasty) of the gingival contour and periodontal maintenance.

Treatment

Treatment for this patient included oral hygiene instructions and supragingival and subgingival scaling followed by reevaluation at four weeks. During the reevaluation appointment, an improvement in oral hygiene technique was noted. However, the gingival enlargement persisted. Therefore, surgical excision of excessive soft tissue was performed via external bevel gingivectomy technique (B). Following the administration of local anesthesia, bleeding points corresponding to the apical extent of the pocket depth were created on the external

gingiva using a periodontal probe (Figure 3.1.6). Using 15C blades, a coronally directed external bevel incision was made starting slightly apical to the bleeding points and coronal to the mucogingival junction. The inner portion of the blade should contact the teeth at the base of the pocket at a position corresponding to the bleeding point. The incision line should be a straight-line incision that begins and ends in the gingival sulcus mesially and distally to the gingival area removed. The detached gingiva was removed with a scaler, and rotary diamond burs were used to reshape the gingival margin to normal physiologic contours, as shown in Figures 3.1.6 and 3.1.7. This reshaping of the gingiva is referred to as gingivoplasty (A). Oral hygiene instructions were reinforced, and the patient was asked not to brush the wounded areas until the next appointment in two weeks and was given a prescription for Peridex rinse and ibuprofen 600 mg for pain control.

The patient was evaluated two weeks post gingivectomy to assess the healing (Figure 3.1.8). Oral hygiene was reinforced, instructing on brushing the area of surgery.

Discussion

Patients undergoing orthodontic treatment may experience various oral clinical manifestations such as sensitivity, increased caries risk, and gingival enlargement [1,2]. Gingival enlargement associated with orthodontic therapy can begin as dental plaque-induced gingivitis followed by gingival enlargement. The

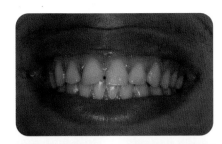
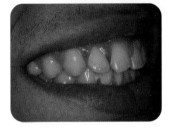
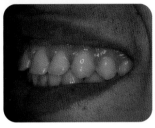

Figure 3.1.8 Two weeks post gingivectomy: full smile frontal and side views.

enlargement is usually associated with an inflammatory response triggered by corrosion of the orthodontic appliances. The most likely component of the brackets creating this response is nickel. Therefore, the condition is frequently classified as nickel allergic contact stomatitis [3]. A study by Gursoy et al. [1] describes the appearance of orthodontic treatment-induced gingival enlargement as a specific fibrous and thickened gingiva, different from the fragile gingiva with marginal gingival redness that is seen in allergic or inflammatory gingival lesions. Histologic analysis of orthodontic-induced gingival enlargement tissues demonstrated an increase in epithelial thickness and a significant increase in epithelial cell proliferation in response to low-dose nickel concentrations, and the in vitro results are suggestive of the continuing low-dose nickel release to epithelium as the initiating factor of gingival enlargement induced by orthodontic treatment [1]. Complete resolution of the gingival enlargement developed during orthodontic treatment may not appear even 3–12 months after the removal of the fixed appliances, as reported by Kouraki et al. [2].

Therefore, because in the present case the gingival enlargement persisted four months after removal of orthodontic appliances and phase 1 therapy, including professional dental cleaning and reinforcement of home care dental hygiene, the surgical excision of excessive gingiva was planned and performed.

External bevel gingivectomy was performed using 15C blades and final reshaping of gingival contours using diamond burs. The postoperative follow-up showed excellent healing as well as a significant

improvement in the esthetic appearance that improved local access for proper oral hygiene. Similar results have been described by Benoist et al. [4] in two cases of gingival enlargement treated with gingivectomy in young Senegalese women undergoing orthodontic treatment with fixed appliances, with improvement in the morphologic conditions of gingiva allowing better plaque control. The same authors emphasized that periodic evaluation of the child and adolescent during orthodontic therapy is required for a healthy periodontium and that collaboration between orthodontist and periodontist is one of the most important keys to successful treatment.

Laser gingivectomy has also been pursued for the removal of excessive gingiva in the case of orthodontic treatment-associated gingival enlargement. In a study by Gama et al. [5], the effect of using the CO_2 laser on the treatment of gingival hyperplasia in orthodontic patients wearing fixed appliances was reported. This study concluded that use of the CO_2 laser was effective in the treatment of gingival hyperplasia. Additionally, use of the Nd:YAG and diode laser in the surgical management of soft tissues related to orthodontic treatment, including recontouring of gingival enlargement, was described in a study by Fornaini et al. [6]. Nonsurgical periodontal treatment with Er:YAG laser has also been shown to promote regression of gingival overgrowth in patients taking cyclosporine [7]. The laser-assisted surgery was particularly beneficial due to reported reduced bleeding during surgery with consequent reduced operating time and rapid postoperative hemostasis, thus eliminating the need for sutures, as well as improved postoperative comfort and healing, which make this technique particularly useful for very young patients [6].

In a comparative study, Liboon et al. [8] evaluated the histologic effects of scalpel, CO_2 laser, electrosurgery, and constant-voltage electrosurgery incisions on the mucosal tissue in a swine model. The results show that the speed of incisions and excisions was fastest with the scalpel and electrosurgery unit, the amount of bleeding was least for electrosurgery and CO_2 laser, and the histologic damage was least with scalpel followed by constant-voltage electrosurgery.

In recent years, the development of new technologies including intraoral scanners, dental software for digital planning and design, and 3D printers has improved and made the digital workflow more accessible. In a clinical report, Revilla-Leon et al. [9] described the use of the digital workflow to design the digital wax-up, plan the surgery and 3D-print a surgical guide for a gingivectomy procedure.

Self-Study Questions

A. What is gingivectomy/gingivoplasty? What are the indications and contraindications for gingivectomy/gingivoplasty?

B. What are the surgical techniques for performing gingivectomy/gingivoplasty?

C. What is the oral hygiene protocol after gingivectomy?

D. What are the expected results and wound healing after gingivectomy?

Answers located at the end of the chapter.

ACKNOWLEDGMENT

The authors thank Dr. Athbi Alquareer for referral and collaboration on the case presented here.

References

1. Gursoy UK, Sokucu O, Uitto V-J, et al. The role of nickel accumulation and epithelial cell proliferation in orthodontic treatment-induced gingival overgrowth. *Eur J Orthod* 2007;29:555–558.
2. Kouraki E, Bissada NF, Palomo JM, Ficara AJ. Gingival enlargement and resolution during and after orthodontic treatment. *N Y State Dent J* 2005;71:34–37.
3. Holmstrup P. Non-plaque induced gingival lesions. *Ann Periodontol* 1999;4:20–29.
4. Benoist HM, Ngom PI, Seck-Diallo A, Diallo PD. Gingival hypertrophy during orthodontic treatment: contribution of external bevel gingivectomy. *Case report. Odontostomatol Trop* 2007;30(120):42–46.
5. Gama SKC, De Araújo TM, Pozza DH, Pinheiro ALB. Use of the CO(2) laser on orthodontic patients suffering from gingival hyperplasia. *Photomed Laser Surg* 2007;25:214–219.
6. Fornaini C, Rocca JP, Bertrand MF, et al. Nd:YAG and diode laser in the surgical management of soft tissues related to orthodontic treatment. *Photomed Laser Surg* 2007;25:381–392.
7. Capodiferro S, Tempesta A, Limongelli L, et al. Nonsurgical periodontal treatment by erbium:YAG laser promotes regression of gingival overgrowth in patient taking cyclosporine A: a case report. *Photobiomodul Photomed Laser Surg* 2019;37:53–56.
8. Liboon J, Funkhouser W, Terris DJ. A comparison of mucosal incisions made by scalpel, CO_2 laser, electrocautery, and constant-voltage electrocautery. *Otolaryngol Head Neck Surg* 1997;116:379–385.
9. Revilla-Leon M, Besne-Torre A, Sanchez-Rubio JL, et al. Digital tools and 3D printing technologies integrated into the workflow of restorative treatment: a clinical report. *J Prosth Dent* 2019;121:3–8.
10. Robicsek S. Ueber das Wesen und Entstehen der Alveolar-Pyorrhoe und deren Behandlung. 1884. The 3rd Annual Report of the Australian Dental Association (reviewed in J Periodontol 1965;36:265).
11. Grant DA, Stern IB, Everett FG, Orban BJ. *Periodontics in the Tradition of Orban and Gotlieb*, 5th edn. St. Louis, MO: Mosby, 1979.
12. Goldman HM. Gingivectomy. *Oral Surg Oral Med Oral Pathol* 1951;4:1136–1157.
13. Mavrogiannis M, Ellis JS, Thomason JM, Seymour RA. The management of drug-induced gingival overgrowth [review]. *J Clin Periodontol* 2006;33:434–439.
14. Engler WO, Ramfjord SP, Hiniker JJ. Healing following simple gingivectomy. A tritiated thymidine radiographic study. I. Epithelialization. *J Periodontol* 1966;37:298–308.
15. Ramfjord SP, Engler SP, Hiniker JJ. A radioautographic study of healing following simple gingivectomy. II. The connective tissue. *J Peridontol* 1966;37:179–189.
16. Listgarten M. Ultrastructure of the dento-gingival junction after gingivectomy. *J Periodontal Res* 1972;7:151–160.
17. Stahl SS, Witkin G, Cantor M, Brown R. Gingival healing II. Clinical and histologic repair sequences following gingivectomy. *J Periodontol* 1968;39:109–118.

TAKE-HOME POINTS

A. The gingivectomy procedure was first recognized by Robicsek [10] (straight incision technique) as an alternative surgical approach to subgingival scaling for pocket therapy. Grant et al. [11] later defined gingivectomy as "the excision of the soft tissue wall of a pathologic periodontal pocket" to eliminate the pocket and restore a physiologic gingival contour.

Gingivoplasty represents reshaping of the gingiva to a so-called physiologic form. Indications for gingivectomy/gingivoplasty include the following.
- To eliminate gingival pockets – suprabony pockets – that persist after completion of oral hygiene instructions, scaling and root planing, and other disease control measures (Figures 3.1.3, 3.1.6, and 3.1.7).
- To reduce gingival enlargements resulting from medications or genetic factors (Figure 3.1.9).
- To create clinical crown length for restorative or endodontic purposes when ostectomy is not required (Figure 3.1.10).
- To eliminate soft tissue craters resulting from disease or subsequent to other surgical procedures (Figure 3.1.11).
- To create an esthetic gingival form in cases of delayed passive eruption.

Contraindications to the performance of gingivectomy are as follows.
- Acute inflamed gingiva.
- Inadequate oral hygiene.
- Inadequate keratinized gingiva: pocket depth is located apical to the mucogingival junction.
- Presence of interdental osseous craters and infrabony defects.
- Inadequate depth of vestibule.
- Presence of large exostoses and osseous ledges.
- When removal of the soft tissue would lead to an undesirable esthetic compromise.

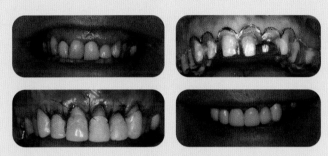

Figure 3.1.10   Clinical example of gingivectomy for restorative and esthetic reasons: smile at the initial presentation (top left); gingival marking using a vacuum-form template prior to gingivectomy (top right); delivery of temporary prosthesis at the end of gingivectomy (bottom left); smile at delivery of the final restoration of teeth #6–#11 at five months post gingivectomy (bottom right).

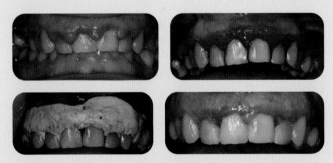

Figure 3.1.9   Clinical example of external bevel gingivectomy for phenytoin-induced gingival enlargement: frontal view in occlusion before gingivectomy (top left); external bevel gingivectomy in the anterior maxilla (top right); periodontal dressing applied at the end of gingivectomy (bottom left); one week after maxillary gingivectomy, after periodontal dressing removal (bottom right).

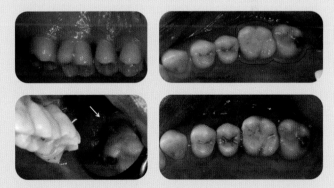

Figure 3.1.11   Clinical example of an inverse bevel distal wedge: palatal preoperative view (top left); outline of the initial scalloped incision and extended into the tuberosity region in a triangular shape (top right); osseous defect from the distal view after removal of the collar of tissue and distal wedge and thorough debridement (bottom left); the flaps positioned and sutured to gain primary closure (bottom right).

• In case of increased rate of caries that jeopardizes maintenance of dentition.

B. Gingivectomy can be performed using the classical external bevel gingivectomy (as described by Goldman in 1951 [12]), internal bevel gingivectomy technique, or distal wedge procedures as well as by the use of electrosurgery, lasers, or chemical gingivectomy. Gingivoplasty can also be performed by using rotary instruments with appropriately shaped coarse diamond stones in addition to using the edge of a round-bladed gingivectomy knife.

External bevel gingivectomy (shown in Figure 3.1.6 for a case of dental plaque-induced gingivitis after orthodontic treatment and in Figure 3.1.9 for a case of phenytoin-induced gingival enlargement, previously detailed in Chapter 1, Case 4) consists of several steps.

1. Pocket marking: placement of a series of bleeding points on the outside of the gingiva that correspond to the apical extent of the pocket using either the periodontal probe or a mechanical device such as the Crane-Kaplan or Goldman-Fox pocket marker; usually three points are marked per tooth (mid-radicular area, mesial, and distal line angles).
2. A primary coronally directed external bevel incision, of about 45 degrees, is next made using an appropriate surgical knife: broad-blade or round-blade gingivectomy knife such as the Goldman-Fox 7/8, or Kirkland 15K/16K, or 15/15C blade that starts slightly apical to the "dotted line" created by the bleeding points but always coronal to the mucogingival junction with an internal end point corresponding to the base of the pocket as indicated by the bleeding points.
3. A secondary interdental incision is made to sever the interproximal portion of the soft tissue pocket using a triangular narrow-blade knife such as the Goldman-Fox 8 or 11 or the Orban 1/2.
4. Removal of the excised soft tissue using a Prichard curette or any sharp universal curette provides a surface that is smooth and free of tags.
5. The exposed root surfaces are examined and instrumented to ensure proper and complete removal of calculus.
6. After debridement, refinement by gingivoplasty of the margins of the gingiva is performed if needed by means of knives or rotary diamond burs.
7. Periodontal dressing can be placed over the incised area during the initial period of healing (10–14 days) (Figure 3.1.9).

Internal bevel gingivectomy generally begins with a scalloped internal bevel incision placed several millimeters apical to the free gingival margin, following a scalloped contour associated with normal gingival margin. The gingival marking for the incision line can be performed by using a previously vacuum-form template representing the final gingival margins fabricated on the patient's cast as shown in Figure 3.1.10 prior to gingivectomy to create clinical crown length for restorative and esthetic purposes.

In the case of internal bevel gingivectomy, a mucoperiosteal flap is produced that can then be positioned and sutured to cover the alveolar bone (Figure 3.1.10, bottom left). This procedure is most frequently referred to as a partial-thickness flap procedure, rather than a true gingivectomy.

The inverse bevel distal wedge technique is usually associated with buccal and palatal inverse bevel access incisions and flap reflection for pocket reduction. Figure 3.1.11 is an example of the distal wedge procedure distal of the second maxillary molar, presenting a preoperative palatal view of the enlarged tuberosity region with excessive probing depth (top left). The procedure included an initial scalloped incision apically to the gingival margin and coronal to mucogingival junction made around the first and second molars and extended into the tuberosity region in a triangular shape (top right). The palatal view shows the underlying bony defect with no distal furcation involvement. Once the distal triangular-shaped wedge was dissected from the underlying bone and removed, thick flaps were thinned and thorough debridement in the area was completed (bottom left). The buccal and palatal flaps are positioned and sutured apically using external vertical mattress sutures obtaining a reduction in soft tissue height in the tuberosity region in addition to the palatal and buccal areas of the first and second molars (bottom right). Often this procedure is combined with osteotomy/ostectomy procedures, detailed in Chapter 3, Case 3.

Electrosurgery (reviewed by Mavrogiannis et al. [13]) and chemical gingivectomy are currently outdated procedures due to delayed healing [8] and poor accuracy in reshaping of gingival tissue, as well as damage to the healthy adjacent hard and soft tissues.

Laser-assisted surgery has been introduced for the treatment of soft tissue, including removal and recontouring of gingiva in cases of persistent gingival enlargement of various etiologies. Various types of laser, such as Nd:YAG, Er:YAG and CO_2, have been used for a variety of intraoral soft tissue procedures, and the overall benefits of laser treatment include reduced bleeding during surgery with consequent reduced operating time and rapid postoperative hemostasis, no need for sutures, and improved postoperative comfort and healing [6,7,13].

C. The critical period for complete healing of a gingivectomy wound is between two and five weeks after the surgery; therefore meticulous oral hygiene is essential for the establishment of a physiologic gingival sulcus [14].

D. The sequence of the wound healing process after gingivectomy has been studied by various methods, in both animal models as well as humans. The initial study by Engler et al. [14] examined epithelialization post gingivectomy in rhesus monkeys using tritiated thymidine radiography and found that migrating epithelial cells start to cover the wound between 12 and 24 hours after surgical excision. Complete healing of the sulcus aspect of the gingivectomy takes four to five weeks, although the surface appears to be healed after two weeks.

Moreover, the same group [15] published a follow-up paper describing the connective tissue aspect of healing and regeneration following simple gingivectomy in three monkeys with histologic and radioautographic techniques. Their results show that connective tissue proliferation is initiated one to two days after the surgery and reaches a peak three to four days after surgery. However, functional arrangement and collagenous maturation of the gingival connective tissue fibers as well as the establishment of a physiologic restoration of a gingival crevice, with a sealing normal epithelial attachment that depends on a firm gingival tone, both require three to five weeks following gingivectomy.

Similarly, Listgarten [16], using an electron microscopic examination of the dentogingival junction after gingivectomy in monkeys, found that epithelial reattachment against morphologically normal and superficially altered cementum may occur in 12 days or less after surgical excision.

Another study [17] investigating clinical and histologic gingival healing in humans following gingivectomy reported that complete surface epithelialization of the gingivectomy wound appears within 7–14 days after surgery; still active connective tissue repair was seen 28 days after gingivectomy, the last time point examined after the surgery.

Case 2

Preprosthetic Hard Tissue and Soft Tissue Crown Lengthening

CASE STORY

The patient was a 29-year-old male who had been referred to the Department of Periodontology for evaluation of the anterior mandibular sextant based on a history of trauma. He had been accidentally hit in the anterior mandible with a racket while playing squash; tooth #24 was extracted subsequent to the accident. His chief complaint was to save and restore as many teeth as possible. Figures 3.2.1–3.2.4 illustrate the clinical situation at the first periodontal examination.

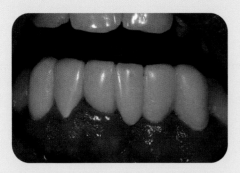

Figure 3.2.1 Preoperative condition with the temporary fixed partial denture, facial view.

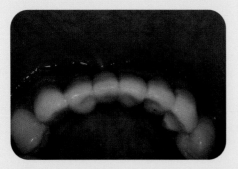

Figure 3.2.2 Preoperative condition with the temporary fixed partial denture, occlusal view.

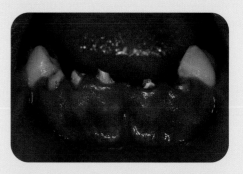

Figure 3.2.3 Preoperative condition without the temporary fixed partial denture, facial view.

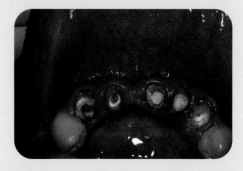

Figure 3.2.4 Preoperative condition without the temporary fixed partial denture, occlusal view.

LEARNING GOALS AND OBJECTIVES

- To identify the indications for crown lengthening
- To understand the prosthetic needs and periodontal requirements to restore altered teeth
- To understand key considerations at the time of surgery

Medical History

The patient was healthy and received a medical examination every year. He did not take medications and did not report any allergies or any medical problems.

Review of Systems

- Vital signs
  - Blood pressure: 123/68 mmHg
  - Pulse rate: 62 beats/minute (regular)

Social History

The patient drank alcohol occasionally. He did not smoke and did not use recreational drugs.

Extraoral Examination

No significant findings were found (Figure 3.2.5). The patient had no masses or swelling, and the temporomandibular joints were within normal limits.

Intraoral Examination

- The soft tissues of the mouth appeared normal. The oral cancer screen was negative.
- The gingival examination revealed a thick and flat periodontium with generalized mild marginal erythema, rolled margins, and blunted papillae in the mandibular anterior sextant (Figures 3.2.1 and 3.2.3).
- A hard tissue examination was completed. There was a small amount of sound tooth structure available for the prosthetic restoration of teeth #22, #23, #25, #26, and #27 (Figures 3.2.3 and 3.2.4).
- The edentulous ridge (site #24) had deformities in the buccolingual and apico-coronal directions (Seibert class 3).

Occlusion

Findings included canine and molar Angle class 1, group function on lateral excursion, and incisal guidance in protrusion.

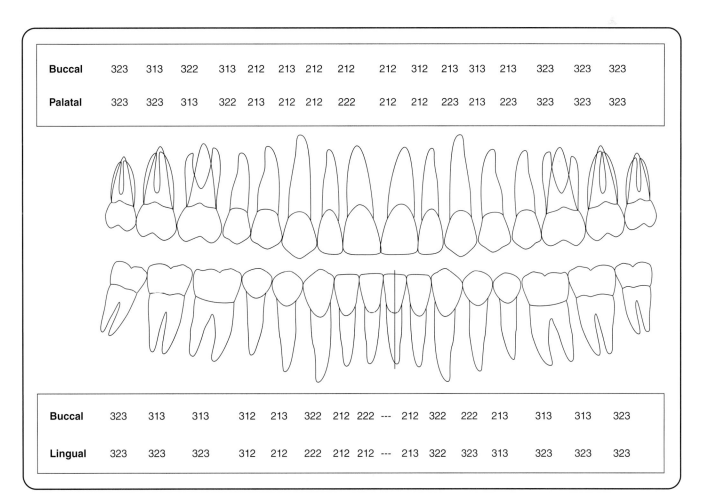

Buccal	323	313	322	313	212	213	212	212	212	312	213	313	213	323	323	323
Palatal	323	323	313	322	213	212	212	222	212	212	223	213	223	323	323	323

Buccal	323	313	313	312	213	322	212	222	---	212	322	222	213	313	313	323
Lingual	323	323	323	312	212	222	212	212	---	213	322	323	313	323	323	323

Figure 3.2.5 Periodontal charting.

Radiographic Examination

Incomplete root canal treatments on teeth #22, #23, #25, #26, and #27 and periapical radiolucencies on #25 and #26 were observed on the periapical radiographs. There was no horizontal bone loss, the lamina dura was visible and continuous, and bone trabeculations appeared normal (Figure 3.2.6).

Diagnosis

Clinical gingival health on an intact periodontium.

Treatment Plan

Periodontal, prosthodontic, and endodontic evaluations were performed to assess the restorability of the teeth. The multidisciplinary team deemed the teeth restorable with an endodontic retreatment for teeth #22, #23, #25, #26, and #27, crown lengthening, cast post and core, PFM crowns #22, #27, and a fixed partial denture (FPD) #23-x-25-26.

Treatment

The patient received oral hygiene instructions and a prophylaxis. The endodontic retreatments were performed (Figure 3.2.7), and a temporary FPD #22-23-x25-26-27 was fabricated (Figure 3.2.8).

Preoperative Consultation

The medical history was reviewed. A clinical and radiographic examination was performed. The amount of sound tooth structure present in the mandibular anterior sextant supragingivally was inadequate, and there was a lack of ferrule (Figure 3.2.3); the restorative margins were subgingival in some areas and were impinging on the supracrestal attachment, formerly known as biologic width (Figure 3.2.4). Upon radiographic examination (Figure 3.2.6), the periodontal support for the incisors and canines was sufficient and could tolerate 3 mm of ostectomy.

The consent form addressing benefits and risks associated with the procedure was reviewed with the patient. Preoperative prescriptions were delivered to the patient: ibuprofen 600 mg (every four to six hours for pain as needed) and Peridex 0.12% (b.i.d.).

Crown Lengthening Procedure

Bilateral mental nerve blocks and local infiltrations were achieved with lidocaine 2% (epinephrine 1:100 000). The temporary FPD was removed (Figures 3.2.8 and 3.2.9). A submarginal incision was performed around #22, #23, #25, #26, and #27 (Figure 3.2.10) to

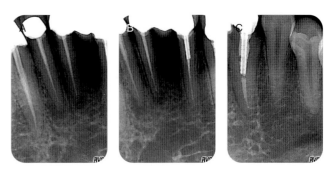

Figure 3.2.6 Periapical radiographs of the mandibular anterior sextant. Incomplete root canal treatments and periapical radiolucencies on #25 and #26 are visible.

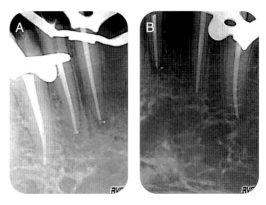

Figure 3.2.7 Periapical radiographs after endodontic therapy. Source: courtesy Dr. Fiza Singh.

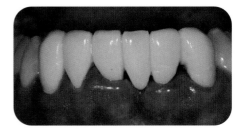

Figure 3.2.8 Preoperative facial view.

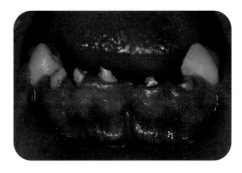

Figure 3.2.9 Preoperative facial view after the temporary fixed partial denture is removed.

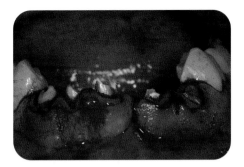

Figure 3.2.10 Submarginal incisions.

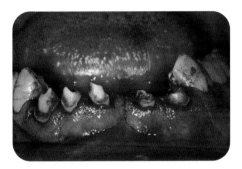

Figure 3.2.11 Gingivectomy.

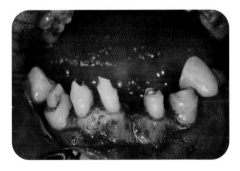

Figure 3.2.12 A full-thickness flap is elevated and cortical bone is exposed.

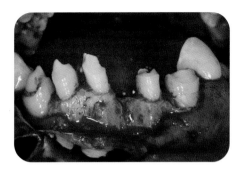

Figure 3.2.13 Ostectomy and osteoplasty allow a greater exposure of sound tooth structure.

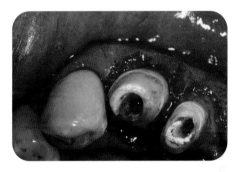

Figure 3.2.14 The embrasure between #21 and #22 is narrow.

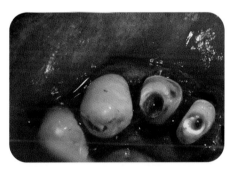

Figure 3.2.15 Odontoplasty of the distal surface of #22 is performed to open the embrasure between #21 and #22.

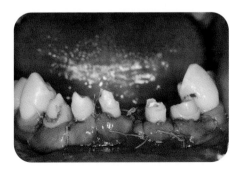

Figure 3.2.16 The flaps are apically positioned and stabilized with vertical mattress sutures.

achieve 2–3 mm of gingivectomy (Figure 3.2.11). Buccal and lingual full-thickness flaps were elevated beyond the mucogingival junction to expose the cortical bone of the mandibular anterior sextant (Figure 3.2.12). Ostectomy was carried out to expose at least 4 mm of sound tooth structure above the crestal bone and allow for 2 mm of biologic width and at least 1.5 mm of ferrule. Osteoplasty allowed the removal of widow's peaks, ledges, and bony irregularities (Figure 3.2.13). Odontoplasty was performed as needed when the embrasure space was too narrow (Figures 3.2.14 and 3.2.15). The buccal and lingual flaps were apically positioned and stabilized with vertical mattress sutures (Figure 3.2.16). The temporary FPD was cemented back (Figure 3.2.17). Postoperative instructions including oral

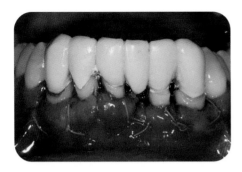

Figure 3.2.17 The temporary FPD is cemented back.

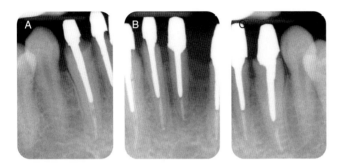

Figure 3.2.18 Periapical radiographs after cementation of the final cast post and core. Source: courtesy of Dr. Priyank Taneja.

hygiene instructions were delivered and an ice pack was placed against the patient's lip.

The patient was seen for a postoperative consultation at seven days and at 21 days after the procedure.

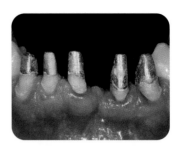

Figure 3.2.19 Final cast post and core. Source: courtesy of Dr. Priyank Taneja.

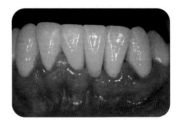

Figure 3.2.20 Permanent FPD.

The prosthetic margins were refined eight weeks after surgery, cast post and core (Figures 3.2.18 and 3.2.19) and final restorations (Figure 3.2.20) were cemented three weeks later.

Self-Study Questions

A. What are the components of the attachment apparatus of a tooth? What does "biologic width" mean?

B. What is the definition of crown lengthening? What are the goals of a crown lengthening procedure?

C. What are the indications and contraindications of crown lengthening?

D. How do you perform a crown lengthening?

E. How does a crown lengthening heal?

F. How does the gingival contour reestablish? How long after crown lengthening should a tooth receive permanent restoration?

Answers located at the end of the chapter.

ACKNOWLEDGMENTS

Thanks to Dr. Priyank Taneja, Department of Prosthodontics, Harvard School of Dental Medicine, and Dr. Fiza Singh, Department of Endodontics, Harvard School of Dental Medicine.

References

1. Ten Cate AR. *Oral Histology: Development, Structure and Function*, 3rd edn. Toronto, Ontario: Mosby, 1989.

2. Gargiulo A, Wentz F, Orban B. Dimensions and relations of the dentogingival junction in humans. *J Periodontol* 1961;32:261–267.

3. Ingber JS, Rose LF, Coslet JG. The "biologic width": a concept in periodontics and restorative dentistry. *Alpha Omegan* 1977;70:62–65.

4. Nevins M, Skurow HM. The intracrevicular restorative margin, the biologic width, and the maintenance of the gingival margin. *Int J Periodontics Restorative Dent* 1984;3:31–49.

5. Rose LF, Genco RJ, Mealey BL. *Periodontics: Medicine, Surgery, and Implants*. St. Louis, MO: Elsevier Mosby, 2004:424–464.

6. Palomo F, Kopczyk RA. Rationale and methods for crown lengthening. *J Am Dent Assoc* 1978;96:257–260.

7. Assif D. Pilo R, Marshak B. Restoring teeth following crown lengthening procedures. *J Prosthet Dent* 1991;65:62–64.

8. Wagenberg B, Eskow R, Langer B. Exposing adequate tooth structure for restorative dentistry. *Int J Periodontics Restorative Dent* 1989;9:323–331.

9. Sorensen JA, Engelman MJ. Ferrule design and fracture resistance of endodontically treated teeth. *J Prosthet Dent* 1990;63:529–536.

10. Gegauff AG. Effect of the crown lengthening and ferrule placement on static load failure of cemented cast post-cores and crowns. *J Prosthet Dent* 2000;84:169–179.

11. Coslet JG, Vanarsdall R, Weisgold A. Diagnosis and classification of delayed passive eruption of the dentogingival junction in the adult. *Alpha Omegan* 1977;70:24–28.

12. Allen EP. Surgical crown lengthening for function and esthetics. *Dent Clin North Am* 1993;37:163–179.

13. Friedman N. Periodontal osseous surgery: osteoplasty and ostectomy. *J Periodontol* 1955;26:257–269.

14. Ochsenbein C. A primer for osseous surgery. *Int J Periodontics Restorative Dent* 1986;6:8–47.

15. Ivey DW, Calhoun RN, Kemp WB, et al. Orthodontic extrusion: its use in restorative dentistry. *J Prosthet Dent* 1980;43:401–407.

16. Lanning SK, Waldrop TC, Gunsolley JC, Maynard JG. Surgical crown lengthening: evaluation of the biological width. *J Periodontol* 2003;74:468–474.

17. Caton JG, Zander HA. The attachment between tooth and gingival tissues after periodic root planing and soft tissue curettage. *J Periodontol* 1979;50:462–466.

18. Waerhaug J. Healing of the dento-epithelial junction following subgingival plaque control. II. As observed on extracted teeth. *J Periodontol* 1978;49:119–134.

19. Van Der Velden U. Regeneration of the interdental soft tissues following denudation procedures. *J Clin Periodontol* 1982;9:455–459.

20. Carnevale G, Sterrantino S, Di Febo G. Soft and hard tissue wound healing following tooth preparation to the alveolar crest. *Int J Periodontics Restorative Dent* 1983;3:37–53.

21. Oakley E, Rhyu IC, Karatzas S, et al. Formation of the biologic width following crown lengthening in nonhuman primate. *Int J Periodontics Restorative Dent* 1999;19:529–541.

22. Schluger S. Osseous resection: a basic principle in periodontal surgery. *Oral Surg Oral Med Oral Pathol* 1949;2:316–325.

23. Levine H, Stahl S. Repair following periodontal flap surgery with the retention of gingival fibers. *J Periodontol* 1972;43:99–103.

24. Lindhe J, Socransky SS, Nyman S, Westfelt F. Dimensional alteration of the periodontal tissues following therapy. *Int J Periodontics Restorative Dent* 1987;7:9–21.

25. Kaldahl WB, Kalkwarf KL, Patil KD, et al. Long-term evaluation of periodontal therapy: I. Response to 4 therapeutic modalities. *J Periodontol* 1996;67:93–102.

26. Pontoriero R, Carnevale J. Surgical crown lengthening: a 12-month clinical wound healing study. *J Periodontol* 2001;72:841–848.

27. Bragger U, Lauchenauer D. Surgical lengthening of the crown. *J Clin Periodontol* 1992;19:58–63.

28. Listgarten MA. Periodontal tissue repair over surgically exposed dentin and cementum surfaces. International Association for Dental Research, 49th General Meeting, 1971, Abstract 473.

TAKE-HOME POINTS

A. The attachment apparatus of a human tooth [1] (Figure 3.2.21) is composed of the following elements.

1. An epithelial attachment that attaches the enamel surface with hemidesmosomes.
2. A connective tissue attachment made of type I collagen fibers and Sharpey fibers inserting into the cementum at a 90-degree angle.
3. Alveolar bone covered by bundle bone on its inner surface and periosteum on its outer surface.
4. A periodontal ligament with type I and III collagen fiber bundles and Sharpey fibers inserted in the alveolar bone and the cementum.
5. Cementum overlying dentin on the root surface. Gargiulo et al. [2] found great consistency in the distance between the bone alveolar crest and the bottom of the sulcus in human dentitions. They called this area of the attachment apparatus of the tooth the *dentogingival junction*, made of an epithelial attachment coronally and a connective tissue attachment apically. Their study determined an average dimension of 0.97 mm for the epithelial attachment and 1.07 mm for the connective tissue attachment. The combined dimension of these two structures was called thereafter *biologic width* [3] and averages 2.04 mm according to the findings of Gargiulo et al. [2]. Nevins and Skurow [4] include the space occupied by the gingival sulcus (at least 1 mm) in addition to the epithelial and connective tissue attachment space and therefore estimate that biologic width measures a minimum of 3 mm.

B. The goals of the crown lengthening procedure include increasing the dimension of the clinical crown, maintaining or re-creating favorable periodontal conditions, establishing appropriate biologic width, creating adequate ferrule effect for anterior teeth, and aiding in the overall delivery of prosthetic restorations. There are two types of crown lengthening: functional and esthetic.

Functional crown lengthening is indicated when the clinical crown is too short to provide sufficient retention for an overlying crown [5] (Figure 3.2.22A). In the absence of crown lengthening, the restorative margin will impinge on the biologic width and produce an inflammatory response, resulting in loss of bone and connective tissue attachment as well as apical migration of the epithelial attachment. The goal of the crown lengthening procedure is to expose more sound tooth structure when wear, caries, or fracture have altered tooth integrity [3,4,6] (Figure 3.2.22B). As a result, the prosthetic margin can be placed supragingivally or intrasulcularly, enhancing the quality of the restoration and facilitating access for oral hygiene (Figure 3.2.22C). To achieve this objective, a space of at least 3 mm

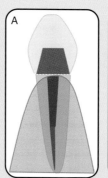
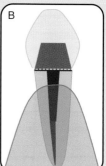
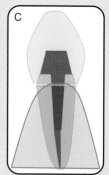

Figure 3.2.22   (A) Initial situation: inadequate prosthetic margin, lack of prosthetic retention. (B) A crown lengthening is performed; some sound tooth structure is exposed. (C) Final situation: the prosthetic margin is moved apically, adequate retention is provided, and the biologic width is preserved.

Figure 3.2.21   The attachment apparatus of a human tooth.

must be created between the preparation margin and the alveolar bony crest; 2 mm are devoted to the reestablishment of the biologic width, and 1 mm of intrasulcular tooth structure is available for crown retention. Many authors advocate the exposure of further tooth surface (4–5 mm) to provide more retention for the restoration [7,8]. In addition, it has been described that the presence of ≥2 mm of tooth structure available for the prosthetic crown to encircle is beneficial to the structural integrity of the tooth. This so-called ferrule effect improves fracture resistance of endodontically treated anterior teeth [9,10] (Figure 3.2.22C).

This ferrule effect is needed for anterior teeth that have an extra component that make the tooth a two-piece unit instead of a one piece, such as a core or a post and core. This 2 mm of solid tooth structure beneath the core will help direct the forces of occlusion toward the periodontal ligament and reduce the stress on the post or core interface, thus preventing cement fatigue of the restoration and dislodgment over time (Figure 3.2.22A–C).

Esthetic crown lengthening has a cosmetic goal. It is performed in the following situations.

1. Short clinical crowns. In this situation, the periodontium and the skeletal bases are normal. The tooth is shorter because of attrition. Sometimes the tooth keeps on erupting as wear reduces its length. Therefore, the width of keratinized tissue continuously increases and results in an excessive gingival display that can be corrected by esthetic crown lengthening [5]. However, if eruption does not happen in conjunction with attrition, a loss of vertical dimension will occur. In this situation, treatment to restore the vertical dimension will be indicated and crown lengthening of a functional rather than an esthetic nature will be required.

2. Excessive gingival display in the esthetic area (also called "gummy smile"). It can be caused by delayed passive eruption when the attachment apparatus fails to establish properly around the tooth [11]. The clinical crown can appear too short because of an excess of keratinized gingiva when the attachment apparatus is positioned too coronally on the anatomic crown or when the two phenomena are combined.

Gingival enlargement induced by medications (such as calcium channel blockers, phenytoin, and

cyclosporine among others) or orthodontic treatment can be surgically managed once the etiology is corrected (replacement of the medication, removal of braces). These situations are managed most of the time with gingivectomy without bone recontouring, the goal of which is both esthetic and functional. Excessive gingival display caused by hereditary gingival fibromatosis and vertical maxillary excess can also be treated with esthetic crown lengthening, although it might not be sufficient to entirely treat the problem. For instance, vertical maxillary excess most of the time requires orthognathic surgery in addition to crown lengthening.

C. Crown lengthening is indicated in the following situations [1,2].

- Caries extending under the gingival line: crown lengthening will provide better access for removing caries and will simplify the restoration (i.e. having a dry field for bonding, having an intrasulcular or supragingival prosthetic margin).
- Tooth fracture: the amount of tooth structure left might be insufficient for retention of the restorative material or the crown.
- Existing restoration impinging on the biologic width: the violation of biologic width generates chronic inflammation that leads to periodontal ligament destruction. Space must be re-created for the establishment of the epithelial and connective tissue attachment and crown retention.
- Lack of available tooth structure for prosthetic retention or lack of ferrule effect.
- Improved esthetic in the presence of short clinical crowns or excessive gingival display. There is not necessarily a functional need.

Crown lengthening is contraindicated in the following situations [12].

- Nonrestorable tooth.
- Unfavorable crown-to-root ratio: this would compromise the long-term prognosis of the tooth and increase the risk of tooth fracture (blunted roots, history of apicoectomies).
- Root proximity: this mainly concerns the interproximal space between the first and second maxillary molar where the distobuccal root of the first molar can be closely located to the mesiobuccal root of the second molar. A thin amount of interproximal bone makes ostectomy infeasible

and increases the chance of damaging the integrity of both roots.

- Exposure of the furcation for multirooted teeth: if the ostectomy generates a furcation involvement, the long-term prognosis of the tooth is compromised. An alternative approach such as root resection or tooth hemisection should be considered.
- Improper oral hygiene and lack of patient cooperation.

D. Crown lengthening can be performed in two different ways.

Surgical Crown Lengthening

1. A preoperative consultation is performed to review the patient's past medical history, detect contraindications to surgery, and determine the restorability of the tooth. Clinical and radiographic findings will allow the practitioner to determine the amount of crown lengthening needed. The tooth should ideally be prepared and have a temporary restoration to better evaluate the final prosthetic margin (Figure 3.2.23A). Premedication (antibiotics, sedative, analgesic medication) should be prescribed as needed.
2. Surgical procedure: the temporary restoration is removed and the excess of cement washed away. An intrasulcular or submarginal incision is performed to the crestal bone (submarginal incision is preferred in the presence of adequate amount of keratinized tissue). A vertical releasing incision might be considered to enhance surgical access.

Then a full-thickness flap is elevated to expose the cortical bone; soft tissue tags are removed if present (Figure 3.2.23B). The distance from the crestal bone to the prosthetic margin is measured to determine where and how much ostectomy is needed (removal of the supporting bone next to a tooth). Ostectomy is performed with an end-cutting bur or bone chisels so that the desired amount of tooth structure is exposed (see Question B) (Figure 3.2.23C). One should ensure that a positive architecture (buccal and/or lingual margin of bone apical to the proximal margin of bone) is maintained or reestablished to prevent pocket formation [13,14]. An osteoplasty (removal of nonsupporting bone) is frequently needed to remove "widow's peaks" and re-create a bony contour favorable to a healthy gingival architecture. Exposed root surfaces should be scaled and root planed. The flap is eventually apically positioned or repositioned at the level of the new bone crest and sutured with vertical mattress sutures that will prevent the movement of the flap in a mesiodistal or apico/coronal direction. The temporary crown is cemented back on the tooth (Figure 3.2.23D). A surgical dressing (e.g. Coe-Pak) can be placed over the surgical site.

3. Postoperative care: postoperative instructions (including oral hygiene instructions) are delivered to the patient and an ice pack is placed adjacent to the surgical site. Pain medications (ibuprofen or acetaminophen) and a 0.12% chlorhexidine mouthwash are prescribed. Antibiotics can also be prescribed, although they are not mandatory

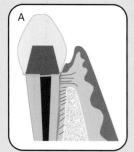 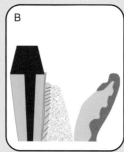 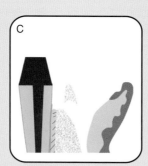 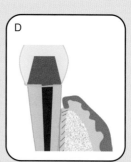 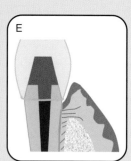

Figure 3.2.23   (A) Preoperative situation: inadequate prosthetic margin, lack of prosthetic retention. (B) A full-thickness flap is elevated, cortical bone is exposed. (C) Ostectomy is performed to expose adequate sound tooth structure. (D) The flap is apically repositioned. (E) Final restoration: the epithelial and connective tissue attachment is reestablished. The prosthetic margin stands on sound tooth structure with adequate retention.

for a healthy patient. The patient should be seen for a postoperative visit and suture removal at 7–10 days post surgery and before the final prosthetic restoration (Figure 3.2.23E).

Orthodontic Extrusion [15]

A bracket is bonded on the crown and vertical forces are applied to force the eruption of the tooth until the appropriate amount of supragingival tooth structure is exposed. This technique is mainly used in the maxillary anterior sextant to preserve the gingival contour.

E. Evidence has shown that biologic width reestablishes after crown lengthening in about six months [16]. However, the biologic mechanisms involved in the re-creation of epithelial and connective tissue attachment after periodontal flap surgery is still not completely understood. There is a substantial consensus regarding reestablishment of the epithelial attachment: a long junctional epithelium will form along the root-planed surface to the apical level of root planing [17,18]. Reestablishment of the connective tissue attachment is more controversial. Some authors believe it re-forms coronal to the apical level of root planing [19], whereas some others consider it re-creates apical to the apical level of root planing by crestal resorption of the alveolar bone [20,21]. This divergence in opinion explains why some authors expose more tooth structure above the crestal bone than others.

In any situation, general principles of osseous resective surgery should be applied to prevent pocket formation [13,22]. Re-creation of a positive architecture and a scalloped bony contour without

ledges, notches, and peaks will allow appropriate soft tissue healing. Widow's peaks should be removed carefully, and the root surface should be root-planed thoroughly to prevent reattachment of the attachment apparatus too coronally [23] which might require retreatment [21].

F. It has been described that the gingival margin tends to move coronally over a year after a flap procedure with bone recontouring [24,25] and crown lengthening [19] to eventually stabilize in this position [25]. In a human study, Pontoriero and Carnevale [26] described a 3-mm coronal displacement of the gingival margin after one year, with most of the coronal displacement occurring within the first month of healing (about 2 mm). Gingival displacement is influenced by multiple parameters including gingival biotype and the magnitude of ostectomy performed [16]. Bragger and Lauchenauer [27] did not observe coronal displacement of the gingival margin over time in most cases and reported that the gingival margin position remained stable from six weeks to six months.

As a consequence, a healing period should be respected before final prosthetic restoration to allow the gingival contour to reestablish and stabilize. The final restoration should not be performed sooner than six weeks post surgery to allow stabilization of the gingival margin [27] and to obtain repair of the attachment apparatus [28]. In certain situations, such as the presence of a thin gingival biotype or an esthetic area, more time might be needed to observe gingival margin stabilization and proceed with the permanent restoration [26,27].

Case 3

Flap Osseous Surgery

CASE STORY

Julie is a 34-year-old women who presented to the Department of Endodontics for assessment of a painful tooth. Following examination a periodontal consult was requested. Prior to this appointment she was seen regularly for hygiene appointments at a community dental clinic.

LEARNING GOALS AND OBJECTIVES

- To diagnose severe periodontal disease and identify the indications for flap osseous surgery (FOS) as opposed to other surgical techniques
- To identify preoperatively any conditions that may compromise the final outcome of this procedure
- To be introduced to a surgical technique used to perform FOS
- Understand postoperative complications and their management

Medical History

The patient was in good health. She indicated that as a child she was diagnosed with a heart murmur. A recent examination by her physician revealed that the murmur was no longer audible and thus no antibiotic prophylaxis was required. A mild allergic reaction to penicillin recently indicated sensitivity to this drug class. She suffered from seasonal allergies and a mild form of asthma for which she did not take any medication. For several months she had been dealing with mild to moderate anxiety.

Review of Systems

- Vital signs
  - Blood pressure: 128/75 mmHg
  - Pulse rate: 70 beats/minute (regular)

Social History

The patient did not drink alcohol nor did she consume recreational drugs. She exercised regularly and was a nonsmoker.

Extraoral Examination

No major significant findings. The patient had no masses or swelling and the temporomandibular joints were within normal limits. Mild tenderness of the left masseter and temporalis muscles was recorded.

Intraoral Examination

- The soft tissues of the mouth including the tongue appeared normal. The oral cancer screen was negative.
- The gingival examination revealed generalized mild to moderate marginal erythema, with areas of severe inflammation (Figure 3.3.1). Bleeding on probing was generalized and significant.
- A hard tissue examination was negative for caries.
- A mild generalized discomfort on percussion of the teeth was noted.
- A full periodontal charting was completed (Figure 3.3.2).

Radiographic Examination

A full-mouth series of radiographs were obtained. There was moderate localized bone loss on the D of tooth #2, localized vertical defects on the distal of teeth #4, #5, and #6 and on the medial of #30 and #31 (Figure 3.3.3).

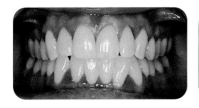
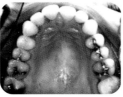

Figure 3.3.1 Intraoral photos of both maxillary and mandibular teeth in occlusion and occlusal view of maxillary arch.

Occlusion

The patient's occlusion was considered class I with no occlusal interferences evident. Crowding of the mandibular anterior teeth was recorded. Mutually protected occlusion was evident upon examination.

Treatment Plan

Recommendations were made to the patient to follow up with her primary care physician regarding her anxiety. Our concern was not only for her mental well-being but also for her clenching and poor oral hygiene that could be a result of this condition.

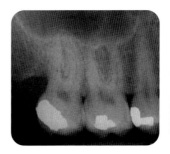
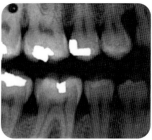

Figure 3.3.3 Preoperative radiographic evaluation (periapical and bitewings in the maxillary right quadrant).

A transitional night guard was provided to the patient and was ultimately replaced with a permanent one following treatment. Endodontic consultations were required to establish a comprehensive treatment plan. Full-mouth radiographs and plaque accumulation analysis (disclosing solution) were performed.

The final treatment plan included extensive periodontal surgical treatment as well as protecting the teeth and periodontium from occlusal trauma.

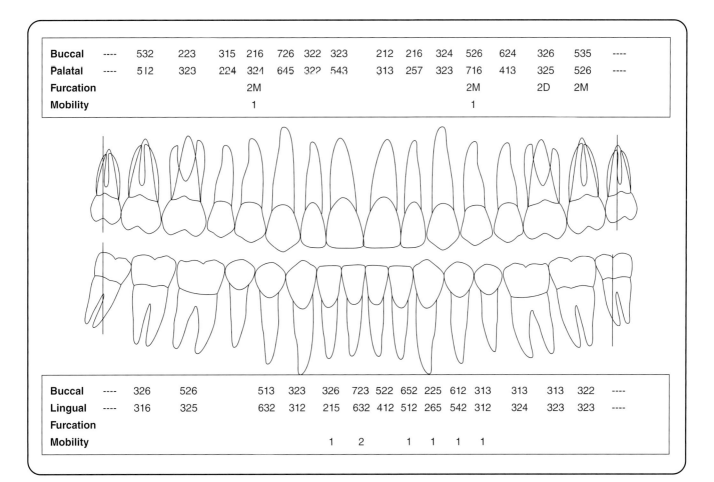

Buccal	----	532	223	315	216	726	322	323	212	216	324	526	624	326	535	----
Palatal	----	512	323	224	324	645	322	543	313	257	323	716	413	325	526	----
Furcation					2M							2M		2D	2M	
Mobility					1							1				

Buccal	----	326	526		513	323	326	723	522	652	225	612	313	313	313	322	----
Lingual	----	316	325		632	312	215	632	412	512	265	542	312	324	323	323	----
Furcation																
Mobility							1	2		1	1	1	1			

Figure 3.3.2 Probing pocket depth measurements (following phase 1 therapy).

Treatment

This patient received oral hygiene instruction and two complete scaling and root planing sessions prior to surgical therapy. A transitional occlusal protective appliance (acrylic) was provided. The patient was reevaluated to determine the effectiveness of phase 1 therapy and to see if she demonstrated good oral hygiene practices. Pocket depths shown were recorded following phase 1 therapy. Surgical therapy then commenced.

Preoperative Consultation

The medical history was reviewed. Her blood pressure was monitored. The consent form addressing benefits and risks associated with the procedure was reviewed with the patient. Accessibility to the surgical site was clinically assessed. Ibuprofen 600 mg (every four to six hours as needed for pain), Vicoden ES (every six hours as needed for pain), and Peridex 0.12% b.i.d. were prescribed.

Flap Osseous Procedure (Figures 3.3.4 and 3.3.5)

A procedural sedation and analgesia, middle superior alveolar nerve block, greater palatine nerve block, and local infiltrations were achieved with lidocaine 2% (epinephrine 1:100 000). Preoperative views of tissues are illustrated in Figure 3.3.6A,B. A submarginal incision was made in a scalloped fashion in all interproximal regions (Figure 3.3.6C,D) A full-thickness flap in the maxillary right quadrant was elevated buccally and lingually from mesial of tooth #6 to distal of #2 (Figure 3.3.6E,F). The teeth in this region were thoroughly scaled and root planed. Complete degranulation of all bony defects followed. A rotary finishing bur was used to reduce the concavity of the furcation on mesial tooth #5 and conservatively recontour surrounding bone to produce a positive architecture (Figure 3.3.6G–J). A distal wedge procedure was performed on tooth #2 (Figure 3.3.6K). The surgical site was thoroughly rinsed with sterile saline and the flap was

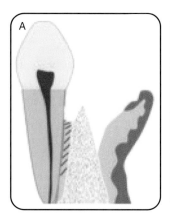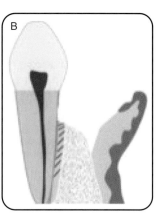

Figure 3.3.5 (A) Exposed alveolar bone demonstrating sharp irregular peaks. (B) Smoothing of the irregular bone structure to provide an environment that promotes pocket reduction.

reapproximated and then sutured (Figure 3.3.6L). External vertical mattress sutures were placed to apically position the tissue. Healing was uneventful thereafter.

Discussion

FOS is a predictable procedure that will reduce pocket depths and provide a healthy architecture (see Figures 3.3.4 and 3.3.5) to the surrounding bone and tissue such that the patient can now access these sites for cleaning.

Healthy architecture can be defined as when alveolar bone is consistently more coronal on the interproximal surfaces than on the facial and lingual surface and there exists a smooth, flowing alveolar bone anatomy such that the interproximal surfaces are flat leading to a spillway buccally and lingually. This technique is most appropriate for patients with early to moderate bone loss (2–3 mm) with moderate-length root trunks [1] that have bony defects with one or two walls. Patients with deep intrabony defects are not candidates for FOS. In order to achieve this positive architecture, excessive bone would have to be removed such that the survival of the teeth could be compromised [2].

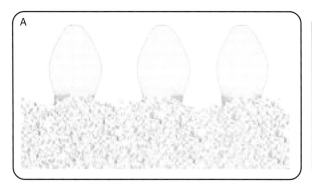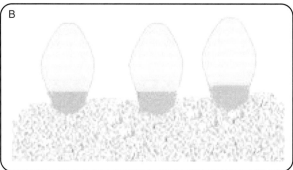

Figure 3.3.4 (A) Exposed alveolar bone and teeth demonstrating negative architecture. (B) Positive architecture created by osteoplasty and ostectomy.

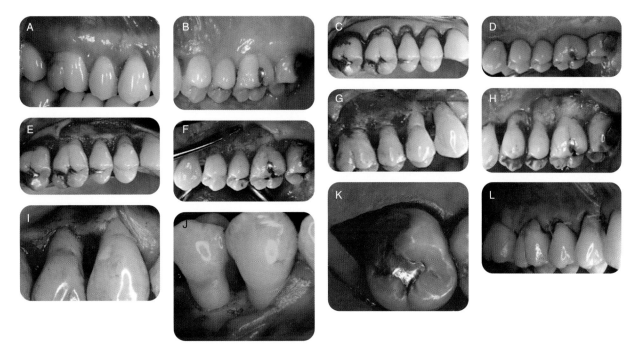

Figure 3.3.6 (A–L) Intraoral surgical photos.

The surgery was uneventful. The patient was seen for postoperative visits at one week to remove the sutures and at six weeks. She did not complain of significant postoperative tooth sensitivity that may occur due to the exposure of root cementum. Following three months of healing a permanent acrylic night guard was provided for the patient.

After six months, periapical and bitewing radiographs were taken to assess this region (Figure 3.3.7). Since regenerative periodontal procedures were performed elsewhere, the radiographs allowed us to assess these areas as well (i.e. opposing arch).

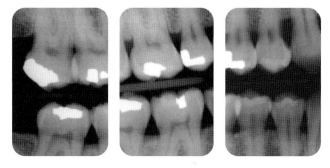

Figure 3.3.7 Vertical bitewings following six months of healing.

Self-Study Questions

A. What is the rationale for performing a FOS?

B. What are the techniques employed?

C. What other procedures are often required at the time of FOS?

D. What are the determinants of success of FOS?

E. What alterations in technique are required due to unique anatomy? How do you manage these?

F. What are the possible major complications associated with FOS? How do you manage these complications?

G. What are the possible minor complications associated with FOS? How do you manage these complications?

Answers located at the end of the chapter.

References

1. Ochsenbein C, Bohannan HM. The palatal approach to osseous surgery. II. Clinical application. *J Periodontol* 1964;35:54–68.
2. Newman MG, Takei HH, Klokkevold PR, Carranza FA (eds). *Carranza's Clinical Periodontology*, 10th edn. St. Louis, MO: Saunders Elsevier, 2006.
3. Easley J. Methods of determining alveolar osseous form. *J Periodontol* 1967;38:112–118.
4. Kaldahl WB, Kalkwarf KL, Patil KD, et al. Long-term evaluation of periodontal therapy. I. Response to four therapeutic modalities. *J Periodontol* 1996;67:93–102.
5. Selipsky HS. Osseous surgery: how much need we compromise? *Dent Clin North Am* 1976;20:79–106.
6. Tibbetts L, Ochsenbein C, Loughlin D. The lingual approach to osseous surgery. *J Periodontol* 1976;20:61–78.
7. Kaldahl WB, Kalkwarf KL, Patil KD, et al. Evaluation of four modalities of periodontal therapy: mean probing depth, probing attachment level and recession changes. *J Periodontol* 1988;59:783–793.
8. Knowles J, Burgett F, Nissle R, et al. Results of periodontal treatment related to pocket depth and attachment level: eight years. *J Periodontol* 1979;50:225–233.
9. Schluger S. Osseous resection: a basic principle in periodontal surgery. *Oral Surg* 1949;2:316–325.
10. Goldman H, Cohen D. The intrabony pocket: classification and treatment. *J Periodontol* 1958;29:272–291.
11. Friedman N. Periodontal osseous surgery: osteoplasty and osteoectomy. *J Periodontol* 1955;26:257–269.
12. Nabers CL. Repositioning the attached gingiva. *J Periodontol* 1954;25:38–39.
13. Donnenfeld OW, Marks RM, Glickman I. The apically repositioned flap: a clinical study. *J Periodontol* 1964;35:381–387.
14. Robinson RE. The distal wedge operation. *Periodontics* 1966;4:256–264.
15. Fracol M, Dorfman R, Janes L, et al. The surgical impact of E-cigarettes: a case report and review of the current literature. *Arch Plast Surg* 2017;44:477–481.
16. Nyman S, Lindhe J, Rosling B. Periodontal surgery in plaque-infected dentitions. *J Clin Periodontol* 1977;4(4):240–249.
17. Froum SJ, Coran M, Thaller B, et al. Periodontal healing following open debridement flap procedures. I. Clinical assessment of soft tissue and osseous repair. *J Periodontol* 1982;53(1):8–14.
18. Black GV. Surgical treatment of pockets. In: Black AD (ed.) *Special Dental Pathology*, 3rd edn. Chicago: Medico Dental, 1917.
19. Garguilo AW, Wentz FM, Orban B. Dimensions and relations of the dentogingival junction in humans. *J Periodontol* 1961;32:261–267.
20. Ochsenbein C, Bohannan HM. The palatal approach to osseous surgery. I. Rationale. *J Periodontol* 1963; 34:60–68.
21. Sachs HA, Farnoush A, Checchi L, Joseph CE. Current status of periodontal dressings. *J Periodontol* 1984;55(12): 689–696.
22. Penmetsa GS, Ramya Teja G, Anudeep M, Chaitanya A. Evaluation of post operative healing response and patient comfort with two periodontal dressings, ResoPac and CoePak, following periodontal flap surgery: a comparative clinical study. *J Biomed Pharm Res* 2017;6(2). https://jbpr.in/index.php/jbpr/article/view/64
23. Mittal S, Jain S. Tooth splinting: an update. *Heal Talk* 2013;5:38–39.

TAKE-HOME POINTS

A. Inflammatory periodontal disease if left untreated will lead to destruction of the tooth-supporting bone. The deformities are rarely uniform and can vary in severity and location from one tooth to the next. As can be appreciated from the images, the soft tissue architecture does not necessarily have to follow the bone architecture. Bone loss can be classified as "horizontal," "vertical," and/or a combination of both. The severity, morphology, and position of the defect will determine the technique of FOS and whether or not regenerative therapy (guided tissue regeneration) should be considered.

Ultimately this loss of bone leads to deep pockets, which then become a harbor for pathogenic bacteria that the patient is unable to access. It has also been suggested that the change in the normal anatomy of the alveolar bone predisposes patients to the recurrence of pocket depth postsurgically [3]. In order to achieve the desired result of pocket depth reduction this technique is usually combined with apical flap repositioning.

In summary, FOS provides pocket depth reduction, access for surgeon and patient to clean the sulcus of pathogenic bacteria, and a positive bone and soft tissue architecture that enhances the ability of the site to be cleaned [4–6]. The literature fully supports the fact that FOS is the most predictable pocket reduction technique [4,7,8].

B. Schluger [9] first introduced the original technique that outlines the surgical principles of FOS in 1949. Prior to this, gingivectomy was the preferred surgical method of dealing with deep pockets.

Goldman and Cohen [10] first classified types of infrabony osseous defect according to the number of remaining walls: three, two or one osseous walls and combinations thereof. In combination defects they determined that the apical parts may have more walls than coronal parts. This classification now allows us to communicate the severity of the infrabony defect and assign the most successful treatment for each category. Variations of this technique have been introduced since then and include lingual ramping of the bone in the posterior mandible [6] and palatal ramping in the posterior maxilla [1].

Bone manipulation in FOS involves osteoplasty and ostectomy (see Figures 3.3.4 and 3.3.5) [11]. Osteoplasty refers to reshaping the bone without removing tooth-supporting bone. Ostectomy includes the removal of tooth-supporting bone. One or both of these procedures may be required for optimal outcomes.

The technique of osseous recontouring involves four basic steps: vertical grooving, radicular blending, flattening of interdental bone, and ostectomy [2].

1. Vertical grooving is the first step of the resective process. It provides continuity from the interproximal surface onto the radicular surface. This step is usually performed with rotary instruments, such as round carbide burs or diamonds.
2. Radicular blending, the second step of the osseous reshaping technique, is an attempt to gradualize the bone over the entire radicular surface. This provides a smooth blended surface for good flap adaptation.
3. Flattening of the interdental bone is indicated when interproximal bone levels vary horizontally.
4. The final step is ostectomy. Bone removal is minimal but necessary to provide a sound, regular base for the gingival tissue to follow. This step involves the removal of small bony discrepancies on the gingival line angles of teeth (widow's peaks).

Following osseous recontouring, the open flaps should be thoroughly rinsed with sterile saline and the flaps apically repositioned [12,13] (see Figure 3.3.6L).

Healing of the surgical site is usually uneventful. Normally the flaps attach to the underlying bone in 14–21 days [2]. Maturation and remodeling can continue for up to six months. The literature supports the idea that six weeks of healing should pass before starting dental restorations [2].

C. Depending on the severity of the bone defect and the amount of remaining keratinized gingiva, a scalloped submarginal incision is made to remove the excess gingival tissue in order to prevent pocket re-formation. Usually this is required on the palatal aspects of maxillary teeth where apical repositioning is not possible. Excess subepithelial connective tissue is often removed from this region in order to facilitate closer adaptation of the tissues to the tooth.

A third procedure often required in this region is the distal wedge [14]. The objectives of this treatment are to obtain access to the bone, to preserve and utilize attached gingival tissue, to eliminate the pocket by wound closure, to decrease the healing period, and to minimize periodontal pocket recurrence of any proximal periodontal pocket (see Figure 3.3.6K). The three classical distal wedge operations include the triangular, the square, and the linear. Each has their own indication but essentially differ on the quantity of attached gingiva that is removed [14].

If it has been determined that the vertical defect is too severe for treatment with FOS, other treatment modalities may have to be added to the procedure in order to facilitate ideal treatment. One may want to consider a regenerative procedure such as guided tissue regeneration or a root resection or hemisection procedure if a particular root is not salvageable or furcation involvement is severe. If the bone loss is too severe, extraction of the tooth may be the only option.

D. Some determinants promoting success have been reported in the literature and include the following.

1. Absence of medical conditions (including systemic diseases such as diabetes, bisphosphonate therapy, irradiation, smoking and vaping) [15]. The patient should be referred to a physician if there is any significant medical condition reported during the preoperative examination.
2. Appropriate patient and site selection are essential for predicable long-term success of FOS.

Thorough debridement of granulation tissue as well as appropriate handling of the hard and soft tissue is critical.

3. Even if all the surgical principles are closely adhered to, if the patient is not competent with their oral hygiene practices this treatment is likely to fail. A study by Nyman et al. [16] covered postoperative results of treatment following five methods of surgical pocket elimination in patients who were not recalled for maintenance. In patients who were unable to meet the requirements for proper oral hygiene, treatment of periodontitis failed irrespective of the surgical technique used for pocket elimination. Other studies looking at the role plaque control plays in the predictability of FOS support these finding [17].

E. However, more than any other surgical technique, osseous resective surgery is performed at the expense of bony tissue and attachment level [2,18,19]. If excessive bone is removed in order to facilitate a positive architecture, there exists no remediation for this error. The patient may then experience significant root sensitivity and mobility. As mentioned earlier, studies demonstrate that we do not have to obtain ideal architecture of the bone if it means compromising adjacent teeth excessively [5,20]. Furthermore, if the furcation is exposed the likelihood of further progression of periodontal disease is assured.

If the surgery involves esthetic regions, FOS may have to be modified to a palatal approach or the patient may have to be treated conservatively with scaling and root planing. If FOS is performed in esthetic regions, "black triangles" can appear between the teeth and these can be very difficult to correct.

Poor suturing technique, such that the tissue is not apically repositioned, may lead to excessive pocket depth again. The only solution to this would be a gingivectomy if the bony architecture has not changed. Some practitioners place a surgical dressing over the surgical site to maintain pressure on the tissue to remain more apical [21,22].

One of the most common complaints following FOS is root sensitivity and tooth mobility. Root sensitivity can generally be treated with over-the-counter toothpastes that contain desensitizers or in-office application of fluoride pastes. Rarely would endodontic treatment be necessary to deal with this issue. As far as tooth mobility is concerned, studies demonstrate that within one year of the surgery the mobility of these teeth will return to their presurgical levels [5].

Food accumulation in the now open embrasures may also be an issue. The patient needs to be instructed on the use of alternative hygiene devices such as the proxy brush in order to effectively clean interproximally.

F.
- Infection: antibiotics such as penicillin, amoxicillin, clindamycin, azithromycin, or metronidazole can be used. If the infection cannot be controlled with antibiotics, referral to the appropriate specialist is necessary. To reduce the chances of postoperative infections it is important to rinse under the flaps with sterile saline in order to remove debris that has accumulated.
- Bleeding: instruct the patient to apply pressure to the area and then reassess. If this is not successful, arrangements should be made to see the patient as soon as possible.
- Nerve paresthesia, dysesthesia: damage to the mental nerve is possible when FOS is performed in the mandible. If the surgeon did not expose the nerve, stretching of the tissue and the nerve in this region is the most likely cause. Follow the patient closely until paresthesia has diminished. At each follow-up appointment a diagram should be made that indicates the regions that have regained feeling.

G.
- Residual root sensitivity: warning the patient of this likely outcome is essential. Topical placement of fluoride varnish and daily use of desensitizing toothpastes have been helpful.
- Mobile teeth: as long as there is at least 50% or more bone coverage over roots, mobility will likely increase following surgery and then tighten up in the months following. If teeth continue to be painful due to the mobility, consideration should be given to temporary extracoronal splinting [23].
- Open embrasures are a permanent and deliberate outcome of FOS to allow for cleansibility. Warn patients of this outcome and that they should use alternative aids such as a proxy brush to help them.

Case 4

Root Resection

CASE STORY

A 65-year-old Caucasian male had been referred by his general dentist with a chief complaint of "pain and bleeding of my gums in the upper right back area with deep pockets." He noted there was bleeding when flossing as well as swelling and pain in this region.

LEARNING GOALS AND OBJECTIVES

■ To gain an understanding of the underlying and contributing etiologic factors resulting in furcation involvement
■ To understand a differential treatment plan and identify teeth suitable for root resection therapy

Medical History

There were no contributing medical problems, and the patient had no known allergies. Upon further questioning the patient reported that he was not taking any prescription medications or naturopathic remedies/supplements.

Review of Systems

• Vital signs
  o Blood pressure: 124/76 mmHg
  o Pulse rate: 68 beats/minute (regular)
  o Respiratory rate: 14 breaths/minute
  o Temperature: 37°C

Social History

The patient drank alcohol "socially" (i.e. at parties and/or one to two drinks on the weekend). The patient had never been a smoker and did not use any tobacco products. The patient did not use recreational or illicit street drugs. He was a retired nurse who presently volunteered at a local hospital.

Extraoral Examination

The patient was obese (body mass index 32), and he did not exhibit any skeletal discrepancies or deformation of extremities. There were no visible or palpable nodal involvements throughout the head and neck region. The patient displayed a unilateral functional clicking of the right temporomandibular joint but no crepitation or tenderness of the masticatory muscles.

Intraoral Examination

All soft tissues of the mouth including mucosal surfaces, oropharynx, tongue surfaces, and floor of the mouth appeared to be within normal limits. The gingiva displayed mild to moderate inflammation and generalized slight/moderate marginal erythema. The patient did not report any tactile sensitivity, discomfort with percussion, or apical palpation tenderness. The patient explained that he had been experiencing sensitivity to hot and cold in the upper left region. Observation of plaque control techniques revealed inadequate brushing and flossing. He demonstrated a scrub technique of brushing, and he did not adapt the floss to the proximal sides of the teeth and line angles [1,2]. Figures 3.4.1 and 3.4.2 offer an overview.

Occlusion

There were no occlusal discrepancies or interferences in working and nonworking excursions. The patient did not report habitual bruxing or clenching, either diurnal or nocturnal, although he displayed mild generalized attrition and wear facets.

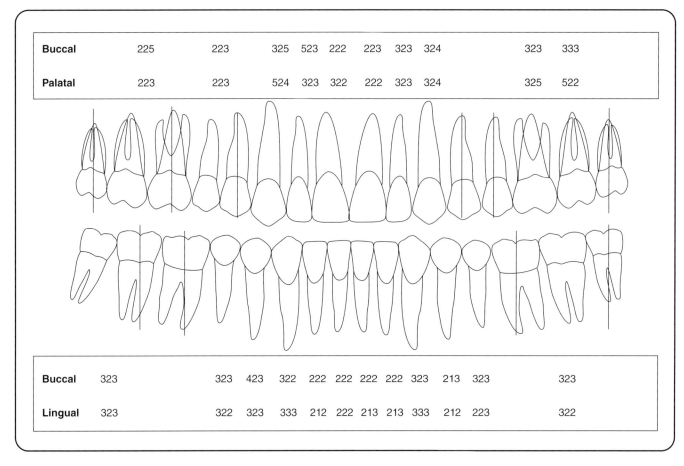

Buccal	225	223	325	523	222	223	323	324		323	333
Palatal	223	223	524	323	322	222	323	324		325	522

Buccal	323		323	423	322	222	222	222	222	323	213	323		323
Lingual	323		322	323	333	212	222	213	213	333	212	223		322

Figure 3.4.1 Periodontal charting.

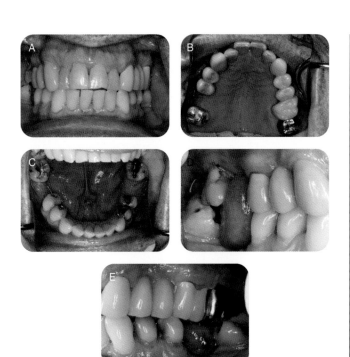

Figure 3.4.2 Intraoral initial visit. (A) frontal view; (B) maxillary view; (C) mandibular view; (D) right lateral; (E) left lateral.

Radiographic Examination

Figures 3.4.3 and 3.4.4 show part of the radiographic examination.

Diagnosis

Using the 2017 Classification of Periodontal and Peri-Implant Diseases and Conditions, the patient exhibited stage 3, grade B periodontitis, recession Cairo type 2 and type 3 (RT2, RT3) defects, and evidence of occlusal trauma (attrition and wear facets). Tooth #14 exhibited an over-contoured crown.

Treatment Plan

Additional consultations were as follows

1. Consultation with the patient's general dentist regarding general restorative needs and specifically the restoration of tooth #14 following root resection therapy.
2. Endodontic evaluation of tooth #14 to confirm the integrity of the existing root canal therapy.

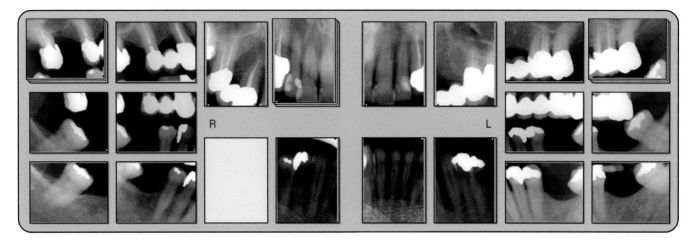

Figure 3.4.3 Complete-mouth series radiographs.

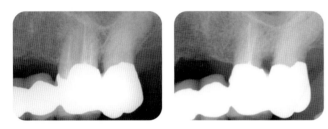

Figure 3.4.4 Radiographs of #14 DB before (left) and after (right) root resection.

Phase 1

The first phase of therapy consisted of plaque control instruction using the Bass technique of brushing and the adapted horizontal flossing technique [1,2]. Scaling and root planing of maxillary right sextant (#6M, #7D) and maxillary left sextant (#14D, #15M), and generalized supragingival scaling and polishing were performed over two months (two or more visits) prior to reevaluation.

Reevaluation included the following.
1. Place the patient on a three-month, or less if needed, periodontal maintenance schedule pending periodontal status following localized scaling and root planing.
2. Consider surgical pocket reducing intervention (phase 2 surgical therapy) if localized areas do not respond adequately to scaling and root planing (i.e. persistent deep pockets).

Phase 2

Perform flap #14 with the following treatment options.
1. Distobuccal root resection of tooth #14.
2. Extraction of tooth #14 with ridge preservation and subsequent implant placement. As the decision to undergo extraction therapy would result in loss of the existing bridge, #11–14, a second implant would be required in the #12 position to create an

implant-supported bridge, #12-x-14, which might require guided bone regeneration in the area of tooth #12.
3. Gingival curettage and locally delivered antibiotic therapy.

Phase 3

The third phase would consist of crown recontouring to accommodate the resection, which would allow for adequate home care by the patient and the sealing of the root canal orifice.

Phase 4

1. Maintenance hygiene therapy
2. Periodic periodontal evaluations
3. Periodic restorative examinations

Treatment
Phase 1

The patient was seen for plaque control technique instruction [1,2] and scaling and root planing. After eight weeks the patient was reevaluated and displayed much improved home care techniques and significantly reduced gingival inflammation. The patient was placed on a three-month dental hygiene maintenance program. Surgical therapy was explained to treat tooth #14, as pocketing was deeper than could be managed with dental plaque removal techniques solely by the patient and, as a result, bleeding on probing persisted. Surgical options of root sectioning, gingival curettage, or extraction were presented to the patient. The patient elected to have flap surgery with sectioning of the distobuccal root of tooth #14. A consent form for surgery for tooth #14 and the adjacent teeth was obtained. The postoperative surgical instructions were explained and given to the patient.

Phase 2

The patient presented for a distobuccal root resection of tooth #14; there was no change in his medical history. His blood pressure was 135/85 mmHg, and clinical examination with a Nabers probe revealed a class II buccal and distal furcation on tooth #14. Anesthesia was obtained with lidocaine 2% (1:100 000 epinephrine) by buccal and palatal infiltration. Intrasulcular incisions were made around teeth #14 and #15 with a vertical releasing incision at the mesiobuccal line angle of tooth #14 (Figure 3.4.5A). A full-thickness mucoperiosteal flap was raised and the area was degranulated with a Younger-Good 7/8 curette. The buccal and distal class II furcation involvement (Figure 3.4.5B) on tooth #14 was visualized, and a fine diamond bur was used to section the distobuccal root at the fornices of the buccal and distal furcations (Figure 3.4.5C,D). After removing a portion of the buccal bony plate, the distobuccal root was removed with an elevator (Figure 3.4.5E–G). Scaling and root planing were performed to remove residual granulation tissue, and osteoplasty was done to assure adequate gingival contour to provide access for hygiene. A complete gutta percha seal was evident at the root canal orifice. Because of the thickness of the palatal mucosa, the underlying connective tissue was thinned. Mineralized freeze-dried bone allograft was placed in the socket, and a collagen membrane covered the graft (Figure 3.4.5H,I) The flaps were coapted with 5-0 chromic gut, single interrupted and vertical mattress sutures. Primary closure could not be achieved (Figure 3.4.5J,K). Postoperative instructions were again reviewed, and the patient appeared to have a good understanding of them. Prescriptions included 0.12% chlorhexidine gluconate 15 ml b.i.d. to be rinsed, plus 800 mg ibuprofen every six hours for the first three days and then as needed for comfort.

The patient presented for a postoperative appointment following root resection of tooth #14 (Figure 3.4.5L). There was no change in the patient's medical or dental history. The patient reported slight pain and swelling for the first few days following the procedure. The patient did not report bleeding, fever, or lymphadenopathy following surgery. The surgical site appeared to be healing normally with minimal inflammation and absence of suppuration. The sutures were removed, and the area was cleansed with 0.12% chlorhexidine. After an endodontic consultation, it was advised to remove a portion of the exposed gutta percha and replace it with a restorative material (glass ionomer: Fuji 2) to accomplish a better seal (Figure 3.4.5M).

Discussion

After a comprehensive intraoral examination and subsequent classification of Glickman class II buccal and distal furcation invasions of tooth #14, consideration was given to the appropriate therapy and the long-term prognosis of the tooth. The presence of a class II furcation involvement presents a distinct barrier for good oral hygiene with normal home care techniques for the patient and must be treated surgically to allow for maintenance. It has consistently been shown that if teeth with interproximal furcation involvements

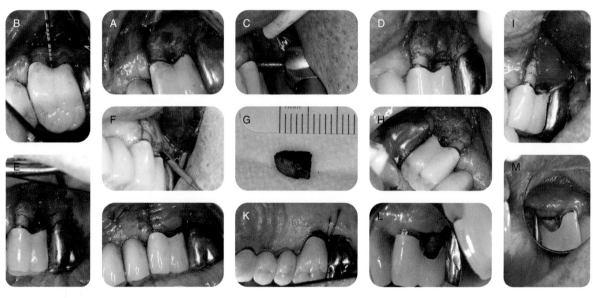

Figure 3.4.5 Root resection #14 DB.

are not treated definitively, the patient's teeth are eventually lost despite the patient's best efforts at home care [3–5].

Despite the numerous advances in guided tissue regeneration (GTR), limited evidence supports predictable regenerative treatment of class II furcation involvements in maxillary molars with respect to various clinical parameters, such as clinical attachment gain and reduced probing depth following therapy [6,7]. Few cases show complete resolution of class II furcations. Improvement to a grade I furcation is more common at best. Although several studies have been successful in showing that class II furcations are amenable to GTR, most are lacking in sample size and a strong level of evidence [8–10]. Additionally, interproximal furcation defects have been shown to be poorly responsive to an array of surgical modalities and less than those located on the buccal aspect [9].

In this case, in addition to considering GTR and root sectioning, the patient was informed of other procedures to treat the tooth, which included closed curettage, open flap debridement, or flap surgery with osseous contouring. The consideration of extraction with or without tooth replacement was discussed. The options for replacement included either removable or fixed partial prostheses (11-x-x-x-15), single implants to replace teeth #12, #13, and #14, or an implant-supported fixed prosthesis (12-x-14). All the procedures were explained in detail to the patient. The patient declined a removable prosthesis. A fixed partial denture was not recommended due to the long span supported by periodontally compromised abutment teeth. Both single implants and an implant-supported prosthesis would require ridge augmentation and a sinus elevation. The patient's choice was to retain the tooth and have root-resective therapy performed. The fact that root canal therapy had already been completed and it was not possible to predictably improve class II furcation defects with GTR indicated that a more predictable approach was that of root resection. Root sectioning therapy is a procedure to remove one of the roots from a multirooted tooth, usually molars. It is undertaken to create a soft tissue morphology that will allow the patient and clinician complete access for plaque removal. Although root-resective therapy can be performed on both maxillary and mandibular molars, greater longevity and lower failure rates have been associated with the maxillary molars [11,12]. When selecting which root is to be amputated, several factors play into the decision and are discussed later in this chapter. Ultimately, the root to be sectioned is the root

showing the least support to the tooth, the greatest attachment loss, and providing the best access for plaque control. In the maxilla, the distobuccal root is the most common, and it is usually the root with the least attachment [13].

It has also been shown that when performing a root resection, having the endodontic therapy completed in advance is favorable as in this case. A so-called nonvital approach is preferable and has been advocated in the literature [14]. If the decision is made to proceed with therapy while the tooth is vital, root canal therapy should be completed within a two-week window to increase the chance of success [15]. Many times, the decision to resect a root is made following flap reflection and degranulation. This affords the best opportunity for the operator to visualize and palpate the extent of the furcation involvement.

Although there are many reasons for failure of root-resected teeth cited in the literature, including root caries, endodontic failure, periodontal breakdown, and prosthetic problems, the most common etiology is root fracture [11,16]. Moreover, studies that have explored the origin of such root fractures reveal that parafunctional habits such as bruxism and clenching often remained unaddressed. This finding further emphasizes the importance of a thorough examination of the patient's occlusion at the initial examination. During the disease control phase, interferences should be eliminated, and habits should be addressed with an occlusal guard before surgical intervention.

Of equal importance to the appropriate occlusal adjustment at the outset of therapy is the contour of the root-resected tooth when it is restored prosthetically [17]. The prosthodontic literature has endorsed the need for full coronal coverage of these teeth due to the predisposition of endodontically treated root-resected teeth to fracture due to a lack of natural tooth support. The unique anatomy following such therapy calls for placement of an appropriately designed crown or the recontouring of an existing crown, as was the case with tooth #14. Reducing the occlusal table buccolingually and reducing cusp steepness is preferable on a root-sectioned tooth. An adequate emergence profile will allow access for the patient's plaque removal techniques. Fractures of root canal-treated teeth relate to the weakening of the tooth as a result of root canal therapy and/or after preparation.

If in this case exploratory flap surgery had revealed caries on the palatal root, grade II mobility following resection, a mesiobuccal root dehiscence, a deep grade II or III furcation involvement with the distobuccal and palatal roots, or other compromising findings, the decision to remove the tooth in an atraumatic fashion would have been taken. The patient had been informed of this possibility in advance of therapy. The patient was aware that in the event the tooth was untreatable, the alternative plan in this circumstance would involve a ridge preservation procedure, involving allograft and barrier membrane, in an effort to minimize future bone resorption, the possibility of a sinus elevation, and the placement of an implant in the future [18] (see Chapter 4).

Although the placement of implants has become a popular approach for replacing questionable teeth, studies have observed equal rates of success in root-resected teeth when compared with similar sites replaced by implant therapy [10]. Such studies empha-size the importance of appropriate case selection and technique in ensuring the high degree of success achieved for both modalities. In this case, the tooth was stable, the furcation invasions were confined primarily to the distobuccal root of tooth #14, and there was little or no furcation involvement of the mesial and palatal root. In addition, root canal therapy had previously been done and was determined to be successful. Although there was a full crown on the tooth before root

sectioning, it could be modified by recontouring and was not an esthetic problem for the patient. Thus, the decision to retain the tooth and do a root resection took into consideration all the parameters just described. It was also a better financial option for the patient than if the tooth were removed, guided bone regeneration (GBR) done, and an implant placed and restored. In addition, because GBR was done to regenerate bone in the socket of the distofacial root, should an implant need to be placed in the future, the bone volume would not be compromised as a result of the root section.

In conclusion, clinicians must look not only at the so-called "ideal or optimal" treatment plan, but rather take into consideration a patient-centered approach to care. Although factors such as the patient's age, finan-cial situation, and insurance do not dictate our therapeu-tic options, we must surely consider these factors in our decision-making criteria. No longer does the physi-cian solely decide upon an intervention, but rather it behooves the clinician to advise their patients of the scope of options available along with the advantages and disadvantages of each. Root amputation, which perhaps has come to be viewed as an antiquated approach, can very well hold a strong place in modern-day care when appropriate case selection is used.

Self-Study Questions

A. What is the difference between root resection, root amputation, and hemisection?

B. How are furcation involvements classified?

C. What are the indications and contraindications for root resections?

D. What is the difference between vital and nonvital resection (i.e. what comes first, the surgery or the endodontic therapy)?

E. What are the criteria for selecting the root that is to be removed and why?

F. Is root resection a predictable therapeutic modality?

G. How does root resection compare with extraction and implant therapy as a treatment option?

H. What is the relationship between periodontal disease, obesity, and systemic disease?

I. Why is it important to seal the canal orifice with a permanent restorative material?

Answers located at the end of the chapter.

References

1. Ausenda F, Jeong N, Arsenault P, et al. The effect of the Bass intrasulcular toothbrushing technique on the reduction of gingival inflammation: a randomized clinical trial. *J Evid Based Dent Pract* 2019;19:106–114.

2. Basali DH. The effect of instructed dental flossing on interdental gingival bleeding: a randomized controlled clinical trial. Master's Thesis, Department of Periodontology, Tufts University School of Dental Medicine, 2019.

3. Goldman MJ, Ross IF, Goteiner D. Effect of periodontal therapy on patients maintained for 15 years or longer. A retrospective study. *J Periodontol* 1986;57:347–353.

4. Hirschfeld L, Wasserman B. A long-term survey of tooth loss in 600 treated periodontal patients. *J Periodontol* 1978;49:225–237.

5. McFall WT Jr. Tooth loss in 100 treated patients with periodontal disease. A long-term study. *J Periodontol* 1982;53:539–549.

6. Metzler DG, Seamons BC, Mellonig JT, et al. Clinical evaluation of guided tissue regeneration in the treatment of maxillary class II molar furcation invasions. *J Periodontol* 1991;62:353–360.

7. Yukna RA, Yukna CN. Six-year clinical evaluation of HTR synthetic bone grafts in human grade II molar furcations. *J Periodontal Res* 1997;32:627–633.

8. Camello M, Nevins ML, Schenk RK, et al. Periodontal regeneration in human class II furcations using purified recombinant human platelet-derived growth factor-BB (rhPDGF-BB) with bone allograft. *Int J Periodontics Restorative Dent* 2003;23:213–225.

9. Pontoriero R, Lindhe J. Guided tissue regeneration in the treatment of degree II furcations in maxillary molars. *J Clin Periodontol* 1995;22:756–763.

10. Rosen PS, Marks MH, Bowers GM. Regenerative therapy in the treatment of maxillary molar class II furcations: case reports. *Int J Periodontics Restorative Dent* 1997;17:516–527.

11. Langer B, Stein SD, Wagenberg B. An evaluation of root resections. A ten-year study. *J Periodontol* 1981;52:719–722.

12. Fugazzotto PA. A comparison of the success of root resected molars and molar position implants in function in a private practice: results of up to 15-plus years. *J Periodontol* 2001;72:1113–1123.

13. Hallmon WM, Carranza FA, Drisko CL, et al. (eds) Etiology and Contributing Factors. Section 4: Furcation anatomy and furcation invasion. In: *Periodontal Literature Reviews.*

    A Summary of Current Knowledge. Chicago, IL: American Academy of Periodontology, 1996:84.

14. Filipowicz F, Umstott P, England M. Vital root resection in maxillary molar teeth: a longitudinal study. *J Endod* 1984;10:264–268.

15. Smukler H, Tagger M. Vital root amputation. *A clinical and histological study J Periodontol* 1976;47:324–330.

16. Carnevale G, Di Febo G, Tonelli MP, et al. A retrospective analysis of the periodontal-prosthetic treatment of molars with interradicular lesions. *Int J Periodontics Restorative Dent* 1991;11:189–205.

17. Gerstein KA. The role of vital root resection in periodontics. *J Periodontol* 1977;48:478–483.

18. Iasella JM, Greenwell H, Miller RL, et al. Ridge preservation with freeze-dried bone allograft and a collagen membrane compared to extraction alone for implant site development: a clinical and histologic study in humans. *J Periodontol* 2003;74:990–999.

19. Hamp SE, Nyman S, Lindhe J. Periodontal treatment of multirooted teeth. Results after 5 years. *J Clin Periodontol* 1975;2:126–135.

20. Glickman I. The treatment of bifurcation and trifurcation involvement. In: *Clinical Periodontology: The Periodontium In Health And Disease*, 2nd edn. Philadelphia, PA: Saunders, 1958:693–704.

21. Basaraba N. Root amputation and tooth hemisection. *Dent Clin North Am* 1969;13:121–132.

22. Haskell EW, Stanley H, Goldman S. A new approach to vital root resection. *J Periodontol* 1980;51:217–224.

23. Buhler H. Evaluation of root-resected teeth. Results after 10 years. *J Periodontol* 1988;59:805–810.

24. Erpenstein H. A 3 year study of hemisectioned molars. *J Clin Periodontol* 1983;10:1–10.

25. Green EN. Hemisection and root amputation. *J Am Dent Assoc* 1986;112:511–518.

26. Ross IF, Thompson RH. A long term study of root retention in the treatment of maxillary molars with furcation involvement *J Periodontol* 1978;49:238–244.

27. Ordovas JM, Shen J. Gene–environment interactions and susceptibility to metabolic syndrome and other chronic diseases. *J Periodontol* 2008;79:1508–1513.

28. Khayat A, Lee SJ, Torabinejad M. Human saliva penetration of coronally unsealed obturated root canals. *J Endod* 1993;19:458–461.

29. Swanson K, Madison S. An evaluation of coronal microleakage in endodontically treated teeth. Part I. Time periods. *J Endod* 1987;13:56–59.

TAKE-HOME POINTS

A. See Table 3.4.1

B. The furcation is defined as the point at which the roots of multirooted teeth divide into separate entities. In a healthy periodontal state the bone surrounding the teeth normally lies coronal to the furcations. When bone loss takes place, as in periodontitis, the furcations can become involved to varying degrees.

A number of classifications exist but the two most common are as follows.

Hamp et al. [19]
Grade I   Horizontal loss <3 mm
Grade II   Horizontal loss >3 mm but not encompassing the total width
Grade III Horizontal through-and-through

Glickman [20]
Grade II   ncipient; pocket is suprabony; no radiographic change
Grade II   Loss of interradicular bone and pocket formation but not extending through to the opposite side; "cul-de-sac" radiographic change may or may not be seen
Grade III Through and through; permits complete passage of a probe
Grade IV   Through and through with gingival recession, "tunnel"; a clearly visible furcation area

C. See Table 3.4.2

D. A vital root resection implies that the root removal takes place before endodontic therapy, whereas nonvital resection indicates that root canal treatment has already been initiated or completed.

Although literature does exist supporting the performance of root resection prior to endodontic intervention [14,15,22], most evidence advocates completion of the root canal therapy before removal of the targeted root [14]. Filipowicz et al. [14] found that almost half of the teeth treated via vital root resection were nonvital at six months and this increased to 87% nonvital at five-year follow-up.

Despite the increased success of resecting a root following endodontic therapy, a significant concern is the possibility that upon flap elevation the tooth is deemed unsuitable for the recommended treatment and requires extraction. A fine balance must be struck by the clinician to ensure that the tooth is amenable to root resection so as to avoid unnecessary endodontic care. If the decision to undertake

Table 3.4.1 Differentiating between root resection, root amputation, and hemisection.

Root resection	Surgical removal of all or a portion of a tooth root [13]
Root amputation	The removal of an entire root from a multirooted tooth [13]
Hemisection	The surgical separation of a multirooted tooth, usually a mandibular molar, through the furcation in such a way that a root and the associated portion of the crown may be removed [13]

Table 3.4.2 Indications and contraindications for root resection.

Indications

- The patient's desire to retain the tooth
- Severe bone loss affecting a single root
- Class II, III, IV furcation(s) [18] where the furcations are not amenable to be treated via odontoplasty
- Unfavorable root proximity with adjacent teeth
- Root fracture, perforation, root caries, or root resorption involving a single root
- When required endodontic therapy of a particular root cannot be performed adequately
- When the tooth has little or no mobility

Contraindications

- Medical condition not allowing surgical intervention
- Insufficient alveolar bone to support remaining root (i.e. poor crown-to-root ratio)
- Unfavorable anatomy, deep concavity distal aspect of mesial root mandibular molar when distal root is to be sectioned
- Fused roots
- Root canal therapy not possible on remaining root following procedure
- Unrestorable remaining tooth
- Postoperative periodontal state compromised or not maintainable
- Significant tooth mobility
- Does not complement the prosthetic plan

Source: Basaraba [21].

vital therapy is made, it is considered prudent to have the subsequent root canal treatment done within two weeks [15].

E. The roots most commonly resected are the distobuccal in maxillary molars and the mesial root of the mandibular molars [13].

Resection therapy is undertaken in multirooted teeth, namely the maxillary and mandibular molars. The clinician must weigh many variables when assessing not only the appropriateness of resection therapy but also which specific root should be removed. Interdisciplinary lines of communication are essential between the surgeon, endodontist, and prosthodontist to increase the efficacy of this modality of therapy. Generally, the maxillary molars are the most common teeth chosen for root sectioning.

Some of the factors to consider in the decision of which root to remove include the following.
1. Removal of the root which eliminates the furcation involvement to the greatest degree, which in essence reduces future periodontal complications.
2. Removal of the most pathologically involved root (i.e. greatest bone defect, attachment loss, caries, etc.).
3. Removal of the root which affords patient the greatest ability to achieve home care and successful maintenance.
4. Removal of the root which facilitates sound prosthetic rehabilitation, whether it be a single crown or abutment tooth.
5. Removal of the root which might pose the greatest challenge to endodontic therapy.
6. Removal of a root that is in very close proximity to a neighboring tooth, creating an interdental space that is difficult or impossible to clean or restore.

F. Historically, prior to the advent of dental implants, root resection was one of the few options that existed to retain teeth with significant furcation involvements and teeth with a periodontally questionable or nontreatable prognosis, which otherwise would require extraction. Many studies have examined the predictability of root sectioning therapy by comparing outcomes to similar teeth with furcation involvements where root sectioning was not done. Reports of failure

rates of root-resected teeth show a large range depending on the authors. Reports varied between 16 and 73% depending on the length of follow-up [11,19,23,24]. These studies show a consistent trend for the failure rate to increase significantly in relation to the length of follow-up [11,23,25]. Patients who were not compliant in attending professional dental hygiene maintenance therapy experienced more failures than maintenance-compliant patients. However, there are two major exceptions. One study by Carnevale et al. [16] found a higher rate of failure between three and six years versus 7–11 years, and a recent study by Fugazzotto [12] showed a success rate comparable with the implant success rate.

In contrast, a classic study [26] maintained 88% of maxillary molars with furcation invasion that did not receive root resection or osseous surgery and rather were maintained via scaling and root planing, gingivectomy, or apically positioned flaps over 5–24 years.

In addition, these same studies sought to investigate the causes behind failures of resected teeth over the long term. The variables that have been associated with failure of teeth undergoing root resection include periodontal disease, caries, and root fracture. Root fracture has been deemed the most common cause for the failure of such teeth. Mandibular molars also tend to have a higher failure rate when compared with maxillary molars [11,19,23,24].

G. Before the advent of osseointegration, there were few options available to those teeth which had been severely compromised due to periodontal disease. Such teeth commonly had furcation involvement that was unable to be maintained by patients or periodontal maintenance and required extraction.

Although many studies indicate a significantly higher success rate for endosteal implants, a recent paper that retrospectively compared implant success with resected molars reported almost identical cumulative success rates of 97.0% and 96.8%, respectively [12]. The author attributes this high rate of success to a variety of factors, including comprehensive management of the patient's occlusion and a thorough and consistent maintenance hygiene program.

H. Chronic periodontal disease and obesity are conditions that produce cytokines responsible for various systemic conditions, including cardiac disease, diabetes, cerebrovascular accidents, rheumatoid arthritis, and others [27]. Achieving periodontal health

can reduce the host's inflammatory response and production of cytokines, which could otherwise contribute to these conditions.

I. Gutta percha does not provide an adequate seal of a root canal-treated tooth exposed to the oral fluids (bacteria). To prevent bacterial contamination, a definitive restorative material such as amalgam or glass ionomer should be placed [28,29].

4

Regenerative Therapy

Case 1: Treatment of Furcations..156
    Soo-Woo Kim, DMD, MS and Myron L. Nevins, DMD, MMSc

Case 2: Treatment of Intrabony Defects Using Allografts.................................164
    Kevin Guze, DMD, DMSc, MSc, FRCD(C), FICOI

Case 3: Treatment of Intrabony Defects Using Growth Factors.........................174
    Marc L. Nevins, DMD, MMSc and Vinicius Souza Rodrigues, DDS, SDD, DMSc

Case 4: Treatment of Intrabony Defects Using Alloplastic Materials..................181
    N. Joseph Laborde III, DDS, MMSc and Giuseppe Intini, DDS, MS, PhD

Case 5: Guided Bone Regeneration...188
    Kevin Guze, DMD, DMSc, MSc, FRCD(C), FICOI and Mohamed A. Maksoud, DMD

Case 1

Treatment of Furcations

CASE STORY

A 47-year-old Caucasian female was referred for periodontal evaluation of the maxillary posterior teeth by a dental hygienist at the office of a general dentist. She was aware of bleeding when brushing but had no other clinical symptoms. However, the hygienist was concerned by gingival distension and the deep probing depth. The patient reported that she brushed her teeth two to three times a day and flossed regularly.

LEARNING GOALS AND OBJECTIVES

■ To be able to diagnose/classify furcation involvement
■ To identify possible etiologic factors
■ To be aware of appropriate treatments for furcation involvement

Medical History

There was no significant medical history. She was not currently taking any medication except multivitamins, and the patient had no known drug or food allergies.

Review of Systems

- Vital signs on the day of initial visit
  - Blood pressure: 128/83 mmHg
  - Pulse rate: 74 beats/minute (regular)
  - Respiratory rate: 16 breaths/minute
- No significant problems were reported.

Social History

The patient was a well-spoken certified public accountant. She denied any use of tobacco, alcohol, or recreational drugs, and reported no parafunctional habits such as clenching, bruxism, tongue thrusting, and mouth breathing.

Extraoral Examination

This articulate patient appeared to be under no apparent distress. The extraoral examination revealed no masses, swelling, or lymphadenopathy. Her temporomandibular joints were in full range of motion and within normal limits.

Intraoral Examination

The oral mucosa including lips, tongue, and palate demonstrated no aberrations. The periodontal examination revealed generalized pink gingiva with localized marginal erythema. There was a deviated papilla, and exudate was present at tooth #14. Periodontal charting was completed (Figure 4.1.1).

Occlusion

There was a minimal discrepancy between centric relation and centric occlusion but no eccentric interferences.

Diagnosis

Review of the full-mouth radiographic survey demonstrated minimal osseous loss excluding tooth #14, giving a diagnosis of type II, grade A periodontitis, generalized. A vertical probing depth of 6 mm and horizontal probing depth of 5 mm were present at the site of the buccal furcation on tooth #14. The palatal root prevented further horizontal probing. The nonsurgical diagnosis of this furcation was a class II furcation involvement in the buccal of #14 according to Glickman's classification.

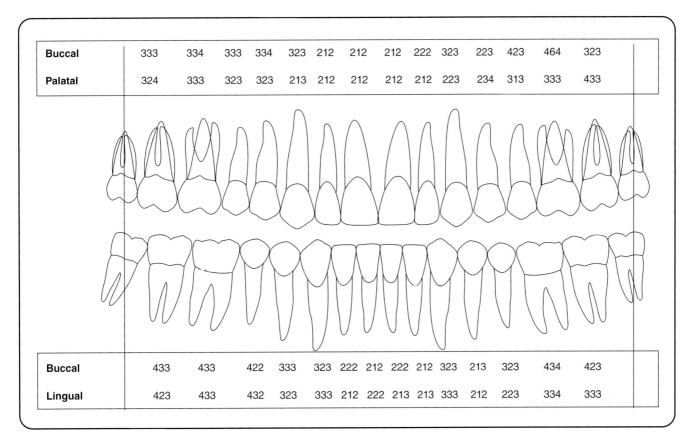

Buccal	333	334	333	334	323	212	212	212	222	323	223	423	464	323
Palatal	324	333	323	323	213	212	212	212	212	223	234	313	333	433

Buccal	433	433	422	333	323	222	212	222	212	323	213	323	434	423
Lingual	423	433	432	323	333	212	222	213	213	333	212	223	334	333

Figure 4.1.1 Periodontal charting.

Treatment Plan

The treatment plan was to address type II, grade A periodontitis, generalized with four quadrants of root planing under local anesthesia complemented by oral hygiene instruction. Surgical intervention would be necessary to treat #14 with the hope that periodontal regeneration could be performed. It was impossible to determine mesial and distal extension of furcation involvement until the time of surgery.

Treatment

The left maxillary quadrant was anesthetized buccally and palatally around #14 with 2% lidocaine with 1:50 000 epinephrine. A full-thickness buccal flap was reflected using mesial and distal vertical incisions to obtain the maximum visibility. All granulation tissue was removed from the affected area, and root planing removed all accretions from the tooth. This was the appropriate time to evaluate any loss of proximal structure between the palatal and two buccal roots. The internal proximal areas were evaluated with a no. 23 explorer and Kramer Nevins no. 4 curette, but there was no proximal extension. We therefore concluded that this problem was limited to the buccal furcation and we could treat the area to achieve periodontal regeneration. A tetracycline slurry was introduced to decontaminate the surface. The area was thoroughly washed with sterile saline. Autogenous bone was harvested with a trephine from an edentulous mandibular posterior site. The cores were ground with a bone mill and adapted to the defect. Ti-reinforced membrane (Gore, Newark, DE, USA) was fitted to cover the defect, apically tacked with a fixation screw, and sutured coronally with 4.0 Gore-Tex suture. Then flap was repositioned coronally to protect the surgical site. The area was reopened to remove the membrane at six months. There was clinical evidence of periodontal regeneration interradicularly and to a lesser extent on the radicular surface of the buccal roots. The patient was under observation at the periodontal office for a year and returned to the family practice (Figure 4.1.2).

Discussion

The interradicular loss of periodontium of a multirooted tooth is referred to as furcation involvement. The compromised furcation is most successfully treated

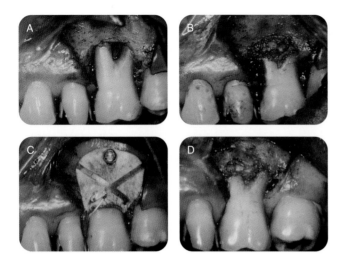

Figure 4.1.2 (A) Full-thickness flap raised showing furcation involvement; (B) autogenous bone in place; (C) membrane with fixation screw; (D) six-month postoperative view.

when its loss of structure is minimal or incipient and is categorized as class I.

The opportunities for successful periodontal regeneration are limited for maxillary molars. The best-case scenario is when the buccal furcation between the two buccal roots is involved. If the loss of attachment has continued between the palatal root and the two buccal roots, the most difficult factor for the regeneration effort is to eliminate the infected granulation tissues and the accretions on the root surface. Standard curettes are frequently larger than the interradicular space, and many clinicians use ultrasonic instruments as a supplement.

If the procedure only requires the treatment of a buccal furcation, the next decision relates to the selection of the osteogenic materials. This tooth was treated with autogenous bone and a nonresorbable membrane, but there are many products available. They include allografts, xenografts, and alloplasts used with or without a barrier membrane. The only treatment regimen that has satisfied the definition of periodontal regeneration for a furcation defect in the form of human histologic evidence is the use of recombinant human platelet-derived growth factor (rhPDGF-BB) in combination with an allograft [1,2].

Self-Study Questions

A. How would you classify/define furcation involvement?

B. What information would you need to make a correct diagnosis of furcation involvement?

C. What etiologic and anatomic factors influence furcation involvement?

D. How would you treat different furcation involvements?

E. What are the factors that affect treatment outcome?

F. What is the long-term prognosis of treatment of furcation involvement?

G. What are possible complications from the treatment of furcation involvement?

H. What would be the maintenance protocol after the treatment of furcation involvement?

Answers located at the end of the chapter.

References

1. Camelo M, Nevins M, Schenk RK, et al. Periodontal regeneration in human class II furcations using purified recombinant human platelet-derived growth factor-BB (rhPDGF-BB) with bone allograft. *Int J Periodontics Restorative Dent* 2003;23:213–225.

2. Nevins M, Camelo M, Nevins ML, et al. Periodontal regeneration in humans using recombinant human platelet-derived growth factor-BB (rhPDGF-BB) and allogenic bone. *J Periodontol* 2003;74:1282–1292.

3. Glickman I. The treatment of bifurcation and trifurcation involvement. In: *Clinical Periodontology: The Periodontium in Health and Disease*, 2nd edn. Philadelphia, PA: Saunders, 1958:693–704.

4. Hamp SE, Nyman S, Lindhe J. Periodontal treatment of multirooted teeth. Results after 5 years. *J Clin Periodontol* 1975;2:126–135.

5. Eskow RN, Kapin SH. Furcation invasions: correlating a classification system with therapeutic considerations. Part I. Examination, diagnosis, and classification. *Compend Contin Educ Dent* 1984;5:479–483, 487.

6. Tarnow D, Fletcher P. Classification of the vertical component of furcation involvement. *J Periodontol* 1984;55:283–284.

7. Ricchetti PA. A furcation classification based on pulp chamber–furcation relationships and vertical radiographic bone loss. *Int J Periodontics Restorative Dent* 1982;2:50–59.

8. Al-Shammari KF, Kazor CE, Wang HL. Molar root anatomy and management of furcation defects. *J Clin Periodontol* 2001;28:730–740.

9. Zappa U, Grosso L, Simona C, et al. Clinical furcation diagnoses and interradicular bone defects. *J Periodontol* 1993;64:219–227.

10. Mealey BL, Neubauer MF, Butzin CA, Waldrop TC. Use of furcal bone sounding to improve accuracy of furcation diagnosis. *J Periodontol* 1994;65:649–657.

11. Abdallah F, Kon S, Ruben MP. The furcation problem: etiology, diagnosis, therapy, and prognosis. *J West Soc Periodontol Periodontal Abstr* 1987;35:129–141.

12. Larato DC. Furcation involvements: incidence and distribution. *J Periodontol* 1970;41:499–501.

13. Tal H. Relationship between the depths of furcal defects and alveolar bone loss. *J Periodontol* 1982;53:631–634.

14. Hermann DW, Gher ME Jr, Dunlap RM, Pelleu GB Jr. The potential attachment area of the maxillary first molar. *J Periodontol* 1983;54:431–434.

15. Bower RC. Furcation morphology relative to periodontal treatment. Furcation entrance architecture. *J Periodontol* 1979;50:23–27.

16. Everett FG, Jump EB, Holder TD, Williams GC. The intermediate bifurcational ridge: a study of the morphology of the bifurcation of the lower first molar. *J Dent Res* 1958;37:162–169.

17. Gutmann JL. Prevalence, location, and patency of accessory canals in the furcation region of permanent molars. *J Periodontol* 1978;49:21–26.

18. Moskow BS, Canut PM. Studies on root enamel (2). Enamel pearls. A review of their morphology, localization, nomenclature, occurrence, classification, histogenesis and incidence. *J Clin Periodontol* 1990;17:275–281.

19. Masters D, Hoskins SW. Projection of cervical enamel into molar furcations. *J Periodontol* 1964;35:49–53.

20. Pontoriero R, Lindhe J. Guided tissue regeneration in the treatment of degree II furcations in maxillary molars. *J Clin Periodontol* 1995;22:756–763.

21. Filipowicz F, Umstott P, England M. Vital root resection in maxillary molar teeth: a longitudinal study. *J Endod* 1984;10:264–268.

22. Langer B, Stein SD, Wagenberg B. An evaluation of root resections. A ten-year study. *J Periodontol* 1981;52:719–722.

23. Newell DH. The role of the prosthodontist in restoring root-resected molars: a study of 70 molar root resections. *J Prosthet Dent* 1991;65:7–15.

24. Nevins M, Langer B. The successful application of osseointegrated implants to the posterior jaw: a long-term retrospective study. *Int J Oral Maxillofac Implants* 1993;8:428–432.

25. Bahat O, Handelsman M. Use of wide implants and double implants in the posterior jaw: a clinical report. *Int J Oral Maxillofac Implants* 1996;11:379–386.

26. Bowers GM, Schallhorn RG, McClain PK, et al. Factors influencing the outcome of regenerative therapy in mandibular Class II furcations: Part I. *J Periodontol* 2003;74:1255–1268.

27. Mellonig JT, Valderrama Mdel P. Histological and clinical evaluation of recombinant human platelet-derived growth factor combined with beta tricalcium phosphate for the treatment of human class III furcation defects. *Int J Periodontics Restorative Dent* 2009;29:169–177.

28. Karring T, Cortellini P. Regenerative therapy: furcation defects. Periodontol 2000 1999;19:115–137.

29. Pontoriero R, Nyman S, Lindhe J. The angular bony defect in the maintenance of the periodontal patient. *J Clin Periodontol* 1988;15:200–204.

30. Huynh-Ba G, Kuonen P, Hofer D, et al. The effect of periodontal therapy on the survival rate and incidence of complications of multirooted teeth with furcation involvement after an observation period of at least 5 years: a systematic review. *J Clin Periodontol* 2009;36:164–176.

TAKE-HOME POINTS

A.

Glickman's Classification of Furcation Involvement [3]

- Grade I: early furcation involvement just into the flute of the furcation is present, but the interradicular bone is intact. There is no significant destruction of bone or connective tissue in the furcation proper.
- Grade II: distinct horizontal destruction of the furcation area including interradicular bone is present. Destruction should not be extended to the other side of furcation. Vertical bone loss may or may not be present.
- Grade III: destruction of interradicular bone and connective tissue all the way through the furcation so that an instrument can be passed through the furcation. The furcation defect is not yet visible clinically.
- Grade IV: severe destruction of interradicular bone and connective tissue all the way through the furcation so that the tunnel is completely visible through the furcation defect when viewed clinically.

Horizontal Furcation Classification [4]

- Degree I: horizontal loss of periodontal tissue support <3 mm.
- Degree II: horizontal loss of support >3 mm but not encompassing the total width of the furcation area.
- Degree III: horizontal "through-and-through" destruction of the periodontal tissue in the furcation.

Vertical Furcation Classification [5,6]

In addition to the horizontal classification:
- Subclass A: probable vertical depth of 1–3 mm from the roof of the furcation apically.
- Subclass B: probable vertical depth of 4–6 mm from the roof of the furcation apically.
- Subclass C: probable vertical depth >7 mm from the roof of the furcation apically.

Horizontal and Vertical Furcation Classification [7]

Ricchetti's furcation classification system divides the molar into buccal, middle, and lingual/palatal thirds. The classifications are as follows.

- Class I: incipient involvement; horizontal involvement just into the interradicular area.
- Class Ia: involvement into approximately the first half of the buccal or lingual third.
- Class II: horizontal involvement beyond class Ia but not into the middle third of the molar.
- Class IIa: horizontal involvement into the middle third of the molar but not beyond halfway.
- Class III: horizontal involvement beyond half of the tooth width.

B.

- Radiographs: may assist in the diagnosis of furcation defects but have a limited value if used as the sole diagnostic tool, especially in early and moderate defects [8].
- Clinical examination: clinical measurements alone also have limited value [9]. However, the combination of radiographic and clinical examinations improves detection to 65% for maxillary molars but only to 23% for mandibular molars. Probing the deepest interradicular site does not measure the true pocket depth or the attachment level of the furcation area. This indicates that the probing measurement records the depth of probe penetrating into the inflamed connective tissue rather than the true pocket depth.
- Bone sounding with local anesthesia may assist in the diagnosis of furcation defects by more accurately determining the underlying bony contours [10].
- Diagnosing furcation invasion is best accomplished using a combination of radiographs, periodontal probing with a curved explorer or Nabers probe, and bone sounding (Figure 4.1.3).

C.

Primary Factors

- Bacterial plaque: the extension of inflammatory periodontal disease into the furcation area leads to interradicular bone resorption and formation of furcation defects [11].
- Age: the average number of furcation involvements increases with age [12].

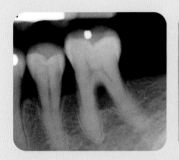
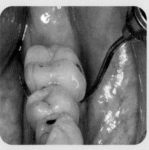

Figure 4.1.3   Mandibular class III furcation involvement showing a probe entering the furcation.

Occlusal Trauma

- Glickman showed that hyperfunction of the rat molar makes the furcation area susceptible to attachment loss. The heavy occlusal load on molar teeth may render them susceptible to increased bone loss in the furcation areas if inflammation is present.

Predisposing Anatomic Factors

- Root trunk length: the distance from the cementoenamel junction (CEJ) to the entrance of the furcation varies by individual. The shorter the trunk length, the less attachment loss before furcation involvement [13].
- Root length: teeth with long root trunks and short roots may have lost most of their support by the time the furcation becomes affected [14].
- Root form
  - Furcation entrance diameter: 81% of entrances on molars are <1 mm in width, and 58% are <0.75 mm, which is less than the diameter of the blade of standard curettes [15]. A small furcation entrance further complicates the proper maintenance of good hygiene.
  - Root concavity [15]
    - Mandibular first molars have concavities in 100% of mesial roots and 99% of distal roots. Deeper concavity is found in the mesial root than the distal root.
    - Maxillary first molars have concavities in 94% of mesiobuccal roots, 31% of distobuccal roots, and 17% of palatal roots. Deepest concavity is found in the mesiobuccal root.
- Interradicular dimension: root proximity can be a precipitating factor. Closely proximated or fused roots can impede complete periodontal treatment

or maintenance once they get involved.
- Anatomy of furcation: the presence of bifurcational ridges, a concavity in the dome [16], and possible accessory canals [17] can complicate appropriate periodontal treatment and maintenance therapy.
- Developmental anomalies: these include enamel pearls (EPs) and cervical enamel projections (CEPs). EPs are larger round deposits of enamel, and CEPs are flat ectopic extensions of enamel beyond the CEJ. EPs are seen in 1–5% of permanent molars [18]. CEPs are seen in 29% of mandibular molars and 17% of maxillary molars [19]. These anatomic structures interfere with the attachment apparatus, making furcation more vulnerable to the disease process.

Other Factors

- Orthodontics: poorly planned orthodontic procedures may make teeth supererupt, exposing furcations.
- Pulpal pathology: when present, especially with accessory canals, it is very likely that furcation would be involved.
- Vertical root fractures: associated with rapid and localized alveolar bone loss.
- Iatrogenic factors: overhanging margin of restorations near furcations can lead to furcation involvement.

D.
Class I

- Limited to the incipient lesions
  - Scaling and root planing in conjunction with debridement. Good root preparation is the key to successful therapy. Efficacy decreases with more roots involved. Presence of precipitating anatomic factors also hinders the success of therapy.
  - Apically positioned flap in conjunction with osteoplasty/ostectomy. This provides an environment for improved oral hygiene application with reduced pocket depth postoperatively.

Class II

- Buccal and lingual mandibular/buccal maxillary furcations

○ Apically positioned flap in conjunction with osteoplasty/ostectomy. A shallow class II mandibular lesion with divergent roots will benefit from this procedure.
○ Guided tissue regeneration (GTR)
  – Combination treatment (debridement + bone graft + membrane) at buccal class II furcations results in decreased probing depth and bone gain and reduces the amount of soft tissue recession above what was accomplished by flap debridement alone [20].
  – Introduction of growth factor. Use of growth factors has permitted the treatment of many mandibular class III defects and maxillary class II defects with a regenerative approach. Nevins et al. [2] used rhPDGF-BB with demineralized freeze-dried bone allograft to successfully treat human class II furcation defects.
○ Root resection (see other chapters)
  – Factors that influence the outcome of root resections include (i) the patency of the root canal system, (ii) occlusal forces, (iii) the length of the edentulous span, and (iv) the length, width, and shape of the root.
  – Root resection in conjunction with endodontic therapy is necessary because long-term survival of vital root resection is poor [21].
  – In the short term of three or four years, this treatment has been highly successful, but after 10 years approximately one-third fail. A substantial number of failures were attributed to recurrent periodontal disease, recurrent caries, root fractures, or endodontic failures [22,23].
○ Extraction and implant (see other chapters)
  – This treatment completely removes etiology and successfully restores the function.
  – It is highly predictable with success rates of 99% [24]. Wide implant (diameter >5 mm) also favors successful treatment of furcation involvements [25].
• Other proximal furcations: access to proximal maxillary furcations must proceed with individual defect analysis based on surgical access.

• It is critical not to allow class II to become class III.

Class III
• Debridement treatment as a maintenance and no invasive therapy.
• Root resection (see other chapters).
• Tunneling
  ○ This treatment will convert grade III and deep grade II furcations into grade IV furcation to improve access for oral hygiene.
  ○ Success is challenged with interradicular caries with limited access to repair; size of pulp chamber is 2 mm or more.
• Extract and implant (see other chapters).
• Regeneration with growth factors
  ○ Studies report favorable results in mandibular class II furcation; less favorable results were found in mandibular class III defects and maxillary class II defects [20,26]. In general, class III has a less favorable outcome than class II.
  ○ Histologic evidence of regeneration in class III furcation is not available yet. Mellonig et al. [27] used rhPDGF-BB with beta tricalcium phosphate for improving human class III furcation defect. However, predictability remains questionable.

E.
The following factors affect treatment outcome [28]
• Patient factors
  ○ Oral hygiene: patient compliance
  ○ Smoking
  ○ Systemic conditions (diabetics, metabolic disorders, etc.)
• Defect factors
  ○ Mandibular versus maxillary teeth
  ○ Location of the defect (buccal class II defects have better prognosis [29])
  ○ Vertical height of the defect (<3 mm of vertical defect: better prognosis)
• Technique factors
  ○ Operator skill (technique sensitive)
  ○ Incomplete removal of etiologic factors
  ○ Postoperative infection control

○ Adjunctive systemic antibiotics (minimal benefits?)

F.

- Depending on diagnostic skills, all these methods have been clinically demonstrated as efficacious; none are exclusive.
- Based on a systematic review [30], good long-term prognosis of multirooted teeth with furcation involvement has been obtained following various therapeutic approaches. The long-term prognosis of the case depends on patient's ability to maintain daily hygiene. To achieve better long-term prognosis, both clinicians and patients have to work as a team. It is the clinician's role to provide the patient with a cleansable environment using surgical or nonsurgical modalities and it is the patient's role to maintain the proper hygiene daily.

G. Possible complications of the treatment of furcation involvement are recurrent caries, recurrent periodontal disease, fracture of the root, and endodontic failure. The most frequent complications are caries development in the furcation area after a tunneling procedure and vertical root fractures and endodontic failure following root resective procedures [30].

H.

- The patient should be seen every three months because they have already demonstrated their susceptibility to periodontal disease.
- Successful treatment resulting in minimal probing depth will benefit both the oral hygienist and the patient.
- Strict oral hygiene with proximal brush for interproximal furcations is a necessity for long-term success of the treatment.

Case 2

Treatment of Intrabony Defects Using Allografts

CASE STORY

The patient was a 63-year-old male who presented to the Department of Periodontology for consultation regarding several "loose teeth" in both the maxilla and mandible. His chief complaint was his missing teeth and his desire to have fixed restorations to replace them (Figure 4.2.1).

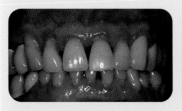
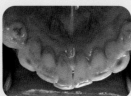

Figure 4.2.1 Intraoral photo of both maxillary and mandibular teeth in occlusion and mandibular arch.

LEARNING GOALS AND OBJECTIVES

- To identify and appropriately diagnose patients requiring guided tissue regeneration (GTR)
- To understand preoperative and postoperative issues that lead to successful GTR therapy
- To be introduced to surgical techniques and biomaterials used to perform GTR

Medical History

The patient had been diagnosed with type 1 hypertension several years ago and had been under treatment with his physician ever since. His physician had prescribed atenolol 50 mg once daily and hydrochlorothiazide 25 mg daily. He regularly monitored his condition and had been stable since prescription treatment began. Otherwise this patient was in good health, did not have any other significant medical problems, and did not report any allergies or history of diabetes.

Review of Systems

- Vital signs
  - Blood pressure: 126/75 mmHg
  - Pulse rate: 58 beats/minute (regular)

Social History

The patient was married with three children. He did not consume alcohol and did not smoke.

Extraoral Examination

No significant findings were noted. The patient had no masses or swelling, and the temporomandibular joints were within normal limits. Figure 4.2.2 shows pocket depth measurements after phase 1 therapy.

Intraoral Examination

- The soft tissues of the mouth including tongue appeared normal. Oral cancer screen was negative.
- The gingival examination revealed a generalized moderate marginal erythema. Several areas of boggy tissue and mobile teeth were noted.
- A hard tissue examination was completed.
- The edentulous ridge in the maxillary right quadrant had deficiencies buccolingually and apico-coronally (Seibert class 3).
- Minimal salivary flow of mucous consistency.

Radiographic Examination

There was mild to moderate horizontal bone loss with some angular defects (as illustrated in the mandibular periapicals) (Figure 4.2.3).

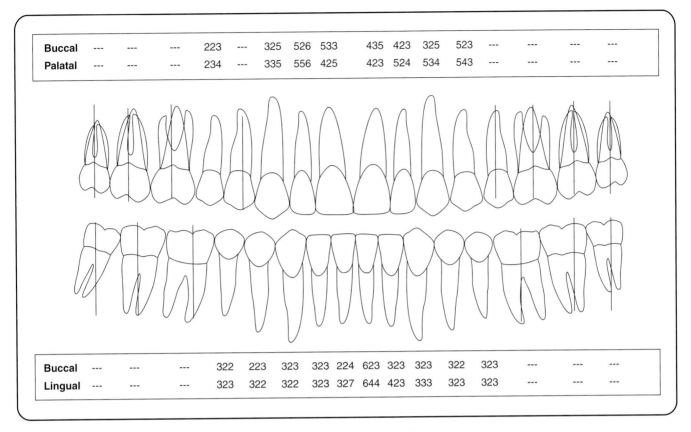

Buccal	---	---	---	223	---	325	526	533	435	423	325	523	---	---	---	---
Palatal	---	---	---	234	---	335	556	425	423	524	534	543	---	---	---	---

Buccal	---	---	---	322	223	323	323	224	623	323	323	322	323	---	---	---
Lingual	---	---	---	323	322	322	323	327	644	423	333	323	323	---	---	---

Figure 4.2.2 Probing pocket depth measurements (following phase 1 therapy).

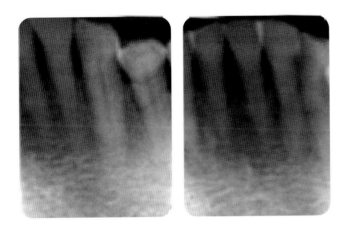

Figure 4.2.3 Radiographic evaluation (periapicals of the mandibular anterior teeth).

Occlusion

There was a lack of posterior support in the right quadrant and unprotected occlusion. First occlusal contacts were on anterior teeth (see Figure 4.2.1).

Treatment Plan

The primary care physician was contacted to obtain comprehensive information regarding the patient's cardiovascular status and to suggest alternative medication to increase salivary flow. Prosthodontic and endodontic consultations were required to establish a comprehensive treatment plan. A cone beam computed tomography scan was ordered for the maxillary and mandibular arch for potential implant placement in edentulous areas.

The final treatment plan included extensive periodontic, prosthetic, and occlusal rehabilitation with implant-supported crowns. GTR procedures involved several teeth including tooth #24. Figure 4.2.4 illustrates the steps involved in GTR surgery.

Treatment

The patient received oral hygiene instructions and three complete scaling and root planing sessions prior to surgical therapy. The patient was placed on a permanent saliva substitute program. Pocket depths (Figure 4.2.2) were recorded following phase 1 therapy.

Preoperative Consultation

The medical history was reviewed. His blood pressure was again monitored. The consent form addressing

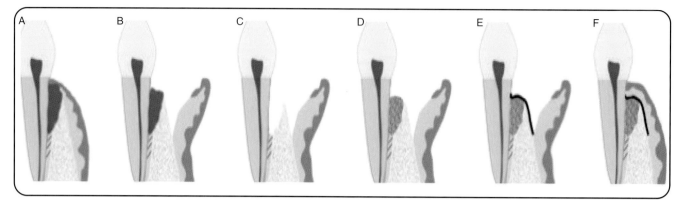

Figure 4.2.4 (A) Vertical defect evident with granulation tissue fill. (B) Sulcular incision is made and tissue is reflected to expose osseous defect. (C) Complete debridement of defect and root planing of root surface. (D) Defect filled with allograft bone. (E) Membrane placed over grafts and endogenous bone. (F) Primary soft tissue closure is obtained and sutured.

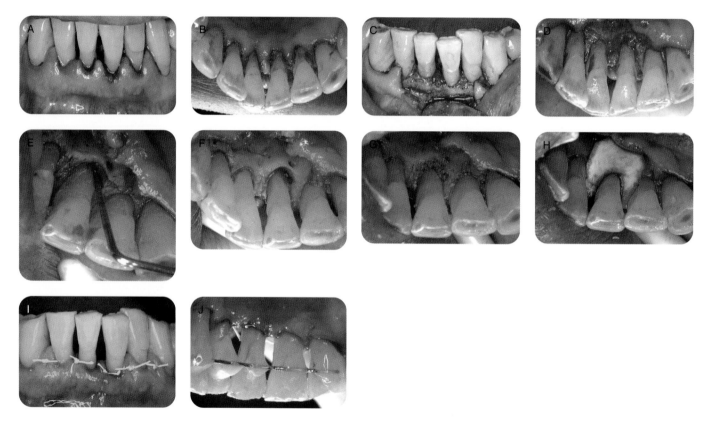

Figure 4.2.5 (A–J) Intraoral surgical photos.

benefits and risks associated with the procedure was reviewed with the patient. Accessibility to the surgical site was clinically assessed. Significant (class II) mobility of tooth #24 was noted. The following prescriptions were delivered to the patient: amoxicillin 500 mg (t.i.d. for 10 days starting 24 hours before the procedure), ibuprofen 600 mg (every four to six hours as needed for pain), and Peridex 0.12% (b.i.d.).

Guided Tissue Regeneration Procedure

Bilateral mental nerve blocks and local lingual infiltration were achieved with lidocaine 2% (epinephrine 1:100 000). A full-thickness flap was elevated buccally and lingually from distal of teeth #23 to mesial #27 to achieve access (Figure 4.2.5A–D). The teeth in this region were thoroughly scaled and root planed, and the osseous defect was completely degranulated

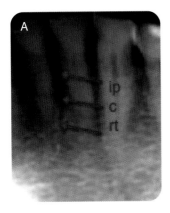
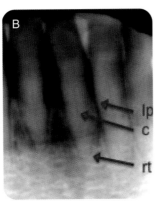

Figure 4.2.6 Periapical radiographs: (A) initial; (B) following six months of healing.

(Figure 4.2.5E,F). A rotary finishing bur was used to remove additional debris and conservatively recontour surrounding bone. Following a thorough rinse of the teeth, rehydrated freeze-dried mineralized bone allograft (FDBA) was placed in the defect to the crest of the surrounding bone (Figure 4.2.5G). A resorbable collagen membrane was placed over the augmented site (Figure 4.2.5H) and the flap was reapproximated to achieve primary closure and then sutured (Figure 4.2.5I). The six mandibular anterior teeth were splinted together with orthodontic wire and composite resin to stabilize the mobile tooth #24 (Figure 4.2.5J). Healing

was uneventful thereafter. Periapical radiographs at six months show bone fill (Figure 4.2.6).

Discussion

GTR is a predictable procedure for regenerating bone adjacent to teeth that was lost due to inflammatory periodontal disease. It is important to understand the limitations of this procedure in order to achieve these results. Successful oral hygiene management as well as appropriate maintenance intervals is an essential part of the treatment. Good communication with the referring general dentist and/or hygienist is necessary in order to provide patients with optimal care.

Although we were unable to change this patient's blood pressure medication, we were able to provide saliva substitutes that will provide an additional defense against future periodontal breakdown.

The surgery was successful and uneventful. The patient was seen for postoperative visits at two weeks to remove the sutures and at three and six weeks for evaluation. After six months the fixed splint was removed from this region and periapical radiographs were taken to assess the amount of bone regenerated (Figure 4.2.5G). Tooth #24 was now only slightly mobile compared with the +2 mobility originally recorded. Final occlusal rehabilitation by the prosthodontist following additional periodontic therapy provided the patient with a stable atraumatic occlusion.

Self-Study Questions

A. What is the rationale for performing GTR as opposed to other available surgical techniques?

B. What are the techniques used in GTR therapy?

C. Which biomaterials can be used in GTR? Is there histologic evidence of bone formation?

D. What are the determinants of success in GTR?

E. Do traumatic occlusal events affect the success of treatment with GTR?

F. What are the complications associated with GTR? How do you manage these complications?

Answers located at the end of the chapter.

References

1. Murphy K, Gunsolley J. Guided tissue regeneration for the treatment of periodontal intrabony and furcation defects. A systematic review. *Ann Periodontol* 2003;8:266–302.

2. Black BS, Gher ME, Sandifer JB, et al. Comparative study of collagen and expanded polytetrafluoroethylene membranes in the treatment of human Class II furcation defects. *J Periodontol* 1994;65:598–604.

3. Yukna CN, Yukna RA. Multi-center evaluation of bioabsorbable collagen membrane for guided tissue regeneration in human Class II furcations. *J Periodontol* 1996;67:650–657.

4. Wang HL, O'Neal RB, MacNeil LM. Regenerative treatment of periodontal defects utilizing a bioresorbable collagen membrane. *Pract Periodontics Aesthet Dent* 1995;7:59–66.

5. Caffesse RG, Smith BA, Duff B, et al. Class II furcations treated by guided tissue regeneration in humans: case reports. *J Periodontol* 1990;61:510–514.

6. Pontoriero R, Nyman S, Lindhe J, et al. Guided tissue regeneration in the treatmentof furcation defects in man. *J Clin Periodontol* 1987;14:618–620.

7. Melcher AH. On the repair potential of periodontal tissues. *J Periodontol* 1976;47:256–260.

8. Becker W, Becker BE, Berg L, et al. New attachment after treatment with root isolation procedures: Report for treated class III and class II furcations and vertical osseous defects. *Int J Periodontics Restorative Dent* 1988;8:8–23.

9. Dahlin C, Linde A, Gottlow J, Nyman S. Healing of bone defects by guided tissue regeneration. *Plast Reconstr Surg* 1988;81:672–676.

10. Garrett JS, Crigger M, Egelberg J. Effects of citric acid on diseased root surfaces. *J Periodontal Res* 1978;13:155–163.

11. Stahl SS, Froum SJ, Kushner L. Healing responses of human intraosseous lesions following the use of debridement, grafting and citric acid root treatment. II. Clinical and histologic observations: one year postsurgery. *J Periodontol* 1983;54:325–338.

12. Albair WB, Cobb CM, Killoy WJ. Connective tissue attachment to periodontally diseased roots after citric acid demineralization. *J Periodontol* 1982;53:515–526.

13. Terranova VP, Franzetti LC, Hic S, et al. A biochemical approach to periodontal regeneration: tetracycline treatment of dentin promotes fibroblast adhesion and growth. *J Periodontal Res* 1986;21:330–337.

14. Blomlöf J, Blomlöf L, Lindskog S. Effect of different concentrations of EDTA on smear removal and collagen exposure in periodontitis-affected root surfaces. *J Clin Periodontol* 1997;24:534–537.

15. Blomlöf J, Jansson L, Blomlöf L, Lindskog S. Root surface etching at neutral pH promotes periodontal healing. *J Clin Periodontol* 1996;23:50–55.

16. Caffesse RG, Kerry GJ, Chaves ES, et al. Clinical evaluation of the use of citric acid and autologous fibronectin in periodontal surgery. *J Periodontol* 1988;59:565–569.

17. Mariotti A. Efficacy of clinical root surface modifiers in the treatment of periodontal disease. A systematic review. *Ann Periodontol* 2003;8:205–226.

18. Newman MG, Takei HH, Klokkevold PR, Carranza FA (eds). *Carranza's Clinical Periodontology*, 10th edn. St. Louis, MO: Saunders Elsevier, 2006.

19. Carranza FA Sr. A technic for reattachment. *J Periodontol* 1954;25:272–278.

20. Moskow BS, Tannenbaum P. Enhanced repair and regeneration of periodontal lesions in tetracycline-treated patients: case reports. *J Periodontol* 1991;62:341–350.

21. Lindhe J, Karring T, Lang NP (eds) *Clinical Periodontology and Implant Dentistry*, 4th edn. Oxford: Wiley-Blackwell, 2003.

22. Zellin G, Gritli-Linde A, Linde A. Healing of mandibular defects with different biodegradable and non-biodegradable membranes: an experimental study in rats. *Biomaterials* 1995;16:601–609.

23. Friedmann A, Strietzel FP, Maretzki B, et al. Histological assessment of augmented jaw bone utilizing a new collagen barrier membrane compared to a standard barrier membrane to protect a granular bone substitute material. *Clin Oral Implant Res* 2002;13:587–594.

24. Sandberg E, Dahlin C, Linde A. Bone regeneration by the osteopromotive technique using bioabsorbable membranes: an experimental study in rats. *Int J Oral Maxillofac Surg* 1993;51:1106–1114.

25. Hollinger JO, Brekke J, Gruskin E, Lee D. Role of bone substitutes. *Clin Orthop Relat Res* 1996;324:55–65.

26. Tolman DE. Reconstructive procedures with endosseous implants in grafted bone: a review of the literature. *Int J Oral Maxillofac Implants* 1995;10:275–294.

27. Mowlem R. Cancellous chip bone grafts: report on 75 cases. *Lancet* 1944;244:746–748.

28. Mellonig JT. Autogenous and allogeneic bone grafts in periodontal therapy. *Crit Rev Oral Biol Med* 1992;3:333–352.

29. Mulliken JB, Glowacki J. Induced osteogenesis for repair and construction in the craniofacial region. *Plast Reconstr Surg* 1980;65:553–560.

30. Cammack GV II, Nevins M, Clem DS III, et al. Histologic evaluation of mineralized and demineralized freeze-dried bone allograft for ridge and sinus augmentations. *Int J Periodontics Restorative Dent* 2005;25:231–237.

31. Simion M, Trisi P, Piattelli A. Vertical ridge augmentation using a membrane technique associated with osseointegrated implants. *Int J Periodontics Restorative Dent* 1994;14:496–511.

32. Cochran DL, Douglas HB. Augmentation of osseous tissue around nonsubmerged endosseous dental implants. *Int J Periodontics Restorative Dent* 1993;13:506–519.

33. Becker W, Becker BE, Caffesse R. A comparison of demineralized freeze-dried bone and autologous bone to induce bone formation in human extraction sockets. *J Periodontol* 1994;65:1128–1133.

34. Becker W, Schenk R, Higuchi K, et al. Variations in bone regeneration adjacent to implants augmented with barrier membranes alone or with demineralized freeze-dried bone or autologous grafts: a study in dogs. *Int J Oral Maxillofac Implants* 1995;10:143–154.

35. Becker W, Urist MR, Tucker LM, et al. Human demineralized freeze-dried bone: inadequate induced bone formation

in athymic mice: a preliminary report. *J Periodontol* 1995;66:822–828.

36. Nabers CL, O'Leary TJ. Autogenous bone transplants in the treatment of osseous defects. *J Periodontol* 1965; 36:5–14.

37. Sanders J, Sepe W, Bowers GM, et al. Clinical evaluation of freeze-dried bone allografts in periodontal osseous defects. III. Composite freeze-dried bone allograft with and without autogenous bone. *J Periodontol* 1983;54:1–8.

28. Sepe W, Bowers G, Lawrence JJ, et al. Clinical evaluation of freeze-dried bone allograft in periodontal osseous defects. *Part II. J Periodontol* 1978;49:9–14.

39. Mellonig JT. Freeze-dried bone allografts in periodontal reconstructive surgery. *Dent Clin North Am* 1991;35:505–520.

40. Mellonig JT, Bowers GM, Bailey RC. Comparison of bone graft materials. Part I. New bone formation with autografts and allografts determined by strontium-85. *J Periodontol* 1981;52:291–296.

41. Mellonig JT, Bowers GM, Cotton WR. Comparison of bone graft materials. Part II. New bone formation with autografts and allografts: a histological evaluation. *J Periodontol* 1981;52:297–302.

42. Libin BM, Ward HL, Fishman L. Decalcified lyophilized bone allografts for use in human periodontal defects. *J Periodontol* 1975;46:51–56.

43. Pearson GE, Rosen S, Deporter DA. Preliminary observations on the usefulness of a decalcified freeze-dried cancellous bone allograft material in periodontal surgery. *J Periodontol* 1981;52:55–59.

44. Quintero G, Mellonig JT, Gambill VM, Pelleu GB Jr. A six-month clinical evaluation of decalcified freeze-dried bone allografts in periodontal osseous defects. *J Periodontol* 1982;53:726–730.

45. Anderegg CR, Martin SJ, Gray JL, et al. Clinical evaluation of the use of decalcified freeze-dried bone allograft with guided tissue regeneration in the treatment of molar furcation invasions. *J Periodontol* 1991;62:264–268.

46. Schallhorn RG, McClain PK. Combined osseous composite grafting, root conditioning, and guided tissue regeneration. *Int J Periodont Restorative Dent* 1988;8:8–31.

47. Magnusson I, Runstad L, Nyman S, Lindhe J. A long junctional epithelium: a locus minoris resistentiae in plaque infection. *J Clin Periodontol* 1983;10:333–340.

48. Cortellini P, Pini Prato G, Tonetti MS. Periodontal regeneration of human infrabony defects. II. Re-entry procedures and bone measures. *J Periodontol* 1993;64:261–268.

49. Selvig KA, Kersten BG, Wikesjö UM. Surgical treatment of intrabony periodontal defects using expanded polytetrafluoroethylene barrier membranes: influence of defect configuration on healing response. *J Periodontol* 1993;64:730–733.

50. Cortellini P, Tonetti M. Radiographic defect angle influences the outcome of GTR therapy in intrabony defects. *J Dent Res* 1999;78:381 (abstract).

51. Anderegg CR, Metzler DG, Nicoll BK. Gingiva thickness in guided tissue regeneration and associated recession at facial furcation defects. *J Periodontol* 1995;66:397–402.

52. Periodontal Literature Reviews, 3rd edn. Chicago, IL: American Academy of Periodontology, 1996.

53. Flezar TJ, Knowles JW, Morrison EC, et al. Tooth mobility and periodontal therapy. *J Clin Periodontol* 1980;7:495–505.

54. Trejo PM, Weltman RL. Favorable periodontal regenerative outcomes from teeth with presurgical mobility: a retrospective study. *J Periodontol* 2004;75:1532–1538.

TAKE-HOME POINTS

A. Regeneration refers our ability to re-create the original healthy periodontal apparatus that has been destroyed because of disease or injury, the goals being to end up with regenerated alveolar bone and cementum and a functional periodontal ligament. The cells responsible for this regeneration are osteoblasts, cementoblasts, and periodontal ligament cells. Fundamental to GTR therapy is the presence of a barrier membrane that prevents the infiltration of epithelial and connective tissue cells (fibroblasts) into the environment adjacent to the root surface and bone such that these three cell types have an opportunity to regenerate their respective tissues. Because epithelial cells and fibroblasts proliferate at a much greater rate, it is essential that this barrier be in place. Following a period of healing of approximately three to six months, the barrier can then be removed if a nonresorbable membrane has been used. GTR differs from other more traditional procedures such as flap osseous surgery in terms of regenerating tissue as opposed to resecting it. GTR has also shown promising results in the treatment of furcation involvement and recession defects, with supporting histologic evidence of bone fill and tissue coverage [1–6].

B. The principles of surgical technique involved in GTR are similar to the general principles of periodontal surgery, with some additional concepts as summarized here (see Figure 4.2.4) [7–9].

- Isolation of the debrided periodontal defect (usually filled with bone material) with a barrier membrane such that the borders of the membrane extend 3–4 mm beyond the confines of the defect in all directions.
- Adaptation of the membrane with sling sutures with respect to the periodontal defect so the defect is isolated from the gingival cellular components and if the membrane is resilient, to achieve the function of space maintenance during wound healing (regeneration).
- Following thorough scaling and root planing of the root surface, many surgeons prefer to use a root surface modifier to enhance attachment and stimulate connective tissue ingrowth. Examples of surface modifiers include citric acid, tetracycline, and ethylenediaminetetraacetic acid (EDTA). Although human studies fail to support these arguments, some animal studies provide evidence of its effectiveness. Histologically, the healing patterns do not result in significant improvement in clinical outcome compared with control sites in human studies [10–17].
- Complete coverage of the mucoperiosteal flap over the membrane.
- Optional coronal displacement of the flap is indicated to further facilitate the delay in the potential migration of gingival cells into the wound area.

Systemic antibiotics are generally used after reconstructive periodontal therapy, although definitive information on the advisability of this measure is still lacking [18]. Case reports have shown extensive reconstruction of periodontal lesions after scaling, root planing, and curettage, with systemic and local treatment using penicillin or tetracycline, in combination with other forms of therapy [19,20].

C. GTR procedures are based on the use of a membrane to prevent epithelial and connective tissue growth into the regenerating site with or without a bone filler that primarily provides a scaffold to which cells can attach. Membranes can be classified as resorbable or nonresorbable.

- Resorbable membranes: can be a tissue, such as connective tissue graft or allogeneic dermal matrix, but usually refers to membranes made of collagen. Synthetic resorbable membranes (polyglactin 910, polylactic acid, polyglycolic acid, polyorthoester, polyurethane, and polybutyrate) are also used.
- Nonresorbable membranes: usually made of polytetrafluoroethylene (PTFE) or expanded PTFE (ePTFE) and can be reinforced by titanium structure to give more stability. Titanium mesh and titanium foil are also nonresorbable membranes used for GTR. Typically, nonresorbable membranes are removed after 6–12 months [21].

The primary advantage of nonresorbable membranes is stabilization of the graft. The disadvantages of a nonresorbable barrier membrane relates to its difficulty in handling and the possibility of its exposure during the healing process. Exposed membranes become contaminated with oral bacteria, which may lead to infection of the site and result in bone loss [18]. It is important to remove these membranes at a designated time during the healing process. If the membrane is removed too early, bone loss can also occur [18].

The advantages of a resorbable membrane are the elimination of surgical reentry for membrane removal as well as reduced complications if the membrane becomes exposed. Disadvantages of using resorbable membranes include the possibility of early degradation prior to completion of bone formation as well as the presence of inflammation brought on by this degradation process [22]. More recently, new developments including cross-linking of collagen to increase resistance to biodegradation have been developed [23]. Fortunately, the mild inflammatory reaction caused by bioresorbable membranes does not seem to interfere with osteogenesis [18]. In addition to these attributes, resorbable membranes are also user friendly. However, their lack of resiliency results in collapse of the membrane into the defect area [24]. Resorbable membranes are best reserved for clinical indications that allow the graft material or hardware (tenting screws, plates) to maintain the space required [18].

Bone Materials

There is adequate clinical and histologic evidence of bone fill and periodontal regeneration to recommend the use of bone replacement grafts in clinical practice. The available sources of bone materials include the following [25].

- Autograft: the patient's own bone.
- Allograft-processed cadaver bone from another human (FDBA) and demineralized freeze-dried bone allograft (DFDBA).
- Alloplast: synthetic bone substitutes such as tricalcium phosphate.
- Xenograft: cadaver bone from an animal source, e.g. bovine or porcine (i.e. Bio-Oss; Geistlich Pharma AG, Wolhusen, Switzerland).

These products are provided in a particulate form of various sizes as well as in block form. Particulate grafts from the preceding list may also be combined [25].

The particulate autograft is still considered the gold standard for most ridge augmentation procedures primarily due to its inherent osteogenic behavior [26,27]. Blood vessels are able to penetrate the spaces between the particles compared with a block graft and thus provide for more rapid ingrowth of blood vessels. Larger osteoconduction surface area, more exposure of osteoinductive growth factors, and easier biologic remodeling are also advantages of the particulate graft [18].

However, autografts have limitations that include donor site morbidity, increased cost, potential resorption, size mismatch, and an inadequate volume of graft material [28,29]. Bone allografts overcome many of the shortfalls of autogenous grafts but are considered primarily osteoconductive and to some degree osteoinductive (DFDBA) in nature. The literature suggests that DFDBA may have greater osteoinductive potential because of the availability of morphogenetic proteins. However, a histologic study comparing FDBA and DFDBA for ridge augmentation demonstrated regeneration of 42% new bone area with no statistical difference between the two materials [30].

Bone allograft is bone collected from a human cadaver that is commercially available from tissue banks. It is obtained from cortical or cancellous bone

within 12 hours of the death of the donor, defatted, cut in pieces, washed in absolute alcohol, and flash frozen. The material may then proceed to be mineralized (FDBA) or demineralized (DFDBA). Both products then are ground and sieved to a particle size of 250–750 μm and freeze-dried. They are then vacuum-sealed in glass vials [18].

The use of particulate allograft bone replacement substitute has been reported for numerous applications, including GTR [31,32]. From a histologic standpoint, biopsies of some studies using bone allografts indicate viable bone cells and visible osteocytes in lacunae, and a nine-month specimen showed no remaining allograft material [10]. However, there are some contradictory results using DFDBA and membrane combinations [33–35].

Several clinical studies by Mellonig, Bowers, and coworkers reported bone fill exceeding 50% in 67% of the defects grafted with FDBA and in 78% of the defects grafted with FDBA plus autogenous bone [36–38]. However, FDBA is considered an osteoconductive material, whereas decalcified FDBA (DFDBA) is considered an osteoinductive graft and thus potentially has greater osteogenic potential. Several studies back up this theory [18,39–41].

In 1975, Libin et al. [42] reported three patients with 4–10 mm of bone regeneration in periodontal osseous defects. Clinical studies were also done that compared cancellous DFDBA and cortical DFDBA [43,44]. The results of these studies demonstrated the superiority of cortical particulate (2.4 mm vs. 1.38 mm of bone fill).

These studies provided strong evidence that DFDBA in periodontal defects results in significant probing depth reduction, attachment level gain, and osseous regeneration. The combination of DFDBA and GTR has also proved to be very successful [45–47].

Even though there are studies that have demonstrated true periodontal regeneration, this issue still remains a topic for discussion because other studies demonstrate a long junctional epithelial (LJE) attachment as opposed to a connective tissue attachment. The question arises as to whether or not LJE is as resistant to disease as connective tissue. In an animal study, Magnusson et al, [47] were able to demonstrate that LJE is not more prone to new pocket formation and reinstitution of disease activity compared with connective tissue.

To enhance the quality and quantity of bone regenerated there is growing interest in growth factors. Products that are now clinically available include recombinant platelet-derived growth factor (rhPDGF-BB; marketed as GEM 21S, Osteohealth Inc., Shirley, NY, USA) and the recombinant human bone morphogenetic protein 2 (rhBMP-2) (Infuse Medtronics Inc., Minneapolis, MN, USA). Platelet-rich growth factors derived from the patient's own blood are compounds rich in different growth factors.

In summary, many well-controlled studies of interdental lesions show pocket depth reductions of up to 4 mm, with associated similar attachment level gains and fill of osseous defects. Reconstructive surgical treatment of furcation lesions has a more moderate result but is still superior to other surgical and nonsurgical therapies. Reports also show that these initial postsurgical gains are maintained for three to five years in patients who comply with normal maintenance schedules [18].

D. Success in GTR therapy relies on several factors that need to be an essential part of preoperative, perioperative, and postoperative treatment.

Preoperative

1. Absence of medical conditions including systemic diseases, bisphosphonate therapy, diabetes, autoimmune disease, irradiation, and smoking. The patient should be referred to a physician if there is any significant medical condition reported during the preoperative examination.
2. The patient's oral hygiene practices and response to phase 1 therapy are important factors to consider before proceeding with treatment.

Perioperative

1. The depth of the infrabony lesion will determine the ultimate amount of regeneration according to well-accepted studies. Two or three wall defects were 95% filled; one wall or hemiseptal defect was 39% filled [48,49].
2. The defect angle was also considered a determinant of success by Cortellini and

colleagues. They found that if the infrabony defect angle was less than 25 degrees (narrow defect) there was 1.5 mm more bone fill compared with a defect over 37 degrees (wide defect) [50].
3. The literature supports rigorous cleaning of both the tooth surface and complete degranulation of the defect.
4. Control of excessive mobility with splint stabilization has been shown to influence success of therapy (refer to Question F).
5. Follow proper technique protocol as outlined in Question B.
6. Tissue thickness has also been indicated as a factor that may affect the success of this procedure [51].

Postoperative

The surgeon should deliver postoperative instructions to the patient emphasizing that the surgical site should not be disturbed with brushing, eating, and so on. It should be stressed that the patient should not pull at the lip or tissues at the surgical site. The patient should also be instructed to take all medications that have been prescribed until finished and apply ice to reduce swelling that may otherwise place excessive stretching forces on the tissue. To help prevent potential adverse events, the patient should be followed over the next six to eight weeks.

E. According to the Periodontal Literature Review (1996), occlusal trauma can be defined as follows [52].

- **Occlusal trauma**: an injury to the attachment apparatus as a result of excessive occlusal force.
- **First-degree occlusal trauma**: injury resulting from excessive occlusal forces applied to a tooth or teeth with normal support.
- **Second-degree occlusal trauma**: injury resulting from normal occlusal forces applied to a tooth or teeth with inadequate support.

According to Flezar et al. [53] pocket reduction of clinically mobile teeth did not respond as well to various forms of periodontal surgery as firm teeth with comparable initial disease severity. In another study, Trejo and Weltman [54] were able to demonstrate that interproximal intraosseous defects of teeth with limited presurgical tooth mobility (i.e.

Miller's class 1 and 2 mobility) will respond favorably to regenerative therapy.

Therefore, before any regenerative procedures, the clinician should consider immobilizing or splinting mobile teeth to remove this possible risk factor.

F. According to the literature, these are some of the complications that have been reported for GTR with allograft.
1. Membrane exposure
2. Inflammatory reaction
3. Infection
4. Incision line opening
5. Loss of graft or reduced graft
6. Potential of disease transfer from the cadaver
   Management of these complications is as follows.

1. **Membrane exposure**: the literature supports the removal of exposed nonresorbable membranes but not before sufficient time has elapsed for bone formation. Often these problems can be managed with good oral hygiene and use of topical 0.12% chlorhexidine rinse until time of removal.
2. **Inflammatory reaction**: with the use of resorbable membrane, a confined inflammatory event does take place upon degradation of the graft. As mentioned earlier this does not seem to affect the result of the augmentation. Surgical trauma can also cause significant inflammation that may put overwhelming pressure on the tissues resulting in suture line opening. To avoid this event a careful

atraumatic surgical technique is required, and the use of steroids such as prednisone may be helpful.
3. **Infection**: careful aseptic surgical technique, including thorough postoperative rinsing of the surgical site with sterile saline, can reduce the chances of infection. Preoperative and postoperative systemic antibiotics have been shown to improve augmentation results. Antibiotics such as penicillin, amoxicillin, clindamycin, azithromycin, or metronidazole can be used. If the infection cannot be controlled with antibiotics, removal of the bone graft may be necessary.
4. **Incision line opening**: as mentioned, a careful atraumatic surgical technique as well as the use of steroids may reduce the likelihood of this happening. More importantly, however, the surgeon must release the flap from the underlying periosteum to ensure tension-free closure.
5. **Loss of graft**: the clinical situation should be reevaluated. The option of performing a second GTR procedure can be discussed.
6. **Potential of disease transfer from the cadaver**: according to the literature, the use of DFDBA includes the possible, although remote, potential of disease transfer from the cadaver [18].

Other complications with performing GTR surgery include ankylosis between bone and tooth that may or may not result in root resorption. Recession of the gingival tissue as a result of bone/graft loss as well as recurrence of deep pockets may also be an issue [18].

Case 3

Treatment of Intrabony Defects Using Growth Factors

CASE STORY

The patient was a 30-year-old female who was referred to private practice/periodontology clinic for examination and consultation. Her chief concern related to the fractured maxillary right lateral incisor. She had been aware of a problem due to the root fragment protruding through the buccal gingival margin (Figure 4.3.1).

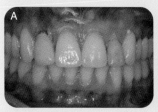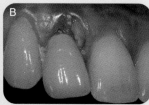

Figure 4.3.1 (A) Initial evaluation. (B) Tooth #7 presents with root fracture.

LEARNING GOALS AND OBJECTIVES

- To understand the use of recombinant human platelet-derived growth factor for implant site development
- To introduce the concepts of growth factor-mediated wound healing for oral regeneration
- To observe the results of a clinical case using novel clinical application of tissue engineering principles

Medical History

The patient was in excellent medical health with a noncontributory medical history (no history of hospitalization, no daily medications, negative smoking history).

Dental History

The dental history provided a report of root canal therapy and crown restoration, approximately 10 years previously. The patient had noted a crack in the tooth (#7) about 14 months ago but had no dental pain and did not understand the need for timely treatment.

Examinations

Extraoral and intraoral examinations were generally within normal limits. Mucogingival defects were noted for teeth #3–12, #14, and #19–31. Probing depths ranged from 2 to 4 mm for maxillary sites, 2–4 mm with localized 9-mm probing depth buccal of tooth #7, and 5 mm mesial of #7 for the buccal and palatal surfaces. Mandibular probing depths ranged from 2 to 4 mm with localized 5-mm probing for the interproximal lingual of teeth #30/31. There was a generalized pattern of gingival recession ranging from 2 to 4 mm. Mobility grade 3 was noted for the maxillary right lateral incisor. Figure 4.3.2 shows the charting for the maxillary right quadrant.

Radiographic Examination

Periapical radiograph revealed 100% bone loss for the maxillary right lateral incisor. There was significant loss of lamina dura for the adjacent canine and central incisor. Vertical fracture was evident in the radiograph, which confirmed a hopeless prognosis for this tooth (Figure 4.3.3).

Treatment Options

Treatment options were presented to the patient, including replacement with a dental implant-supported crown restoration, a fixed partial denture, and a

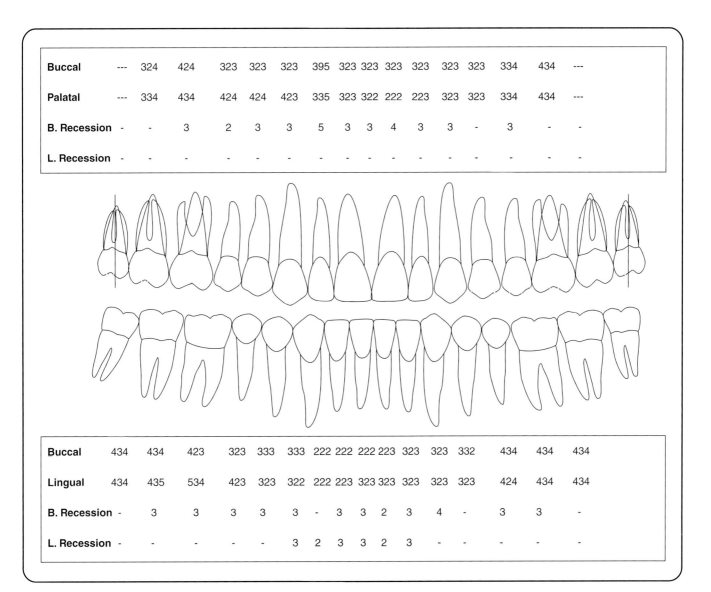

Buccal	---	324	424	323	323	323	395	323	323	323	323	323	323	334	434	---
Palatal	---	334	434	424	424	423	335	323	322	222	223	323	323	334	434	---
B. Recession	-	-	3	2	3	3	5	3	3	4	3	3	-	3	-	-
L. Recession	-	-	-	-	-	-	-	-	-	-	-	-	-	-	-	-

Buccal	434	434	423	323	333	333	222	222	222	223	323	323	332	434	434	434
Lingual	434	435	534	423	323	322	222	223	323	323	323	323	323	424	434	434
B. Recession	-	3	3	3	3	3	-	3	3	2	3	4	-	3	3	-
L. Recession	-	-	-	-	-	3	2	3	3	2	3	-	-	-	-	-

Figure 4.3.2 Initial probing depths and periodontal measurements (mm).

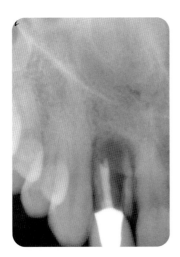

Figure 4.3.3 Periapical radiography revealed root fracture with bone loss.

removable partial denture. The patient was highly motivated to have a fixed restoration and wanted an implant-supported crown.

This case presents challenges for obtaining a healthy foundation for a dental implant and an esthetic result for this patient, whose smile displays the free gingival margin of the papilla in the esthetic zone.

- There is vertical and horizontal loss of alveolar bone including the complete buccal plate.
- There is gingival recession and no attached gingiva, with approximately 1 mm keratinized tissue for the lateral incisor.
- There is the need to regenerate the bone support for the adjacent teeth to improve their prognosis.
- There is the challenge of providing ridge augmentation procedures and maintaining the gingival papillae.

- Due to the gingival recession, the adjacent teeth would benefit from a root coverage procedure.

  The standard approach to dental implant replacement would include the following three alternatives.

1. Extraction of tooth #7

- Because of the advanced bone loss, extraction alone will cause resorption of remaining bone and shrinkage of papilla during healing. Once this tissue is lost, it may be difficult to recover.
- Subsequent graft procedures may be able to reestablish the necessary amount of bone tissue for implant placement, but this may not be sufficient to achieve esthetic goals due to increased clinical crown length.
- Surgical extraction with ridge augmentation advancing the buccal flap for closure presents a challenge: there is poor quality of buccal tissue, which will be unpredictable when trying to achieve primary closure. This technique would also decrease the vestibule space and advance the mucogingival junction.

2. Flapless extraction and grafting

- Placement of passive bone replacement material in such a noncontained defect is generally unpredictable.

3. Growth factor-enhanced therapy

This should be considered to enhance the healing for the above standard procedures in an attempt to improve the final outcome.

- The goal of the proposed therapy is to use a minimally invasive approach to stimulate bone regeneration through the use of a growth factor-enhanced matrix, combining recombinant human platelet-derived growth factor BB (rhPDGF-BB) with mineralized freeze-dried bone allograft (FDBA). The growth factor upregulates the wound healing process to a clinically significant level, allowing for improved healing.
- The goal of the preservation procedure performed at the time of extraction is to recover the vertical bone height without flap surgery and with preservation of the esthetic form of the gingival tissues and papillae. Therefore, even if there is the need for additional lateral ridge augmentation, the case can be converted to a less complex problem, which is more predictable to treat than a vertical defect.
- The patient is advised there may be multiple steps of bone augmentation and that the site will be evaluated with three-dimensional tomography to determine the bone available for implant placement. Soft tissue grafting is planned to be combined with dental implant placement, once it is determined to be adequate bone, with connective tissue grafting for the implant site and the adjacent natural teeth.

Treatment

Extraction and ridge preservation with growth factor-enhanced matrix rhPDGF-BB and FDBA (Figure 4.3.4).

- With local anesthesia the lateral incisor is extracted and the extraction socket debrided and degranulated. A periapical radiograph is exposed to confirm removal of all the root fragments.
- 0.5 ml rhPDGF-BB (0.3 mg/ml) is combined with 0.5 g FDBA (growth factor-enhanced matrix) and allowed to bind for approximately 10 minutes prior to being condensed incrementally into the socket.
- The site is overfilled to the level of the gingival margin and a collagen membrane (BioGide; Osteohealth, Inc., Shirley, NY, USA) is placed over the coronal aspect of the graft and stabilized with medical adhesive (PeryAcryl; GluStitch, Delta, BC, Canada). The patient is provided with a removable "Essix" appliance for two weeks to allow healing, avoiding any disturbance to the wound; then a removable partial denture is delivered to provide the provisional tooth replacement during the remaining healing period. It is important that there is no pressure on the edentulous ridge during the early healing period (Figure 4.3.5).

  The site is allowed to heal for five months and then a cone beam computed tomography (CT) scan is obtained to evaluate the bone available for dental implant

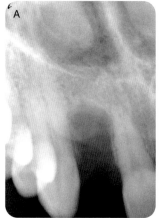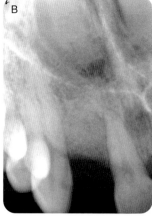

Figure 4.3.4 (A) Intraoperative radiograph reveals removal of all root fragments and preservation of the fragile interproximal periodontium for the adjacent teeth. (B) Periapical radiograph four months post grafting with evidence of significant bone formation.

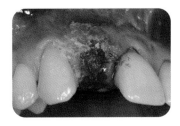

Figure 4.3.5 Immediate postoperative view of extraction socket grafted with growth factor-enhanced matrix combining rhPDGF-BB with FDBA protected by a collagen membrane and a medical adhesive.

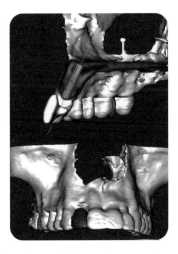

Figure 4.3.6 Cone beam CT scan five months postoperatively is used to determine if there is adequate bone for implant placement. The barium stent guides the surgical plan. (Top) Sagittal view with projection of the planned implant at ideal placement position. (Bottom) Anterior view with barium stent highlighted.

placement (Figure 4.3.6). The CT scan is taken with the patient wearing a barium stent to identify the tooth position of the future implant-supported crown. This allows for analysis as to whether the potential implant position is adequate to meet the restorative goals. The implant is planned using a viewing software (SimPlant; Materialise Dental, Plymouth, MI, USA), and in the three-dimensional view it is readily visible that the implant can be placed in the proper position. It is interesting to note the lack of bone width throughout the patient's maxilla, observed from the protuberance of the roots of the other anterior teeth.

A procedure is planned consisting of a dental implant placement combined with soft tissue grafting – a connective tissue graft – to provide root coverage for the adjacent teeth and to enhance the soft tissue profile of the dental implant site for function and esthetics. Additional particulate bone grafting can also be used to

provide contour grafting to the edentulous ridge if necessary during the same procedure. The procedure is provided utilizing the barium stent as a guide to implant placement and a 4.0 × 13 mm implant is placed in a submerged fashion. A connective tissue graft harvested from the palate is placed to provide root coverage for the maxillary right canine extending mesially to the right central incisor and the buccal flap is advanced for closure over the grafted sites.

The implant is allowed to heal for five months before providing second-stage surgery with placement of a healing abutment with a modified punch technique. The tissues were allowed to heal for four weeks prior to beginning the restorative procedures (Figure 4.3.7).

The maintenance of tissue height and width provides an esthetic framework for the design of an esthetic implant-supported crown restoration. The final restoration meets the patient's functional and esthetic needs (Figure 4.3.8).

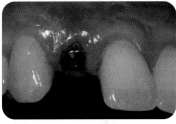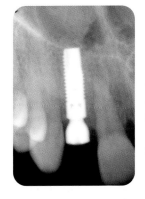

Figure 4.3.7 Implant after second-stage surgery. Note the tissue height preservation.

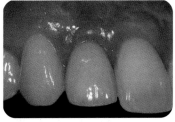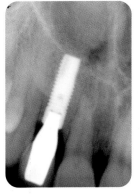

Figure 4.3.8 Definitive crown delivered to the patient. Note the improved gingival margin and the decreased gingival recession. Prosthodontist: Nancy S. Arbree, DDS, FACP, MS. Dental technician: Paul Chen.

Self-Study Questions

A. What are the benefits of growth-factors, such as PDGF, for implant site development?

B. What are the esthetic challenges for predictable esthetic outcomes?

C. What is the biologic effect of PDGF?

Answers located at the end of the chapter.

References

1. Bassir SH, Alhareky M, Wangsrimongkol B, et al. Systematic review and meta-analysis of hard tissue outcomes of alveolar ridge preservation. *Int J Oral Maxillofac Implants* 2018;33(5):979–994.
2. Khoshkam V, Chan H-L, Lin G-H, et al. Outcomes of regenerative treatment with rh PDGF-BB and rhFGF-2 for periodontal intra-bony defects: a systematic review and meta-analysis. *J Clin Periodontol* 2015;42:272–280.
3. Simion M, Rocchietta I, Kim D, et al. Vertical ridge augmentation by means of deproteinized bovine bone block and recombinant human platelet-derived growth factor-BB: a histologic study in a dog model. *Int J Periodontics Restorative Dent* 2006;26:415–423.
4. Simion M, Nevins M, Rocchietta I, et al. Vertical ridge augmentation using an equine block infused with recombinant human platelet-derived growth factor-BB: a histologic study in a canine model. *Int J Periodontics Restorative Dent* 2009;29:245–255.
5. Nevins ML, Camelo M, Nevins M, et al. Minimally invasive alveolar ridge augmentation procedure (tunneling technique) using rhPDGF-BB in combination with three matrices: a case series. *Int J Periodontics Restorative Dent* 2009; 29:371–383.
6. Nevins ML, Camelo M, Schupbach P, et al. Human histologic evaluation of mineralized collagen bone substitute and recombinant platelet-derived growth factor-BB to create bone for implant placement in extraction socket defects at 4 and 6 months: a case series. *Int J Periodontics Restorative Dent* 2009;29:129–139.
7. Buser D, Sennerby L, De Bruyn H. Modern implant dentistry based on osseointegration: 50 years of progress, current trends and open questions. *Periodontol 2000* 2017; 73(1):7–21.
8. Nevins ML, Said S. Minimally invasive esthetic ridge preservation with growth-factor enhanced bone matrix. *J Esthet Restor Dent* 2018;30(3):180–186.
9. Hollinger JO, Hart CE, Hirsch SN, et al. Recombinant human platelet-derived growth factor: biology and clinical applications. *J Bone Joint Surg Am* 2008;90(Suppl 1):48–54.
10. Homsi J, Daud AI. Spectrum of activity and mechanism of action of VEGF/PDGF inhibitors. *Cancer Control* 2007; 14:285–294.
11. Matsuda N, Lin WL, Kumar NM, et al. Mitogenic, chemotactic, and synthetic responses of rat periodontal ligament fibroblastic cells to polypeptide growth factors in vitro. *J Periodontol* 1992;63:515–525.
12. Oates TW, Rouse CA, Cochran DL. Mitogenic effects of growth factors on human periodontal ligament cells in vitro. *J Periodontol* 1993;64:142–148.
13. Sarment DP, Cooke JW, Miller SE, et al. Effect of rhPDGF-BB on bone turnover during periodontal repair. *J Clin Periodontol* 2006;33:135–140.
14. Cooke JW, Sarment DP, Whitesman LA, et al. Effect of rhPDGF-BB delivery on mediators of periodontal wound repair. *Tissue Eng* 2006;12:1441–1450.
15. Nevins M, Giannobile WV, McGuire MK, et al. Platelet-derived growth factor stimulates bone fill and rate of attachment level gain: results of a large multicenter randomized controlled trial. *J Periodontol* 2005;76:2205–2215.

TAKE-HOME POINTS

A. Growth factors have been used for enhancement of wound healing of multiple tissues for many years, with varying degrees of improvement on their clinical outcomes. Their uses in ridge preservation have been shown to improve the outcomes of such techniques [1]. Among these, bone morphogenetic protein (BMP)-2 has been extensively studied for osseous regeneration, while PDGF-BB and fibroblast growth factor (FGF)-2 have been used for soft and hard tissue regeneration, especially dentoalveolar tissues [2]. Preclinical studies and case reports provide proof of principle that rhPDGF-BB, when combined with other graft matrices, can support improved bone formation and wound healing in alveolar ridge reconstruction and implant therapy. Simion et al. [3] reported a canine study that demonstrated the potential for a deproteinized cancellous bovine block, which when infused with rhPDGF-BB regenerated significant amounts of new bone in severe mandibular vertical ridge defects without placement of a barrier membrane. The xenogeneic block grafts were infused with rhPDGF-BB and stabilized in alveolar defects using two dental implants with or without collagen membranes. The histologic findings revealed robust osteogenesis throughout the block graft, with significant graft resorption and replacement. In contrast, alveolar ridge defects treated with traditional guided bone regeneration without the growth factor supported little or no bone formation.

Simion et al. [4] also reported similar findings using rhPDGF-BB in combination with a novel equine hydroxyapatite and collagen (eHAC) bone block in the canine model. Moreover, recent case reports demonstrate that FDBA and anorganic bovine bone can serve as effective scaffolds to deliver rhPDGF-BB for lateral ridge augmentation and reconstruction, following extraction for implant placement [5,6].

B. Extraction socket grafting presents the dilemma as to whether to raise a flap or proceed with a flapless approach. Often there is the need for flap elevation to be able to debride the defect thoroughly. Alternative techniques such as a submarginal incision may preserve the gingival form and allow access to a periapical defect with the limitation of secondary healing at the coronal aspect of the socket. For sockets with a complete loss of the buccal plate flap, advancement will provide primary closure and the best protection of the bone graft. However this requires surgical skill and experience, and the soft tissues must be managed to prevent wound dehiscence that can result in tissue volume shrinkage and loss of interdental papillae, which can be difficult to recover in the future. The use of procedures combining hard and soft tissue grafting can result in optimal preservation of ridge form. The soft tissues are often supported by the root prominence, and there is the need for additional volume of tissue beyond that easily regenerated with the bone graft procedure. These combined procedures are performed for optimal esthetic preservation.

In the case of flapless socket preservation, additional soft tissue thickness can be provided to enhance the tissue biotype either at the time of extraction with tunneling techniques or at the time of implant placement using flap access. This will minimize the need for additional surgery after the implant has integrated by diagnosing and intercepting this, so that the tissue thickness is augmented in combination with the implant placement procedure.

Overall there are significant dimensional changes on the alveolar socket that may compromise esthetics and the availability of support for future implant placement, but minimization of such dimensional loss has been associated with ridge preservation, especially with the adjunct use of growth factors [1]. An overall appraisal of other issues of concern with esthetic and functional outcomes for dental implants, including current trends of treatment associated with improvement of these, are discussed in the literature [7]. Further detailed discussion of the use of growth factors to maximize the esthetic outcomes of ridge preservation is provided in the review by Nevins and Said [8].

C. PDGF exerts potent stimulatory effects as a chemoattractant and mitogen for mesenchymal cells (including osteogenic cells), as well as a promoter of angiogenesis, complementing the actions of endogenous vascular endothelial growth factor (VEGF) [9,10]. PDGF-BB has been shown to enhance the chemotactic and mitogenic activity of periodontal ligament cells at concentrations as low as 1 ng/ml [11,12]. PDGF-BB triggers a cascade of biologic and cellular events at the surgical wound during the initial postoperative period that lasts for weeks, as documented in human clinical trials [13]. These events are characterized by the recruitment and differentiation of mesenchymal cell populations, as well as new vessel formation, ultimately supporting wound healing and regeneration [9].

Cooke et al. [14] examined the effects of PGDF-BB on levels of VEGF and bone turnover in periodontal wound fluid in 16 patients who were randomized to receive treatment of intrabony defects with β-tricalcium phosphate (TCP) carrier alone, β-TCP plus 0.3 mg/ml rhPDGF-BB, or β-TCP plus 1.0 mg/ml rhPDGF-BB. These patients had participated in a large clinical trial evaluating the efficacy and safety of PDGF-BB in the treatment of intraosseous periodontal defects [15]. Pyridinoline cross-linked carboxy-terminal telopeptide of type I collagen (ICTP) is an indicator of osseous metabolic activity and provided a marker of bone turnover. Low-dose rhPDGF-BB application was found to elicit increases in ICTP at three to five days in the wound healing process, with the 1.0 mg/ml rhPDGF-BB group showing the most pronounced difference in VEGF at three weeks. Thus a single dose of rhPDGF-BB exhibited demonstrable, sustained metabolic actions at the clinical site of application.

Case 4

Treatment of Intrabony Defects Using Alloplastic Materials

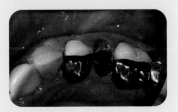
Medical History

The patient's medical history was reviewed with no significant findings. She was taking no medications other than a daily multivitamin. She had no known drug allergies.

Review of Systems

• Vital signs
  o Blood pressure: 114/68 mmHg
  o Pulse rate: 62 beats/minute
  o Respiratory rate: 12 breaths/minute

Social History

The patient did not use tobacco products. She drank alcohol socially and reported drinking one to three drinks per week. She was married with two children who were currently in college. She was an elementary school teacher.

Extraoral Examination

There were no significant findings. The patient had no masses or swelling and the temporomandibular joint evaluation showed parameters within normal limits.

Intraoral Examination

• The soft tissues of the mouth including tongue appeared normal. Oral cancer screen was negative.
• A gingival examination revealed coral pink tissue with stippling and knife-edge margins. Mild plaque accumulation was present on the buccal surfaces of the maxillary second molars with mild marginal inflammation.
• A periodontal charting was completed (Figure 4.4.2).

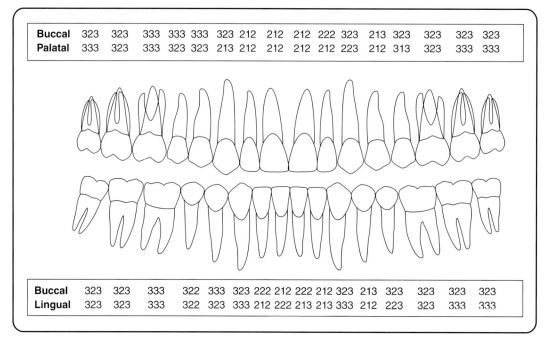

| Buccal | 323 | 323 | 333 | 333 | 333 | 323 | 212 | 212 | 212 | 222 | 323 | 213 | 323 | 323 | 323 | 323 |
| Palatal | 333 | 323 | 333 | 323 | 323 | 213 | 212 | 212 | 212 | 212 | 223 | 212 | 313 | 323 | 333 | 333 |

| Buccal | 323 | 323 | 333 | 322 | 333 | 323 | 222 | 212 | 222 | 212 | 323 | 213 | 323 | 323 | 323 | 323 |
| Lingual | 323 | 323 | 333 | 322 | 323 | 333 | 212 | 222 | 213 | 213 | 333 | 212 | 223 | 323 | 333 | 333 |

Figure 4.4.2 Probing pocket depth measurements.

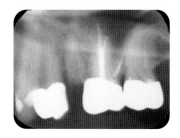

Figure 4.4.3 Periapical radiograph depicting the fractured root and the interproximal bone levels.

Occlusion

There were no occlusal discrepancies or interferences.

Radiographic Examination

A periapical radiograph was ordered (Figure 4.4.3).

Diagnosis

Tooth #13 was diagnosed with a localized tooth-related factor (fracture) that modifies or predisposes to plaque-induced gingival diseases/periodontitis. It was determined nonrestorable due to the amount of tooth structure lost. Teeth #1, #2, #3, #14, #15, and #16 were diagnosed with localized dental plaque biofilm-induced gingivitis on an intact periodontium.

Treatment Plan

The treatment plan for this patient included treatment of the localized dental plaque biofilm-induced gingivitis (not shown) and subsequent atraumatic extraction of tooth #13 with immediate implant placement and simultaneous osteotome sinus augmentation.

Treatment

Prior to surgery, a surgical guide was fabricated (Figure 4.4.4A) and a periapical radiograph was taken (Figure 4.4.4B). Immediately prior to surgery, 20 ml of blood were withdrawn and processed for the preparation of 1 ml of platelet-rich plasma (PRP). After local infiltration with lidocaine 2% and epinephrine 1:50 000, the root was gently extracted using periotomes and forceps, minimizing trauma to the soft and hard tissues (Figure 4.4.4C,D). No flaps were elevated. After degranulation of the extraction socket, a 3-mm elevation of the sinus floor was achieved with osteotomes and the site was prepared for implant placement. Subsequently, one endosteal implant of 13 mm, 3.75 mm was placed (tapered Screw-Vent MP-1 HA Dual Transition Surface; Centerpulse Dental Inc., Carlsbad, CA, USA). A preparation of calcium sulfate and PRP (CS-PRP) [1] was used to fill the residual gap between the socket wall and the implant body (Figure 4.4.4F,G). A barrier of pure calcium sulfate was used to cover the head of the implant and the grafted area. A Vicryl 5-0 suture was used to hold

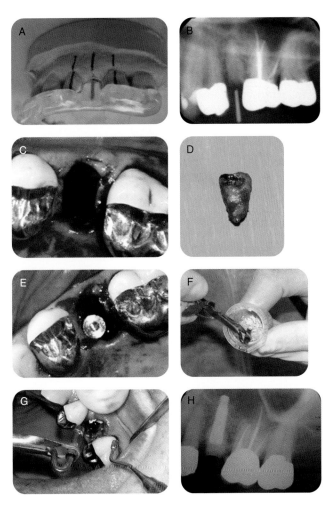

Figure 4.4.4   Surgical procedure.

the barrier in place. No attempt was made to cover the calcium sulfate barrier with soft tissue. The immediate postoperative radiograph revealed the presence of grafted material both apical to, and around the neck of, the implant (Figure 4.4.4H). The patient was prescribed a seven-day course of amoxicillin 250 mg t.i.d. starting one day before the surgery.

Self-Study Questions

A. What is an alloplast?

B. What are some of the commonly used alloplast materials?

C. What are the indications for using an alloplast?

D. Do alloplast materials influence regeneration and repair?

E. Why would a practitioner choose an alloplast over an autograft, allograft, or xenograft?

F. What is the diagnosis of this case according to the American Academy of Periodontology (AAP) classification system?

G. Describe the differences between at least two different prognosis systems.

H. To establish a correct prognosis, what information should be gathered?

I. What are the treatment options for this clinical case?

J. How would you perform socket preservation in this clinical case?

K. How do you measure treatment success for this clinical case?

L. What is the correct maintenance protocol for the presented clinical case?

Answers located at the end of the chapter.

References

1. Intini G, Andreana S, Intini FE, et al. Calcium sulfate and platelet-rich plasma make a novel osteoinductive biomaterial for bone regeneration. *J Transl Med* 2007;5:13.
2. Lindhe J, Lang N (eds) *Clinical Periodontology and Implant Dentistry*, 6th edn. Oxford: Wiley Blackwell, 2015.
3. Nasr HF, Aichelmann-Reidy ME, Yukna RA. Bone and bone substitutes. Periodontol 2000 1999;19:74–86.
4. Meffert RM, Thomas JR, Hamilton KM, Brownstein CN. Hydroxylapatite as an alloplastic graft in treatment of human periodontal osseous defects. *J Periodontol* 1985;56:63–73.
5. Snyder AJ, Levin MP, Cutright DE. Alloplastic implants of tricalcium phosphate ceramic in human periodontal osseous defects. *J Periodontol* 1984;55:273–277.
6. Froum SJ, Weinberg MA, Tarnow D. Comparison of bioactive glass synthetic bone graft particles and open debridement in the treatment of human periodontal defects. A clinical study. *J Periodontol* 1998;69:698–709.
7. Froum SJ, Kusher L, Scopp IW, Stahl SS. Human clinical and histologic responses to Durapatite implants in intraosseous lesions. *J Periondontol* 1982;53:719–725.
8. Froum S, Stahl SS. Human intraosseous healing responses to the placement of tricalcium phosphate ceramic implants. II. 13 to 18 months. *J Periodontol* 1987;58:103–109.
9. Garrett S. Periodontal regeneration around natural teeth. *Ann Periodontol* 1996;1:621–666; followed by Consensus report, 667–670.
10. Darby I, Chen S, Buser D. Ridge preservation techniques for implant therapy. *Int J Oral Maxillofac Implants* 2009;24(Suppl):260–271.
11. Caton JG, Armitage G, Berglundh T, et al. A new classification scheme for periodontal and peri-implant diseases and conditions: introduction and key changes from the 1999 classification. *J Periodontol* 2018;89(Suppl 1):S1–S8.
12. Becker W, Berg L, Becker BE. The long term evaluation of periodontal treatment and maintenance in 95 patients. *Int J Periodontics Restorative Dent* 1984;4:54–71.
13. McGuire MK, Nunn ME. Prognosis versus actual outcome. II. The effectiveness of clinical parameters in developing an accurate prognosis. *J Periodontol* 1996;67:658–665.
14. Kwok V, Caton JG. Prognosis revisited: a system for assigning periodontal prognosis. *J Periodontol* 2007;78:2063–2071.
15. Albrektsson T, Zarb G, Worthington P, Eriksson AR. The long-term efficacy of currently used dental implants: a review and proposed criteria of success. *Int J Oral Maxillofac Implants* 1986;1:11–25.
16. Research, Science and Therapy Committee of the American Academy of Periodontology. Position paper: Dental implants in periodontal therapy. *J Periodontol* 2000; 71: 1934–1942.

TAKE-HOME POINTS

A. Alloplastic materials are synthetic, inorganic, biocompatible, and/or bioactive bone graft substitutes that are claimed to promote bone healing through osteoconduction [2].

B. Hydroxyapatite (HA): three forms are available for periodontal use. These include a solid particulate nonresorbable form, a porous nonresorbable form derived from the exoskeleton of coral, and a resorbable nonceramic form.
- β-Tricalcium phosphate (β-TCP): a porous form of calcium phosphate.
- Polymers: include polyhydroxyethylmethacrylate (PHEMA), often referred to as HTR (hard tissue replacement).
- Bioactive glasses (bio-glasses): these are composed of SiO_2, NaO_2, and P_2O_5 and are resorbable or nonresorbable depending on the relative proportion of these components. When bio-glasses are exposed to tissue fluids, a double layer of silica gel and calcium phosphate is formed on the surface. The material promotes absorption and concentration of proteins through this layer, allowing the osteoblasts to form extracellular bone matrix that theoretically may promote bone formation [3].
- Calcium sulfate (plaster of Paris): biocompatible and porous, thereby allowing fluid exchange, which prevents flap necrosis. The material resorbs completely in two to three weeks and is osteoconductive [1]. A combination of calcium sulfate and platelet-rich plasma presents with osteoinductive qualities that may turn useful in bone regenerative procedures [1].

C. Alloplasts can be used in place of autografts, allografts, or xenografts when performing bone grafts in the oral cavity. The periodontal literature is replete with studies that have examined the clinical and histologic outcomes of alloplastic materials used to treat periodontal intrabony defects. When compared with open flap debridement, materials such as HA, β-TCP, and bioactive glass all showed significant gains in clinical attachment levels [4–6]. When results were examined histologically, the graft particles were often encapsulated in fibrous connective tissue with pocket closure primarily through long junctional epithelium [7,8]. The 1996 World Workshop in Periodontics concluded that "synthetic graft materials function primarily as defect fillers. If regeneration is the desired treatment outcome, other materials are recommended" [9]. Alloplastic materials can also be used successfully for ridge augmentation or sinus augmentation procedures. Histologic samples of bone grafting with different alloplastic materials show varying amounts of bone regeneration [10]. Particles of nonresorbable alloplasts usually become encapsulated by connective tissue, which may interfere with osseointegration of a dental implant if that is the desired goal of the grafting procedure. To avoid encapsulation of the alloplast by connective tissue, a completely resorbable alloplast is preferred to an nonresorbable one.

D. When the periodontium is damaged by inflammation or as a result of surgical treatment, the defect heals through either periodontal regeneration or repair. In periodontal regeneration, healing occurs through the reconstitution of a new periodontium, which involves the formation of alveolar bone, periodontal ligament, and new cementum in an area where the periodontium has been lost. Repair is healing by replacement with epithelium or connective tissue, or both, that matures into various nonfunctional types of scar tissue, termed *new attachment*. Histologically, patterns of repair include long junctional epithelium, new connective tissue adhesion, and/or ankylosis. Fully resorbable alloplast may favor regeneration, whereas nonresorbable alloplast tends to favor repair.

E. Several factors may influence a practitioner to choose an alloplast as a graft material. Alloplastic materials are synthetically derived so there is an unlimited supply with no risk of disease transmission or antigens that initiate cross-reactivity. Alloplastic materials are also a viable option for patients who have moral or religious objections to using human- or animal-derived graft materials.

F. In November 2017, the World Workshop on the Classification of Periodontal and Peri-implant Diseases and Conditions was held and a new classification system for periodontal diseases was generated [11]. According to this classification, a root fracture (such as the one shown on tooth #13) is classified within the "Prostheses and tooth-related factors that modify or predispose to plaque-induced gingival diseases/periodontitis" group and defined as a "localized tooth-related factor." Moreover, according to this new classification, the gingivitis detected on the buccal aspects of the maxillary molars is classified as localized dental plaque biofilm-induced gingivitis on an intact periodontium (since no previous loss of periodontal tissue has occurred for these teeth).

G. In 1984 Becker et al. [12] proposed a classification with three categories: good, questionable, and hopeless. In their studies, this system correctly predicted most of the prognoses in well-maintained patients. However, it was unable to predict outcomes in poorly maintained patients.

McGuire and Nunn [13] subsequently developed a more detailed prognostication system with five different categories: good, fair, poor, questionable, and hopeless. A tooth with a fair prognosis presents with approximately 25% attachment loss; a tooth with a poor prognosis presents with 50% attachment loss; a tooth with a questionable prognosis presents with attachment loss >50%; and a tooth with hopeless prognosis presents with inadequate attachment to maintain the tooth in health, comfort, and function.

More recently, Kwok and Caton [14], arguing that tooth loss is influenced by natural and iatrogenic reasons, proposed a prognostication system based on the probability of disease progression. Four categories are proposed: favorable, when future loss of periodontal supporting tissue is unlikely; questionable, when future periodontal breakdown may occur if the periodontium is not stabilized with comprehensive periodontal care; unfavorable, when periodontal

breakdown is likely to occur even with comprehensive periodontal care; and hopeless, when the tooth must be extracted.

H. Practitioners use several factors when assessing the prognosis of individual teeth and the overall case. McGuire evaluates prognosis based on the amount of periodontal support or clinical attachment loss of each tooth. Additional factors considered include the elimination or control of the disease etiology, patient compliance and ability to maintain the tooth, crown-to-root ratio and root form, furcation involvement, and mobility. To restore the tooth under consideration, a root canal, post and core, and a crown would be necessary. Crown lengthening would be required to achieve adequate biologic width and ferrule. The amount of ostectomy required to achieve the treatment goals would result in a greater compromise of support of the fractured tooth as well as the adjacent teeth. See Chapter 3 for a detailed discussion on crown lengthening. Based on these criteria the tooth is given a hopeless prognosis.

I. Whenever a tooth has been given a hopeless diagnosis, the patient should be presented with all viable treatment options. This includes leaving the space unrestored. If the patient prefers this option, he or she must be informed of the sequelae involved with a missing tooth, such as supereruption of mandibular teeth. The patient can have a fixed or removable partial denture. Or the patient can have an implant placed. If the patient elects to pursue implant therapy, a delayed or immediate placement option can be discussed with the patient. In this particular case, due to proximity to the maxillary sinus, a sinus elevation procedure will likely be needed to accommodate a dental implant.

J. In case socket preservation was selected as treatment alternative, after atraumatic extraction of the tooth, the extraction site should be thoroughly debrided, ensuring the removal of all granulomatous tissue and irrigated with sterile saline. To preserve the ridge width, a bone graft material should be placed into the site. The practitioner has the option of a variety of grafting materials with different properties. These options include autograft harvested from another site, allograft, xenograft, or alloplast. Factors that influence the decision on what material to use include the desire to have a material that is osteoinductive, osteoconductive, or osteogenic. For additional information on socket preservation see Chapter 7, Case 3.

K. The established criteria for successful implant treatment include the following.
1. The absence of persistent signs or symptoms such as pain, infection, neuropathies, paresthesias, and violation of vital structures.
2. Implant immobility.

3. No continuous peri-implant radiolucency.
4. Negligible progressive bone loss (<0.2 mm annually after physiologic remodeling during the first year of function).
5. Patient/dentist satisfaction with the implant-supported restoration [15].

L. Patients should be on a regular recall schedule to monitor the maintenance, including plaque control, of the implant-supported prosthesis. Maintenance programs should be designed individually because there is a lack of data detailing precise recall intervals, methods of plaque and calculus removal, and appropriate antimicrobial agents for maintenance around implants [16].

Case 5

Guided Bone Regeneration

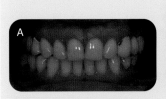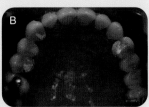
Medical History

There were no significant medical problems and the patient had no known allergies. She had been previously diagnosed with depression but was no longer on any medication for this condition. The only medications she was currently taking were oral contraceptives.

Review of Systems

- Vital signs
  - Blood pressure: 128/79 mmHg
  - Pulse rate: 68 beats/minute (regular)

Social History

The patient was of Hispanic descent and married with three children. She did not drink alcohol, smoke, or use recreational drugs.

Extraoral Examination

No significant findings were noted. The patient had no masses or swelling, and the temporomandibular joints were within normal limits.

Intraoral Examination

- The oral cancer screen was negative.
- The gingival examination revealed generalized mild marginal erythema.
- A hard tissue examination was completed.
- The edentulous ridges in the maxillary right and left quadrant were deformed in the buccolingual and apico-coronal directions (Seibert class 3) (Figure 4.5.1).
- The tongue was serrated laterally.
- Saliva was of normal flow and consistency.
- Amalgam tattoo was present on ridge in #18 region.
- Slightly inflamed palatal tonsils were noted.
- A periodontal charting was completed (Figure 4.5.2).

Occlusion

- Supereruption #14, distoversion #19 leading to left posterior bite collapse.
- No significant mobility or traumatic occlusion was noted.

Radiographic Examination

Periapical radiographs of the maxillary left posterior teeth were taken (Figure 4.5.3).

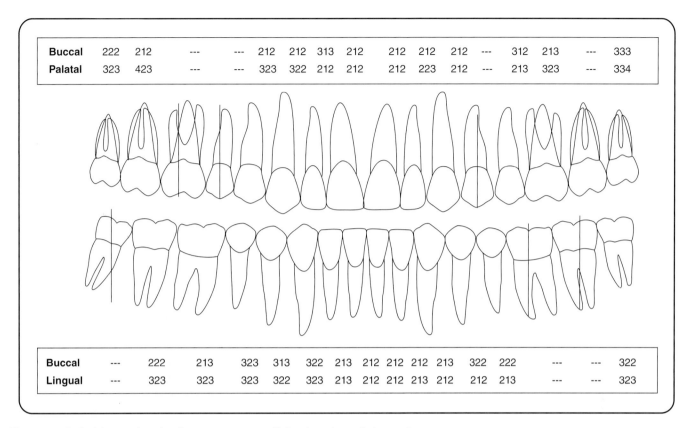

Buccal	222	212	---	---	212	212	313	212	212	212	212	---	312	213	---	333
Palatal	323	423	---	---	323	322	212	212	212	223	212	---	213	323	---	334

Buccal	---	222	213	323	313	322	213	212	212	212	213	322	222	---	---	322
Lingual	---	323	323	323	322	323	213	212	212	213	212	212	213	---	---	323

Figure 4.5.2 Probing pocket depth measurements (following phase 1 therapy).

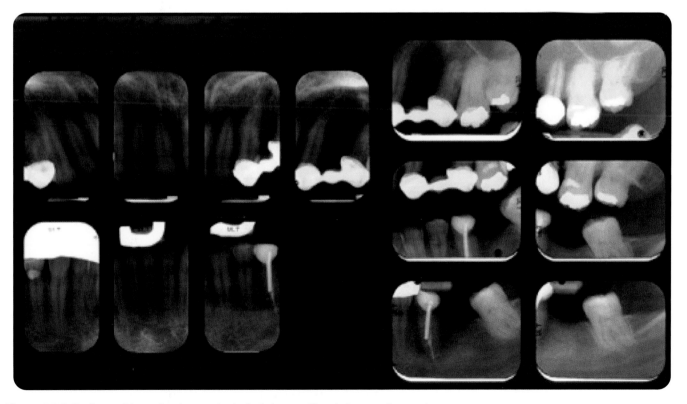

Figure 4.5.3 Radiographic evaluation: periapical of the maxillary left posterior teeth.

Treatment Plan

Prosthodontic, endodontic, and orthodontic consultations were required to establish a comprehensive treatment plan. A cone beam computed tomography (CT) scan was ordered for the maxillary arch to understand the anatomy, the condition of the deficient ridges, and the proximity of the maxillary sinus (Figure 4.5.4).

The CT clearly indicates sufficient bone in the vertical dimension. However, to accommodate the appropriate implant for this site, 6–7 mm of width is required.

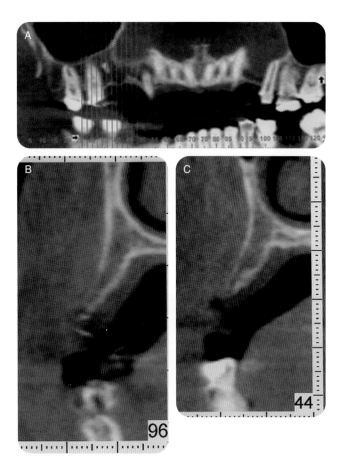

Figure 4.5.4 CT scans displaying horizontal ridge deficiency in #12 region.

The final treatment plan for this region included GBR, and prosthetic and occlusal rehabilitation including an implant-supported fixed partial denture #4-x-6 (Figure 4.5.5).

Treatment

The patient received oral hygiene instructions and a prophylaxis eight weeks prior to surgery.

Preoperative Consultation

The medical history was assessed. The consent form addressing benefits and risks associated with the procedure was reviewed with the patient. The patient was apprehensive about the procedure. Following a full disclosure of the treatment procedure, the patient became more comfortable. Accessibility to the surgical site was acceptable. The CT scan demonstrated that <3 mm of bone was present horizontally at edentulous site #12. No major anatomic obstacles were present. The site was significantly deficient in osseous width so a GBR technique involving tenting screws and a rigid resorbable membrane was selected. The following prescriptions were delivered to the patient: amoxicillin 500 mg (t.i.d. for 10 days starting 24 hours before the procedure), ibuprofen 600 mg (every four to six hours as needed), Vicodin ES (every six hours), and Peridex 0.12% (b.i.d.).

Guided Bone Regeneration Procedure

A posterior superior alveolar, middle superior alveolar, greater palatine nerve block, and local infiltrations were achieved with lidocaine 2% (epinephrine 1:100 000). A full-thickness flap was elevated in the maxilla right quadrant to expose the cortical bone (Figure 4.5.6A–C).

Two vertical relaxing incisions were made to improve visibility and reduce the possibility of tissue tearing. Following surgical access to the region, the buccal aspects of the deficient ridge were decorticated with a round diamond bur to enhance osseous bleeding. Two 10-mm tenting screws were placed and deemed immobile (Figure 4.5.6D). Rehydrated mineralized

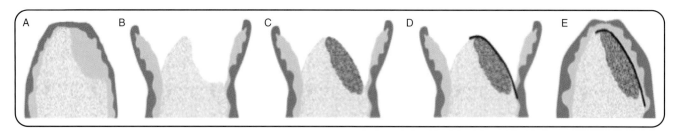

Figure 4.5.5 (A) Horizontal defect evident with soft tissue fill. (B) Crestal incision is made and the tissue is reflected to expose the osseous defect. (C) Defect filled with allograft bone. (D) Membrane placed over grafts and endogenous bone. (E) Primary soft tissue closure is obtained and then sutured.

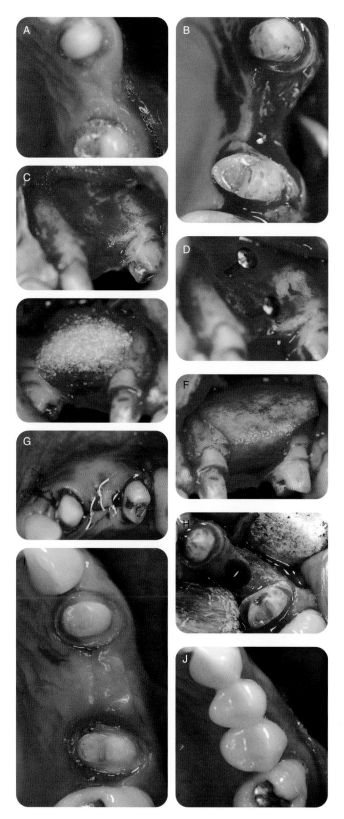

Figure 4.5.6 (A–J) Intraoral surgical photos.

freeze-dried bone allograft (FDBA) was then placed in excess onto this site (Figure 4.5.6E).

A rigid resorbable collagen membrane (OsseoGuard; Collagen Matrix, Inc., Oakland, NJ, USA) was placed over the bone allograft (Figure 4.5.6F), and the flap was repositioned and sutured back to its initial position (Figure 4.5.6G). Healing was uneventful. Six months following GBR the site was anesthetized and exposed. A 4.1-mm osteotomy was performed allowing for sufficient buccal and lingual bone to assure long-term stability of tissues and prevent recession (Figure 4.5.6H). Photographs taken prior to finalization with permanent fixed implant crowns demonstrate significant improvement in ridge width (Figure 4.5.6I,J). Figure 4.5.7 shows the radiograph taken on the day of the procedure.

Discussion

GBR is a predictable procedure for regenerating bone in a deficient maxillary or mandibular ridge, provided the determinants of success and the potential risk factors are identified. The degree of postoperative bone loss determines the technique the clinician chooses. There are certain tenets of tissue engineering that must be enforced for successful predictable augmentation. A scaffold is required (bone particles) for the patient's bone cells to attach to, a blood supply to the site is required (decorticate the patient's bone), the graft must be separated from the soft tissue to prevent fibroblast and squamous cell infiltration (membrane), and the graft must be stabilized. Larger defects can be treated with the technique described or with a titanium reinforced nonresorbable membrane to stabilize the graft. Autogenous bone may also be added to the bone mixture in such a situation to provide more of the patient's own bone-producing cells.

The healing for this procedure was uneventful. The tenting screws were removed and the permanent dental implant placed five months following the GBR procedure.

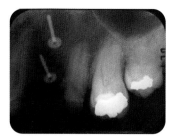

Figure 4.5.7 Radiograph on the day of the procedure.

Self-Study Questions

A. Define the Seibert classification system for edentulous ridge osseous defects.

B. What is the rationale for performing GBR?

C. When is GBR indicated? When is it contraindicated?

D. Which biomaterials can be used in a GBR? Is there histologic evidence of bone formation?

E. What are the techniques used for GBR therapy?

F. Are implants placed in GBR site as successful as implants placed in pristine bone? Does the surgical technique have an influence on the implant survival rate in the long term?

G. What are the complications associated with GBR? How do you manage these complications?

Answers located at the end of the chapter.

References

1. Seibert J, Nyman S. Localized ridge augmentation in dogs: a pilot study using membranes and hydroxyapatite. *J Periodontol* 1990;61:157–165.
2. Seibert JS. Reconstruction of deformed, partially edentulous ridges, using full thickness onlay grafts. Part I. Technique and wound healing. *Compend Contin Educ Dent* 1983;4:437–453.
3. Chiapasco M, Zaniboni M. Clinical outcomes of GBR procedures to correct peri-implant dehiscences and fenestrations: a systematic review. *Clin Oral Implants Res* 2009;20(Suppl 4):113–123.
4. Shanaman RH. The use of guided tissue regeneration to facilitate ideal prosthetic placement of implants. *Int J Periodontics Restorative Dent* 1992;12:256–265.
5. Wachtel HC, Langford A, Bernimoulin JP, Reichart P. Guided bone regeneration next to osseointegrated implants in humans. *Int J Oral Maxillofac Implants* 1991;6:127–135.
6. Fiorellini JP, Nevins ML. Localized ridge augmentation/preservation. A systematic review. *Ann Periodontol* 2003;8:321–327.
7. Li J, Wang HL. Common implant-related advanced bone grafting complications: classification, etiology, and management. *Implant Dent* 2008;17:389–401.
8. Newman MG, Takei HH, Klokkevold PR, Carranza FA (eds). *Carranza's Clinical Periodontology*, 10th edn. St. Louis, MO: Saunders Elsevier, 2006.
9. Zellin G, Gritli-Linde A, Linde A. Healing of mandibular defects with different biodegradable and non-biodegradable membranes: an experimental study in rats. *Biomaterials* 1995;16:601–609.
10. Friedmann A, Strietzel FP, Maretzki B, et al. Histological assessment of augmented jaw bone utilizing a new collagen barrier membrane compared to a standard barrier membrane to protect a granular bone substitute material. *Clin Oral Implant Res* 2002;13:587–594.
11. Sandberg E, Dahlin C, Linde A. Bone regeneration by the osteopromotive technique using bioabsorbable membranes: an experimental study in rats. *Int J Oral Maxillofac Surg* 1993;51:1106–1114.
12. Lindhe J, Karring T, Lang NP (eds) *Clinical Periodontology and Implant Dentistry*, 4th edn. Copenhagen: Blackell Munksgaard, 2003.
13. Hollinger JO, Brekke J, Gruskin E, Lee D. Role of bone substitutes. *Clin Orthop* 1996;324:55–65.
14. Tolman DE. Reconstructive procedures with endosseous implants in grafted bone: a review of the literature. *Int J Oral Maxillofac Implants* 1995;10:275–294.
15. Mowlem R. Cancellous chip bone grafts: report on 75 cases. *Lancet* 1944;244:746–748.
16. Mellonig JT. Autogenous and allogeneic bone grafts in periodontal therapy. *Crit Rev Oral Biol Med* 1992;3:333–352.
17. Mulliken JB, Glowacki J. Induced osteogenesis for repair and construction in the craniofacial region. *Plast Reconstr Surg* 1980;65:553–560.
18. Cammack GV II, Nevins M, Clem DS III, et al. Histologic evaluation of mineralized and demineralized freeze-dried bone allograft for ridge and sinus augmentations. *Int J Periodontics Restorative Dent* 2005;25:231–237.
19. Simion M, Trisi P, Piattelli A. Vertical ridge augmentation using a membrane technique associated with osseointegrated implants. *Int J Periodontics Restorative Dent* 1994;14:496–511.
20. Cochran DL, Douglas HB. Augmentation of osseous tissue around nonsubmerged endosseous dental implants. *Int J Periodontics Restorative Dent* 1993;13:506–519.
21. Mellonig JT, Nevins M. Guided bone regeneration of bone defects associated with implants: an evidence-based outcome assessment. *Int J Periodontics Restorative Dent* 1995;15:168–185.
22. Proussaefs P, Lozada J, Kleinman A, et al. The use of titanium mesh in conjunction with autogenous bone graft and inorganic bovine bone mineral (Bio-Oss) for localized

alveolar ridge augmentation: a human study. *Int J Periodontics Restorative Dent* 2003;23:185–195.

23. Becker W, Becker BE, Caffesse R. A comparison of demineralized freeze-dried bone and autologous bone to induce bone formation in human extraction sockets. *J Periodontol* 1994;65:1128–1133.

24. Becker W, Schenk R, Higuchi K, et al. Variations in bone regeneration adjacent to implants augmented with barrier membranes alone or with demineralized freeze-dried bone or autologous grafts: a study in dogs. *Int J Oral Maxillofac Implants* 1995;10:143–154.

25. Becker W, Urist MR, Tucker LM, et al. Human demineralized freeze-dried bone: inadequate induced bone formation in athymic mice. A preliminary report. *J Periodontol* 1995;66:822–828.

26. Landsberg C, Grosskopf A, Weinreb M. Clinical and biological observations of demineralized freeze-dried bone allografts in augmentation procedures around dental implants. *Int J Oral Maxillofac Implants* 1994;9:586–592.

27. Carranza FA Sr. A technic for reattachment. *J Periodontol* 1954;25:272–278.

28. Moskow BS, Tannenbaum P. Enhanced repair and regeneration of periodontal lesions in tetracycline-treated patients: case reports. *J Periodontol* 1991;62:341–350.

29. Esposito M, Grusovin MG, Kwan S, et al. Interventions for replacing missing teeth: horizontal and vertical bone augmentation techniques for dental implant treatment. *Cochrane Database Syst Rev* 2009;(3):CD003607.

30. Meijndert L, Meijer HJ, Stellingsma K, et al. Evaluation of aesthetics of implant-supported single-tooth replacements using different bone augmentation procedures: a prospective randomized clinical study. *Clin Oral Implants Res* 2007;18:715–719.

31. Donos N, Mardas N, Chadha V. Clinical outcomes of implants following lateral bone augmentation: systematic assessment of available options (barrier membranes, bone grafts, split osteotomy). *J Clin Periodontol* 2008;35(8 Suppl):173–202.

32. Chiapasco M, Abati S, Romeo E, Vogel G. Clinical outcome of autogenous bone blocks or guided bone regeneration with e-PTFE membranes for the reconstruction of narrow edentulous ridges. *Clin Oral Implants Res* 1999;10:278–288.

33. Urban IA, Monje A, Lozada JL, Wang H-L. Long-term evaluation of peri-implant bone level after reconstruction of severely atrophic edentulous maxilla via vertical and horizontal guided bone regeneration in combination with sinus augmentation: a case series with 1 to 15 years of loading. *Clin Implant Dent Related Res* 2017;19:46–55.

34. Tran, DT, Gay IC, Diaz-Rodriguez J, et al. Survival of dental implants placed in grafted and nongrafted bone: A retrospective study in a university setting . *Int J Oral Maxillofac Implants* 2016;31:310–317.

35. Simion M, Ferrantino L, Idotta E, Zarone F. Turned implants in vertical augmented bone: a retrospective study with 13 to 21 years follow-up. *Int J Periodontics Restorative Dent* 2016;36:309–317.

36. Rominger JW, Triplett RG. The use of guided tissue regeneration to improve implant osseointegration. *J Oral Maxillofac Surg* 1994;52:106–112.

TAKE-HOME POINTS

A. The Seibert classification was developed to facilitate communication between clinicians as to the severity of ridge deformities as well as indicate the potential outcome of regenerative procedures based on their value within the classification system [1,2].

- Class I: buccolingual loss of tissue with normal apico-coronal ridge height.
- Class II: apico-coronal loss of tissue with normal buccolingual ridge width.
- Class III: combination of buccolingual and apico-coronal loss of tissue, resulting in loss of normal height and width of the ridge.

Typically, the higher the Seibert class, the more difficult it is to regenerate the ridge to its original form. There is a caveat to this rule, however. Not always do we require vertical and/or horizontal augmentation to place implants. If the remaining ridge displays sufficient bone for implant placement, no regenerative procedure may be necessary. Furthermore, when placing an implant in an esthetic area such as the maxillary anterior region, augmentation may be necessary for esthetic reasons only.

B. According to Chiapasco and Zaniboni, in a systematic review in 2009, GBR is a procedure that allows spaces maintained by a barrier membrane to be filled with bone [3]. Bone loss can be a result of several factors: tooth loss, traumatic extractions, periodontal disease, infection, and so on. Thus the rationale for GBR procedures is to re-create the osseous ridge for either esthetic or functional reasons. Primarily, this procedure is used to rebuild the ridge for eventual implant placement. Most importantly, the implant should be placed so the eventual restoration is in the original tooth position and provides a natural emergence of the tooth from the soft tissues (prosthetically driven) [4].

The term "guided bone regeneration" was initially coined by Wachtel et al. [5] to describe the principles of guided tissue regeneration (GTR) applied to bone structures. Other authors contributed greatly to the early understanding of GBR [1].

C. According to the 2003 Periodontal World Workshop, GBR is indicated for patients who have had previous bone loss/destruction such that insufficient bone remains for implant placement [6].

There are no absolute contraindications for GBR, but the following conditions may present more risk of complications [7].
- Elderly patients: commonly present systemic conditions that may compromise healing.
- Bisphosphonates
  o Intravenous: great risk of osteonecrosis of the jaws.
  o Oral: low risk of osteonecrosis.
- Diabetes: uncontrolled diabetes is associated with delayed healing, failure of bone grafts, and further bone loss.
- Radiation: risk of osteoradionecrosis but is apparently low. Probably more risk after the first year post exposure.
- Alcoholism: risk of more adverse results.
- Severe bone loss, especially in the vertical dimension: limited and unpredictable results. In the anterior region this condition can lead to multiple surgeries that may negatively affect esthetics.
- Active infectious oral disease, especially periodontal disease: may promote infection, including patients with poor oral hygiene and poor compliance.
- All other conditions that would be a contraindication for any oral surgery, such as uncontrolled high blood pressure, cancer, or blood dyscrasias.

D. The GBR procedure is based on the use of a membrane to prevent epithelial and connective tissue growth into the regenerating site and a bone filler that primarily provides a scaffold where cells can attach. Membranes can be classified as resorbable or nonresorbable.

Resorbable Membranes
Can be a tissue, such as a connective tissue graft or allogeneic dermal matrix, but usually refers to

membranes made of collagen (BioGuide) and polylactic acid (e.g. Atrisorb, Guidor) [8,9]. Polyglycolic acid, polyorthoester, polyurethane, and polyhydroxybutyrate are also synthetic membranes used for GBR.

The advantages of a resorbable membrane are the elimination of surgical reentry for membrane removal as well as reduced complications if membrane becomes exposed. Disadvantages of using resorbable membranes include the possibility of early degradation prior to completion of bone formation as well as the presence of inflammation brought on by this degradation process [9]. More recently, new developments including cross-linking of collagen to increase resistance to biodegradation have been developed [10]. Fortunately, the mild inflammatory reaction caused by bioresorbable membranes does not seem to interfere with osteogenesis [8]. In addition to these attributes, resorbable membranes are also user friendly. However, their lack of resiliency results in a collapse of the membrane into the defect area [11]. Resorbable membranes are best reserved for clinical indications that allow the graft material or hardware (tenting screws, plates) to maintain the space required [8].

Nonresorbable Membranes
Usually made of polytetrafluoroethylene (PTFE) or expanded PTFE (ePTFE), and can be reinforced by titanium structure to give more stability. Titanium mesh and titanium foil are also occasionally used. Typically, nonresorbable membranes are removed after 6–12 months [12].

The primary advantage of nonresorbable membranes is stabilization of the graft. The disadvantages relate to its difficulty in handling and the possibility of its exposure during the healing process. Exposed membranes become contaminated with oral bacteria, which may lead to infection of the site and result in bone loss [8]. It is important to remove these membranes at a designated time during the healing process. If the membrane is removed too early, bone loss can also occur [8].

The available sources of bone materials include the following [13].
- Autograft: patient's own bone.
- Allograft-processed cadaver bone from another

human (FDBA) and demineralized freeze-dried bone allograft (DFDBA).
- Alloplast: synthetic bone substitutes such as tricalcium phosphate.
- Xenograft: cadaver bone from an animal source, e.g. bovine or porcine.

These products are provided in a particulate form of various sizes as well as in block form. Particulate grafts from the preceding list may also be combined [13].

The particulate autograft is still considered the gold standard for most ridge augmentation procedures primarily due to its inherent osteogenic behavior [14,15]. Blood vessels are able to penetrate the spaces between the particles compared with a block graft and thus provide for more rapid ingrowth of blood vessels. A larger osteoconduction surface area, more exposure of osteoinductive growth factors, and easier biologic remodeling are also advantages of the particulate graft [8].

However, autografts have limitations that include donor site morbidity, increased cost, potential resorption, size mismatch, and an inadequate volume of graft material [16,17]. Bone allografts overcome many of the shortfalls of autogenous grafts but are considered primarily osteoconductive and to some degree osteoinductive (DFDBA) in nature. The literature suggests that DFDBA may have greater osteoinductive potential because of the availability of morphogenetic proteins. However, a histologic study comparing FDBA with DFDBA for ridge augmentation demonstrated regeneration of 42% new bone area with no statistical difference between the two materials [18].

Bone allograft is bone collected from a human cadaver that is commercially available from tissue banks. It is obtained from cortical or cancellous bone within 12 hours of death of the donor, defatted, cut in pieces, washed in absolute alcohol, and deep frozen. The material may then proceed to be mineralized (FDBA) or demineralized (DFDBA). Both products then are ground and sieved to a particle size of 250–750 μm and freeze-dried. They are then vacuum-sealed in glass vials [8]. The use of particulate allograft bone replacement substitute has been reported for numerous applications, including ridge augmentation [19,20].

Successful horizontal ridge augmentation has been described with the use of a variety of different techniques and materials including allograft bone [14,21]. Vertical ridge augmentation with bone allograft has proven to be more difficult primarily due to the problem of osteogenic cells and blood vessels gaining access to the far reaches of the graft. Success was demonstrated using titanium mesh with autogenous particulate grafts [22].

From a histologic standpoint, biopsies from some studies using bone allografts indicate viable bone cells and visible osteocytes in lacunae, and a nine-month specimen showed no remaining allograft material [8]. However, there are some contradictory results using DFDBA and membrane combinations [23–25].

To enhance the quality and quantity of bone regenerated there is growing interest in growth factors. Products that are now clinically available include recombinant platelet-derived growth factor (rhPDGF-BB; marketed as GEM 21S, Osteohealth Inc., Shirley, NY, USA) and the recombinant human bone morphogenetic protein 2 (rhBMP-2; Infuse Medtronics Inc., Minneapolis, MN, USA). Platelet-rich growth factors derived from the patient's own blood are compounds rich in different growth factors.

E. GBR encompasses a variety of different applications including socket preservation, sinus elevation, peri-implant GBR, and ridge augmentation. Our focus is on ridge augmentation.

Typically the surgery begins with a crestal incision within the keratinized tissue. A full-thickness buccal and lingual flap is elevated to completely expose the osseous defect (Figure 4.5.5A,B). The exposed cortical bone is then perforated (decorticated) to allow for the osteogenic potential of the autogenous bone, including blood supply, osteoblasts, and growth factors, to enter into the graft (Figure 4.5.5B). Bone allograft is then placed with slight overfill to compensate for some bone resorption during the healing phase (Figure 4.5.5C). The membrane is then placed confirming that it overlaps the existing ridge (Figure 4.5.5D). To achieve primary closure, a periosteal releasing incision is necessary (Figure 4.5.5E) to achieve tension-free closure [26]. Most reports suggest removing sutures approximately 10–14 days after surgery. It is also suggested that no prosthesis be inserted for two to three weeks after surgery, to avoid pressure over the wound during the early healing period.

Additional concepts for flap management associated with ridge augmentation include the following [8]. It is desirable to make incisions remote relative to the placement of barrier membranes (e.g. vertical releasing incisions at least one tooth away from the site to be grafted). In the anterior maxilla, keeping vertical incisions remote is also an esthetic advantage [8].

Systemic antibiotics are generally used after regenerative periodontal therapy, even though studies to support their use are minimal. There have been some case reports that have demonstrated rebuilding of periodontal lesions after scaling, root planing, and curettage, with systemic and local treatment using penicillin or tetracycline, in combination with other forms of therapy [27,28].

F. Conclusions from a recent meta-analysis of randomized controlled clinical trials looking at different bone grafting studies for ridge augmentation suggest there are too few studies, and most have insufficient numbers of subjects. Even though various techniques are effective in augmenting bone horizontally and vertically, it is unclear which are the most efficient [29].

According to the literature, vertical ridge augmentation using bone allograft does not demonstrate predictable results and is often associated with more complications, including implant failure [12]. Lindhe et al. [12] suggested that "short implants appear to be a better alternative to vertical bone grafting of resorbed mandibles." According to Simion et al. [19], vertical bone augmentation was limited to approximately 4 mm with autogenous particulate bone.

Meijndert et al. [30] provided the best evidence for the success of horizontal ridge augmentation. This group demonstrated implant success when they were placed in augmented ridges with block grafts and particulate grafts (Bio-Oss). This finding is consistent with a systematic review by Donos et al. [31], who also concluded that the stability of these grafts and implants placed in them appears to

be similar to pristine bone. In terms of the membranes, the results of this study also indicated that both resorbable and nonresorbable demonstrated good results.

The review by Donos et al. concluded that "The implant survival at the augmented sites irrespective of the procedure used varied from 91.7% to 100% and from 93.2% to 100% at the control sites for a period between 12 and 59.1 months." These results include implants placed at the same time of augmentation [31]. An earlier review [6] had concluded that "Significant increase of the ridge dimensions (87–95%) can be expected for this procedure and block grafts appear to be slightly better" [30,32].

Further evidence to support these conclusions is illustrated in a systematic review of survival rates of dental implants after ridge augmentation therapy by Fiorellini and Nevins [6]. They reported that the survival rates for implants placed in augmented bone using several GBR procedures were similar to implants placed in native bone. Other researchers have examined the data of implants collected from multiple sources and concluded that patients receiving implants in augmented sites displayed higher variability and lower predictability in terms of peri-implantitis compared with patients receiving implants in pristine sites [33–35].

G. A systematic review by Li and Wang [7] reported that the complications most reported for particulate GBR are as follows.

1. Membrane exposure
2. Inflammatory reaction
3. Flap sloughing (associated with use of nonabsorbable membrane)
4. Infection
5. Incision line opening
6. Loss of graft or reduced graft
7. Sublingual edema

Management of these complications is as follows.

1. **Membrane exposure**: in a study where implants were placed in conjunction with nonresorbable barrier membranes and FDBA, a success rate of 96.8% was achieved with complete bone fill. This study reported an exposure rate of 29% of the membranes, but little effect on bone regeneration

was noted [6,8,36]. The literature supports the removal of the exposed nonresorbable membranes but not before sufficient time has elapsed for bone formation. Often these problems can be managed with good oral hygiene and use of topical 0.12% chlorhexidine rinses until that time.

2. **Inflammatory reaction**: with the use of resorbable membrane a confined inflammatory event does occur upon degradation of the graft. As mentioned earlier this does not seem to affect the result of the augmentation. Surgical trauma can also cause significant inflammation that may put overwhelming pressure on the tissues, resulting in suture line opening. To avoid this event, a careful atraumatic surgical technique is required and the use of steroids such as prednisone may be helpful.

3. **Flap sloughing**: because there is no blood supply below the flap when using nonresorbable membranes, a compromised environment exists. It is essential to maintain an appropriate thickness of the flap as well as a good base blood supply to minimize this possibility.

4. **Infection**: careful aseptic surgical technique, including thorough postoperative rinsing of the surgical site with sterile saline, can reduce the chances of infection. Preoperative and postoperative systemic antibiotics have been shown to improve augmentation results. Antibiotics such as penicillin, amoxicillin, clindamycin, azithromycin, or metronidazole can be used. If the infection cannot be controlled with antibiotics, removal of the bone graft may be necessary.

5. **Incision line opening**: as mentioned, a careful atraumatic surgical technique as well as the use of steroids may reduce the likelihood of this happening. More importantly, however, the surgeon must release the flap from the underlying periosteum for tension-free closure.

6. **Loss of graft or reduced graft**: the clinical situation should be reevaluated. The options of placing shorter implants or performing a complementary GBR can be discussed.

7. **Sublingual edema/bleeding**: some drawbacks of GBR are that the augmentation procedures, especially in the vertical dimension, can result in more serious complications (including life-threatening sublingual edema and bleeding), major discomfort, and pain. Pressure can be applied on the bleeding point with gauze until hemostasis is observed (tamponade). Vessel ligature and electrocautery have also been reported, although they need to be used with caution.

5

Mucogingival Therapy

Case 1: Pedicle Flaps 200
N. Joseph Laborde III, DDS and Kasumi Kuse Barouch, DDS, PhD, CAGS

Case 2: Connective Tissue Grafts. 206
Ronny S. Taschner, DDS and Jennifer F. Taschner, DDS, MMSc

Case 3: Free Gingival Grafts 214
Ronald M. Fried, DMD, MMSc and Maria Dona, DMD, MSD, DMSc

Case 4: Allografts (Alloderm) for Mucogingival Therapy. 228
Livia Valverde, DDS, MS, PhD, DMSc and Sarah D. Shih, DDS, MS, DMSc

Case 5: Frenectomy and Vestibuloplasty. 235
*Daniel Kuan-te Ho, DMD, DMSc, MSc, Satheesh Elangovan, BDS, DSc, DMSc, and
Sarah D. Shih, DDS, MS, DMSc*

Case 6: Minimally Invasive Coronally Advanced Flap Techniques .242
Samar Shaikh, BDS, MS, Pooyan Refahi, DMD, MS, and Irina F. Dragan, DDS, DMD, MS

Clinical Cases in Periodontics, Second Edition. Edited by Nadeem Karimbux.
© 2022 John Wiley & Sons, Inc. Published 2022 by John Wiley & Sons, Inc.
Companion website: www.wiley.com/go/karimbux/periodontics

Case 1

Pedicle Flaps

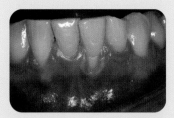
Medical History

There were no significant findings on reviewing the patient's medical history. She did not report taking any medications or supplements. The patient reported having no known drug allergies. She had had an annual physical with her primary care physician.

Review of Systems

- Vital signs
  - Blood pressure: 121/70 mmHg
  - Pulse rate: 70 beats/minute (regular)
  - Respiratory rate: 15 breaths/minute

Dental History

The patient reported that she saw her general dentist twice yearly for a cleaning and checkup. She had received orthodontic treatment as a teenager to correct crowding of her maxillary and mandibular arches. She reported brushing twice daily with a medium-bristle toothbrush. The patient tried to floss daily but sometimes she forgot.

Social History

The patient had been born and raised in Massachusetts. She currently resided in Boston with her husband and four-year-old daughter. The patient was a high-school English teacher. She reported drinking alcohol socially and had between one and three drinks per week and denied the use of tobacco products.

Extraoral Examination

The patient had no detectable lesions, masses, or swelling, and the temporomandibular joint was within normal limits.

Intraoral Examination

There were no detectable masses or lesions of the tongue, floor of the mouth, hard/soft palate, or buccal mucosa. Oral cancer screening was negative.

Hard Tissue Examination

The patient had no carious lesions. The restorations were intact on radiographic and clinical examination.

Periodontal Examination

- The full-mouth charting revealed probing depths of 1–3 mm with some bleeding on probing in the posterior quadrants.
- Mild gingival inflammation was present in the posterior quadrants adjacent to the second molars.
- An isolated recession defect was present on tooth #24 measuring 3 mm from the cementoenamel junction (CEJ).
- There was a minimal amount of attached keratinized tissue adjacent to the recession defect with mild localized marginal inflammation.

Occlusion

There were no occlusal discrepancies or interferences.

Radiographic Examination

- A recent full-mouth series revealed no carious lesions or pathologic findings.
- The bone levels appeared to be within normal limits with intact crestal lamina dura.

Diagnosis

According to the American Academy of Periodontology, the patient's gingival condition is classified under periodontal developmental and acquired deformities and conditions [1,2].

The recession defect can be also classified according to the Miller Classification System of gingival recession defects [3]. This defect is a Miller class 1 because it does not extend beyond the mucogingival junction and there is no interproximal bone loss. For a more in-depth discussion of classification of gingival recession, refer to Chapter 5, Case 3.

Treatment Plan

The proposed treatment plan for this patient involves dental prophylaxis including oral hygiene instructions. After establishing proper home care, the recession will be treated with a pedicle graft to repair the isolated gingival defect.

Discussion

Prior to treatment of gingival recession it is important to identify the possible etiology of the defect. The patient received orthodontic treatment, which can result in gingival recession if the teeth are moved labially beyond their bony housing. The patient also has a thin biotype, which is characterized by a thin scalloped gingiva and buccal plate that make the patient more prone to recession. Improper toothbrushing technique, such as overzealous brushing with a medium or hard-bristle toothbrush, can also lead to gingival recession. Once a dental prophylaxis was completed and the patient demonstrated the ability to maintain proper oral hygiene, treatment of the recession defect could proceed.

In this case the desired treatment outcome was to achieve root coverage and increase the width of attached tissue around tooth #24. After considering the possible treatment options, the decision to use a laterally positioned pedicle graft was made (refer to Question D to review the indications for laterally positioned pedicel graft).

The lateral pedicle graft was performed under local anesthesia with no complications (see Question C for a step-by-step guide to the procedure). The patient was seen for postoperative appointments at two, four, and six weeks. At six weeks there was almost full root coverage, with an increase in the amount of attached keratinized tissue around #24. The patient also reported a decrease in sensitivity in her lower front teeth (Figure 5.1.2).

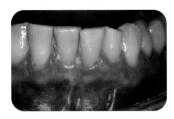

Figure 5.1.2 Six-week postoperative picture. Source: courtesy of David S. Greenfield, DMD.

Self-Study Questions

A. What is a pedicle graft?

B. What are the surgical techniques that use pedicle grafts for root coverage?

C. How is a laterally positioned pedicle flap performed?

D. What are the indications/contraindications for using these techniques?

E. What are the benefits/limitations of using pedicle flaps compared with free autogenous grafts?

F. How else can pedicle flaps be used in the oral cavity?

Answers located at the end of the chapter.

References

1. Cortellini P, Bissada NF. Mucogingival conditions in the natural dentition: narrative review, case definitions, and diagnostic considerations. *J Periodontol* 2018;89(Suppl 1):S204–S213.
2. Cairo F, Nieri M, Cincinelli S, Cincinelli S, et al. The interproximal clinical attachment level to classify gingival recessions and predict root coverage outcomes: an explorative and reliability study. *J Clin Periodontol* 2011;38:661–666.
3. Miller PD Jr. Root coverage using the free soft tissue autograft citric acid application. III. A successful and predictable procedure in areas of deep-wide recession. *Int J Periodontics Restorative Dent* 1985;5(2):14–37.
4. Grupe HE, Warren RF Jr. Repair of gingival defects by a sliding flap operation. *J Periodontol* 1956;27:92–95.
5. Cohen DW, Ross SE. The double papillae repositioned flap in periodontics. *J Periodontol* 1968;39:65–70.
6. Harris R. The connective tissue and partial thickness double pedicle graft: a predictable method of obtaining root coverage. *J Periodontol* 1992;63:447–486.
7. Mariotti A. Efficacy of chemical root surface modifiers in the treatment of periodontal disease. A systematic review. *Ann Periodontol* 2003;8:205–226.
8. Rose LF, Mealy BL, Genco RJ, Cohen DW. *Periodontics: Medicine, Surgery and Implants.* St. Louis, MO: Elsevier Mosby, 2004:432.
9. Rose LF, Mealy BL, Genco RJ, Cohen DW. *Periodontics: Medicine, Surgery and Implants.* St. Louis, MO: Elsevier Mosby, 2004:432–434.
10. Wennstrom JL. Mucogingival therapy. *Ann Periodontol* 1996;1:671–701.
11. Fugazzotto PA. Maintenance of soft issue closure following guided bone regeneration: technical considerations and report of 723 cases. *J Periodontol* 1999;70:1085–1097.
12. Nemcovsky CE, Zvi A, Moses O, Gelernter I. Healing of dehiscence defects at delayed-immediate implant sites primarily closed by a rotating palatal flap following extraction. *Int J Oral Maxillofac Implants* 2000;15(4):550–558.

TAKE-HOME POINTS

A. A pedicle graft (also called pedicle flap) is a full- or split-thickness flap designed in such a way that it remains connected at its base. The flap can then be rotated or positioned at an adjacent location while still maintaining its own blood supply through its connection. The blood supply nourishes the graft and facilitates the vascular union with the recipient site. This differs from a free autogenous tissue graft that is completely severed from its blood supply but can be attached to another part of the oral cavity.

B.
- **Laterally positioned flap**: this technique, first described by Grupe and Warren in 1956, uses donor gingiva from a healthy tooth to cover the exposed root of an adjacent tooth [4].
- **Double papilla flap**: this technique, described by Cohen and Ross in 1968, is used to cover defects where there is an inadequate amount of gingiva on the adjacent area for a laterally positioned flap [5]. In this method, the papillae from each side of the problem tooth are reflected and rotated over the midfacial aspect of the recipient tooth and sutured. Harris described a modification of this technique by placing a subepithelial connective tissue graft under the double pedicle flaps [6].
- **Coronally positioned flap**: this technique can be used when there is an adequate amount of keratinized tissue and thickness of gingiva adjacent to the recession defect. The gingiva is released and advanced coronally to cover the recession defect. The procedure can be performed with or without vertical releasing incisions and it is often used in combination with other mucogingival techniques.

C. Before beginning the procedure, the bone level on the facial of the donor site should be evaluated with bone sounding. If the distance from the bone to the CEJ is >2 mm, there is a risk of recession on the donor tooth. Leaving a collar of tissue at the donor site can reduce this risk. The root surface where coverage will be attempted should be thoroughly planed and smoothed to remove surface irregularities or defects. Some practitioners might use chemicals

such as ethylenediaminetetraacetic acid (EDTA), citric acid, or tetracycline to condition the root surface. However, there is no definitive evidence in humans that chemically treated roots are more biologically acceptable than mechanically prepared surfaces for soft tissue grafting [7].

The first incisions are made to prepare the recipient site for the donor tissue. An incision starting in the papilla between the donor and recipient site is made from the level of the CEJ continuing at an oblique angle beyond the base of the defect. A small horizontal incision at the level of the expected root coverage is made on the opposite side of the recipient site and then extended apically to meet the first incision. The epithelium between these incisions is removed in preparation to receive the pedicle graft.

The next incision is made from the line angle of the tooth adjacent to the donor site and extended parallel to the first incision. The following incision extends across the donor site connecting the first and third incision. This incision can be sulcular, or if there is a concern of recession, this incision can be made so a collar of tissue remains. The tissue collar should have at least 0.5 mm of attached tissue (Figure 5.1.3).

The flap is reflected with a split-thickness dissection. Full-thickness dissection may be necessary in some portions to maintain adequate flap thickness and prevent perforations. The flap can now be mobilized and rotated to the recipient site. If there is tension on the flap at the recipient site, additional release of the tissue may be done (Figure 5.1.4).

Once the pedicle flap is in the correct position and tension free, it is sutured in place using 5-0 or 6-0 simple interrupted sutures. The leading edge of the

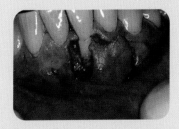

Figure 5.1.3 Incision design for lateral pedicle flap.
Source: courtesy of David S. Greenfield, DMD.

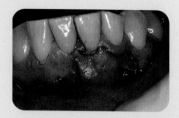

Figure 5.1.4 Rotation of pedicle flap. Source: courtesy of David S. Greenfield, DMD.

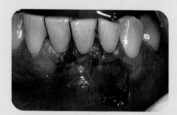

Figure 5.1.5 Flap sutured to recipient site. Source: courtesy of David S. Greenfield, DMD.

flap is secured first with sutures in the papilla and mucosa. The trailing edge is secured with a suture in the papilla. If there is periosteum left intact from the split-thickness dissection, additional sutures can be placed to stabilize the flap (Figure 5.1.5).

The graft should be stable and immobile, which can be confirmed by movement of the lip. If desired, a periodontal dressing can be applied to the area [8].

D. Indications for the use of pedicle grafts for root coverage include the following [9].

- An isolated area of recession with no bone loss on the proximal surface.
- A donor site with adequate soft tissue width and thickness, sufficient vestibular depth, and adequate bone thickness with no dehiscence.

Contraindications for the procedure include the following.

1. A donor site with thin tissue is not recommended because it is prone to future recession.
2. If the distance from the crest of bone to the CEJ on the facial surface of the donor tooth is >2 mm, there is a risk of recession after the tissue is rotated.

E.

1. There is only one surgical site with a pedicle graft (palatal donor site not needed), which limits the risk of postoperative morbidity.
2. The pedicle maintains its own blood supply, which increases the chance for graft survival and root coverage.

3. There is a harmonious blend of tissue color and contour after healing compared with free autogenous tissue grafts that can have less esthetic results.
4. It is more difficult to treat multiple teeth using pedicle grafting techniques compared with free autogenous grafts, which can be harvested according to the size needed.
5. There is less risk of recession from the donor site of free autogenous grafts compared with pedicle flaps.
6. Root coverage is less predictable using pedicle grafting techniques, with a mean root coverage of 62.5% for laterally positioned or double papilla flaps. The mean root coverage for connective tissue grafts in combination with various flap techniques is 89.3% [10].

F. A variety of surgical techniques using pedicle grafts are described in the dental literature. Fugazzotto reported a technique using a rotated palatal pedicle graft to help obtain primary closure in guided bone regeneration procedures [11]. After palatal reflection, a layer of connective tissue is dissected away from the base (apical) of the flap while maintaining its connection at the coronal portion. This method helps achieve tension-free primary closure over the grafted site. Nemcovsky et al. have demonstrated a technique that uses rotated palatal tissue to achieve primary tissue closure over extraction sites [12]. They reported the use of full- and partial-thickness rotated palatal flaps to cover extraction sites as well as coverage of immediate implants placed in the maxilla. In the technique demonstrated here, a subepithelial connective tissue graft is harvested adjacent to and one tooth distal from the extraction site. This graft is rotated to cover the grafted extraction site while maintaining its attachment adjacent to the area. This technique helps achieve primary closure to aid in the formation of adequate bone and soft tissue formation (Figures 5.1.6–5.1.8).

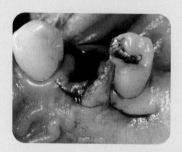

Figure 5.1.6 Connective tissue harvested from palate. Source: courtesy of Kasumi Barouch, DDS.

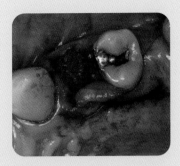

Figure 5.1.7 Allograft placed in extraction socket and connective tissue rotated under sulcular tissue on palate. Source: courtesy of Kasumi Barouch, DDS.

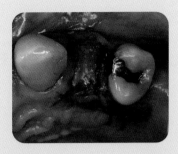

Figure 5.1.8 Connective tissue sutured in place while maintaining connection at base of graft. Source: courtesy of Kasumi Barouch, DDS.

Case 2

Connective Tissue Grafts

CASE STORY

The patient was a 36-year-old male whose general dentist had noticed that the recession on teeth #3, #4, and #5 was progressing and had referred him to a periodontist. The dentist had also been concerned with the cervical abrasion/erosion, lack of keratinized tissue, and associated frenum close to the gingival margin on tooth #5 (Figure 5.2.1).

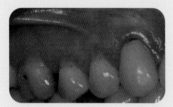

Figure 5.2.1 Preoperative clinical presentation.

LEARNING GOALS AND OBJECTIVES

■ To identify the indications and rationales for soft tissue grafting
■ To understand the surgical technique for subepithelial connective tissue grafting, including:
  ○ Zucchelli incision designs and technique for multiple recession sites
  ○ Root preparation
  ○ Harvesting of donor tissue
  ○ Suturing of graft and flap
■ To understand the rationale for root preparation
■ To understand the presurgical and postsurgical considerations

Medical History

The patient's medical history was not significant. The patient was not taking any medications and denied having any allergies.

Review of Systems

• Vital signs
  ○ Blood pressure: 128/76 mmHg
  ○ Pulse rate: 68 beats/minute
  ○ Respiratory rate: 14 breaths/minute

Social History

The patient admitted to smoking cigarettes as a young adult but had not smoked for at least 10 years. He denied using chewing tobacco. He was a social drinker and admitted to drinking one or two alcoholic beverages three to four times a week.

Dental History

The patient had received fairly regular dental care throughout most of his childhood and adult years, with periodic cleanings and examinations approximately every six months. He had had orthodontic care as a teenager; treatment lasted approximately two years.

Oral Hygiene Status

The patient brushed his teeth three to four times a day, using a medium or soft brush, and admitted to brushing somewhat "aggressively." He flossed three to four times a week.

Family History

One of his parents had been treated for recession, but both parents had all or most of their own teeth.

Extraoral Examination

No significant findings were present.

Intraoral Examination

- Oral cancer screening was negative. Soft tissues including buccal mucosa, hard and soft palate, floor of the mouth, and tongue all appeared normal.
- There was generally an adequate amount of attached keratinized gingiva present on all remaining teeth (Table 5.2.1).
- The patient had excellent oral hygiene with a minimal amount of plaque accumulation and gingival inflammation.

- See Figure 5.2.2 for periodontal charting.
- There was some mild clinical attachment loss with no probing depths >3 mm, no tooth mobility, and no furcation invasion.
- Tissue color, contour, and consistency: generalized pink color with normal contour except for recession as noted below. Consistency was firm with normal stippling.
- Bleeding on probing was localized and very slight.

Table 5.2.1 Keratinized/attached gingiva.

Tooth #	1	2	3	4	5	6	7	8
Recession (mm)	X	2	3	2	4	0	0	0
Width of keratinized tissue (mm)	X	4	3	4	1	4	4	4
Width of attached gingiva (mm)	X	2	1	2	0	2	2	2

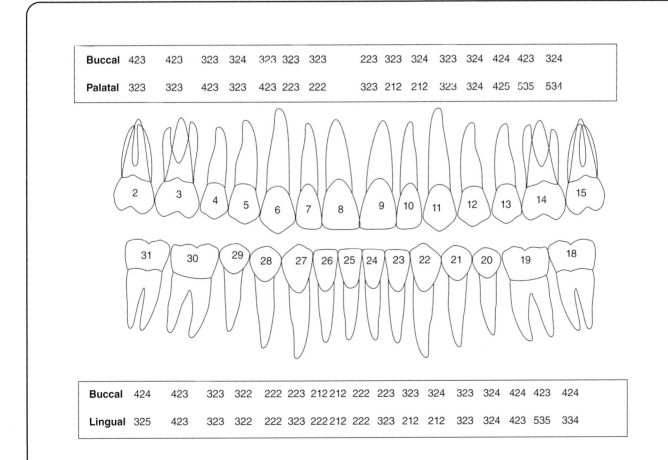

Figure 5.2.2 Probing pocket depth/recession measurements during initial visit.

Radiographic Examination

There was no bone loss evident on radiographic examination.

Diagnosis

- Recession with inadequate attached gingiva, localized #3 and #5.
- Cervical abrasion/erosion, #3–#5.

Treatment Plan

- Oral hygiene instructions to modify traumatic brushing technique.
- Subepithelial connective tissue graft, #3, #4, and #5.
- Discuss possible dietary influence on cervical erosion.

Treatment

After evaluation of the thickness and anatomy of the palate by "sounding," administration of local anesthetic, and evaluation of the amount of keratinized tissue present on the facial of teeth #3–5, treatment of #3–5 with a subepithelial connective tissue graft (SCTG) using the right palate as a donor site was recommended.

A decision was made to reposition the overlying flap coronally to completely or almost completely cover the graft. Because there was still a small width of keratinized tissue on #5 and 2–3 mm of keratinized tissue on #2, #3, and #4, the cosmetic result would be better than it would be if several millimeters of connective tissue was left exposed.

With the Zucchelli technique [1] (Figure 5.2.3), the incisions are made at an angle extending from the cementoenamel junction (CEJ) of one tooth to the height of the recession on the adjacent tooth. Where multiple teeth are involved, a tooth in the middle is designated and the incisions are angled apically from the mesial and distal at the level of the CEJ to the height of recession of the tooth to the mesial and to the tooth to the distal.

The purpose of this design is to (i) avoid vertical releasing incisions and (ii) create papillary shapes that, when coronally repositioned, will rotate mesially or distally and cover the de-epithelialized papillae and the underlying connective tissue graft.

In this case, tooth #5 was selected (Figure 5.2.4A), and Zucchelli incisions were made mesial and distal

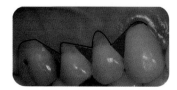

Figure 5.2.3 Zucchelli technique.

starting at the CEJ. Additional incisions were made starting at the distal CEJ of #4, angling to the apical extent of the recession of #3. Another similar incision was made starting at the distal cervical of tooth #3.

A partial-thickness flap was reflected (Figure 5.2.4B), freeing the flap apically to allow the flap to easily be coronally repositioned. To avoid perforating the flap with sharp dissection, it may be necessary to elevate carefully over any exostoses.

The papillae are carefully de-epithelialized (Figure 5.2.4C) using a 12b scalpel blade. The amount of tissue removed is approximately 1 mm or less, leaving as much of the underlying connective tissue papilla as possible.

Root Preparation

1. Root plane to smooth the roots and remove or "round out" any grooves, at times creating a saddle shape (Figure 5.2.5). It may be necessary to use a high-

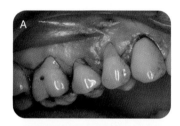

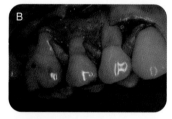

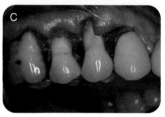

Figure 5.2.4 (A) Initial incisions; (B) reflection; (C) de-epithelialization of the papillae.

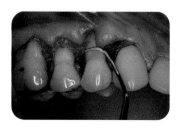

Figure 5.2.5 Root planing.

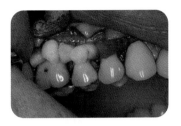

Figure 5.2.6 Application of EDTA solution.

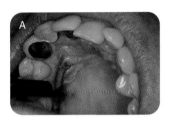

Figure 5.2.7 (A) Harvesting of the graft; (B) trimming of the graft.

speed handpiece lightly and carefully with football-shaped diamond finishing burs (medium, fine, and extra-fine) if the grooving on the root is severe or if an existing restoration needs to be removed.

2. Chemically treat the root with ethylenediaminetetraacetic acid (EDTA) solution 17% (Pulpdent) for two minutes by applying saturated cotton pellets or burnishing with a saturated cotton pellet for 45 seconds (Figure 5.2.6).

3. After measuring the length of graft needed to cover the roots, mark the approximate positions at the beginning and end of the graft on the palate with the point of the probe.

4. Make the first incision 4 mm from the gingival margin. Make the second incision 1–2 mm closer to the tooth and parallel to the first incision (Figure 5.2.7A).

5. The depth of the incisions can safely extend 7 mm from the CEJ on a shallow palate, 12 mm on an average palate, and 17 mm on a high palate [2].

6. If the palate is thin, it may be necessary to elevate the graft from the palatal bone instead of making a second incision.

7. At the apical extent of the incision, angle the scalpel toward the palate to free the graft. Do the same at the mesial and distal borders of the graft.

8. Remove the epithelium by trimming it with a sharp scalpel (Figure 5.2.7B).

Suturing

Suture the graft with individual sling sutures using 5-0 chromic gut suture. Tie on the lingual, if possible, to allow for better flap-to-graft contact (Figure 5.2.8A). Suture the flap with 6-0 monofilament nylon or Gore

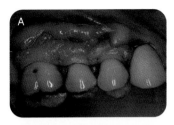

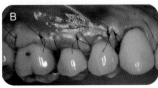

Figure 5.2.8 (A) Suturing of the connective tissue graft; (B) suturing of flap.

CV-6 suture. Use one sling suture per tooth (Figure 5.2.8B).

Enter the flap from the facial about 3 mm from the gingival margin, approximately at the mesial line angle of the tooth. Proceed interproximally, not engaging the interproximal connective tissue papilla but going coronal to it, wrapping around the lingual, passing through the distal embrasure to the facial, again keeping the suture coronal to the papilla. Pass the suture needle through the facial flap 3 mm apical to the gingival margin at the distal line angle, pass through the distal embrasure coronal to the papilla, wrap around the lingual to the mesial embrasure, pass through it, and tie the suture on the facial. Repeat for each tooth. Also place a sling suture to secure the gingival flap one tooth mesial and one tooth distal to the graft.

Postoperative Instructions

- Ice the area for 24–48 hours, 20 minutes on and 20 minutes off.
- Sleep on back with head slightly elevated.
- Rinse with chlorhexidine 0.12% rinse b.i.d.
- Avoid brushing or flossing for two to four weeks.
- Eat a soft diet and try to avoid eating on the side of the surgery.
- After two weeks use an ultra-soft brush to gently remove debris with roll technique.

Prescriptions

- Motrin 800 mg, one tablet t.i.d. starting one hour before procedure.
- Vicodin 5/500, one to two tablets every four to six hours as needed for pain.
- Doxycycline 100 mg, one tablet b.i.d. day of surgery, then one tablet every day for 10 days.
- Chlorhexidine rinse 0.12%: rinse for 30–60 seconds b.i.d.

Postoperative Follow-up

Patients should be seen 7–14 days after the surgery to remove dressing/sutures (Figure 5.2.9A). Additional follow-up to observe patient home care and healing should be planned accordingly (Figure 5.2.9B).

Discussion

Indications

The need for an adequate band of attached gingiva has been a topic in the periodontal literature for at least 50 years. It has been argued that without an adequate band of attached gingiva, the stability of the gingival margin would be at risk with the potential for further attachment loss, recession, pocket formation, and inflammation.

The amount of attached gingiva needed to prevent further recession and attachment loss has also been debated and is unclear. Early papers suggested that 5–6 mm of keratinized tissue with a probing depth of 2–3 mm would result in a functional band of attached gingiva of 2–3 mm that was necessary to obtain stability of the marginal gingiva. Lang and Löe [3] stated that most areas (80%) with 2 mm or more keratinized gingiva and 1 mm attached gingiva remained healthy while inflammation persisted in areas with <2 mm keratinized gingiva and 1 mm attached gingiva even with good oral hygiene. Several other studies found that areas with minimal width of keratinized gingiva were no more prone to inflammatory changes.

The 1989 World Workshop [4] concluded there were several parameters that should be considered when determining if an adequate zone of attached gingiva is present and the minimum amount of attached gingiva that is acceptable.

The American Academy of Periodontology Consensus Statement on Mucogingival Conditions [5] defines an inadequate amount of keratinized tissue as <2 mm of width, of which <1 mm is attached gingiva. It states that a minimal amount or absence of attached gingiva alone is not a justification for gingival augmentation. The presence of "recession, loss of supporting bone, absence or reduction of keratinized tissue, and probing depths extending beyond the mucogingival junction" must be considered as well as resulting "root sensitivity, loss of tooth structure (abrasion), increased length of the clinical crown, and inflammation and bleeding of the marginal tissue." Ultimately, the clinician's best judgment must be used to determine whether or not to treat mucogingival conditions [5].

The 2017 World Workshop [6] agrees with the American Academy of Periodontology Consensus Statement on Mucogingival Conditions [5] regarding the amount of keratinized and attached gingiva needed as noted above. However, the indications for treatment have been revised and are based on classification of periodontal biotypes, gingival recession, and root surface conditions. The treatment considerations are divided into two main groups: (i) teeth with absence of gingival recession and (ii) teeth with gingival recession. Within each of these groups, there are two case types.

- *Teeth without gingival recession*: there are two case types, labeled "Case a" and "Case b," which are differentiated by thick (Case a) and thin (Case b) biotypes. In the Case a group, prevention is recommended through good oral hygiene and monitoring. In the Case b group, an increased level of monitoring is recommended. In addition, mucogingival surgery could be considered, if implants, restorations with subgingival margins or orthodontics is planned.

- *Teeth with gingival recession*: there are also two case types, labeled "Case c" and "Case d." In the Case c group, monitoring and charting the recession and the amount of keratinized tissue is recommended. If increased recession or root wear or sensitivity develops, then, treatment may be considered. In the Case d group, a treatment-oriented approach is considered. These include cases with gingival recession, thin biotypes, and patient concerns or complaints of hypersensitivity or esthetic compromise. Also included in this group are teeth with recession, thin biotype, cervical caries, and non-carious cervical lesions.

With these considerations in mind, gingival grafting to increase the width of attached gingiva may be indicated if there is (i) <2 mm width of keratinized tissue in which <1 mm is attached gingiva, (ii) the recession is progressive, (iii) the gingival margin would be stressed by a restorative margin at or below the gingival margin, (iv) a removable partial denture would stress the gingival margin, (v) orthodontic treatment is planned (and the teeth are to be moved labially), in progress or completed, or (vi) an inability to maintain the gingival margin free of inflammation, bleeding, and/or plaque accumulation [4]. Grafting for root coverage should also be considered when recession has resulted

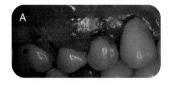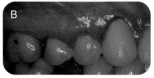

Figure 5.2.9 (A) Suture removal at two weeks; (B) eight weeks post surgery.

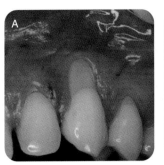
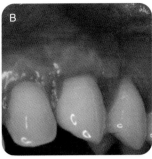

Figure 5.2.10 (A, B) Inadequate attached gingiva with recession.

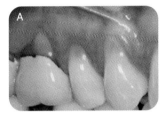
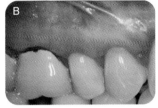

Figure 5.2.11 (A, B) Treatment with subepithelial connective tissue graft.

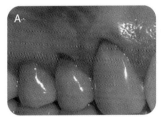
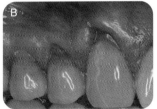

Figure 5.2.12 (A, B) Progressive recession.

in root abrasion, root sensitivity, and/or compromised esthetics.

There are several reasons for performing connective tissue grafts. These include areas where there is inadequate attached gingiva (Figure 5.2.10) in order to improve esthetics, decrease root sensitivity, improve cleanability, and reduce the exposure of furcations (Figure 5.2.11), stop progressive recession (Figure 5.2.12), treat root wear/erosion/cervical abrasion (Figure 5.2.13), cover exposed crown margins (Figure 5.2.14), cover an exposed implant collar (Figure 5.2.15), cover lingual recession (Figure 5.2.16), and for root coverage and ridge augmentation prior to a fixed bridge (Figure 5.2.17).

Treatment with SCTG can accomplish the following (see Figures 5.2.3 and 5.2.4):

• Improve esthetics
• Decrease root sensitivity
• Improve cleanability
• Reduce exposure of furcations (improving long-term prognosis).

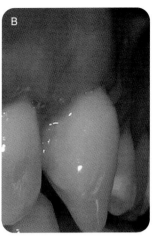
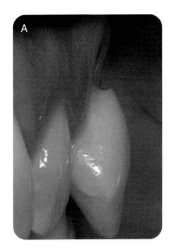

Figure 5.2.13 (A, B) Root wear/erosion/cervical abrasion.

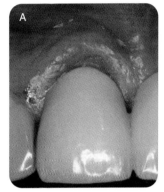
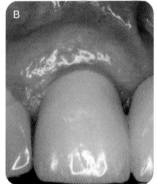

Figure 5.2.14 (A, B) Covering exposed crown margins.

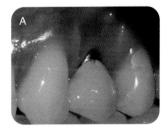
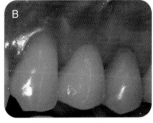

Figure 5.2.15 (A, B) Covering an exposed implant collar.

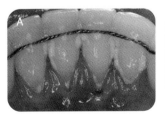
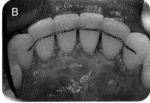

Figure 5.2.16 (A, B) Covering lingual recession.

Techniques

The early procedures developed to augment the zone of attached gingiva included denudation of the bone, denudation of the periosteum, apically repositioned flap,

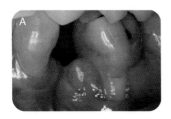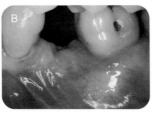

Figure 5.2.17 (A, B) Root coverage and ridge augmentation prior to a fixed bridge.

and free gingival grafts. The bone denudation procedure produced a beautiful result but also caused attachment loss and significant morbidity, taking months to heal with the need to wear periodontal packing for most of the time. Leaving exposed periosteum decreased the bone loss, but the morbidly and healing period were still significant. Free gingival grafts, using the stratified squamous epithelium and the underlying connective tissue from the palate as donor material, decreased morbidity at the recipient site, but morbidity at the palatal donor site gave free gingival grafts an unpleasant reputation among patients.

All these procedures were quite successful in creating adequate zones of attached gingiva and eliminating or minimizing the risk of further recession. However, these procedures were not indicated for root coverage, and there was little that could be done to correct the recession that often resulted in unsatisfactory esthetics, root sensitivity, chemical erosion, mechanical abrasion, and caries. Pedicle flap procedures were developed and used successfully to obtain root coverage, but an adequate adjacent donor site was needed and not always available, limiting the use of this procedure.

Root coverage with a free gingival graft was described by Holbrook and Ochsenbein [7] in 1983. The procedure required taking a rather large graft from the surface of the palate, often measuring 12–15 mm in the vertical dimension, and suturing the graft in place with a complex pattern of mattress sutures to closely adapt the graft to the root and periosteum apical and lateral to the root. Root coverage was fairly predictable with this procedure, but an acrylic appliance was needed to cover the donor area because of the large palatal wound. However, even with the best attempts at wound coverage, postoperative morbidity was prolonged.

The SCTG was developed by Langer and Langer [8] to create an increased zone of attached gingiva and to partially or completely cover roots, improving esthetic outcomes, decreasing root sensitivity, covering areas of

erosion and abrasion, and protecting the root from additional root wear.

The SCTG has become the standard of care for treatment of recession. The techniques used for SCTGs are varied, and well-publicized modifications of the Langer technique have been developed by P. D. Miller [9], John Bruno, and Pat Allen, among others.

Conclusion

As the demand for esthetics in dentistry has increased, SCTGs have increasingly become an integral component of periodontal therapy. Although the purest indication for soft tissue grafting is a lack of attached gingiva, indications for SCTGs have grown to include root coverage, either partial or complete, for many reasons including improving esthetics, root sensitivity, cervical abrasion, and covering a crown margin or an exposed implant collar.

All the various techniques, although similar, have subtle differences in outcomes and indications. The technique presented here is ideal for achieving uniform esthetic tissue contours and rarely requires a second procedure of gingivoplasty. Because the existing keratinized tissue is coronally repositioned over the connective tissue graft to the level of the CEJ, the sometimes unsightly line, demarcating where the flap and connective tissue joined, is absent.

Langer's technique can result in horizontal suture lines at the base of the papillae that require a soft tissue plasty. Bruno's technique requires a second procedure to reposition the mucosa apically that was coronally advanced to completely cover the connective tissue graft. This second procedure exposes the connective tissue that then matures into a beautiful band of keratinized attached gingiva.

In the future, we will see further evolution of materials and techniques for increasing zones of attached gingiva, covering roots and implants, and reconstructing lost papillae. Periodontal plastic surgery continues to be a challenging and exciting area of the specialty of periodontology. Together with restorative procedures, periodontal plastic surgery helps us get closer to achieving our goal of restoring our patients' dentition to its most natural and esthetic potential.

References

1. Zucchelli G, De Sanctis M. Treatment of multiple recession-type defects in patients with esthetic demands. *J Periodontol* 2000;71:1506–1514.
2. Reiser G, Bruno JF, Mahan PE, Larkin LH. The subepithelial connective tissue graft palatal donor site: anatomic

considerations for surgeons. *Int J Peridontics Restorative Dent* 1996;16:130–137.

3. Lang NP, Löe H. The relationship between the width of attached gingiva and gingival health. *J Periodontol* 1972;43:623–627.

4. Nevins M, Becker N, *Kornman K (eds) World Workshop in Clinical Periodontics*. Chicago, IL: American Academy of Periodontology, 1989:7–10.

5. American Academy of Periodontology Consensus Statement on Mucogingival Conditions, May 2009. Available at https://www.gepi-mattout.com/wp-content/uploads/2017/02/aap-consensus.pdf

6. Cotellini, P, Bissada, NF. Mucogingival conditions in the natural dentition: narrative review, case definitions and diagnostic considerations. *J Periodontol* 2018;89(Suppl 1):S204–S213.

7. Holbrook T, Ochsenbein C. Complete coverage of the denuded root surface with a one-stage gingival graft. *Int J Periodontics Restorative Dent* 1983;3:8–27.

8. Langer B, Langer L. Subepithelial connective tissue graft technique for root coverage. *J Periodontol* 1985;56:715–720.

9. Miller PD Jr. A classification of marginal tissue recession. *Int J Periodontics Restorative Dent* 1985;5:8–13.

Case 3

Free Gingival Grafts

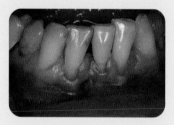
Medical History

The patient reported a history of hyperthyroidism that had been treated with one course of radiation 30 years ago, and she was currently on Levothroid for subsequent hypothyroidism. There were no other significant medical problems, and the patient had no known allergies.

Dental History

The patient reported a history of nonsurgical periodontal treatment and periodontal surgery in the maxillary right quadrant 16 years ago and subsequent three-month recalls. The patient had a history of multiple restorations and extraction of teeth #1, #2, #16, #17, #25, and #32 in her teenage years. Tooth #25 was possibly extracted due to crowding, but no orthodontic treatment was rendered.

Social History

The patient did not drink alcohol and she was a former cigarette smoker. The patient smoked 12 pack-years and stopped smoking 25 years ago.

Oral Hygiene

The patient reported toothbrushing at least once a day using an electric soft toothbrush that was replaced every six to eight weeks. She said she flossed twice a day.

Extraoral and Intraoral Examinations

- There were no significant findings. The patient had no extraoral or intraoral masses or swelling, and the temporomandibular joint was within normal limits.
- A periodontal examination revealed localized mild marginal gingival erythema, with rolled margins, edematous papillae, and bleeding on probing in area #23–24, #26, and #27. There was gingival recession

Probing Buccal	-	-	222	222	323	312	212	223	323	313	213	323	323	333	223	-
Recession	-	-	1	1	2	3	-	1	-	3	3	2	2	3	3	-
Keratinized gingiva	-	-	4	4	3	1	2	3	3	1	1	2	2	3	3	-
Probing Palatal	-	-	323	323	323	323	211	222	212	222	222	322	222	323	323	-

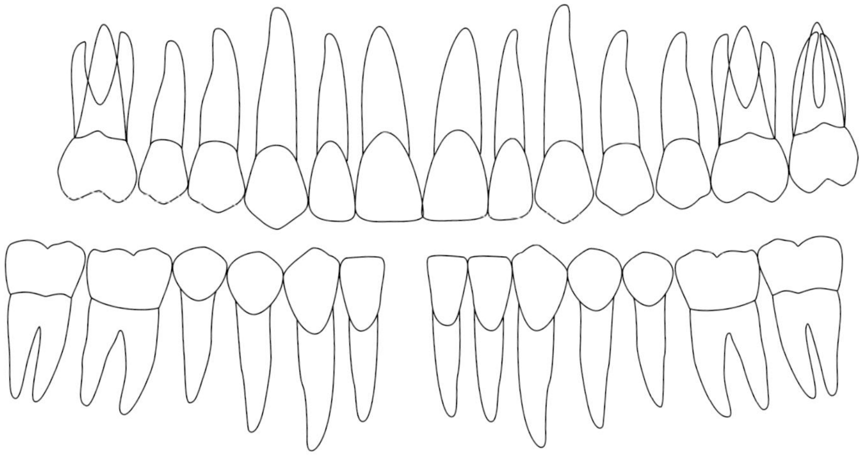

Probing Buccal	-	323	323	323	323	323	322	-	222	222	222	222	223	323	323	-
Recession	-	2	3	-	2	-	2	-	2	3	1	3	-	3	-	-
Keratinized gingiva	-	2	2	2	2	2	1	-	2	1	1	1	1	1	1	-
Probing Lingual	-	323	323	323	323	323	222	-	222	222	222	323	323	333	333	-

Figure 5.3.2 Probing pocket depth, keratinized gingiva, and recession measurements.

present on the buccal aspect of teeth #4–6, #10, #11, #19, #21–24, #26, #28, #30, and #31, with probing depths ranging from 1 to 3 mm throughout, no mobility present, keratinized gingiva ranging from 1 to 4 mm with generalized lack of attached gingiva (Figures 5.3.1 and 5.3.2). Aberrant inferior labial frenum was found.

- Edentulous sites #1, #2, #16, #17, #25, and #32: there were numerous restorations and discolored anterior composites present.
- The remaining soft tissues of the mouth appeared within normal limits.

Occlusion

Angle class I occlusion on left side and Angle class III occlusion on right side.

Radiographic Examination

Periapical radiographs of the mandibular incisor area are presented in Figure 5.3.3 depicting mild horizontal bone loss localized to the anterior mandibular teeth.

Diagnosis

After reviewing the history and the clinical and radiographic examinations, the patient was diagnosed with localized gingivitis on a reduced periodontium and mucogingival defects: gingival recession, decreased vestibular depth, and aberrant frenum attachment.

Treatment Plan

The treatment plan included surgical treatment for correction of the mucogingival defects, followed by periodontal maintenance every three months.

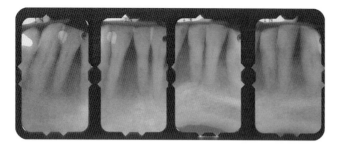

Figure 5.3.3 Periapical radiographs depicting the interproximal bone levels.

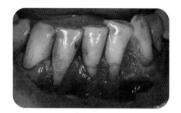

Figure 5.3.4 Preparation of the recipient site.

Treatment

Surgical treatment for this patient included an FGG in area #23-24-x-26, with simultaneous vestibuloplasty, and a labial frenectomy. Topical anesthetic was applied, and 5.4 ml of 0.5% Marcaine plus 1:200 000 epinephrine were locally infiltrated in the buccal and lingual area #22–27, and 1.8 ml of 2% lidocaine plus 1:100 000 epinephrine were given via left greater palatine and nasopalatine blocks.

Preparation of Recipient Site

1. Scaling and root planing of teeth #22–24 and #26 using hand and rotary instruments was completed.
2. Horizontal incisions were made just coronal to the mucogingival junction at the level of the buccal recession from the mesial of #22 to the distal of #26 (Figure 5.3.4).
3. Vertical incisions were made at the mesial and distal aspects of the horizontal incision short of the mesial line angles of #22 and #27 and 3 mm apical to the mucogingival junction.
4. A split-thickness flap was dissected providing for deepening of the vestibule, a labial frenectomy, and the appropriate size of the recipient graft bed, followed by de-epithelialization of the keratinized tissue coronal to the horizontal incision, including the interdental papillae.
5. The residual flap was excised and loose underlying connective tissue removed, preserving the periosteum, to provide a uniform firm bed.

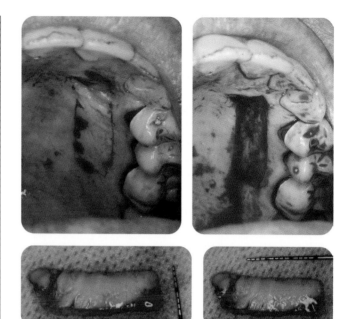

Figure 5.3.5 Harvesting of epithelio-connective tissue graft from the palatal donor site.

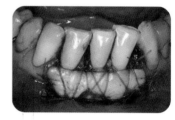

Figure 5.3.6 Epithelio-connective tissue graft sutured to the recipient bed.

Harvesting of Palatal Epithelial–Connective Tissue Graft (Figure 5.3.5)

1. The recipient site was measured for anticipated graft size.
2. Using a no. 15 blade, a 22 × 8 × 1.5 mm epithelio-connective tissue graft was harvested from the donor area: palatal from D of #10 to middle of #14 starting approximately 3 mm apical to cementoenamel junction (CEJ) of teeth.
3. Gelfoam was applied over the donor site and sutured over with 4-0 chromic gut, and hemostasis was obtained.
4. Coe-Pak periodontal dressing was placed over and secured to the palatal teeth surfaces.

Graft Stabilization (Figure 5.3.6)

1. Single interrupted 5-0 chromic gut sutures (P-3 needle) were used to stabilize the flap apically to the periosteum.

2. The graft was positioned coronally to partially cover the recession on the mandibular incisors.
3. Single interrupted sutures engaged the lateral border of the graft to stabilize it to the adjacent mucosa.
4. Continuous compressing cross-mattress sutures were placed over the graft, without engaging the graft, but engaging the apical periosteum and slung around the lingual of the incisors to immobilize the graft and compress it against the underlying vascular bed and root surfaces.
5. Moist gauze was used to compress the graft to ensure intimate adaption to the bed and development of a minimal clot.
6. Periodontal dressing (Coe-Pak) was placed over the recipient site, covering the sutured graft (Figure 5.3.7).
7. The patient tolerated the procedure well.
8. Postoperative instructions (oral and written), ice packs, and prescriptions for Tylenol #3 (#15) and Peridex were given.

The patient was followed postoperatively to monitor healing at two weeks, one month, four months, and one year (Figure 5.3.8).

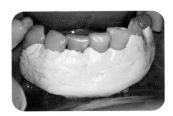
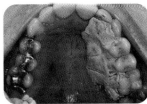

Figure 5.3.7 Recipient and donor sites were protected with periodontal dressing.

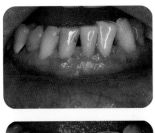
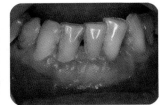
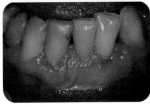
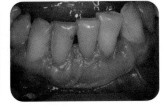

Figure 5.3.8 Postoperative follow-up: (A) two weeks; (B) one month; (C) four months; (D) one year.

Discussion

The FGG belongs to a broader category of gingival reconstructive surgery termed mucogingival surgery or periodontal plastic surgery (A). FGG for gingival augmentation has been used for more than 40 years [1]. These procedures are designed to correct, prevent, or ameliorate mucogingival defects defined as "deviations from the normal anatomic relationship between the gingival margin and the mucogingival junction" (C) [2]. The most common mucogingival deformity is gingival recession, although the rationale for its treatment continues to evolve and be debated. When recession is associated with the absence or lack of keratinized tissue, this defect is considered more vulnerable to progressive attachment loss. Although with adequate plaque control and professional follow-up these defects may be able to be maintained, evidence has demonstrated that without regular dental care, untreated mucogingival defects are more likely to progress than treated ones [3]. Having <1 mm of attached keratinized tissue is generally recognized as a mucogingival defect [2,4]. This finding, coupled with progressive recession, a need for cervical margin restorative care, or inadequate plaque control, indicates a need for treatment (C). Aberrant frenum attachment, planned orthodontic treatment, root abrasion, and sensitivity in conjunction with inadequate keratinized tissue can also be considered indications for treatment (E). The absence of keratinized tissue around dental implants has been shown to be associated with both recession and bone loss (D). It is evident from recent data that both the maintenance of marginal tissue and the preservation of alveolar bone about implants are aided by the presence of marginal keratinized tissue. Gingival augmentation is routinely used to enhance esthetics through root coverage, correction of ridge deformities, and socket preservation.

In this case, to correct or minimize the soft tissue defects found in the mandibular anterior area, including multiple areas of recession, aberrant labial frenum, and reduced vestibular depth, an autogenous free gingival tissue graft was chosen to optimally treat this area (E). The choice of an FGG will provide the opportunity of simultaneously carrying out a labial frenectomy and increasing the zone of attached gingiva, deepening of the vestibule, and establishing improved contours for plaque control by obtaining partial root coverage. The recession found on teeth #23, #24, and #26 correspond to Cairo Recession type 2 (RT2), previously considered Miller class III recession defects; therefore only partial root coverage can be expected [5,6]. In the case of RT1 defects, complete root coverage can be obtained with a one-stage FGG procedure. Bernimoulin et al. [7] demonstrated a second surgical procedure to provide complete root coverage by coronally positioning a mature FGG with a pedicle flap. A later study by Laney et al. [8] compared the relative success of soft tissue coverage of denuded roots (RT1) using two surgical procedures – autogenous FGG and a second-stage coronally positioned flap (CPF) – but could not demonstrate a significant difference in success between FGG and CPF at three months. Livingston [9] reported successful coverage of multiple and adjacent denuded root surfaces with a free gingival autograft. The surgical case presented in this chapter successfully achieved the multiple goals outlined here. Careful attention to each step in the surgical protocol can provide superior outcomes. By harvesting a thick palatal graft, the following are

expected: significant enhancement in the predictability of root coverage (K) [10], augmentation in gingival dimensions with resultant increased resistance to further recession, increase in vestibular depth as well as greater primary contraction but less secondary contraction compared with thin grafts [1]. Furthermore, using a thick palatal graft can likely lead to creeping attachment (I) [11] between one month and one year after the surgery, with no significant difference between one and five years, as reported later by Matter [12]. The periodontal dressing placed on both the donor and recipient sites provided comfort to the patient in the first few days after the surgery (K).

To summarize, the conducted treatment significantly improved the patient's oral health, hygiene, function, and esthetics. Continued periodontal recall and maintenance along with proper plaque control has to be followed to maintain the obtained results.

Self-Study Questions

A. What is a mucogingival defect?

B. What is the etiology of a gingival recession?

C. What is the rationale for the treatment of mucogingival defects?

D. Do we need keratinized tissue about dental implants?

E. What are the indications and contraindications for using an FGG?

F. What are the advantages and disadvantages of using an FGG?

G. What is Cairo's (and Miller's) classification of recessions, and how can they aid in predicting the potential for root coverage?

H. What are the critical anatomic considerations in donor tissue harvesting? What is the anticipated result in case of free gingival grafts of different thicknesses?

I. What healing is expected after an FGG?

J. Is chemical root treatment necessary for successful root coverage with an FGG?

K. What are the possible complications after the surgery, and how can we prevent them? How can smoking affect the treatment result?

L. What other surgical techniques can be used in place of free soft tissue grafting?

Answers located at the end of the chapter.

References

1. Sullivan HC, Atkins JH. Free autogenous gingival grafts. 1. Principles of successful grafting. *Periodontics* 1968;6:5–13.
2. American Academy of Periodontology Consensus Statement on Mucogingival Conditions, May 2009. Available at https://
www.gepi-mattout.com/wp-content/uploads/2017/02/aap-consensus.pdf
3. Kennedy JE, Bird WC, Palcanis KG, Dorfman HS. A longitudinal evaluation of varying widths of attached gingiva. *J Clin Periodontol* 1985;12:667–675.

4. Lang NP, Löe H. The relationship between the width of keratinized gingiva and gingival health. *J Periodontol* 1972;43:623–627.

5. Miller PD Jr. A classification of marginal tissue recession. *Int J Periodontics Restorative Dent* 1985;5:8–13.

6. Cairo F, Nieri M, Cincinelli S, et al. The interproximal clinical attachment level to classify gingival recessions and predict root coverage outcomes: an explorative and reliability study. *J Clin Periodontol* 2011;38:661–666.

7. Bernimoulin JP, Lüscher B, Mühlemann HR. Coronally repositioned periodontal flap. Clinical evaluation after one year. *J Clin Periodontol* 1975;2:1–13.

8. Laney JB, Saunders VG, Garnick JJ. A comparison of two techniques for attaining root coverage. *J Periodontol* 1992;63:19–23.

9. Livingston HL. Total coverage of multiple and adjacent denuded root surfaces with a free gingival autograft. A case report. *J Periodontol* 1975;46:209–216.

10. Miller PD Jr. Root coverage using a free soft tissue autograft following citric acid application. Part 1: Technique. *Int J Periodontics Restorative Dent* 1982;2:65–70.

11. Matter J, Cimasoni G. Creeping attachment after free gingival grafts. *J Periodontol* 1976;7:574–579.

12. Matter J. Creeping attachment of free gingival grafts. A five-year follow-up study. *J Periodontol* 1980;51:682–685.

13. Miller PD Jr. Regenerative and reconstructive periodontal plastic surgery. *Mucogingival surgery. Dent Clin North Am* 1988;32.287–306.

14. Consensus report. Mucogingival therapy. *Ann Periodontol* 1996;1:702–706.

15. Camargo PM, Melnick PR, Kenney EB. The use of free gingival grafts for aesthetic purposes. *Periodontol 2000* 2001;27:72–96.

16. Levin L, Samorodnitzky-Naveh GR, Machtei EE. The association of orthodontic treatment and fixed retainers with gingival health. *J Periodontol* 2008;79:2087–2092.

17. Maynard JG Jr, Wilson RD. Physiologic dimensions of the periodontium significant to the restorative dentist. *J Periodontol* 1979;50:170–174.

18. Ericsson I, Lindhe J. Recession in sites with inadequate width of the keratinized gingiva. An experimental study in the dog. *J Clin Periodontol* 1984;11:95–103.

19. Zigdon H, Machtei EE. The dimensions of keratinized mucosa (KM) around implants affect clinical and immunological parameters. *Clin Oral Implant Res* 2008;19:387–392.

20. Schrott AR, Jimenez M, Hwang J-W, et al. Five-year evaluation of the influence of keratinized mucosa on peri-implant soft-tissue health and stability around implants supporting full-arch mandibular fixed prostheses. *Clin Oral Implants Res* 2009;20:1170–1177.

21. Karring T, Lang NP, Löe H. The role of gingival connective tissue in determining epithelial differentiation. *J Periodontal Res* 1975;10:1–11.

22. Agudio G, Nieri M, Rotundo R, et al. Free gingival grafts to increase keratinized tissue: a retrospective long-term evaluation (10 to 25 years) of outcomes. *J Periodontol* 2008;79:587–594.

23. Paolantonio M, di Murro C, Cattabriga A, Cattabriga M. Subpedicle connective tissue graft versus free gingival graft in the coverage of exposed root surfaces. A 5-year clinical study. *J Clin Periodontol* 1997;24:51–56.

24. Cortellini P, Bissada N. Mucogingival conditions in the natural dentition: narrative review, case definitions, and diagnostic considerations. *J Periodontol* 2018;89(Suppl 1):S204–S213.

25. Reiser GM, Bruno JF, Mahan PE, Larkin LH. The subepithelial connective tissue graft palatal donor site: anatomic considerations for surgeons. *Int J Periodontics Restorative Dent* 1996;16:130–137.

26. Mörmann W, Schaer F, Firestone AR. The relationship between success of free gingival grafts and transplant thickness. Revascularization and shrinkage: a one year clinical study. *J Periodontol* 1981;52:74–80.

27. Orsini M, Orsini G, Benlloch D, et al. Esthetic and dimensional evaluation of free connective tissue grafts in prosthetically treated patients: a 1-year clinical study. *J Periodontol* 2004;75:470–477.

28. Greenwell H, Fiorellini J, Giannobile W, et al. Oral reconstructive and corrective considerations in periodontal therapy. *J Periodontol* 2005;76:1588–1600.

29. Oliver RC, Löe H, Karring T. Microscopic evaluation of the healing and revascularization of free gingival grafts. *J Periodontal Res* 1968;3:84–95.

30. Pasquinelli KL. The histology of new attachment utilizing a thick autogenous soft tissue graft in an area of deep recession: a case report. *Int J Periodontics Restorative Dent* 1995;15:248–257.

31. Miller PD Jr. Root coverage with the free gingival graft. Factors associated with incomplete coverage. *J Periodontol* 1987;58:674–681.

32. Ruggeri A Jr, Prati C, Mazzoni A, et al. Effects of citric acid and EDTA conditioning on exposed root dentin: an immunohistochemical analysis of collagen and proteoglycans. *Arch Oral Biol* 2007;52:1–8.

33. Vanheusden AJ, Goffinet G, Zahedi S, et al. In vitro stimulation of human gingival epithelial cell attachment to dentin by surface conditioning. *J Periodontol* 1999;70:594–603.

34. Baker DL, Stanley Pavlow SA, Wikesjö UME. Fibrin clot adhesion to dentin conditioned with protein constructs: an in vitro proof-of-principle study. *J Clin Periodontol* 2005;32:561–566.

35. Kassab MM, Cohen RE, Andreana S, Dentino AR. The effect of EDTA in attachment gain and root coverage. *Compend Contin Educ Dent* 2006;27:353–360.

36. Ibbott CG, Oles RD, Laverty WH. Effects of citric acid treatment on autogenous free graft coverage of localized recession. *J Periodontol* 1985;56:662–665.

37. Brasher W, Rees T, Boyce WA. Complications of free grafts of masticatory mucosa. *J Periodontol* 1975;46:133–138.

38. Griffin TJ, Cheung WS, Zavras AY, Damoulis PD. Postoperative complications following gingival augmentation procedures. *J Periodontol* 2006;77:2070–2079.

39. Rossmann JA, Rees TD. A comparative evaluation of hemostatic agents in the management of soft tissue graft donor site bleeding. *J Periodontol* 1999;70:1369–1375.

TAKE-HOME POINTS

A. A mucogingival defect is generally defined as any significant deviation from the normal anatomic relationship between the gingival margin and the mucogingival junction [2]. The most common defects present as gingival recession, minimal keratinized marginal tissue (gingiva), a shallow vestibule, and aberrant frenum attachment. Most associate the term mucogingival defect with absence of an adequate zone of attached keratinized tissue (<1 mm of attached gingiva). The amount of attached gingiva is determined by measuring from the free gingival margin to the mucogingival junction and then subtracting the sulcular probing depth from it.

Periodontal plastic surgery [13] is defined as a means of treatment for mucogingival problems with the intent to prevent or correct anatomic, developmental, and traumatic or plaque disease-induced defects of the gingiva, alveolar mucosa, or bone. The goal is the creation of form and appearance that are acceptable and pleasing to the patient and the therapist [14]. The final results following mucogingival surgical therapy should be an increase in the apico-coronal and buccolingual dimensions of the gingival tissues and in the establishment of proper vestibular depth where necessary. When performed for root coverage, mucogingival procedures should additionally result in coverage of the previously denuded root surface to the level of the CEJ and also include biologic attachment between the grafted tissue and the root surface, resulting in a shallow sulcus [15].

B. The most common reason for gingival recession is generally attributed to mechanical trauma/aggressive brushing in an anatomically susceptible site. The anatomic position of the tooth in relation to the bony envelope of the jaw is an important factor in the patient's susceptibility to recession. Teeth with prominent roots extending outside the envelope of the alveolar process and teeth in buccal version generally demonstrate recession.

Progressive periodontal disease can also lead to recession; some evidence indicates that orthodontic therapy can promote recession if the arches are expanded or plaque control is poor [16]. Restorative dentistry that is significantly subgingival, overcontoured, or with poor marginal integrity can contribute to recession [17]. Occlusal trauma such as bruxism can sometimes be associated with recession.

C. The rationale for the treatment of mucogingival defects can be divided into two categories: (i) treatment for esthetic criteria and (ii) treatment to prevent progressive attachment loss. Although the FGG can be used to cover roots and correct ridge deformities, other procedures such as the subepithelial connective tissue graft (SCTG) have supplanted its use due to superior esthetics. When <1 mm of attached keratinized tissue is noted in conjunction with recession, treatment for gingival augmentation should be strongly considered. The study by Kennedy et al. [3] demonstrated that it is possible to maintain periodontal health and attachment for a period of six years through rigorous control of gingival inflammation via scaling, root planing, oral hygiene, and maintenance at three- to six-month intervals despite the absence of attached gingiva. In patients who had discontinued participation in this study for a period of five years, reestablishment of gingival inflammation associated with additional recession was revealed. In the same study, in the experimental sites, where FGG was performed in areas with recession and inadequate or no attached gingiva, the dimension of keratinized and attached gingiva increased. A reduction in recession and gain in clinical attachment was also exhibited and was stable for more than six years. In these patients who were treated by an FGG and discontinued participation in the study, no gingival inflammation and additional recession were observed in areas treated by a free graft as compared with the untreated sites [3].

Other parameters also influence the need for treatment, such as the level of plaque control and the patient's maintenance schedule. The need for restorative treatment or orthodontics in conjunction with a mucogingival defect can indicate treatment. Maynard and Wilson [17] suggested that if intracrevicular margins, defined as those placed into and confined within the

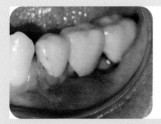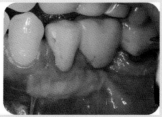

Figure 5.3.9 (A) Preoperative site demonstrating unfavorable soft tissue anatomy. (B) Postoperative site with increased vestibular depth, keratinized tissue, and access for plaque control.

gingival crevice, are planned for a restorative procedure, keratinized tissue is necessary (Figure 5.3.9). Additionally, Ericsson and Lindhe [18] demonstrated that submarginal metal strips caused increased gingival recession in areas with minimal keratinized tissue in beagle dogs. The patient's age, susceptibility to periodontitis, and medical health are other important factors to consider.

D. Having marginal keratinized mucosa (KM) around implants appears to impart significant benefits. Zigdon and Machtei [19] found in their retrospective study that KM around dental implants affects both the clinical and the immunologic parameters at these sites.
- There was negative correlation between mucosal thickness and mucosal recession (mucosal margin to the implant–abutment interface) as well as between KM width and mucosal recession, periodontal attachment level, and prostaglandin E_2 levels.
- Similarly, a thick mucosa (>1 mm) was associated with lesser recession compared with a thin (<1 mm) mucosa.

In patients exercising good oral hygiene and receiving regular implant maintenance therapy, implants with a reduced width (<2 mm) of peri-implant KM were more prone to lingual plaque accumulation and bleeding as well as buccal soft tissue recession over a period of five years [20]. Figure 5.3.10 demonstrates the addition of keratinized tissue and thickening of the soft tissue prior to implant placement.

Additionally, more soreness to plaque control measures and to food impaction is reported by patients with an absence of keratinized tissue adjacent to implants. Figure 5.3.11 shows examples of use of FGG to re-create lost attached gingiva and deepening of the vestibule around previously placed implants. An epithelio-connective tissue palatal pedicle graft can also be performed during a second-stage implant to re-create keratinized tissue around implants soon to be restored (Figure 5.3.12).

E. Since the advent of the SCTG, the indications for use of the FGG have greatly diminished. However, there remain multiple important indications for its use. In regions where a very shallow vestibule exists and coronal manipulation of the gingival flap would exacerbate this situation and possibly hinder future plaque control, an FGG should be considered. Presence of a coronally positioned frenum may also compromise the use of an SCTG, and an FGG can be considered. These situations occur most frequently in the mandibular anterior region. Because these sites are also less esthetically critical, an FGG may become a superior choice.

In addition to the superior esthetics of the SCTG, the postoperative healing of the donor site occurs with significantly less discomfort and time post SCTG. This factor can be taken advantage of by combining a portion of both techniques (Figures 5.3.13 and 5.3.14). A traditional FGG recipient site bed can be made, but the harvesting of the graft can be done with an SCTG technique. This will allow one to take advantage of the superior healing of the palate. The SCTG will produce a keratinized graft as the epithelial coverage is dictated by the underlying connective tissue [21]. The main disadvantage of using just connective tissue is that shrinkage of the graft is extensive. The way to avoid this and also increase the handling properties of the graft is to harvest a "composite" graft containing a portion of only connective tissue graft and a portion of epithelial and connective tissue, comprising a wide band of keratinized tissue. A 3-mm band of keratinized tissue with the rest being connective tissue is generally adequate. Importantly, partial closure of the palatal site can be obtained and the discomfort associated with this technique is no different than with the classical harvest of SCTG.

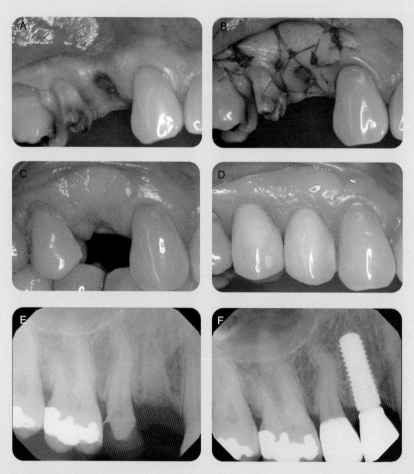

Figure 5.3.10 (A) Implant site with deficient keratinized tissue. (B) FGG placed prior to implant placement. (C) Healed site. (D) Implant placed and restored. (E) Preoperative radiograph. (F) Postoperative radiograph.

FGGs have few contraindications, mostly related to systemic and/or anatomic constraints such as the following.
- Bleeding/coagulation disorders or medications (i.e. use of acetylsalicylic acid-based medication) that can produce uncontrolled bleeding.
- Impingement on critical anatomy such as the mental foramen.
- Improper access to donor (i.e. reduced mouth opening) or recipient sites.

F.
Advantages of FGG
- Predictable procedure to provide an adequate band of keratinized tissue and stable for up to 25 years of follow-up [22].
- Technically less demanding and the procedure is shorter compared with SCTG.

- Will not compromise vestibular depth and also provides an increase in vestibular depth.
- Can be used in conjunction with frenectomy.
- Can be used for root coverage [10].

Disadvantages of FGG
- Percentage of root coverage is less than with SCTG [23].
- Can be perceived as less esthetic than SCTG.
- Increased soreness from donor site than with SCTG, pedicle, and acellular dermal graft.
- Limitation in quantity and quality of donor tissue.
- Limitations for reconstruction of interdental papilla.

As mentioned earlier, better esthetics can be achieved with the SCTG. FGG generally appears significantly paler than adjacent tissue. In most cases this has to do with the contrast of the adjacent mucosa and not the adjacent keratinized tissue.

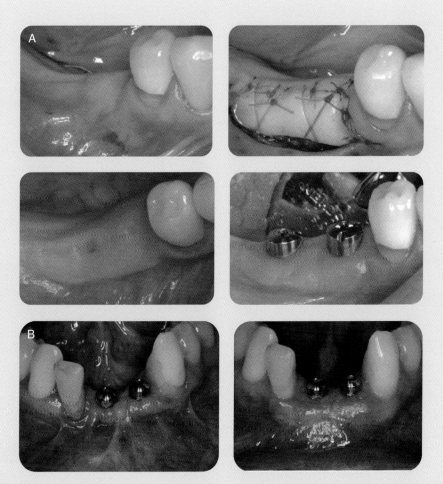

Figure 5.3.11 (A, B) FGG after implant placement, but prior to implant restorations to re-create lost attached gingiva and deepen the vestibule.

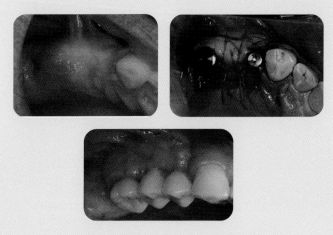

Figure 5.3.12 Epithelio-connective tissue palatal pedicle graft performed during second-stage implant: preoperative, immediate, and five-month postoperative photographs.

In general, the best area to harvest keratinized tissue for grafting is the hard palate. Because of anatomic constraints, this tissue could be limited (H). To date, reconstruction of a lost interdental papilla could not be achieved with an FGG.

G. In the 2017 World Workshop on the Classification of Periodontal and Peri-Implant Diseases and Conditions [24], recession defects were classified using the system delineated by Cairo et al. [6].
• Recession type 1 (RT1): recession with no loss of interproximal attachment. Interproximal CEJ is clinically not detectable on the mesial and distal aspects of the tooth; 100% root coverage can be achieved (Figure 5.3.15).

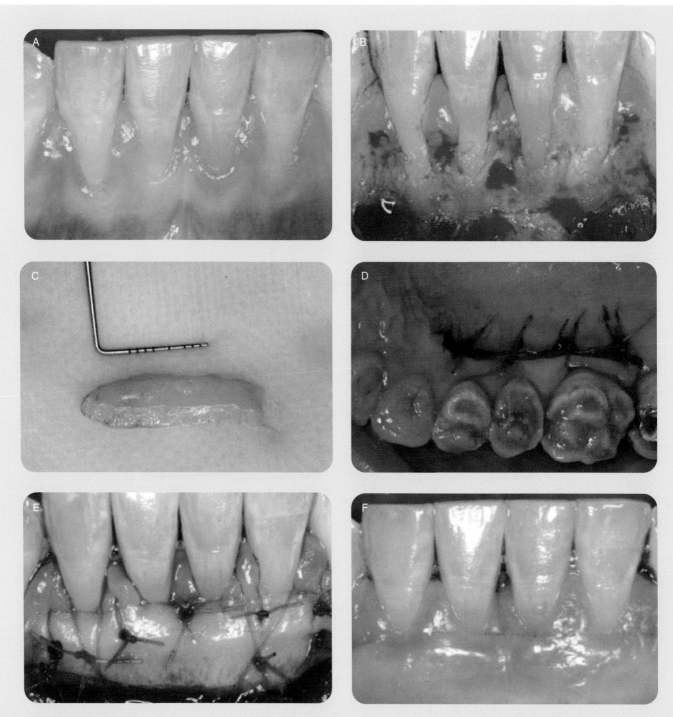

Figure 5.3.13 Connective tissue used as a free graft. (A) Recession associated with mucogingival involvement on the buccal of #23–26. (B) Recipient site prepared. (C) Connective tissue harvested from palate and used as a free graft; 2–3 mm of margin of keratinized tissue. (D) Harvest site on palate sutured. (E) Suturing of graft to recipient site. (F) Healing with keratinization and significant root coverage.

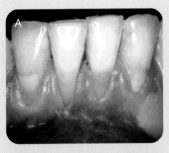

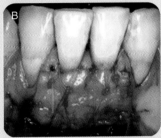

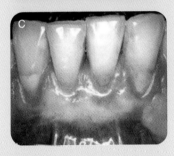

Figure 5.3.14 Connective tissue used as a free graft. (A) Recession associated with mucogingival involvement on the buccal of #24 and #25. (B) Connective tissue harvested from palate and used as a free graft. (C) Healing with keratinization and significant root coverage. Note the approximately 40% shrinkage of the vertical height of the graft but minimal horizontal shrinkage.

- Recession type 2 (RT2): gingival recession associated with loss of interproximal attachment. The amount of interproximal attachment loss (measured from the interproximal CEJ to the depth of the interproximal sulcus/pocket) is less than or equal to the buccal attachment loss (measured from the buccal CEJ to the depth of the sulcus/pocket). Full root coverage may be possible but presently not predictable.
- Recession type 3 (RT3): gingival recession associated with loss of interproximal attachment greater than the buccal attachment loss. Full root coverage is not possible.

The above classification has replaced the Miller classification [5] of marginal tissue recession

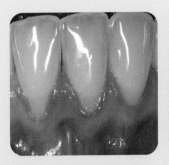

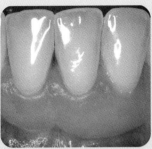

Figure 5.3.15 Root coverage with FGG. (A) Recession and mucogingival involvement #24 and #25. (B) Site healed at eight weeks with root coverage, and elimination of mucogingival defect.

which has been in use since 1985 and is outlined below.
- Class 1: recession does not extend to mucogingival junction, no interdental bone or soft tissue loss; 100% coverage expected.
- Class 2: recession to or beyond mucogingival junction but no interdental bone or soft tissue loss; 100% coverage anticipated.
- Class 3: recession extends to or beyond mucogingival junction; loss of interdental bone or soft tissue, apical to the CEJ but coronal to the level of the recession defect; partial root coverage anticipated.
- Class 4: recession extends to or beyond mucogingival junction with loss of interdental bone or soft tissue apical to the level of the recession defect; no root coverage can be anticipated.

H. The surgeon must be completely familiar with the anatomy of the palatal donor as well as recipient sites for appropriate surgical treatment. Reiser et al. [25] found variations in the size and shape of the hard palate and identified the average location of the neurovascular bundle from the CEJ of the maxillary premolars and molars to vary with the palatal height:
- High palatal vault to 17 mm
- Average palatal vault to 12 mm
- Shallow palatal vault to 7 mm

Additionally, the same authors using cadaver dissection demonstrated that the surgeon can gain substantial donor tissue thickness in the area from the mesial line angle of the palatal root of the first molar to the distal line angle of the canine. Palatal exosis can be encountered over the molar palatal area, thus limiting the thickness of the graft. By extending the harvesting area anteriorly from the distal line angle of the canine, palatal rugae can be encountered with subsequent less esthetic results (see Figure 5.3.5).

The thickness of the graft has a direct effect on its healing behavior. Gingival grafts demonstrated 25–50% shrinkage in vertical height over one year [25]. The thinner the graft, the more vertical shrinkage has occurred [26]. Connective tissue used as a free graft showed more than 43% vertical shrinkage over one year [27]. Thinner gingival grafts (approximately 1 mm) worked predictably when placed over the vascular bed but achieved very poor results with root coverage [28]. Thick grafts (1.5–2 mm) proved to be the better choice for substantial root coverage [9]. These thicker grafts also required a larger vascular bed for predictable root coverage. Generally, 75–80% of the graft needed to be in close apposition to the vascular bed.

I. Sullivan and Atkins [1] described the initial stages of graft maturation after a free autogenous gingival graft as follows.

- Days 0–2: plasmatic circulation (direct diffusion of nutrients from its host bed).
- Days 2–8: reestablishment of vascularization.
- Days 4–10: organic connective tissue union (fibrous tissue attachment) between the graft and its bed.

At histologic evaluation following FGGs, Oliver et al. [29] found complete epithelialization by 14 days and keratinization by 28 days. In a case report histologic study in humans, Pasquinelli [30] reported on new attachment and new bone growth, with minimal sulcus depth of 1 mm, after 10.5 months following treatment of a deep buccal recession with a thick (1.5 mm) free autogenous gingival graft.

Creeping attachment following an FGG was described by Matter and Cimasoni [11] and Matter [12] as a postoperative coronal migration of gingival marginal tissue resulting in partial or total coverage of a previously denuded root, with firm tissue attached to root surface and probing that does not show any sulcular depth. Creeping attachment occurred between one month and one year after surgery, and none was observed after one year

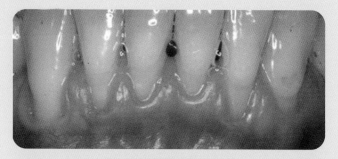
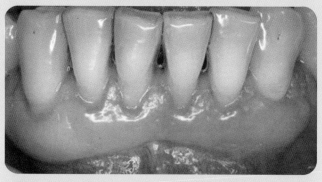
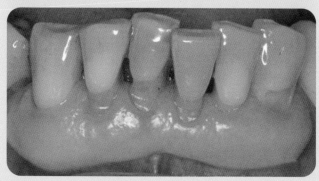

Figure 5.3.16 Long-term stability (over 15 years) of FGG #22–27. Note buccal abrasion but with stable gingival margins, slight gingival creep #27 buccal.

(Figure 5.3.16). In addition, the authors listed various factors that seem to significantly influence creeping attachment, including the width of the recession, position and thickness of the graft, bone resorption, position of the tooth, and hygiene of the patient [11].

J. Root conditioning for enhancing root coverage continues to be controversial. Many agents have been advocated to condition roots before gingival grafting, including citric acid, tetracycline-HCl, and EDTA. Miller [10,31] advocated this from an anecdotal clinical standpoint. Citric acid and EDTA have been shown to expose collagen fibrils and sound dentin while preserving the structural and biochemical properties of the dentin matrix [32]. Enhanced cell attachment was observed after chemical root conditioning in an in vitro study by Vanheusden et al. [33]. Citric acid removes the smear layer that may aid in healing [34]. Using EDTA has more recently been shown to enhance root coverage [35]. However, a study by Ibbott et al. [36] showed there is no significant improvement in root coverage with citric acid pretreatment. Because of the limitations of any definitive studies, root conditioning continues to be debated.

K. Although complications are generally limited after FGG surgery, the most common ones are excessive hemorrhage at donor site, swelling, and discomfort [37,38]. To avoid postoperative bleeding, several measures have been described: use of compressing suture (placed proximal to the bleeding site) [25], hemostatic agents [39], periodontal dressing (suggested to cover the donor site for two weeks) [38], and use of a palatal stent or denture, or a combination of them. By using a periodontal dressing or palatal stent, the bleeding is prevented by the mechanical pressure as well as by protecting the area from direct trauma to the open wound left behind for healing by secondary intention, thus having less sensitivity associated with direct trauma. In addition, in patients who have coagulation disorders or use acetylsalicylic acid-based medication before or during the initial healing process, the likelihood of bleeding is increased [37]. Duration of the procedure was positively associated with postoperative pain and swelling after FGG [38].

The study by Miller [5] showed that smoking interfered with complete root coverage after FGG surgery. Heavy smoking, in excess of 10 cigarettes per day, correlated 100% with failure to obtain root coverage; patients who were "light" or "occasional" smokers (five cigarettes or fewer per day) responded as favorably as the nonsmokers to root coverage using FGGs. A successful protocol was followed consisting of patients refraining from smoking during the initial two weeks of healing after the surgery subsequently resulting in root coverage comparable with nonsmokers. Furthermore, patients who were smokers were found to have three times more postoperative swelling as reported by Griffin et al. [38].

L. In addition to FGG, various techniques can be used to treat mucogingival problems and recession: SCTG, lateral pedicle graft, coronally advanced pedicle flap, guided tissue regeneration, and acellular dermal allograft.

Case 4

Allografts (Alloderm) for Mucogingival Therapy

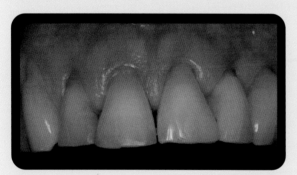
LEARNING GOALS AND OBJECTIVES

- To be able to diagnose gingival recession and inadequate attached gingiva
- To identify the possible treatments and prediction of outcomes for situations where a patient presents with soft tissue recession and interproximal bone loss
- To understand the importance of oral preventive treatment in such cases

Medical History

The patient presented with a history of stroke, knee replacement, thrombocytopenia, depression, and high body mass index (BMI). Because of the previous history of stroke, she presented with limited movements on the left side of her upper body. Medication list included anagrelide, folic acid, omeprazole, bupropion, naproxen, and citalopram hydrobromide. Patient was also allergic to iodine, latex and sulfa drugs.

Review of Systems

- Vital signs
  - Blood pressure: 141/82 mmHg
  - Pulse rate: 59 beats/minute (regular)
  - Respiratory rate: 16 breaths/minute

Social History

The patient drank alcohol socially (once a week) and had a previous history of smoking.

Extraoral Examination

No significant findings were noted. The patient had no masses or swelling, and the temporomandibular joint was within normal limits.

Oral Hygiene

The patient reported brushing twice daily using an electric toothbrush and flossing once daily using dental floss picks. On clinical examination, the patient's hygiene was found to be good with less than 10% on bleeding on probing and plaque-free score of 85%.

Intraoral Examination

- The soft tissues of the mouth (except gingiva) including the tongue appeared normal.

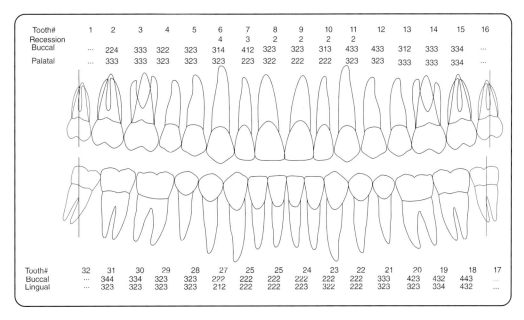

Tooth#	1	2	3	4	5	6	7	8	9	10	11	12	13	14	15	16
Recession						4	3	2	2	2	2					
Buccal	...	224	333	322	323	314	412	323	323	313	433	433	312	333	334	...
Palatal		333	333	323	323	323	223	322	222	222	323	323	333	333	334	

Tooth#	32	31	30	29	28	27	25	25	24	23	22	21	20	19	18	17
Buccal	...	344	334	323	323	222	222	222	222	222	222	333	423	432	443	...
Lingual	...	323	323	323	323	212	222	222	223	322	222	323	323	334	432	...

Figure 5.4.2 Probing pocket depths and recession measurements.

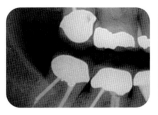
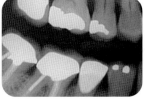
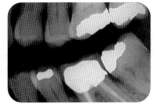
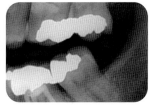

Figure 5.4.3 Bitewing radiographs.

- A gingival examination revealed generalized pyramidal papillae with knife-edged margins and gingival recession on teeth #6–11.
- A periodontal charting was completed (Figure 5.4.2).

Occlusion
There were no occlusal discrepancies or interferences.

Radiographic Examination
Bitewing and localized periapical radiographs were updated (Figures 5.4.3 and 5.4.4). Note the generalized mild horizontal bone loss detected radiographically.

Diagnosis and Treatment Plan
After reviewing the patient's history and clinical examination, it was concluded that her gingival recession was likely secondary to a history of aggressive oral hygiene habits and a thin biotype. The treatment plan includes an initial phase of scaling and polishing with oral hygiene instruction and modification of brushing and flossing techniques.

Overall, the patient's extensive areas of recession could be classified as a combination of Miller class II and

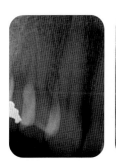
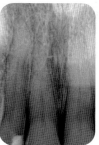
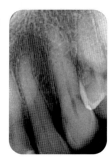

Figure 5.4.4 Periapical radiographs of area of teeth #6–11.

III [1]. The papillae were broad but blunted and recession on the canines extended to the mucogingival junction. Given these clinical findings, and due to the patient's request to avoid use of autogenous tissue, a decision was made to use an acellular dermal matrix (ADM) for root coverage of the maxillary anterior sextant.

Based on the clinical and radiographic examinations, the patient had an American Dental Association (ADA) overall diagnosis of type I gingivitis and an American Academy of Periodontology (AAP) diagnosis of clinical health on a reduced periodontium in a stable periodontitis patient with mucogingival deformities and conditions comprising gingival recession [2].

Treatment

The patient received a scaling and polishing with oral hygiene instruction. Modification of her oral hygiene habits was discussed, including using a soft electric toothbrush and applying minimal pressure against her gingival soft tissues by using a nontraumatic brushing technique.

After phase 1 therapy, the grafting procedures proceeded in the maxillary anterior sextant. After local anesthetic was administered, intrasulcular incisions were made at teeth #6–11 leaving the papillae attached to the palatal aspects (Figure 5.4.5). A split-thickness flap was prepared into the vestibule to allow the flap to sit passively over the teeth (Figures 5.4.6 and 5.4.7).

The ADM graft was rehydrated according to the manufacturer's instructions and contoured to fit the area appropriately. It was then inserted under the tunneled flap with the connective tissue side down (Figure 5.4.8).

The site was sutured using the subpapillary continuous sling suturing method, which combines securing the graft and the margins of the tunneled flap with one continuous sling suture [3]. A single interrupted suture was necessary around tooth #10 to repair a small tissue tear (Figure 5.4.9).

One-week Follow-up Visit

The patient reported minimal postoperative discomfort, swelling and bruising. Healing was within normal limits with mild erythema and the sutures were securely in place (Figures 5.4.10 and 5.4.11).

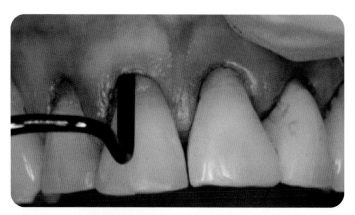

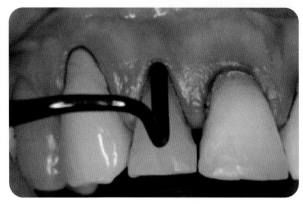

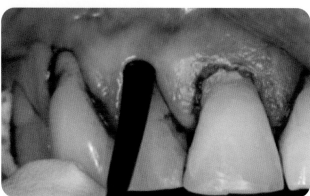

Figure 5.4.5 Initial incisions and tunneling procedure.

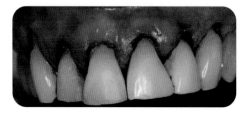

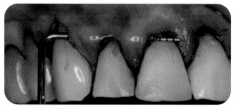

Figure 5.4.6 Tunneling procedure complete and full release of the buccal flap.

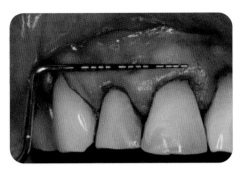
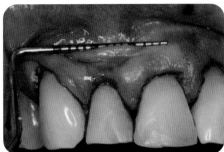

Figure 5.4.7 Passive placement of buccal flap.

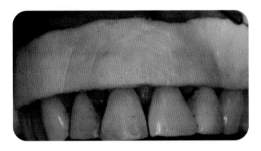
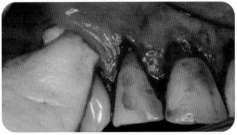

Figure 5.4.8 Contouring ADM try-in on area of teeth #6–11 and being inserted into the tunnel.

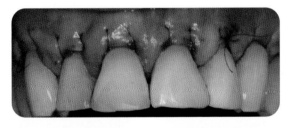

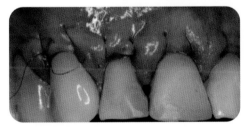
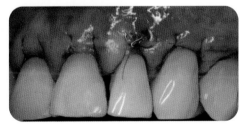

Figure 5.4.9 Subpapillary continuous sling suturing method completed.

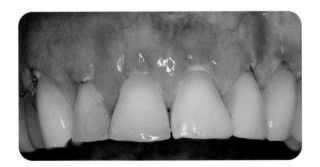

Figure 5.4.10 One-week follow-up visit, frontal view.

Six-week Follow-up Visit

The surgical site was healing well with an increased zone of attached gingiva and approximately 1 mm of residual root exposure. The sutures were removed at this visit (Figures 5.4.12 and 5.4.13).

Four-month Follow-up Visit

At four months, the site had healed well and appeared natural-looking. The patient was pleased with the result (Figure 5.4.14).

Discussion

This patient presented with a chief complaint of recession in the maxillary anterior sextant. On examination, her oral hygiene was observed to be excellent, probing depths were normal, and there was mild interproximal bone loss detected radiographically. Occlusion was evaluated, and there were no interferences on protrusion or lateral excursions. Given these findings, it was established that the patient's recession was likely secondary to her aggressive hygiene habits. The recession could be classified as Miller's class II or III; hence it would be reasonable to anticipate partial to full root coverage with soft tissue grafting. The patient was presented with soft tissue grafting options, which included connective tissue autografts, or ADM matrix allografts. ADM was chosen for grafting because the patient preferred not to have her palatal tissue used as the donor site.

After review of appropriate oral hygiene practices, the patient was prepared for her grafting surgeries. When evaluating the tissues in planning for her allograft procedure, some important elements were examined. Although the papillae were blunted, they were adequately wide at the base to allow for sufficient blood

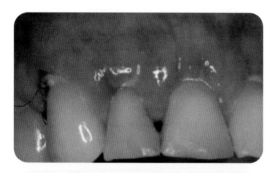

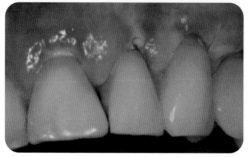

Figure 5.4.11 One-week follow-up visit, right and left side views.

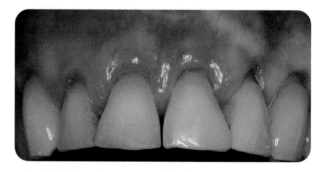

Figure 5.4.12 Six-week follow-up visit, frontal view.

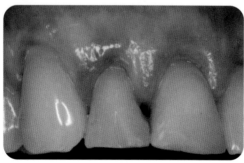

Figure 5.4.13 Six-week follow-up visit, right and left side views.

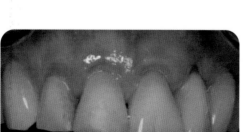

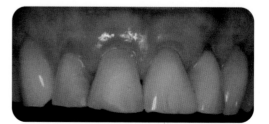

Figure 5.4.14 Four-month follow-up visit.

supply to the graft. In addition, there was adequate vestibular depth and the frenal attachments were not involved, which could potentially make coronal repositioning and stabilization of the flap quite difficult.

For any patient with recession, it is imperative to identify the cause of such lesions and attempt necessary functional and/or behavioral adjustments before any surgical intervention. If not addressed, such factors could lead to long-term recurrence of recession, even subsequent to surgical grafting procedures. Untreated buccal recession defects have been shown to have a tendency to progress over time [4].

Self-Study Questions

A. What is ADM and how is it processed?

B. How does ADM work?

C. What types of procedures can ADM allograft be used for?

D. What are the advantages/disadvantages of using ADM versus a connective tissue graft?

E. What are the long-term results of grafting using an ADM allograft?

Answers located at the end of the chapter.

References

1. Miller PD Jr. A classification of marginal tissue recession. *Int J Periodontics Restorative Dent* 1985;5(2):8–13.
2. Caton J, Armitage G, Berglundh T, et al. A new classification scheme for periodontal and peri-implant diseases and conditions: introduction and key changes from the 1999 classification. *J Periodontol* 2018;89(Suppl 1):S1–S8.
3. Allen EP. Subpapillary continuous sling suturing method for soft tissue grafting with the tunneling technique. *Int J Periodontics Restorative Dent* 2010;30:479–485.
4. Chambrone L, Tatakis DN Long-term outcomes of untreated buccal gingival recessions: a systematic review and meta-analysis. *J Periodontol* 2016;87:796–808.
5. Gapski R, Parks CA, Wang H-L. Acellular dermal matrix for mucogingival surgery: a meta-analysis. *J Periodontol* 2005;76:1814–1822.
6. Mahajan A, Dixxit J, Verma UP. A patient-centered evaluation of acellular dermal matrix graft in the treatment of gingival recession defects. *J Periodontol* 2007;12:2348–2355.
7. Santos A, Goumenos G, Pascual A. Management of gingival recession by the use of an acellullar dermal graft material: a 12-case series. *J Periodontol* 2005;76:1982–1990.
8. Luczyszyn SM, Papalexiou V, Novaes AB Jr, et al. Acellular dermal matrix and hydroxyapatite in prevention of ridge deformities after tooth extraction. *Implant Dent* 2005;14:176–184.
9. Cummings LC, Kaldahl WB, Allen EP. Histologic evaluation of autogenous connective tissue and acellular dermal matrix grafts in humans. *J Periodontol* 2005;76:178–186.
10. Harris RJ. A comparative study of root coverage obtained with an acellular dermal matrix versus a connective tissue graft. *J Periodontol* 2000;20:51–59.
11. Langer G, Langer L. Subepithelial connective tissue graft technique for root coverage. *J Periodontol* 1985;56:715–720.
12. Harris RJ. A short-term and long-term comparison of root coverage with an acellular dermal matrix and a subepithelial graft. *J Periodontol* 2004;75:734–743.
13. Tal H, Moses Ofer, Zohar R, et al. Root coverage of advanced gingival recession: a comparative study between acellular dermal matrix allograft and subepithelial connective tissue grafts. *J Periodontol* 2002;73:1405–1411.
14. Hirsch A, Goldstein M, Goultschin J, et al. A 2-year follow-up of root coverage using subpedicle acellular dermal matrix allografts and subepithelial connective tissue autografts. *J Periodontol* 2005;76:1323–1328.

TAKE-HOME POINTS

A. ADM is derived from prescreened donated human tissue that undergoes multiple steps of processing before its use in the mouth. First, the donated tissue is treated with a buffered salt solution to separate and eliminate the epidermis. It then undergoes a series of washes with a mild detergent to eliminate all remaining cells. The processed tissue is then freeze dried until it is ready to be used clinically.

B. Once the ADM is prepared, any cells that might lead to tissue rejection by the patient are removed. The remaining regenerative matrix consists only of collagens, elastin, vascular channels, and proteins that remain biologically active and are therefore recognized as human tissue. These remaining elements provide scaffolding so the patient's blood can infiltrate, bringing host cells into the area. These cells subsequently adhere to the proteins still found in the ADM and support repopulation and revascularization of the area, ultimately remodeling the ADM into the patient's own tissue.

C. ADM was first introduced into medicine in 1995 for use on burn patients. Since that time, its use has grown exponentially, encompassing many fields including urology, orthopedics, and dentistry. Given that ADM is still a relatively novel material for use by dental specialists (since 1997), there have been limited randomized controlled clinical trials available for comprehensive meta-analysis of ADM procedures versus commonly used mucogingival surgical procedures [5]. Clinical trends, however, have revealed that ADM can be successfully used in mucogingival procedures for root coverage [6,7], soft tissue augmentation, as well as acting as a barrier membrane for extraction socket grafting and guided bone regeneration [8]. One human histologic study found that, when compared with connective tissue graft, ADM has only a slightly different histologic presentation but was able to successfully cover roots with similar attachments to that of connective tissue grafts [9].

D. The advantages and disadvantages of using ADM versus connective tissue grafting are as follows.

Advantages

- Ability to treat multiple sites in a single surgery.
- Good handling properties (easy to use).
- Can be obtained in varying thicknesses (currently available in 0.3–1.8 mm) and sizes.
- Ability to treat patients who have inadequate harvestable tissue.
- Eliminates the need for a second surgical site (donor site).
- Avoids postoperative morbidity associated with harvesting palatal connective tissue.
- Esthetic results are comparable with those from connective tissue grafting [10].

Disadvantages

- Technique sensitive: the consensus clinical practice/opinion is to attempt complete coverage of ADM. Connective tissue grafts, in contrast, can be left slightly exposed [11].
- Some literature has shown that root coverage with subepithelial grafts had better stability over time versus coverage with ADM (these results are not universal) [12].
- Some studies have demonstrated that autogenous grafting can result in greater gain of keratinized gingiva when compared with ADM [12].

E. Given that ADM has only been used for dental purposes since the mid-1990s, long-term results for treatment are limited. Most available literature has shown that when compared with connective tissue grafting for root coverage, procedures using ADM are predictable and stable postoperatively [14].

Case 5

Frenectomy and Vestibuloplasty

CASE STORY

A 20-year-old African American male presented with a chief complaint of "I was told that I need to have some tissues removed between my two upper front teeth before orthodontic treatment." The patient had been referred from his orthodontist, who requested a periodontal consultation regarding the removal of maxillary labial frenum before orthodontic closure of the patient's midline diastema (Figure 5.5.1).

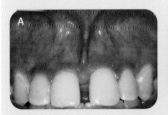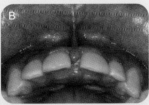

Figure 5.5.1 Preoperative presentation: (A) buccal view; (B) occlusal view.

LEARNING GOALS AND OBJECTIVES

■ To be able to identify the clinical appearance of abnormal frenal attachments and shallow vestibules
■ To understand the potential complications associated with abnormal frenal attachments and shallow vestibules
■ To have a basic understanding of the surgical approaches of frenectomy and vestibuloplasty

Medical History

The patient denied any medical conditions and reported good general health. He was not taking any medications and had no known drug allergies.

Review of Systems

- Vital signs
  - Blood pressure: 136/82 mmHg
  - Pulse rate: 77 beats/minute
  - Respiratory rate: 15 breaths/minute

Social History

The patient had never smoked but occasionally drank beer. He denied using recreational drugs

Extraoral Examination

No abnormal swellings and masses were detected. Examination of temporomandibular joint and muscles of mastication appeared normal.

Intraoral Examination

- Soft tissue including buccal mucosa, tongue, floor of the mouth, and hard/soft palate all appeared within normal limits.
- A high maxillary labial frenal attachment between teeth #8 and #9 was observed; the frenum attached to the papilla between the two central incisors.
- Gingiva in general was healthy with stippling present, and there was adequate amount of attached keratinized gingiva. The papilla between #8 and #9 was blunt.
- Periodontal charting showed no probing depths >3 mm. No tooth mobility, furcal involvement or gingival recession were detected (Figure 5.5.2).

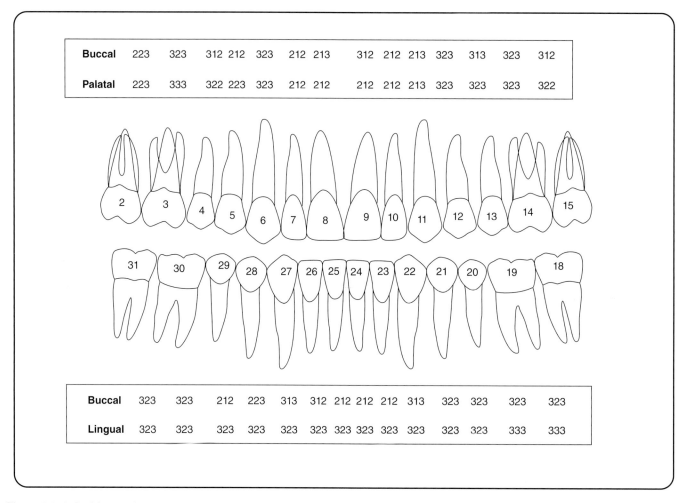

Buccal	223	323		312	212	323		212	213		312	212	213	323		313		323		312
Palatal	223	333		322	223	323		212	212		212	212	213	323		323		323		322

Buccal	323	323		212	223		313		312	212	212	212	313		323	323		323		323
Lingual	323	323		323	323		323		323	323	323	323	323		323	323		333		333

Figure 5.5.2 Probing pocket depth measurements during initial visit.

Occlusion

There was no occlusal disharmony detected.

Radiographic Examination

A panoramic and full-mouth radiographic series were taken. No abnormal findings were detected radiographically.

Diagnosis and Prognosis

Based on the clinical and radiographic examinations, the patient has an American Dental Association (ADA) overall diagnosis of type I gingivitis and an American Academy of Periodontology (AAP) diagnosis of gingivitis associated with dental biofilm alone and a mucogingival deformity comprising an aberrant frenum between the maxillary central incisors [1].

Treatment Plan

The following treatment plan and treatment sequence were discussed with the patient.

- Diagnostic phase: comprehensive periodontal examination, radiographic examination, study casts.
- Disease control phase: oral hygiene instruction, adult prophylaxis.
- Surgical phase: maxillary labial frenectomy.
- Reevaluation phase: follow-up on healing of frenectomy.
- Orthodontic treatment phase: closure of diastema.

Treatment

After the disease control phase had been completed and the patient's oral hygiene optimized, a maxillary frenectomy was performed (Figure 5.5.3 provides detailed description of frenectomy). Once local anesthesia was obtained, a single interrupted suture was made at the base of the frenum in the vestibule. A horizontal incision to bone was then made just coronal to the suturing line to detach the frenum from the vestibule. Using a sharp 15C blade, the frenum and all its underlying muscle fibers were then removed. Multiple single interrupted

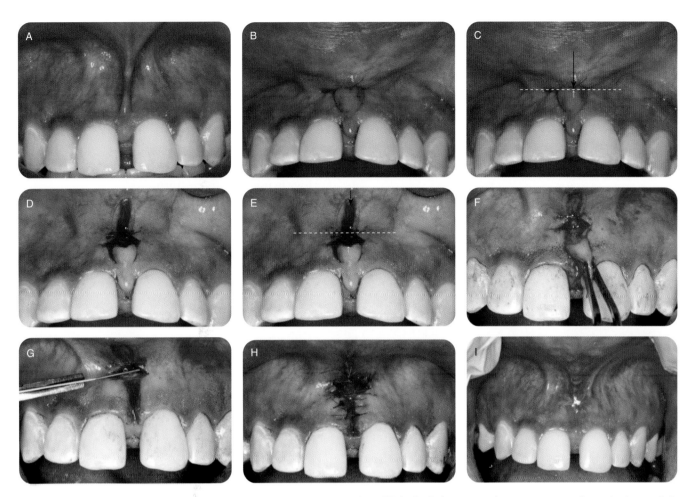

Figure 5.5.3 Maxillary labial frenectomy. (A) Preoperative presentation. (B) A single interrupted suture was made at the base of the frenum in the vestibule. (C) Note the position of the arrow tip (white dotted line represents single interrupted suture). (D) A horizontal incision to bone was made just coronal to the suturing line (i.e. white dotted line seen in C and E). (E) This incision frees the buccal mucosa, which is pulled away from the frenum (note the new position that the black arrow tip is pointing to) while the position of the frenal base remains unchanged. (F) Frenum and all its underlying muscle fibers were removed. (G) An incision was made at the base of frenum to ensure total detachment of muscle fibers from the frenum. (H) Multiple single interrupted sutures were used to suture alveolar mucosa to the underlying periosteum. (I) Three-week postoperative presentation showed removal of maxillary labial frenum pull. Source: courtesy of Dr. Daniel Ho.

sutures were then used to suture the alveolar mucosa to the underlying periosteum to prevent recurrence of the high frenal attachment. Hemostasis was achieved. Postoperative instructions were given. Chlorhexidine mouthwash was prescribed and over-the-counter analgesics were recommended. The patient presented at three weeks postoperatively for a follow-up. Clinically, soft tissues healed well with evidence of epithelialization, and the tension on the papilla between the maxillary central incisors was eliminated.

Discussion

The presence of abnormal maxillary labial frenal attachments often hinders the orthodontist from closing a midline diastema for patients. Even if the diastema can be closed in these situations, patients often observe a relapse after orthodontic treatment [2]. Not only does frenectomy done prior to diastema closure allow orthodontists to easily close the gap, but it helps prevent orthodontic relapse. Depending on the size of the diastema and the extent of the frenal attachment, frenectomy can be done either at the start of the comprehensive orthodontic treatment or in the later phase of treatment just prior to the need for closure. A period of two to three weeks is required for the soft tissue to heal after frenectomy before the orthodontist can start moving teeth again.

Self-Study Questions

A. What is a frenum and what are the complications associated with abnormal frenal attachment?

B. What is the vestibule and what are the clinical implications of a shallow vestibule?

C. What is meant by frenectomy, fiberotomy, and vestibuloplasty?

D. What other tools can be used to perform frenectomy?

E. How is vestibuloplasty performed?

F. How is fiberotomy performed?

Answers located at the end of the chapter.

ACKNOWLEDGMENT

We would like to thank Dr. Maria Dona for providing Figure 5.5.5.

References

1. Caton J, Armitage G, Berglundh T, et al. A new classification scheme for periodontal and peri-implant diseases and conditions: introduction and key changes from the 1999 classification. *J Periodontol* 2018;89(Suppl 1):S1–S8.
2. Edwards JG. The diastema, the frenum, the frenectomy: a clinical study. *Am J Orthod* 1977;71:489–508.
3. Fletcher SG, Meldrum JR. Lingual function and relative length of the lingual frenulum. *J Speech Hear Res* 1968;11:382–390.
4. Ballard JL, Auer CE, Khoury JC. Ankyloglossia: assessment, incidence, and effect of frenuloplasty on the breastfeeding dyad. *Pediatrics* 2002;110:e63–69.
5. Mason C, Hopper C. The use of CO_2 laser in the treatment of gingival fibromatosis: a case report. *Int J Paediatr Dent* 1994;4:105–109.
6. Morosolli AR, Veeck EB, Niccoli-Filho W, et al. Healing process after surgical treatment with scalpel, electrocautery and laser radiation: histomorphologic and histomorphometric analysis. *Lasers Med Sci* 2010;25:93–100.
7. Haytac MC, Ozcelik O. Evaluation of patient perceptions after frenectomy operations: a comparison of carbon dioxide laser and scalpel techniques. *J Periodontol* 2006;77:1815–1819.
8. Shetty K, Trajtenberg C, Patel C, Streckfus C. Maxillary frenectomy using a carbon dioxide laser in a pediatric patient: a case report. *Gen Dent* 2008;56:60–63.
9. Kalkwarf KL, Krejci RF, Shaw DH, Edison AR. Histologic evaluation of gingival response to an electrosurgical blade. *J Oral Maxillofac Surg* 1987;45:671–674.
10. Krejci RF, Kalkwarf KL, Krause-Hohenstein U. Electrosurgery: a biological approach. *J Clin Periodontol* 1987;14:557–563.
11. Flocken JE. Electrosurgical management of soft tissues and restorative dentistry. *Dent Clin North Am* 1980;24:247–269.
12. Wade AB. Vestibular deepening by the technique of Edlan and Mejchar. *J Periodontal Res* 1969;4:300–313.
13. Bohannan HM. Studies in the alteration of vestibular depth. *III. Vestibular incision. J Periodontol* 1963;34:209–215.
14. Edwards JG. A Long term prospective evaluation of the circumferential supracrestal fiberotomy in alleviating orthodontic relapse. *Am J Orthod* 1988;93:380–387.

TAKE-HOME POINTS

A. The frenum is a fold of tissue that consists predominantly of muscle fibers and is covered externally by oral mucosa. High frenal attachments are implicated in midline diastema formation and gingival recession due to frenal pull (especially in a thin biotype gingival apparatus). A high frenal attachment also acts as a barrier for thorough toothbrushing and other oral hygiene measures, leading to accumulation of plaque followed by gingival inflammation. Moreover, high frenal attachments in edentulous patients may affect denture stability, and hence frenum removal is required to improve the stability and retention of dentures.

In addition, a short lingual frenum may result in ankyloglossia, a congenital tongue anomaly associated with decreased tongue mobility and potential speech disturbance resulting in poor articulation [3]. Patients with ankyloglossia resulting from a short lingual frenum may also have poor feeding ability as well as unfavorable mechanical (e.g. playing wind instruments) and social well-being [4].

All these conditions associated with abnormal frenal attachments are indications for frenectomy (Figure 5.5.4).

B. The oral cavity is divided anatomically into the oral cavity proper and the vestibule. The narrow area surrounded by the lips on one side and the dentition on the other is called the vestibule. The area bounded by teeth with palate above and the floor of the mouth and tongue below is called the oral cavity proper.

Adequate vestibular depth aids in proper toothbrushing and allows one to effectively perform various other oral hygiene measures such as the use

of interdental brushes. A shallow vestibule prevents proper positioning of toothbrushes. In addition, a shallow vestibule is an important factor that has to be taken into account when procedures affecting the final vestibular depth are planned. In procedures such as coronally positioned flap for root coverage as well as guided bone regeneration procedure where the buccal flap is overstretched, patients with a shallow vestibule may end up losing the whole vestibule after the procedures.

Apart from its implications in oral hygiene and periodontal surgery, shallow vestibules are not prosthetically favorable, especially in edentulous patients receiving complete or partial dentures. The flanges of the denture will not seat properly leading to poor retention of the prosthesis. All these conditions require vestibuloplasty.

C. Frenectomy is the complete surgical removal of abnormal frenal attachment including its band of tissues attaching to the bone. This procedure often involves incisions extending to the palate (in the maxillary anterior region). One of the serious drawbacks of this procedure is the potential loss of papillary height leading to compromised esthetics in the maxillary anterior region.

Fiberotomy or supracrestal fiberotomy is a minor surgical procedure performed in teeth that have undergone orthodontic rotational movement. Orthodontically, rotated teeth are more prone to relapse, and this procedure if done appropriately will prevent relapse.

Vestibuloplasty is a procedure performed to restore the relative height of the alveolar ridge by apically positioning the muscle/fiber attachments into the vestibule (as opposed to restoring the absolute height of the alveolar ridge in a guided bone regeneration ridge augmentation technique).

D. Laser surgery and electrosurgery are other tools that can be used to perform frenectomy apart from using scalpel blades. The major advantages of using laser surgery for intraoral soft tissue procedures are hemostasis, improved visibility of the surgical field, less severe scarring, and less postoperative pain

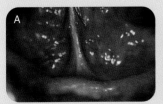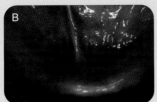

Figure 5.5.4 Mandibular lingual frenectomy: (A) preoperative presentation; (B) four-week postoperative presentation.

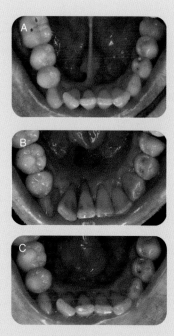

Figure 5.5.5 Mandibular lingual frenectomy using carbon dioxide laser surgery: (A) preoperative presentation; (B) during surgery; (C) two weeks postoperatively. Source: courtesy of Dr. Maria Dona.

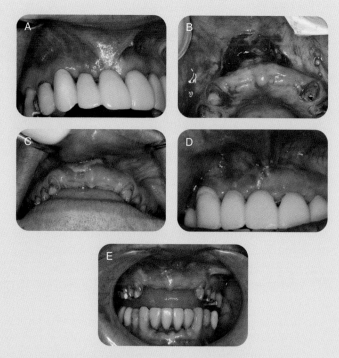

Figure 5.5.6 Vestibuloplasty clinical photos taken (A) preoperatively; (B) during surgery; (C) one week postoperatively; (D) two weeks postoperatively; and (E) four weeks postoperatively.

and swelling [5,6]. Some recent studies have reported that frenectomies done with laser are usually more acceptable to patients, especially in the pediatric population [7,8]. Lasers have been shown to seal blood vessels, and with precise control of the depth it is an ideal surgical tool for soft tissue procedures. The major disadvantage associated with laser surgery is the delayed healing. It has been shown that wounds created by lasers tend to heal one to two weeks later than healing of wounds following conventional techniques [5] (Figure 5.5.5).

Electrosurgery uses electric current delivered via a metal instrument to sever the tissues. The heat generated by the electric current allows electrosurgical instruments to denature the tissue cells and to create a thin layer of coagulated tissue [9,10]. The main advantages of using electrosurgery over conventional surgical techniques are hemostatic control with better visibility of the surgical field, minimized bacterial infection at the incision site, less postoperative discomfort, less scar formation, reduction of chair time, and increased operative efficiency [11]. However, electrosurgery produces an unpleasant odor and is contraindicated in patients

having some types of cardiac pacemaker [11].

E. Vestibuloplasty can be performed using a variety of different techniques [12]. One way is simply to reposition the buccal flap apically by making a partial-thickness horizontal incision either at or slightly coronal to the mucogingival junction. Once the buccal flap is moved to a more apical position, the flap is then secured to this new position by sutures, leaving the underlying tissue coronal to it exposed. A period of two weeks is allowed for the tissue to heal. The patient should be informed of discomfort expected after the surgery because some soft tissues are left exposed in the oral cavity. The soft tissue healing occurs via secondary intention (Figure 5.5.6).

Another way to perform vestibuloplasty is to deepen the vestibule by using gingival grafts. Typically harvested from the palate, the gingival graft is placed in the area where the vestibule is to be deepened. Bohannan [13] showed that vestibuloplasty done using gingival grafts has more predictable long-term result when compared with those done without. An apically repositioned flap in vestibuloplasty done without gingival grafts has the tendency to migrate coronally over time, resulting in a shallower vestibule.

F. Fiberotomy is performed using a scalpel blade that will be inserted into the sulcus of the teeth, severing the epithelial and connective tissue attachments including gingivodental fibers and transseptal fibers. Fiberotomy is not recommended during active orthodontic tooth movement as well as in the presence of gingival inflammation. Fiberotomy has been shown to be more effective in treating teeth in the maxillary anterior region than teeth in other sextants of the mouth [14]. Fiberotomy is highly successful in mitigating rotational relapses rather than labiolingual relapses [14].

Case 6

Minimally Invasive Coronally Advanced Flap Techniques

CASE STORY

A 63-year-old Caucasian female presented with the chief complaint of "My gums are receding and I would like to have it treated." The patient stated she did not like the appearance of her teeth. Upon questioning, she reported no sensitivity to cold.

LEARNING GOALS AND OBJECTIVES

- To recognize and diagnose mucogingival deformities
- To identify possible treatment options and select the approach that best meets the chief complaint
- To compare and contrast the differences between mucogingival therapy carried out with and without soft tissue alternatives

Medical History

The patient reported that she took over-the-counter vitamin D supplements once daily. She also reported to have allergies to sulfa drugs and had been diagnosed with hay fever.

Review of Systems

- Vital signs
  - Blood pressure: 125/87 mmHg
  - Pulse rate: 70 beats/minute
  - Respiratory rate: 15 breaths/minute

Social History

The patient stated she consumed alcohol socially (one glass of wine per week) and reported no history of smoking or recreational drugs.

Extraoral Examination

Extraoral examination revealed no pathologic findings. No significant findings were noted. The patient had no enlargement or swelling, and the temporomandibular joint was within normal limits.

Intraoral Examination (Figures 5.6.1 and 5.6.2)

- Tongue, floor of mouth, and buccal mucosa were within normal limits.
- Periodontal examination:
  - Gingival contour: generalized recession with pyramidal papillae with knife-edged margins.
  - Consistency: generalized firm, stippling present.
  - Plaque and calculus: generalized mild supragingival and subgingival plaque.

Radiographic Examination

Full-mouth radiographs (Figure 5.6.3) showed the following features:

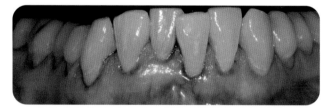

Figure 5.6.1 Clinical presentation.

Parameter	32	31	30	29	28	27	26	25	24	23	22	21	20	19	18	17
BL/SUP																
Calculus					CCC	CCC	CCC		CCC	CCC	CCC					
MOBILITY		N	N	N	N	N	N	N	N	N	N	N	N	N	N	
PLAQUE																
FURCA																
ATTACH		000	000	000	101	000	000	000	000	000	000	000	000	000	000	
FGM		+3+2+3	+3+2+3	+2+1+2	+1+1+1	+1+1+1	+1+1+1	+1+1+1	+1+1+1	+1+1+1	+1+1+1	+2+1+2	+2+1+2	+3+2+3	+3+2+3	
P.D.		323	323	212	212	111	111	111	111	111	111	212	212	323	323	
Tooth	32	31	30	29	28	27	26	25	24	23	22	21	20	19	18	17
BL/SUP																
MGDEF																
Calculus																
FURCA																
PLAQUE																
ATTACH		326	544	444	444	444	254	343	342	342	333	353	143	223	333	
FGM		003	332	232	232	232	132	221	221	231	221	231	010	000	000	
P.D.		323	212	212	212	212	122	122	121	111	112	122	133	223	333	

Figure 5.6.2 Periodontal chart.

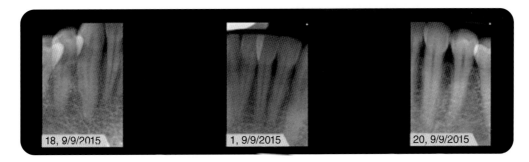

Figure 5.6.3 Periapical radiographs.

- Crestal bone levels within normal limits
- No periapical pathology
- No caries detected

Diagnosis

According to the most recent EFP/AAP classification [1] this case can be diagnosed as:
- Localized plaque-induced gingivitis
- Mucogingival condition with gingival recession at individual sites (relevant condition: tooth position); Cairo RT1/Miller class I classification

Treatment Plan

After reviewing the patient's history and clinical examination, it was concluded that her gingival recession was likely secondary to a history of aggressive oral hygiene habits. The treatment plan included an initial phase of adult prophylaxis with oral hygiene instruction and modification of brushing and flossing techniques. Taking into consideration the clinical findings, number of teeth that needed to be treated, and the patient's request of not using autogenous tissue for grafting, a decision was made to use an acellular dermal matrix (ADM) for root coverage of the maxillary and mandibular arches. This chapter focuses on the treatment for teeth #21–30 utilizing the vestibular incision subperiosteal tunnel access (VISTA) approach.

Treatment

The patient completed phase 1 therapy which included adult prophylaxis with oral hygiene instruction and modification of brushing and flossing techniques. The surgical site (#21–30) was anesthetized via local infiltration with local anesthetic agent. A 5–6 mm vertical vestibular incision was made in the mandibular buccal frenum between #24 and #25 (Figure 5.6.4). VISTA instruments were used to perform a subperiosteal tunnel through the vestibular incision and allow for coronal advancement of the tissue without tension (Figure 5.6.5). ADM was hydrated per the manufacturer's instructions. The graft was measured according to the length of the recipient site and trimmed (Figure 5.6.6). The graft was inserted through the vestibular incision and placed at the level of the cementoenamel junction (CEJ). The flaps

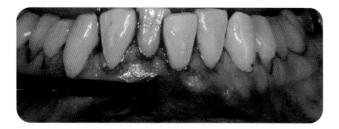

Figure 5.6.4 Vertical vestibular incision to provide access.

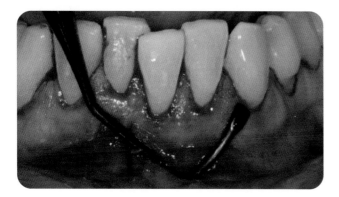

Figure 5.6.5 Use of specific instruments designed for the VISTA procedure.

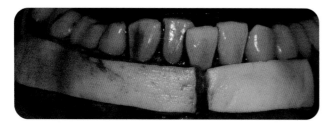

Figure 5.6.6 Preparing and adapting the soft tissue alternative (ADM).

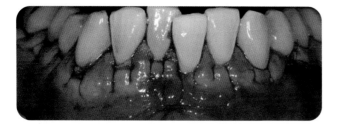

Figure 5.6.7 Subpapillary suturing technique.

were sutured at the level of the CEJ using 6-0 polypropyl-ene sutures utilizing a continuous subpapillary suturing technique (Figure 5.6.7). Postoperative instructions were given to avoid brushing and flossing in the surgical site and the patient was prescribed chlorhexidine 0.12% mouthwash to be used twice daily for one minute, ibuprofen 800 mg t.i.d., and amoxicillin 500 mg t.i.d. for seven days. Healing was uneventful. Tissue appeared

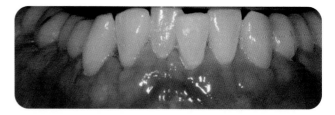

Figure 5.6.8 Presentation at four weeks post surgery.

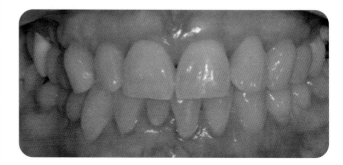

Figure 5.6.9 Presentation at 12 weeks post surgery.

slightly erythematous initially, but appeared to be healing within normal limits. Sutures were intact and retained at two weeks, and were planned to be removed at four weeks (Figure 5.6.8). Figure 5.6.9 shows the result at 12 weeks after surgery.

Discussion

Gingival recession could pose a threat to the stability of a tooth if not treated. It could cause increased root sensitivity, root caries, and esthetic concerns. Serino et al. [2] reported that 3-mm recession worsened 67% of the time and 4-mm recession worsened 98% of the time. However, the treatment would not be completely successful if the etiology is not addressed. The most common etiologic factors associated with recession are bacterial plaque and traumatic toothbrushing habits, along with predisposing factors such as lack of attached gingiva, orthodontic tooth movement, and frenum pull.

The patient presented with a chief complaint of receding gingiva in the maxillary and mandibular arches. The patient's primary concern was esthetics and fear of losing her teeth. Upon clinical examination, the patient had probing depths ranging from 1 to 3 mm with no interproximal bone loss. The patient's oral hygiene was fair and therefore we reinforced oral hygiene instruc-tions. Occlusion was evaluated and patient had no interferences on excursive movements. She was diagnosed with plaque-induced gingivitis with general-ized soft tissue recession. The soft tissue recession was due to traumatic toothbrushing habits in the maxillary and mandibular anterior region.

After reviewing oral hygiene instructions and modifying her toothbrushing habit to a stationary bristle technique, the recession sites were evaluated for soft tissue grafting procedures. Because of lack of interproximal bone loss, the recession was diagnosed as Cairo RT1 recession, which would almost certainly allow for 100% root coverage. The large areas of recession and the patient's preference not to have a donor site on the palate informed a decision to utilize ADM as an alternative.

On evaluation of the recession site, the patient appeared to have a thick gingival phenotype, with adequate gingival thickness and wide papillae. This would allow for adequate blood supply to the graft and increase the chances of a successful procedure. It was decided to address the prominent frenum attachment during the surgery to prevent additional pull during the healing period.

Along with above-mentioned intraoperative factors, postsurgical care and patient compliance are also imperative to achieve success with soft tissue grafting procedures. Avoiding pulling the lip, soft toothbrushing habits, and reducing swelling with the help of anti-inflammatory drugs and ice application could help obtain successful results. ADM has been shown to demonstrate similar results to a connective tissue graft and has reported stability for up to five years and the surgical method was not related to relapse. Long-term follow-up studies are needed to report on the use of ADM with the VISTA technique.

Self-Study Questions

A. What is the sequence of treatment in a case that presents with both mucogingival deformities and malalignment/malocclusion?

B. What is the VISTA technique?

C. What are types of soft tissue alternatives available and why was ADM used in this case?

D. What are the advantages/disadvantages of using a VISTA procedure with ADM in this particular situation?

E. What is the level of evidence supporting this treatment approach?

Answers located at the end of the chapter.

ACKNOWLEDGMENT
We thank Dr. Esra Faden for help in case documentation and for taking some of the postoperative images when the patient was in her care.

References

1. Jepsen S, Caton JG, Albandar JM, et al. Periodontal manifestations of systemic diseases and developmental and acquired conditions: Consensus report of workgroup 3 of the 2017 World Workshop on the Classification of Periodontal and Peri-Implant Diseases and Conditions. *J Periodontol* 2018;89(Suppl 1):S237–S248.
2. Serino G, Wennstrom JL, Lindhe J, Eneroth L. The prevalence and distribution of gingival recession in subjects with a high standard of oral hygiene. *J Clin Periodontol* 1994;21:57–63.

TAKE-HOME POINTS

A. In patients with malalignment – if the teeth are to be moved labially – it is advisable to perform a mucogingival procedure prior to orthodontic treatment. However, if the tooth is being moved lingually, there could be increase in gingiva on the facial aspect by orthodontic treatment alone.

B. VISTA stands for vestibular incision subperiosteal tunnel access. It is a minimally invasive technique which entails making an access incision in the frenum, followed by elevation of a subperiosteal tunnel. VISTA allows for access as well as an opportunity to coronally reposition the gingival margins of all involved teeth.

C. Soft tissue alternatives could be xenograft such as collagen matrix, ADM, and biologics. The reason that ADM was used in this case was because of the patient's request to avoid using her own tissue and creating another surgical site.

Studies have recorded that ADM has demonstrated mean defect coverage of up to 86%, with up to five years of follow-up studies.

D.

Advantages of VISTA

- Minimally invasive
- Maintains papilla integrity
- Less trauma to sulcular tissue
- No chance of donor site morbidity
- Enhances wound stability

Disadvantages of VISTA

- Inability to access bony topography
- Instrumentation
- Surgical experience
- Indirect visualization

E. The level of evidence is limited to case reports and case series and one randomized controlled trial with limited follow-up.

6

Interdisciplinary Treatment

Case 1: Periodontics–Endodontics 248
Paul A. Levi Jr., DMD and Campo E. Perez Jr., DDS

Case 2: Periodontics–Prosthodontics 260
Kevin Guze, DMD, DMSc, MSc, FRCD(C), FICOI and Ryan D. Blissett, DMD, MMSc

Case 3: Periodontics–Orthodontics: Part I. 268
Athbi Alqareer, BDM, DMSc, Shankar Rengasamy Venugopalan, BDS, DDS, PhD, DMSc,
and Veerasathpurush Allareddy, BDS, MBA, MHA, PhD, MMSc

Case 4: Periodontics–Orthodontics: Part II 276
Camille Neste Laboy, DDS, MPH, Soroan Akyalcin, DDS, PhD, and Irina F. Dragan, DDS, DMD, MS

Case 5: Occlusion–Periodontology 284
Mohamed H. Hassan, BDS, DMD, MS, FICD, Irina F. Dragan, DDS, DMD, MS, and
Rory O'Neil, DMD, BDS, MSc

Case 6: Periodontics–Pediatric Dentistry. 289
Nadeem Karimbux, DMD, MMSc, Roslayn Sulyanto, DMD, MS, and Soo-Woo Kim, DMD, MS

Case 1

Periodontics–Endodontics

CASE STORY

In March 2013, a 61-year-old female patient presented for her regular three-month professional dental hygiene therapy. She mentioned to the hygienist that she was experiencing moderate pain from time to time in her upper right bridge, especially when chewing. She stated that when she "got at it" with her water irrigating device on high pressure, the pain would dissipate (Figures 6.1.1 and 6.1.2). As a result of her chief concern at this maintenance hygiene visit, a comprehensive periodontal examination was scheduled for the following day.

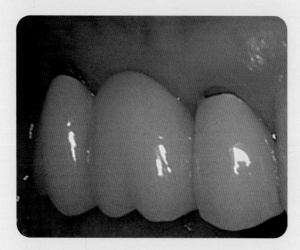

Figure 6.1.1 Initial picture of the bridge.

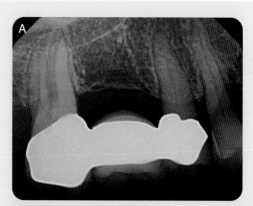

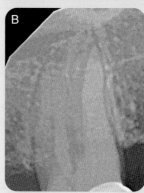

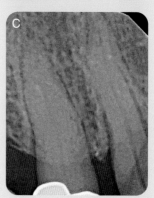

Figure 6.1.2 Periapical radiographs: (A) teeth #2–5; (B) tooth #2; (C) tooth #5.

LEARNING GOALS AND OBJECTIVES

■ To be able to differentiate between periodontal and endodontic pain and to generate a differential diagnosis

■ To identify the possible etiology or etiologies for the problem and to perform the appropriate therapy

■ To understand the multifactorial processes of periodontal diseases and endodontic disease and their treatment

Medical History

- The patient had no systemic conditions that would affect her dental health.
- She was never a smoker and her alcohol consumption included a daily glass of red wine.
- She denied the use of recreational drugs, but took a multivitamin daily.
- She exercised daily.

Dental History

Sixteen years previously the patient presented with stage 2 grade B periodontitis and was treated successfully with the following comprehensive periodontal therapy.

- Plaque control technique instruction comprising:
  - ○ Bass intrasulcular technique of brushing using a soft multi-tufted straight-cut hand toothbrush (Oral-B) [1]
  - ○ Dental tape (J&J Reach) using an adapted "C" shape with an occluso-apical and buccolingual buffing motion [2].
- Subgingival scaling and root planing.
- Pocket-reducing flap surgery with osseous contouring for the posterior sextants.
- The extraction of tooth #3 was due to nonrestorable dental caries.
- A post-extraction evaluation and a treatment plan was performed by her restorative dentist for a fixed bridge utilizing teeth #2 and #4 as abutments (the patient declined implant therapy).
- Maintenance dental hygiene therapy every three months, alternating between her periodontist and her restorative dentist.
- Periodic periodontal and restorative evaluations were done at each maintenance dental hygiene visit and a comprehensive periodontal examination was done every five years.
- Radiographs were exposed after surgical therapy/maintenance (Figure 6.1.3).

Review of Systems

- Vital signs
  - ○ Blood pressure: 104/60 mmHg
  - ○ Pulse rate: 82 beats/minute (regular)
  - ○ Respiratory rate: 15 breaths/minute
  - ○ Temperature: 37°C
- Height: 1.63 m
- Weight: 52 kg

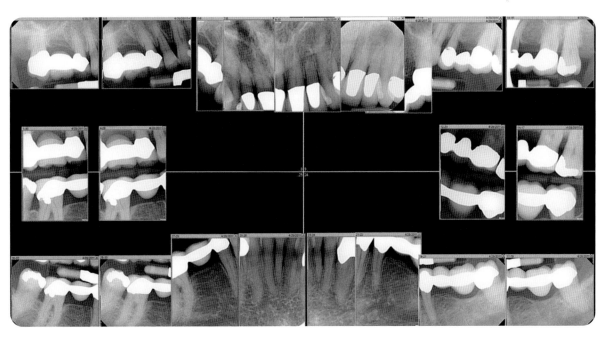

Figure 6.1.3 Complete mouth series of radiographs taken a year following the periodontal surgical therapy.

Extraoral Examination

The patient had no masses or swelling, and the temporomandibular joint appeared to be normal on palpation.

Intraoral Examination

- The patient demonstrated adequate intrasulcular brushing and flossing techniques as described above and was now using a Sonicare electric toothbrush with a Bass technique of brushing as she had previously used with a manual toothbrush.
- The previous day the patient had presented for professional dental hygiene therapy with virtually no plaque and slight supragingival calculus associated with the lingual of the mandibular incisors.
- The soft tissues, lips, buccal mucosa, hard/soft palate, floor of the mouth, and tongue appeared normal in color, shape, texture, and consistency.
- There was no evidence of dental caries.
- Probing depths were normal (2–3 mm). There was a 4-mm pocket distal of tooth #2 associated with thick tuberosity tissue (Figure 6.1.4).
- There were a few areas of slight bleeding on probing around teeth with crowns. There was no purulence with probing.

- The gingiva exhibited very slight marginal gingival inflammation around some of the crowns (Figure 6.1.5).
- Tooth mobility was normal.
- There was no pain on percussion.

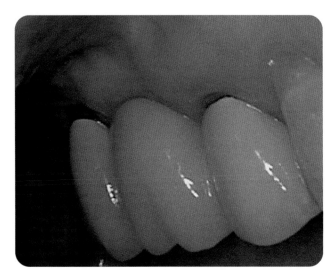

Figure 6.1.5 Initial picture of the maxillary right bridge of teeth #2–4.

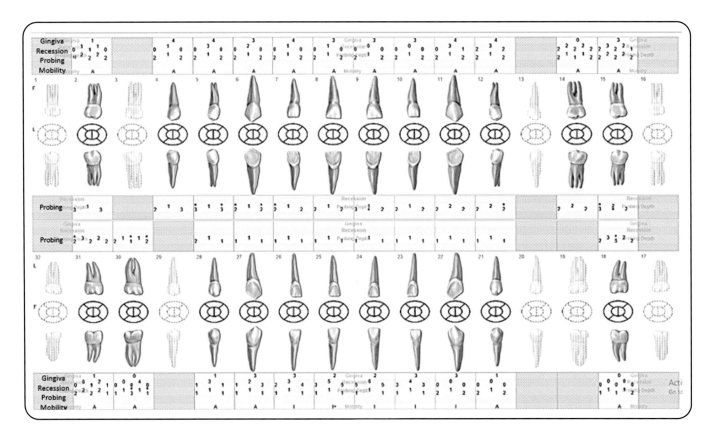

Figure 6.1.4 Periodontal chart illustrating the full-mouth probing depth measurements after the discovery of a 10-mm pocket on the distal of tooth #2 following scaling and curettage.

Occlusion

- There were nonworking side contacts on tooth #2, and pontic for tooth #3 and tooth #4.
- There was no fremitus.
- There was no centric prematurity (CR : CO discrepancy) nor slide.
- There was slight attrition associated with the mandibular anterior teeth.
- The patient was unaware of bruxism or clenching.

Radiographic Examination

The periapical radiographs (Figure 6.1.2) revealed the following.

- Interproximal horizontal bone loss in the coronal third of the teeth.
- Normal crestal bone densities were present, although there was somewhat less density crestally on the mesial of tooth #5.
- Restorations with no marginal discrepancies.
- A furcation arrow seen on the distal of tooth #2.
- Widening of the periodontal ligament (PDL) on tooth #5.
- No evidence of caries.
- No evidence of periapical radiolucencies or breaks in the periapical lamina duras.

Diagnoses

After reviewing the clinical history and performing the clinical–radiographic examination, the diagnoses of this patient were as follows.

Differential Diagnosis for Tooth #2

1. Pulpal inflammation associated with occlusal trauma on teeth #2 and #4 secondary to bruxism.
2. Primary endodontic lesion without discernible periapical radiolucencies.
3. Primary periodontal lesion secondary to the 4-mm distal pocket and furcation involvement on tooth #2.
4. Combined periodontal–endodontic lesion possibly associated with a lateral canal or canals.
5. Vertical fracture of tooth #2 or #4.

Definitive Diagnoses

1. Periodontal health on a reduced periodontium
2. Primary occlusal traumatism

Treatment Plan
Phase 1

- Occlusal adjustment of teeth #2 and #4. This was done at the time of the complete periodontal examination the day following the dental hygiene maintenance

visit when the chief concern of pain associated with the maxillary right bridge was elicited.
- Endodontic evaluation of teeth #2 and #4 with treatment if discomfort persisted following the occlusal adjustment.

Phase 4 (periodic restorative and periodontal evaluations)

- Maintenance dental hygiene therapy every three months:
  - Oral hygiene instruction.
  - Scaling with root planing (if needed).
  - Evaluation of endodontic treatment and periodontal conditions.

Treatment

The next day (a Saturday) following the occlusal adjustment of teeth #2–4 the pain increased in the maxillary right. The patient saw her endodontist that Saturday for evaluation of teeth #2 and #4. The endodontist stated that the pain was of periodontal origin as there was a 4–5 mm pocket on the distal of tooth #2. The following Monday the patient returned to the periodontal practice for therapy. The periodontist placed a gutta percha point in the pocket on the distal of tooth #2 and exposed a radiograph (Figure 6.1.6).

Under injectable local anesthetic (lidocaine 2%, 1:100 000 epinephrine) scaling, root planing, and gingival curettage were performed on the distal of tooth #2 using Younger-Good 7/8 and Gracey 13/14 (Hu-Friedy) hand curettes and a piezoelectric (Acteon Satelec) ultrasonic scaler. The toe of the hand curettes and the

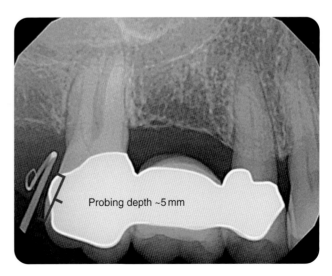

Figure 6.1.6 Periapical radiograph depicting the gutta percha in the distal 4–5 mm pocket of tooth #2 on initial presentation.

tips of the ultrasonic scalers were placed to the crest of the alveolar bone to remove any granulation tissue.

The patient returned for a postoperative visit four days following the scaling and curettage, which was a week after the comprehensive periodontal examination. She reported that the pain was no longer present. The distal of tooth #2 was probed and 10 mm of pocket was found. A gutta percha point was placed in the distal pocket (Figures 6.1.7 and 6.1.8).

The patient was referred to the endodontist that day and root canal therapy was performed When the pulpal tissue was extirpated, the endodontist stated that there appeared to be normal tissue in the palatal canal and

what appeared to be necrotic tissue in the mesiobuccal canals. All canals were filled with the warm gutta percha technique and the access cavity was filled with a composite.

Following the root canal treatment (Figures 6.1.9 and 6.1.10), maintenance dental hygiene therapy was continued every three months. A six-year chronologic sequence of radiographs is presented in Figure 6.1.11. In 2018, at her routine dental hygiene visit a pocket was again found on the distal of tooth #2. No discomfort was reported. A periapical radiograph was exposed with a gutta percha point in the distal pocket (Figures 6.1.12 and 6.1.13). There was no pathology

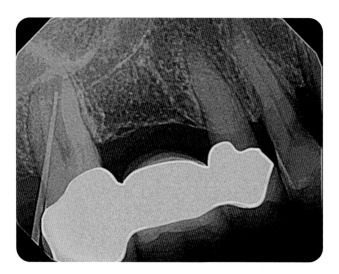

Figure 6.1.7 Periapical radiograph of the right-side molar region depicting the 10-mm pocket with the gutta percha on tooth #2.

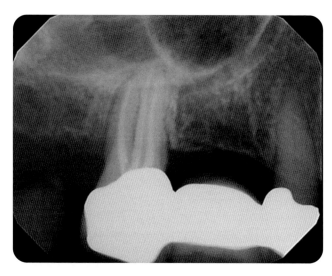

Figure 6.1.9 Periapical radiograph of the right-side molar region following root canal therapy.

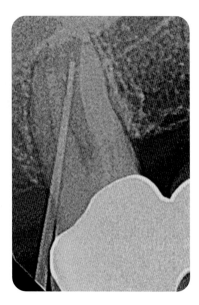

Figure 6.1.8 Periapical radiograph of tooth #2.

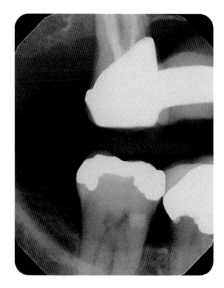

Figure 6.1.10 Bitewing radiograph of the right-side molar region one year after root canal therapy. No discomfort was present. No further bone loss is evident on the distal.

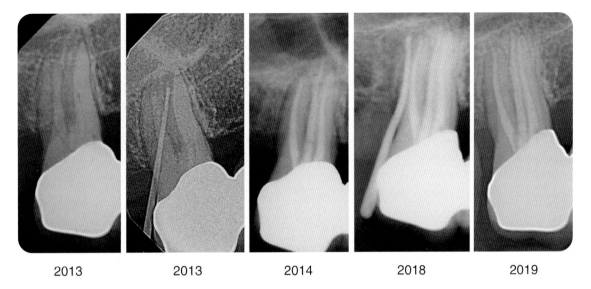

| 2013 | 2013 | 2014 | 2018 | 2019 |

Figure 6.1.11 Chronologic six-year sequence showing no apparent radiographic changes.

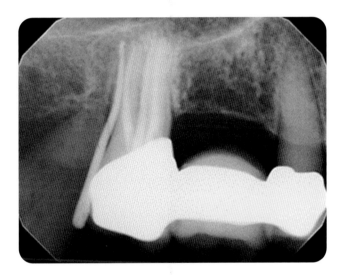

Figure 6.1.12 Tooth #2 with a 10-mm pocket in the distal with a gutta percha point now tracing to the distofacial root five years following initial endodontic therapy.

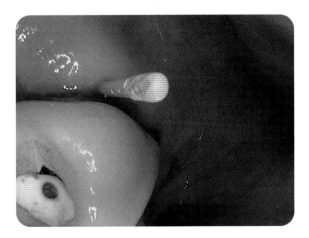

Figure 6.1.13 Clinical picture with gutta percha point.

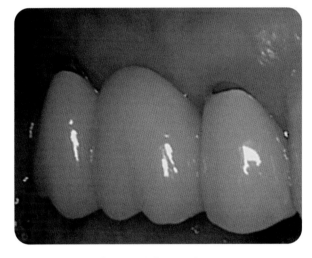

Figure 6.1.14 No soft tissue inflammation.

noted on the buccal (Figure 6.1.14). Unlike six years previously, the gutta percha point now traced to the distobuccal root. The patient was referred to the endodontist who stated that the endodontic treatment was not the problem and made a clinical diagnosis of root fracture on tooth #2.

A treatment consultation was then done with the patient and the following options were explained.

- Flap surgery to determine if the tooth was fractured, and if it were:
  - A root section could be done if the roots were not fused.
  - The bridge could be sectioned at the distal of tooth #4 and tooth #2 could be extracted with ridge preservation and the eventual placement of an implant. Guided bone regeneration would

be done at the same time for the edentulous area of tooth #3.
  ○ Alternatively, the bridge could be sectioned as explained above and no replacement of teeth #2 and #3.

The patient's choice was to retain the tooth as it was not painful and not to undergo any further treatment. She stated that if the problem became acute again, she would decide what she would do at that time. She was informed that with a deep pocket that she could not access for plaque removal, there would be a persistent chronic inflammation which could negatively affect her systemically.

Discussion

This is an unusual presentation of a dental problem. When a patient presents with a chief concern of dental pain, in order to arrive at a correct diagnosis, the clinician elicits a complete history of the symptoms, takes an accurate medical, dental, and social history, and completes a comprehensive periodontal and endodontic evaluation. The examinations include an extraoral evaluation to assess the patient's general appearance that may involve the observation of localized skin redness, facial asymmetry, swelling, a sinus tract, tender or enlarged lymph nodes, or tenderness or discomfort upon palpation or movement of the temporomandibular joint. The intraoral examination consists of a visual and digital assessment of the teeth, gingiva, and other oral mucosa to detect areas of discoloration of the soft tissues, inflammation, ulcerations, swelling, and sinus tract formation. The dental examination includes an assessment for tooth color changes, fractures, abrasion, erosion, caries, large restorations, past endodontic therapy, posts, and other abnormalities. Clinical tests with the objective of discovering the affected tooth or teeth will then be done. These clinical tests include periradicular tests (percussion and palpation), pulp vitality tests (cold, heat, electric, and test cavity) [3], or occlusal tests for a fracture with a bite stick (Tooth Slooth®). A comprehensive periodontal examination encompasses observation of the patient's home care techniques and measurements of probing depth, bleeding, clinical attachment levels, plaque, calculus, gingival recession, furcation involvement, tooth mobility, and mucogingival deformities. Finally, the occlusion is evaluated for fremitus, premature contacts in centric relation occlusion, nonworking contacts or interferences, and wear facets, which can indicate parafunctional habits [4]. In addition to these measurements, parallel technique periapical radiographs are a necessary adjunct to a thorough periodontal and endodontic examination [3,4].

Four main types of noxious stimuli are common causes of pulpal inflammation (Figures 6.1.15–6.1.19).
1. Mechanical damage due to dental procedures, attrition (signifying parafunctional habits), abrasion, and barometric changes.
2. Thermal injury due to large uninsulated metallic restorations, cavity preparation, polishing, and chemical reaction of dental materials.
3. Chemical irritation due to erosion or inappropriate use of acidic dental materials.
4. Bacterial effects causing damage to the pulp through toxins or directly after extension from caries or transportation via the vasculature (anachoresis) [5–7].

Communication between the periodontium and the pulp tissue can occur through many channels or pathways

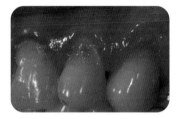

Figure 6.1.15 Abrasion.

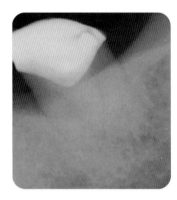

Figure 6.1.16 Thermal injury: large uninsulated metallic restoration.

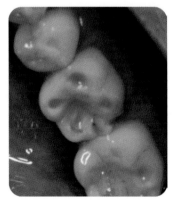

Figure 6.1.17 Chemical irritation.

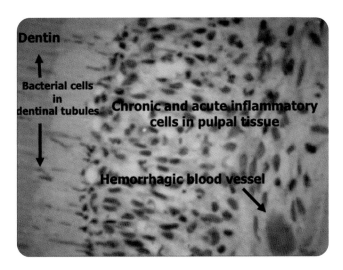

Figure 6.1.18 Bacterial effect: caries. Source: courtesy of Dr. Victor Ratkus.

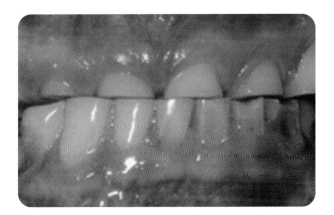

Figure 6.1.19 Bruxism (parafunctional habit).

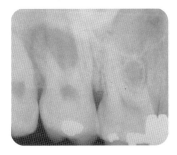

Figure 6.1.20 Apical foramen communication.

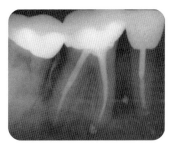

Figure 6.1.21 Lateral accessory canal. Source: courtesy of Dr. Victor Ratkus.

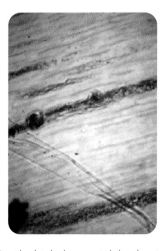

Figure 6.1.22 Dentinal tubules containing bacterial organisms. Source: courtesy of Dr. Victor Ratkus.

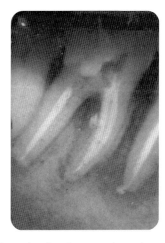

Figure 6.1.23 Furcation involvement lateral canal. Source: courtesy of Dr. Victor Ratkus.

that might be involved in extending pulpal infections (Figures 6.1.20–6.1.23). These include apical foramina (principal route of communication), lateral and accessory canals, and dentinal tubules [3,8–10]. When pulp tests indicate necrosis and when a sinus tract can be traced to the lateral portion of a root, a lateral canal might be the cause of a radiolucency in the PDL space or in the furcation [8]. It is estimated that 30–40% of all teeth have lateral canals principally in the apical third of the root. The incidence of lateral canals in the furcations of molars might vary from 23 to 76% [9].

Likewise, other possible pathways have been mentioned in the literature: lingual grooves, root fractures, cemental agenesis/hypoplasia, root anomalies,

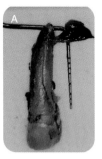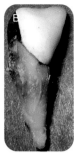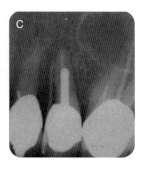

Figure 6.1.24 (A–C) Cracked teeth (roots) and vertical fracture.

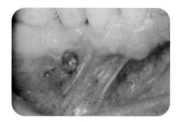

Figure 6.1.25 Draining sinus tract.

intermediate bifurcation ridges, and trauma-induced root resorption [10] (Figure 6.1.24).

Pulpal infection is a polymicrobial process caused mainly by endogenous opportunistic pathogens such as *Eubacterium*, *Peptostreptococcus*, *Fusobacterium*, *Porphyromonas*, *Prevotella*, *Streptococcus*, *Lactobacillus*, *Wolinella*, *Actinomyces* [7], and spirochetes. Acute exacerbations of chronic periapical infections are frequently associated with *Porphyromonas gingivalis* and *Porphyromonas endodontalis* [8–10]. Other microorganisms such as fungi and viruses have been documented in association with endodontic infections [9].

The pulpal–periodontal lesion is a process that involves the interaction of diseases of the pulp and of the periodontium. The etiology, diagnosis, and prognosis help to classify these lesions.

- *Pulpal lesions*: strictly of pulpal origin but may mimic combined lesions with signs and symptoms and will resolve with root canal treatment alone.
- *Periodontal lesions*: strictly of periodontal origin but may also simulate a combined lesion with signs especially, and at times with symptoms. Periodontal lesions can only resolve with periodontal treatment alone.
- *Combined lesions*: there are three types: (i) primary pulpal lesions, (ii) primary periodontal lesions, and (iii) both pulpal and periodontal lesions. The primary pulpal lesions may extend into the periapical PDL and allows secondary periodontitis. The primary periodontal lesion affects the pulpal tissue due to bacterial migration through the dentinal tubules into the pulpal tissue or the periodontal lesion encompassing the apex of the tooth (Figure 6.1.22) and creating secondary pulpitis. The pulpal and periodontal lesion encompasses both diseases, existing independently in both tissues at the same time [3,7–10].

A pulpal lesion or a primary endodontic lesion manifests a necrotic pulp with a chronic apical periodontitis and might have a sinus tract. Usually it is asymptomatic and the suppurative process may drain along the PDL

space and exit at the apical aspect of the sulcus, or it can also perforate the cortical bone close to the apex creating a sinus tract [8] (Figure 6.1.25).

Likewise, multirooted teeth might have a sinus tract along the PDL space that can drain into the furcation area, creating bone loss and exiting through the sulcus (pocket) [6]. Clinically, in primary pulpal lesions where there is no concomitant periodontitis, periodontal probing is within normal limits on the specific tooth and often throughout the patient's mouth. Also, assuming there is no associated generalized periodontal disease, radiographs will often show that the osseous destruction involves only the one tooth in question. If a buccal or lingual swelling appears, a lateral canal should be considered. Confirmation of the diagnosis generally comes from negative pulp vitality readings. The electrical and thermal tests and a test cavity usually reveal no response [8].

The diagnosis of pulpitis might be easily correlated with a diseased tooth; however, the origin of pulpal pain is frequently difficult to identify. It can be referred from arch to arch on the same side, which necessitates pulp testing several teeth. Disorders such as myofascial pain, trigeminal neuralgia, atypical facial neuralgia, migraine headaches, cluster headaches, nasal or sinus pathoses, angina pectoris, and referred cardiac pain in the left mandible have been reported to mimic pulpitis in some patients [5]. Clinical signs and symptoms generally help to determine the classification of pulpal disease. Numerous investigations have shown a lack of correlation between histopathologic findings and clinical symptoms [5,7]. The percentage of spirochetes seen by dark-field microscopy might be of value in the differential diagnosis of periodontal and endodontic abscesses, with a greater number of spirochetes seen in periodontal abscesses. Coccoid cells dominate in endodontic lesions [10].

Initial treatment consists of root canal therapy, which may be performed with multiple appointments so reevaluation of the healing process between the completion of root canal debridement and obturation visits can be made. Most commonly, a sinus tract heals after endodontic instrumentation and irrigation of the root canal. The closure of that tract and the elimination of probing depth indicate that the root canal has been completely cleansed. In the presence of a periodontal pocket, where a primary endodontic lesion is suspected, periodontal root planing should not be done until the endodontic therapy is completed regardless of the original pocket depth. It is important to preserve the PDL fibers so reattachment can occur. Healing is usually accomplished within three to six months, often with complete resolution of the pocket. The prognosis is then excellent [8]. However, the healing of periapical lesions may take up to four years [11].

When there is no periapical pathology, endodontic therapy has a success rate of more than 96% with both vital and nonvital pulps. However, in cases with pulpal necrosis and periapical radiolucencies, only 86% show apical healing. A much lower success rate of 60% is seen with retreatment of previous root canal therapy [8].

For the patient described here the diagnosis was unclear at the initial examination. The following questions will help to understand the etiology and diagnosis, which then leads to the correct therapy.

Self-Study Questions

A. What effect did the patient's excellent hygiene therapy have on the presentation of pain from time to time?

B. Why did the symptoms listed in Question A disappear following the patient's use of a water irrigating device?

C. What caused the symptoms to reappear after the patient used her water irrigating device?

D. Why was the 10-mm pocket apparent following the scaling, root planing, and curettage when it was not detected a week previously or at the time of scaling, root planing, and gingival curettage?

E. Explain the development of the 10-mm pocket on the facial of tooth #2 pointing to the apex of the mesial root.

F. What is the significance of a deep periodontal pocket on one surface of a *single* tooth in a generally periodontal disease-free mouth?

G. What are the reasons that the pain the patient experienced is from a primary *endodontic* origin rather due to periodontitis when there was a furcation involvement on the distal of tooth #2 and a history of past periodontitis?

H. Generally what issue should be treated first in a combination lesion, the endodontic problem or the periodontal problem, and why?

I. What was the possible reason why a periapical radiolucency was not present at the apex of tooth #2?

J. What are the common clinical features of a periodontal abscess?

Answers located at the end of the chapter.

ACKNOWLEDGMENTS

We thank Michael A. Kahn, DDS, past Chairman, Department of Oral and Maxillofacial Pathology, Tufts University School of Dental Medicine, and Kanchan M. Ganda, MD, Director, Division of Medicine, Tufts University School of Dental Medicine.

References

1. Ausenda F, Jeong N, Arsenault P, et al. The effect of the Bass intrasulcular toothbrushing technique on the reduction of gingival inflammation: a randomized clinical trial. *J Evid Based Dent Pract* 2019;19:106–114.
2. Harris-Basali D. The effect of instructed dental flossing on interdental gingival bleeding: a randomized controlled clinical trial. Masters thesis, Tufts University School of Dental Medicine, 2019.

3. American Association of Endodontists. Endodontics. Pulpal/periodontal relationships. Endodontics: Colleagues for Excellence, Spring/Summer 2001. Available at https://f3f142zs0k2w1kg84k5p9i1o-wpengine.netdna-ssl.com/specialty/wp-content/uploads/sites/2/2017/05/ss01ecfe.pdf

4. Armitage GC. The complete periodontal examination. Periodontol 2000 2004;34:22–33.

5. Neville BW, Damm DD, Allen C, Bouquot J. Oral and Maxillofacial Pathology, 3rd edn. St. Louis, MO: Saunders Elsevier, 2009. Chapter 3 pp120–123, 130–132, 698–700, 669–670.

6. Lindhe J, Lang NP (eds) Clinical Periodontology and Implant Dentistry, 5th edn, Vol. 2. Oxford: Wiley Blackwell, 2008:848–874.

7. Newman MG, Takei H, Klokkevold PR, Carranza FA (eds) Carranza's Clinical Periodontology, 10th edn. St. Louis, MO: Saunders Elsevier, 2006:871–880.

8. Rose LF, Mealy BL, Genco RJ, Cohen DW (eds) Periodontics: Medicine, Surgery and Implants. Philadelphia: Mosby, 2004: 773–788.

9. Rotstein I, Simon JH. The endo-perio lesion: a critical appraisal of the disease condition. Endod Topics 2006;13:34–56.

10. Meng HX. Periodontic–endodontic lesions. Ann Periodontol 1999;4:84–89.

11. Orstavik D. Time-course and risk analyses of the development and healing of chronic apical periodontitis in man. Int Endod J 1996;29(3):150–155.

12. Armitage G. A brief history of periodontics in the United States of America: pioneers and thought-leaders of the past, and current challenges. Periodontol 2000 2020;82: 12–25.

TAKE-HOME POINTS

A. Gingivitis and periodontitis are common inflammatory diseases strongly associated with poor oral hygiene. This patient showed excellent plaque control and stable periodontal health following therapy 16 years previously. There was no bleeding on probing on the distal of tooth #2; therefore, she had an intact attachment apparatus, allowing the epithelial attachment to seal the drainage from the apical infection and the inability of the periodontist to probe the sinus tract.

B. With the drainage blocked by the sealed epithelial attachment, the patient exhibited pain due to pressure from the exudative products of the necrotic pulp of the mesiobuccal canals creating apical inflammation. When she used the water irrigating device at high pressure, and when gingival curettage was done by the periodontist, the epithelial attachment was disrupted allowing drainage and relieving the pain. The epithelial attachment is a mucopolysaccharide protein (glycocalyx) secreted through the hemidesmosomes attaching the epithelial cells to the tooth.

C. The origin of the deep probing was a sinus tract created by the drainage along the facial of tooth #2 due to the infection from necrotic pulpal tissue in the mesiobuccal canals. When the drainage was blocked by the seal of the epithelial attachment due to the patient's excellent dental hygiene, the symptoms reappeared.

D. Scaling, root planing, and gingival curettage opened the sinus tract by disrupting the epithelial attachment at the apical portion of the sulcus/pocket. Following physical removal of the supracrestal soft tissue attachment by the curette tip and the ultrasonic instrumentation, it takes about five to seven days to reestablish the epithelial attachment. Thus, the pocket could be accessed four to five days following the therapy.

E. In an acute endodontic lesion, the pressure of the exudative process leads to tissue destruction, creating a pathway for drainage (sinus tract). The drainage in some instances may follow the PDL space along the root or supraperiostally. It will follow the path of least resistance and may exit through the sulcus, creating a narrow three-walled pocket, or through the soft tissue creating a sinus tract (Figure 6.1.25).

F. Periodontitis with deep pockets is a chronic infection caused by dysbiotic bacterial communities and likely eukaryotic viruses [12]. Periodontitis is usually found associated with more than one tooth in a mouth and commonly on more than one surface of a tooth. A single deep periodontal pocket is an important finding that helps to generate a differential diagnosis, because a single deep periodontal pocket may be found associated with a tooth with a necrotic pulp, a cracked tooth, or a tooth that has sustained physical trauma such as a tooth proximal to an impacted third molar.

Overhanging restorations, open interproximal contacts with food impaction, enamel projections, or enamel pearls can also cause isolated deep periodontal pockets, and one should evaluate the area for the findings just described. However, pocketing caused by a periodontal origin are usually wider at the coronal portion than if the origin of the inflammation emanated from the pulp.

G. The distal furcation involvement was the result of the previous stage 2 grade B periodontitis that was treated and had been stable due to the patient's excellent plaque control. With a stable periodontal situation, it is very unlikely that a patient would develop a periodontal abscess. Additionally, a periodontitis-induced infection is usually attended with classical signs of gingival inflammation, erythema, edema, and sponginess combined with pocketing. None of the clinical signs of inflammation were present on a thorough examination. The 4–5 mm pocket on the distal of tooth #2 did not enter the distal furcation (see Figure 6.1.6). It is likely that the necrotic pulp was related to the previous restorative therapy, the crown preparation, and prior restorations. As the patient was susceptible to dental caries and her long-time past plaque removal was inconsistent and ineffective, the pulpal necrosis was likely the result of past pulpal trauma stemming from past caries and restorations along with the past periodontal infection. The introduction of bacteria into a canal with necrotic pulpal tissue is likely to have allowed the acute abscess to occur.

H. The diagnosis here is a primary endodontic lesion. Thus, the conservative approach, treating the endodontic problem first, should always be considered for the initial treatment. Conversely, treating the periodontal problem with scaling and root planing before the endodontic therapy might prevent or lessen the amount of reattachment. Several authors have demonstrated the effectiveness of treating the endodontic problem first to achieve complete pocket reduction and allow for the restitution of a healthy periodontium without additional periodontal therapy [6–8]. In cases of combined periodontal–endodontic lesions, when the deep pocket and furcation involvement remain after endodontic therapy, the residual periodontal defect would then be addressed with resective or regenerative therapy.

I. In most instances of periapical periodontitis there is a radiographic break in the apical lamina dura; on some occasions the drainage and pressure of the tissue can develop in the facial or lingual aspect and the usual radiographic findings might not be observed. For this patient, it appears that the infection drained along the facial, and as the tooth is more radiodense than the bone, the radiographic appearance of bone loss was blocked.

J. Discomfort, swelling in the mid-part of the gingiva, furcation invasion, purulent exudate, bleeding and significant pain on probing. Because this patient was asymptomatic other than her reported paroxysmal stimulated pain when masticating on her bridge, and that she did not show common signs of a periodontal infection, the initial differential diagnosis of endodontic origin was established. Additionally, supporting this differential diagnosis was the presence of a crown on the tooth, the likelihood that the tooth had been previously restored before the crown was placed, and evidence of many dental restorations throughout the mouth.

Case 2

Periodontics–Prosthodontics

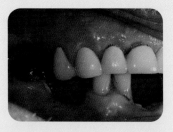

Figure 6.2.1 Preoperative right view of centric occlusion.

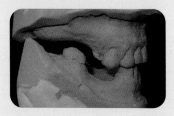

Figure 6.2.2 Preoperative photo of articulated diagnostic casts.

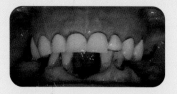

Figure 6.2.3 Preoperative frontal view of centric occlusion.

Medical History

The patient reported a negative review of systems, other than an allergy to penicillin. There were no contraindications to elective dental treatment.

Review of Systems

- Vital signs
  - Blood pressure: 128/88 mmHg
  - Pulse rate: 84 beats/minute (regular)
  - Respiratory rate: 18 breaths/minute

Social History

The patient reported a 25 pack-year smoking history. He currently smoked half a pack of cigarettes per day. There was no reported history of alcohol or substance abuse.

Extraoral Examination

There was no history of temporomandibular joint disorder (TMD) or occlusal orthosis. Temporomandibular joint examination revealed a normal range of motion with no clicking, crepitus, deviation, deflection, muscle tenderness to palpation, frequent headaches, or history of trauma to the face. The patient was unaware of clenching, bruxism, or other parafunctional habits. There was no lymphadenopathy.

Intraoral Examination

There was a negative oral cancer screen. A small epulis fissuratum was present in the edentulous area of tooth #24 from an ill-fitting interim partial denture.

Hyperkeratosis was present in the posterior mandible on the edentulous ridge crests. A small papule was noted on the left lateral tongue border, which the patient and his former dentist had been monitoring for many years. Multiple 4-mm pseudo-pockets were noted in the periodontal charting. No tooth mobility was present. Fremitus was noted on all anterior teeth. Significant atrophy of alveolar bone in the mandible could be visualized clinically. Tooth #31 had supraerupted (Figures 6.2.4–6.2.6).

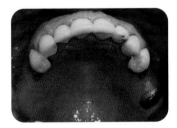

Figure 6.2.4 Preoperative occlusal view of maxilla.

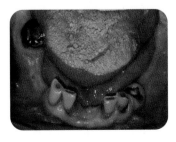

Figure 6.2.5 Preoperative occlusal view of mandible.

Occlusion

There were many noteworthy findings upon occlusal analysis:

- Lack of posterior occlusal contacts
- Fremitus
- Supraeruption of tooth #31 into maxillary dental space
- Loss of VDO
- Vertical maxillary excess

Esthetics

The patient was dissatisfied with the appearance of his recently finished crowns, specifically how short and wide they appeared. The patient reported that his maxillary anterior teeth had begun to develop spacing as his bite began to collapse prior to initiating treatment. He displayed 100% of the maxillary teeth and 3 mm of gingival tissues upon maximal smiling.

Radiographic Examination

The series revealed multiple endodontically treated teeth (Figure 6.2.7). There were favorable crown-to-root ratios on most teeth, with the exception of teeth #23 and #26, which exhibited mesial bone loss but had good bony support on the distal aspect. Both of these teeth displayed widened periodontal ligament (PDL) spaces and fremitus. There was no tooth mobility. Both maxillary sinuses were pneumatized and would require elevation with bone grafting for implant placement. Significant alveolar atrophy was present in the mandibular edentulous areas.

Problem List

- Poor oral hygiene
- Smoking habit
- Gingivitis with associated pseudo-pocketing
- Fremitus
- Widened PDL spaces
- Advanced alveolar atrophy in edentulous spaces
- Loss of VDO associated with bite collapse
- Lack of posterior support
- Lack of interarch space secondary to supraeruption of tooth #31 dentoalveolar complex
- Unsatisfactory esthetics
- Vertical maxillary excess
- Significant caries

Treatment Planning and Sequence Overview
Diagnostics

- History, examination, radiographs, clinical photographs, properly articulated diagnostic casts, diagnostic wax-up

Buccal	xxx	xxx	xxx	xxx	334	314	313	313	314	314	413	314	xxx	xxx	323	xxx
Palatal	xxx	xxx	xxx	xxx	223	323	413	313	323	323	313	213	xxx	xxx	223	xxx

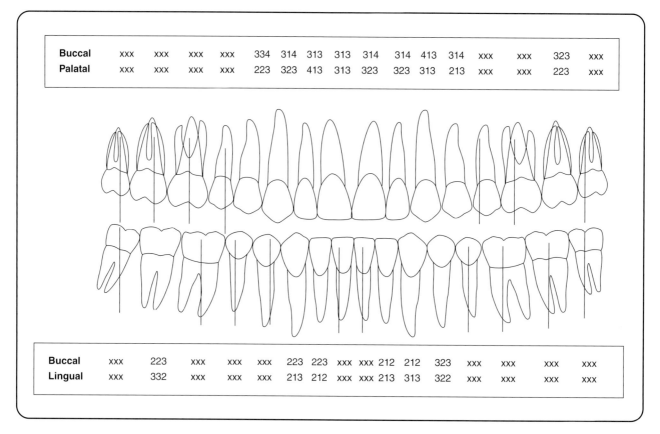

Buccal	xxx	223	xxx	xxx	xxx	223	223	xxx	xxx	212	212	323	xxx	xxx	xxx	xxx
Lingual	xxx	332	xxx	xxx	xxx	213	212	xxx	xxx	213	313	322	xxx	xxx	xxx	xxx

Figure 6.2.6 Initial periodontal probing measurements.

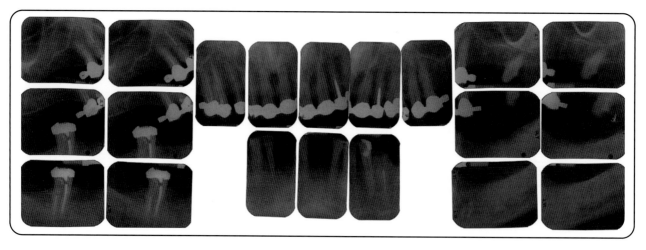

Figure 6.2.7 Preoperative full-mouth series radiographs.

- Computed tomography (CT) scan with radiographic template based on wax-up
- Present treatment options and make financial arrangements

Phase 1 (Figure 6.2.8)

- Prophylaxis with localized scaling and root planing
- Six-week reevaluation of periodontal status and hygiene compliance

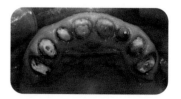

Figure 6.2.8 Occlusal view of maxillary teeth on removal of crowns. Note short clinical crowns, caries, and high degree of total occlusal convergence.

- Smoking cessation program initiated
- Aggressive caries control
- Prepare teeth and place provisional restorations
- Reevaluate abutment prognosis
- Evaluate patient tolerance of restored VDO
- Evaluate phonetics and esthetics
- Prescription fluoride toothpaste

Phase 2

- Surgical treatment: crown lengthening of all maxillary teeth to improve resistance and retention form, esthetics, occlusal plane, interarch space, and correct total occlusal convergence (Figure 6.2.9)
- Surgical template provided by prosthodontist that follows diagnostic wax-up

Phase 3

- Prosthetic rehabilitation (Figures 6.2.10–6.2.15)

Maintenance

- Regular prophylaxis and periodontal reevaluation
- Regular reevaluation of removable partial denture stability with appropriate reline procedures
- Occlusal orthosis
- Fluoride trays

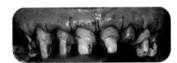

Figure 6.2.9 Maxillary teeth immediately following crown lengthening.

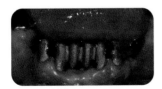

Figure 6.2.10 Clinical view of gold dome coping at time of solder relation.

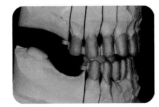

Figure 6.2.11 Right view of metal frameworks showing tooth #31 shortened and restored with gold dome coping. Note ERA attachments.

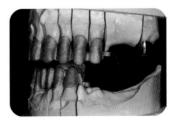

Figure 6.2.12 Left view of metal frameworks showing gold dome coping on tooth #15 for additional posterior support.

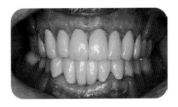

Figure 6.2.13 Facial postoperative view.

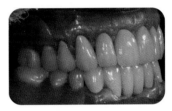

Figure 6.2.14 Right postoperative view.

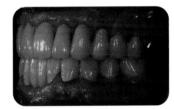

Figure 6.2.15 Left postoperative view.

Discussion

It is not uncommon for specialists to encounter clinical situations similar to this case. In most instances, the common cause for a failure of this magnitude is inadequate treatment planning. Understanding basic principles of dentistry is essential to formulating a comprehensive problem list and treatment plan. Architects draft blueprints and assemble models before beginning any project. The same planning and attention to detail in dentistry will greatly improve the quality of dentistry in your practice and its predictability [1]. It is the responsibility of each practitioner to respect the limitations of his or her knowledge and clinical experience and refer cases to specialists when appropriate.

Self-Study Questions

A. What information is essential when planning a complex dental treatment?

B. What steps should be performed before proceeding to definitive restorations?

C. What risks does one assume when finishing one arch of a dental rehabilitation without first placing provisional restorations in both arches?

D. Which clinical situations may require a clinician to perform crown lengthening in the course of a prosthetic treatment?

E. Other than crown lengthening, which procedures are available to create additional interarch space for restorative materials?

Answers located at the end of the chapter.

ACKNOWLEDGMENT

The presented case was completed by students in the Teaching Practice at the Harvard School of Dental Medicine, Boston, Massachusetts.

References

1. Beck CM, Kaiser DA, Goldfogel MH. Evolution of removable partial denture design. *J Prosthodont* 1994;3:158–166.
2. De Van MM. The nature of the partial denture foundation: suggestions for its preservation. *J Prosthet Dent* 1952;2:210–218.
3. Rudd K. Making diagnostic cast is not a waste of time. *J Prosthet Dent* 1968;20:93–100.
4. Morgan DW, Comella MC, Staffanou RS. A diagnostic wax-up technique. *J Prosthet Dent* 1975;33:169–177.
5. Balshi TJ, Mingledorff EB, Olbrys BH, Cantor SJ. Restorative occlusion utilizing a custom incisal guide table. *J Prosthet Dent* 1976;36:468–471.
6. Gargiulo A, Krajewski J, Gargiulo M. Defining biologic width in crown lengthening. *CDS Rev* 1995;88:20–23.
7. Kois JC. The restorative–periodontal interface: biological parameters. *Periodontol 2000* 1996;11:29–38.
8. Libman WJ, Nicholls JI. Load fatigue of teeth restored with cast posts and cores and complete crowns. *Int J Prosthodont* 1995;8:155–161.
9. Turrell AJW. Clinical assessment of vertical dimension. *J Prosthet Dent* 1972;28:238–246.
10. Lytle RB. Vertical relation of occlusion by the patient's neuromuscular perception. *J Prosthet Dent* 1964;14:12–21.
11. Silverman MM. Accurate measurement of vertical dimension by phonetics and the speaking centric space. *Dent Dig* 1951;57:261–265.
12. Ismail YH, George WA. The consistency of the swallowing technique in determining occlusal vertical dimension in edentulous patients. *J Prosthet Dent* 1968;19:230–236.
13. Sheppard IM, Sheppard SM. Vertical dimension measurements. *J Prosthet Dent* 1975;34:269–277.
14. Wagner A. Comparison of four methods to determine rest position of the mandible. *J Prosthet Dent* 1971;25:506–514.
15. McGee G. Use of facial measurements in determining vertical dimension. *J Am Dent Assoc* 1947;35:342–350.
16. Silverman SI. Vertical dimension record: a three dimensional phenomenon. *Part I. J Prosthet Dent* 1985;53:420–425.
17. Boos RH. Intermaxillary relation established by biting power. *J Am Dent Assoc* 1940;27:1192–1199.
18. Pound E. Controlling anomalies of vertical dimension and speech. *J Prosthet Dent* 1976;36:124–135.
19. Lord JL. The overdenture: patient selection, use of copings and follow-up evaluation. *J Prosthet Dent* 1974;32:41–51.
20. Morrow RM, Feldmann EE, Rudd KD, Trovillion HM. Tooth-supported complete dentures: an approach to preventive prosthodontics. *J Prosthet Dent* 1969;21:513–522.
21. Brewer A, Morrow R. Overdentures. St. Louis, MO: Mosby, 1975.
22. Crum RJ, Rooney GE Jr. Alveolar bone loss in overdentures: a five year study. *J Prosthet Dent* 1978;40:610–613.
23. Holmes JB. Influence of impression procedures and occlusal loading on partial denture movement. *J Prosthet Dent* 1965;15:474–481.
24. Leupold RJ, Kratochvil FJ. An altered cast procedure to improve tissue support for removable partial dentures. *J Prosthet Dent* 1965;15:672–678.
25. Leupold RJ. A comparative study of impression procedures for distal extension removable partial dentures. *J Prosthet Dent* 1966;16:708–720.

TAKE-HOME POINTS

A. Before any treatment begins, a thorough diagnosis must be established. This involves a comprehensive medical history, history of past dental treatment and conditions, eliciting a chief complaint, extraoral examination, oral cancer screen, periodontal examination [2], clinical dental examination with appropriate testing of pulp status, radiographic examination including full-mouth series radiographs (and panoramic radiograph and/or CT scan when appropriate), diagnostic photographs, diagnostic casts [3], diagnostic wax-up [4], and referrals to other specialists.

Prior to considering crown lengthening procedures it is essential that the practitioner assess radiologically the root length, root width, and root pathology. Furthermore, soft tissue examination should include confirming the presence of adequate keratinized tissue and smile line analysis to avoid visible poor gingival contours that may result.

Once a list of diagnoses is established, a problem list is generated. This will aid in contingency planning. All possible contingencies must be anticipated. In the event that the chosen plan cannot be accomplished, a smooth transition into the best possible outcome can be achieved. Your problem list will help you formulate treatment plans with the most predictable outcomes.

Always formulate an ideal treatment plan. This plan should propose the best possible outcome available within the anatomic limitations of the patient and current dental technology. Many patients cannot choose this plan because of financial or health constraints. This ideal plan will serve as a reference for a number of secondary plans, one of which may better suit the individual goals of the patient. Once the patient is informed of all foreseeable risks and benefits, a financial arrangement is made and treatment can begin.

B. A diagnostic wax-up is a critical step in planning any complex treatment. This allows direct visualization of ideal conditions within the patient's anatomic constraints.

When this patient presented to the clinic, it was apparent that the maxillary arch had been addressed before much attention was given to the mandible. Moving to phase 3 treatment in one arch before completing phase 1 in another is not advised, particularly in a case of this complexity. This resulted in a situation that could not be corrected without removing the definitive crowns. If provisional restorations had been placed in both arches with interim removable partial dentures, it would have been recognized that the treatment plan was in need of revision while still in phase 1. This would have saved both the dentist and the patient a considerable amount of time, expense, and frustration.

If the VDO is to be reestablished, provisional restorations allow an opportunity to ensure the proposed VDO is physiologic and tolerated by the patient. Once the clinician and the patient agree that the provisional restorations are appropriate, their form should be captured in an impression and used as a guide for the definitive restorations. Creating a custom anterior guide table on the articulator ensures that the functional guidance of the provisional restorations will be duplicated in the definitive prostheses [5].

C. When addressing a dental rehabilitation, it is sometimes advantageous to finish in segments, for financial feasibility, for biologic reasons, or simply for the ease of the clinician. However, it can be risky to finish one segment of an extensive treatment without first placing provisional restorations on all teeth involved in the rehabilitation. One may encounter problems with esthetics, phonetics, function, restorative space, tooth position, or a host of other conditions that may make it difficult or impossible to finish as envisioned during the planning phase. As demonstrated in this case, an oversight like this can have devastating consequences for the patient and your practice.

D.
- **Invasion of the biologic width (BW):** if the finish line of the tooth preparation encroaches on the periodontal attachment apparatus, osseous

recontouring will be required for proper soft tissue healing. Gargiulo et al. [6] determined that the BW included 1 mm connective tissue, 1 mm junctional epithelium, and 1 mm gingival sulcus, which equals 3 mm from the crest to crown margin. If there is violation of the BW on the facial or lingual surface and the alveolar bone is thin, bone resorption and gingival recession develops, ultimately ending up with esthetic problems. If violation of the BW occurs in the interproximal region (where the bone is thick), bone resorption eventually develops leading to chronically inflamed gingival tissue [7].

- **Short clinical crown**: when tooth preparation provides adequate reduction for restorative materials, there may be insufficient coronal tooth structure above the gingival crest for adequate retention and resistance form. If tooth modifications cannot compensate for these shortcomings, crown lengthening will provide additional supragingival tooth structure to fulfill restorative needs.
- **Lack of ferrule**: if ≤1.5 mm of natural tooth structure exists supragingivally, crown lengthening provides additional natural tooth structure for retention of crowns [8]. This can be supplemented by artificial tooth structure, such as a core buildup or post and core. If one forgoes this procedure, the probability of the artificial buildup material dislodging increases significantly.
- **Lack of interarch space**: if an unopposed tooth is allowed to supraerupt for a significant period of time, it can migrate to a position that makes it difficult to restore the missing tooth in its proper position. The supraerupted tooth may require crown lengthening and/or endodontic therapy to bring it back into the correct occlusal plane. This procedure can also be accomplished with orthodontic intrusion, which has been greatly facilitated in recent years with the advent of temporary anchorage devices.
- **Esthetic considerations**: in many situations, patients may find their tooth proportions or uneven gingival margins unattractive. In these cases, an elective procedure known as esthetic crown lengthening can be performed to provide an ideal gingival architecture. If the

discrepancy is minor, this can often be done as gingivoplasty, which does not require osseous recontouring.

E.
- **Orthodontic intrusion**: in most instances, an orthodontist can provide the least invasive answer to discrepancies in occlusion. Patients often decline this option because of the additional expense, the lengthy treatment time of orthodontics, or anxiety related to wearing braces as an adult. However, if this is the best option, it is our duty to educate the patient and guide him or her to the best long-term decision.
- **Alveoloplasty**: if an opposing arch is edentulous and has an abundance of alveolar bone and/or soft tissue, this tissue can be surgically recontoured to create space for restorative materials. This is frequently done in the posterior maxilla as tuberosity reduction surgery.
- **Alteration of VDO**: if other methods will not create adequate restorative space, or it is apparent that VDO has been lost over time [6–15], reestablishing VDO to an appropriate position is a very effective method for creating interarch space. This procedure should be used judiciously because it can result in catastrophe if not done within physiologic tolerance. If the freeway space is violated, a new clinical challenge will rapidly emerge because the patient will not tolerate the change. Functional, esthetic, phonetic, and/or TMD complications may arise.
- **Extraction of supraerupted teeth with simultaneous alveoloplasty**: if an unopposed tooth is supraerupted so far out of its natural position, it may not be possible to salvage it as part of the global treatment plan. In these situations, the offending teeth are extracted and, using a surgical guide, the alveolus is recontoured to a position that will optimize implant position or removable prosthesis design. This requires careful planning, particularly in the case of implants, where three-dimensional position is so critical to success.
- **Reduction of endodontically treated teeth**: as demonstrated in this case, a tooth can be shortened to accommodate the occlusal plane. This

tooth may not function in full capacity, but it may provide vertical support with a dome coping [16,17], retention with an attachment or telescopic coping [18], or simply serve to retain bone if reduced subgingivally. These teeth can be extracted at a later date when implant placement is planned. Planning in this capacity can help avoid bone grafting and/or sinus elevation procedures [19].

By adding support under a distal extension removable partial denture, the functional Kennedy classification of the prosthesis can be modified. Both prostheses presented earlier are considered Kennedy class II, modification I removable partial overdentures. Altered cast impressions should be made on distal extension prostheses to allow fabrication of prostheses with the most physiologic soft tissue support [20–25].

Case 3

Periodontics–Orthodontics: Part I

CASE STORY

A 14-year, 9-month-old Caucasian female presented with a chief complaint of "I have a tooth that is rotated 180 degrees." A quick intraoral examination revealed that her maxillary left lateral incisor was severely rotated, there was spacing in the maxillary anterior segment, and both the maxillary canines were unerupted. Following the clinical examination, an appointment was scheduled to obtain more diagnostic records including orthodontic study casts, intraoral and extraoral photographs, lateral cephalogram, panoramic radiograph, and a full-mouth radiographic series to aid in treatment planning.

LEARNING GOALS AND OBJECTIVES

■ To become familiar with the epidemiology and etiology of palatally displaced canines
■ To know the various surgical techniques to expose palatally displaced canines
■ To understand the sequencing (periodontics and orthodontics) of treating palatally displaced canines

Medical History

The patient reported no significant medical history and no known allergies to food or drugs.

Review of Systems

- Vital signs
  - Blood pressure: 110/70 mmHg
  - Pulse rate: 62 beats/minute (normal)
  - Respiratory rate: 14 breaths/minute

Dental History

The patient reported that she underwent cleanings every six months and had been to a dentist's office for periodic scaling three months ago. She was currently free of caries. She had a Herbst (functional) appliance for one month two years ago.

Family History

The patient's father had a similar malocclusion. Her mother also had malocclusion and had undergone orthodontic treatment as an adolescent.

Social History

The patient reported no use of tobacco, alcohol, or recreational drugs.

Growth and Development

- The patient's height was 1.7 m (5 feet 7 inches; had menarche at the age of 12 years)
- Father's height was 1.9 m (6 feet 3 inches)
- Mother's height was 1.65 m (5 feet 5 inches)

Extraoral Examination

Extraoral examination revealed no significant pathologic findings. The patient had a round, grossly symmetric face with thin competent lips. There was no tenderness in the temporomandibular joints or of the facial muscles. There were no masses or swellings. Range of motion of the mandible was within the normal range. The centric occlusion and maximum intercuspal position were coincident. On smiling, she showed 100% of her maxillary incisors, 80% of mandibular incisors, and 2 mm of maxillary gingiva. She had a mildly convex profile, slightly retruded mandibular lip, deep mentolabial sulcus, and reduced lower facial height.

Intraoral Examination (Figures 6.3.1–6.3.5)

- Negative to oral cancer screening
- Tongue, floor of mouth, and buccal mucosa were within normal limits
- Enamel opacities were present in teeth #8 and #9
- Unerupted teeth #6 and #11
- Occlusion:
  - Overjet is 3 mm
  - Overbite is 6 mm (90% overlap of mandibular incisors)
  - Rotated teeth #5, #10, and #12
  - Coincident dental midlines
  - Class II molar relationship (third/fourth cusp on both sides)
  - Curve of Spee on both right and left sides was 1 mm
  - Palatally displaced canines in maxillary arch (canine bulges were palpable on the anterior aspect of palate)
  - Presence of torus palatinus in maxillary arch

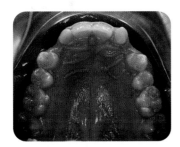

Figure 6.3.1 Maxillary occlusal view.

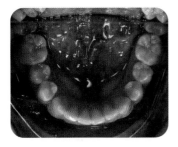

Figure 6.3.2 Mandibular occlusal view.

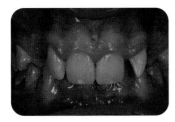

Figure 6.3.3 Intraoral frontal view.

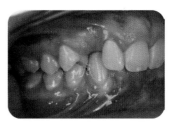

Figure 6.3.4 Intraoral right buccal view.

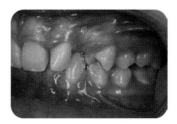

Figure 6.3.5 Intraoral left buccal view.

- Periodontal examination:
  - Gingival color: localized erythema
  - Gingival contour: generalized scalloped
  - Consistency: generalized firm, stippling present
  - Plaque and calculus: generalized mild supragingival and subgingival plaque

  Table 6.3.1 shows the periodontal chart.

Radiographic Examination

Panoramic radiograph (Figure 6.3.6), lateral cephalogram (Figure 6.3.7), and a full-mouth series were requested.

Findings from the panoramic radiograph are summarized below.

- Bone level was within normal limits
- Palatally displaced canines in maxillary arch: this was diagnosed by the SLOB (same lingual opposite buccal) rule using periapical radiographs
- There was no resorption of roots of teeth #7, #8, #9, and #10
- There was a slight anterior flattening of the left condyle
- Third molars in maxillary and mandibular arches were developing

Findings from the lateral cephalogram are summarized below.

- Mild skeletal class II pattern
- Hypodivergent mandible
- Retruded mandible
- Retroclined maxillary incisors

Diagnosis

Class II, division 2 malocclusion with palatally displaced maxillary canines.

Table 6.3.1 Periodontal charting.

Tooth #	1	2	3	4	5	6	7	8	9	10	11	12	13	14	15	16
Facial probing	X	213	222	323	222	X	312	212	212	222	X	312	211	222	312	X
Lingual probing	X	212	212	212	212	X	212	213	222	211	X	213	322	222	212	X
Attached gingiva	X	5	3.5	3	1.5	X	4	4	4	3	X	1.5	4	3.5	4	X
Recession	X	0	0	0	0	X	0	0	0	0	X	0	0	0	0	X
Mobility	X	0	0	0	0	X	0	0	0	0	X	0	0	0	0	X
Tooth #	**32**	**31**	**30**	**29**	**28**	**27**	**26**	**25**	**24**	**23**	**22**	**21**	**20**	**19**	**18**	**17**
Facial probing	X	323	323	312	212	213	212	212	212	212	212	212	312	222	314	X
Lingual probing	X	323	323	323	312	212	212	212	212	212	212	222	323	323	323	X
Attached gingiva	X	2	2	2.5	2	2	3	3	2.5	2.5	1.5	1.5	1.5	2	2	X
Recession	X	0	0	0	0	0	0	0	0	0	0	0	0	0	0	X
Mobility	X	0	0	0	0	1	1	1	1	1	0	0	0	0	0	X

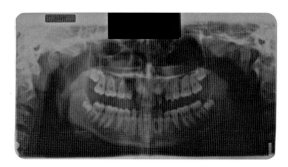

Figure 6.3.6 Panoramic radiograph.

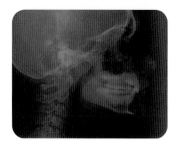

Figure 6.3.7 Lateral cephalogram.

Treatment Plan

Comprehensive orthodontic treatment plan with extractions of teeth #5 and #12 and surgical exposure of teeth #6 and #11.

Treatment Objectives

- Erupt palatally displaced canines and achieve healthy periodontium around them
- Establish mutually protected occlusion
- Achieve class I canine and class II molar occlusion
- Resolve deep bite
- Align teeth

Phase 1

- Oral hygiene instructions
- Prophylaxis
- Reevaluation

Phase 2

- Initiate orthodontic treatment
- Maxillary canines exposure
- Extraction of teeth #5 and #12

Phase 3

- Complete orthodontic treatment
- Retention

Phase 4

- Periodontal and oral hygiene maintenance

Treatment

The relative advantages and disadvantages of the various treatment plans were discussed. The patient opted for the comprehensive orthodontic treatment plan with extraction of teeth #5 and #12 and surgical exposure of teeth #6 and #11. Following informed consent from the patient, the first phase of treatment that included oral hygiene instructions and prophylaxis was initiated (Figure 6.3.8). Then orthodontic treatment was started. The first step was to place bands on the maxillary first and second molars followed by bonding of all other teeth in the maxillary arch. Nickel titanium wires were used to obtain the initial alignment of teeth (Figure 6.3.9).

Approximately eight weeks after the banding/bonding of the maxillary arch, the maxillary canines were surgically exposed by the periodontist. In this appointment,

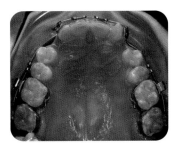

Figure 6.3.8 Start of orthodontic treatment.

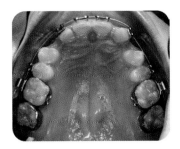

Figure 6.3.9 Four weeks later.

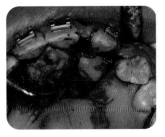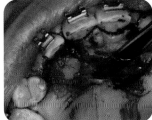

Figure 6.3.10 Canine exposure.

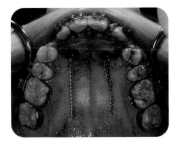

Figure 6.3.11 Gold chains attached to exposed canines.

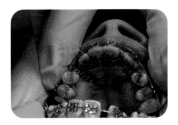

Figure 6.3.12 Gold chains ligated to the maxillary archwires.

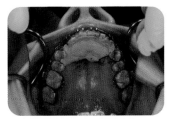

Figure 6.3.13 Periodontal pack placed over the exposure.

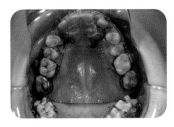

Figure 6.3.14 One-week follow-up.

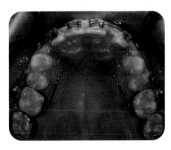

Figure 6.3.15 Two-week follow-up.

buttons were bonded to the exposed canines, and gold chains were attached to these buttons. The free ends of the gold chains were then ligated to the maxillary archwire. The exposure site was then covered with a periodontal pack (Figures 6.3.10–6.3.15).

Four weeks after exposure of the maxillary arch canines, the mandibular arch was bonded (Figure 6.3.16). Three weeks after the mandibular arch was bonded, the maxillary first premolars were extracted. Following the extractions, the patient was seen periodically at four-week intervals and the maxillary canines were retracted into the premolar extraction space using power chains. The orthodontic treatment mechanics to align and level in the mandibular arches were continued simultaneously. Periodic orthodontic treatment was continued for 16 months, at which point the canines were fully retracted into the extraction space in the maxillary arch (Figure 6.3.17).

The next step in orthodontic treatment would be to retract the maxillary anterior segment (lateral incisor to lateral incisor) to obtain class I canine occlusion and good intercuspation of the buccal occlusion. This would then be followed by finishing and retention phases.

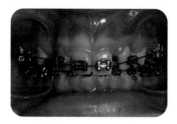

Figure 6.3.16   Both maxillary and mandibular arches are bonded.

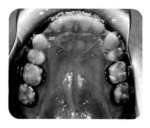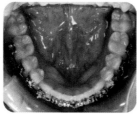

Figure 6.3.17   Retraction of palatally displaced canines and occlusal view of mandibular arch.

Following comprehensive orthodontic treatment, the patient would be debonded and then placed on periodic recall visits to follow up on retention and oral hygiene.

Discussion

In the literature, two main canine exposure techniques are discussed. The first technique is a closed technique where minimal bone removal is done and an attachment is placed on the canines at the time of exposure. Orthodontic treatment usually begins before the exposure, and traction on the canine is started soon after exposure. The advantages with this technique are the conservative bone removal and minimal surgical trauma and some degree of control over the eruption path of the canine. The disadvantages are the limited visibility of the canine during traction and demanding moisture control during attachment placement.

The second technique involves early uncovering and spontaneous canine eruption [1]. Exposure is done before orthodontic treatment or very early on during treatment. The crown of the unerupted canine is usually fully exposed from bone and left exposed after flap closure. After the canine erupts on its own, orthodontic attachments are placed for alignment. The advantages of this technique include better visibility of the canine and better moisture control at the time of placing orthodontic attachments. The disadvantages are the aggressive bone removal and lack of precise control over the eruption path of the canine. Although it is being debated in the literature, trying to establish which technique is ultimately better is somewhat simplistic. The evidence that exists at the moment is not unequivocal. The prudent clinician realizes there is not necessarily a technique that is better in all cases. Emphasis should be placed on clinical diagnosis and individualized treatment planning. Clinical judgment should always be used to select the best technique for every patient.

In this patient a closed eruption technique was used for two main reasons. First, precise control over the path of eruption of the canine was desired to avoid injury to the lateral incisors. Second, the orthodontist wanted to verify that the canines were moving before extraction of the first premolars. No bone removal was needed in this case.

Self-Study Questions

A. What is the difference between impacted teeth and displaced teeth?

B. What is the frequency of occurrence of impacted canines?

C. Enumerate the possible etiologies of palatally impacted canines.

D. What are some aids to determine the position of displaced canines?

E. How useful are cone beam computed tomography (CBCT) images for treating impacted teeth?

F. Describe various surgical techniques to expose displaced canines.

G. Discuss the possible side effects of exposing canines and retracting them into the arch.

H. What are some possible consequences of not treating an impacted maxillary canine?

I. Should impacted teeth always be brought into the arch with orthodontic treatment?

Answers located at the end of the chapter.

References

1. Schmidt AD, Kokich VG. Periodontal response to early uncovering, autonomous eruption, and orthodontic alignment of palatally impacted maxillary canines. *Am J Orthod Dentofacial Orthop* 2007;131:449–455.
2. Suri L, Gagari E, Vastardis H. Delayed tooth eruption: pathogenesis, diagnosis, and treatment. A literature review. *Am J Orthod Dentofacial Orthop* 2004;126:432–445.
3. Peck S, Peck L, Kataja M. The palatally displaced canine as a dental anomaly of genetic origin. *Angle Orthod* 1994;64: 249–256.
4. Becker A. *The Orthodontic Treatment of Impacted Teeth*, 2nd edn. Abington, UK: Informa Healthcare, 2007:93–142.
5. Becker A. Etiology of maxillary canine impactions. *Am J Orthod* 1984;37:437–438.
6. Brin I, Solomon Y, Zilberman Y. Trauma as a possible etiologic factor in maxillary canine impaction. *Am J Orthod Dentofacial Orthop* 1993;104:132–137.
7. Wisth PJ, Nordervall K, Boe OE. Periodontal status of orthodontically treated impacted maxillary canines. *Angle Orthod* 1976;46:69–76.
8. Woloshyn H, Artun J, Kennedy DB, Joondeph DR. Pulpal and periodontal reactions to orthodontic alignment of palatally impacted canines. *Angle Orthod* 1994;64: 257–264.

TAKE-HOME POINTS

A. Impacted teeth are those that are prevented from erupting due to the presence of a physical barrier in their path of eruption [2]. Displacement refers to positional variation of teeth. Displacement may lead to impaction if corrective measures are not taken [3].

B. Depending on the population studied, prevalence rates of palatally impacted canines range from 0.27 to 3% [2,3]. There is a stronger preponderance toward females compared with males [2,3].

C. A considerable body of evidence suggests an association between palatally displaced canines and the following factors [2–5]:

- Severe tooth size and arch length discrepancy
- Heredity (familial tendency)
- Retained deciduous canines
- Missing or anomalous lateral incisors
- Nonresorption deciduous canine roots
- Trauma

D. Maxillary canines should erupt in the oral cavity around 11–12 years of age. They can be palpated labially over the deciduous canines usually at eight to nine years of age [4]. Nonemergence of maxillary canine beyond 11–12 years of age should warrant further examination using tools such as periapical, occlusal radiographs, and panoramic radiographs. Currently CBCT is used to accurately determine the position of canines and also to examine any effects of the displaced canines on the adjacent teeth (Figures 6.3.18 and 6.3.19).

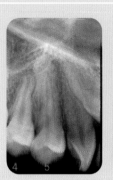
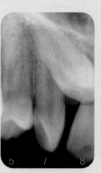
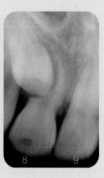

Figure 6.3.18   Periapical radiographs showing a displaced right maxillary canine.

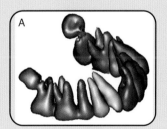
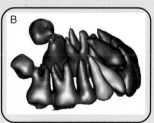

Figure 6.3.19   A three-dimensional reconstructed image of the patient's teeth from Figure 6.3.18 with and without the canine in view.

E. Recent advances in CBCT technology have facilitated image acquisition with limited field (just one arch; Figure 6.3.19) or very limited field (one segment of arch) and these have been especially useful for diagnosis of impacted teeth without significant radiation exposure. CBCT images help us to localize impacted teeth and adjacent structures very precisely

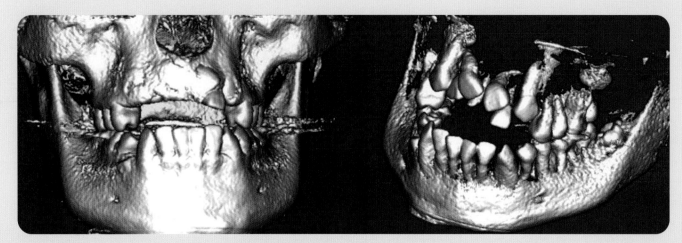

Figure 6.3.20   CBCT images of a patient with impacted maxillary anterior teeth. The image can be manipulated (with or without bone) in multiple ways to enable better visualization of impacted teeth.

and consequently help us to place ideal orthodontic forces in the appropriate direction. Furthermore, with CBCT images we can better identify if root resorption (especially on palatal/lateral aspects of root) is already present prior to orthodontic traction. Figure 6.3.20 shows how CBCT images can be used for better visualization of position of impacted teeth.

F. *Closed eruption technique* involves partial exposure of the crown, immediate attachment placement, and early application of orthodontic force. *Open eruption technique* involves early uncovering, complete exposure of the clinical crown, and spontaneous eruption. Orthodontic force is applied late, after autonomous eruption.

G. Trauma due to surgery [6]:
- Infections at the exposed sites are common.
- Etching materials used during the bonding procedure may spill over onto the surrounding soft tissues and cause localized reactions.
- Bonding failure of attachments (including buttons and brackets) to the exposed canines.
- Poor biomechanics during orthodontic retraction into the arch may lead to resorption of the roots of adjacent teeth.
- Periodontal health of the retracted canines may be compromised. Retracted canines have been shown to exhibit bone loss and increased pocket depths [7].
- Pulpal changes and discoloration of retracted canines have also been reported in the literature [8].

H. Nontreatment of impacted maxillary canine may lead to several adverse consequences, including cystic changes leading to dentigerous cysts, replacement resorption of the crowns of impacted canines, and resorption of roots of adjacent permanent teeth [4].

I. Infrequently, teeth can become impacted in an unfavorable position that precludes use of orthodontic traction for treatment. For example, Figure 6.3.21 is a CBCT image of a patient with impacted maxillary central incisors. It is obvious

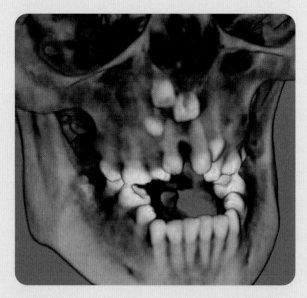

Figure 6.3.21   CBCT image showing impacted maxillary central incisors with poor prognosis due to their position.

that both maxillary central incisors are impacted and positioned very high in the maxilla. Furthermore, their crowns are directly over the roots of lateral incisor teeth which have erupted into the arch and are in good health. In such a situation, a pragmatic approach would be to extract the impacted maxillary central incisors and perform orthodontic treatment to place the maxillary lateral incisors in the position of central incisors (lateral incisor substitution for central incisors) and canines in the place of lateral incisors (canine substitution for lateral incisors).

Case 4

Periodontics–Orthodontics: Part II

CASE STORY

A 15-year, 9-month-old African-American female presented with a chief complaint of "My teeth are crooked." A quick intraoral and extraoral examination revealed that she had a convex profile, increased mandibular divergency, severe crowding in both arches, a 5-mm discrepancy in her dental midlines, and the mandibular left canine was unerupted (Figure 6.4.1).

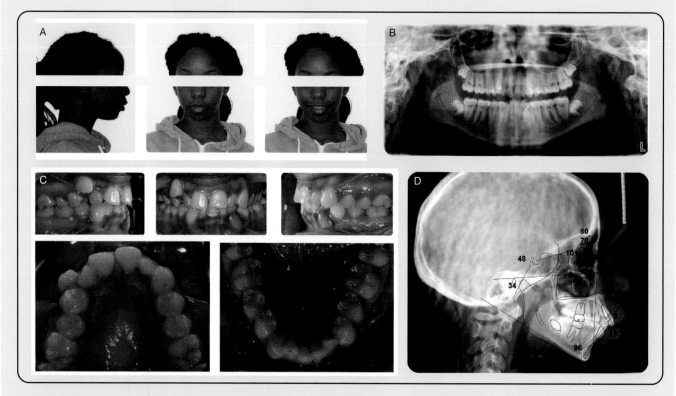

Figure 6.4.1 Initial examination: (A) extraoral images; (B) panoramic radiograph; (C) intraoral photographs; (D) lateral cephalometric radiograph.

Medical History

A complete medical history revealed a healthy patient with no systemic conditions. No temporomandibular joint (TMJ) symptoms were detected during initial examination nor reported by the patient.

Review of Systems

• Vital signs
  o Blood pressure: 110/75 mmHg
  o Pulse rate: 68 beats/minute (regular)
  o Respiratory rate: 16 breaths/minute.
• Height: 1.63 m (5 feet 4 inches; had menarche at age 12 years)
• Cervical vertebral maturation index: stage VI, indicating no significant further growth

Family History

The patient reported no significant family history of any particular orthodontic malocclusions or periodontal conditions.

Social History

The patient reported no use of tobacco, alcohol, or recreational drugs.

Oral Hygiene

The patient reported using a regular brush and an interproximal brush twice per day. On clinical examination despite the orthodontic appliances present, patient was maintaining good plaque control.

Dental History

The patient reported that she underwent dental checks annually and recare visits. However, she presented with incipient caries lesions on teeth #3, #5, #14, and #30. She was initially treated in the orthodontics department and presented for evaluation to the periodontology department when the orthodontic treatment was almost completed (Figure 6.4.2). As the orthodontic therapy progressed, the major concern was the root prominence and limited amount of alveolar mucosa in the areas of #22, #24, #25, and #27. The orthodontist was concerned that if not corrected, the long-term prognosis of #22, #24, #25, and #27 was not favorable.

Extraoral Examination

Extraoral examination revealed no pathologic findings. The patient had an oval, slightly asymmetric face with thick competent lips. There was no tenderness in the TMJ or of the facial muscles. There were no masses or swellings. Range of motion of the mandible was within the normal range. The centric occlusion and maximum intercuspal position were coincident. During a spontaneous smile, she showed 80% of her maxillary incisors and 10% of mandibular incisors. She had a fairly convex profile, weak chin, protrusive lips, acute nasolabial angle, and increased lower facial height.

Intraoral Examination

• Tongue, floor of mouth, and buccal mucosa were within normal limits.
• Mild enamel hypocalcifications were noted on #3, #5, and #14.
• Rudimentary maxillary left lateral incisor.
• Periodontal examination:
  o Gingival color: pigmentations.
  o Gingival contour: generalized scalloped with gingival margins inconsistent (gingival zenith locations differ between #6, #11 and #8, #9).

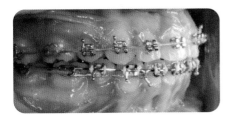 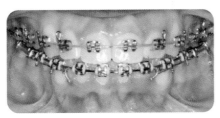 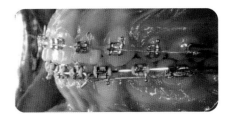

Figure 6.4.2 Intraoral photographs.

○ Alveolar mucosa: root prominences are visible in the areas of #22, #24, #25 and #27.

○ Plaque and calculus: generalized mild supragingival and subgingival plaque.

○ Probing depths: within normal limits.

○ Bleeding on probing: localized.

Occlusion

Before orthodontic therapy:

• Overjet is 3 mm.

• Overbite is 3.5 mm (60% overlap of mandibular incisors).

• Rotated teeth #5, #20, and #29.

• Discrepancy of 5 mm between upper (UDML) and lower (LDML) dental midlines: UDML 3 mm to the right, LDML 2 mm left of the facial midline.

• End-on class II molar relationship on the right.

• Curve of Spee on both right and left sides was fairly leveled.

Radiographic Examination

Summary of findings from panoramic radiograph (see Figure 6.4.1B):

• Bone level was within normal limits.

• Mandibular left canine appeared to be impacted between the lateral and first bicuspid.

• No issued were detected with root development.

• Third molars in maxillary and mandibular arches were developing.

• Condyles appeared to be round, healthy and symmetric.

Summary of findings from cephalometric radiograph (see Figure 6.4.1D):

• Skeletal class II pattern

• Increased mandibular divergency

• Retruded mandible

• Severely protruded mandibular incisors

• Narrow/thin symphysis

Diagnosis

• According to the most recent EFP/AAP classification [1] this case can be diagnosed as:

○ Localized plaque-induced gingivitis.

○ Mucogingival conditions without gingival recession at individual sites (relevant condition: tooth position).

• Angle class II subdivision.

• Hyperdivergent patient with severe crowding and limited alveolar bone housing.

Treatment Plan

Comprehensive orthodontic treatment plan with full-fixed appliances and extraction of teeth #5, #12, #21, and #29.

Treatment Objectives

In addition to projected canine and molar movements from the dental visual treatment objective (VTO), the following treatment objectives were established.

• Erupt lower left canine.

• Resolve the size issue of maxillary left lateral incisor with temporary composite buildup.

• Achieve healthy periodontium around the mandibular incisors with adjunct periodontal treatment.

• Establish mutually protected class I canine and molar occlusion.

• Achieve midline correction and archform coordination.

• Maintain vertical position of posterior teeth.

• Improve smile arc relationship.

During the orthodontic treatment, the development of mucogingival conditions without gingival recession at individual sites #22, #24, #25 and #27 was noted.

The periodontist was contacted and the case was further evaluated. As part of the evaluation by the periodontist, the position of the mandibular incisors was confirmed together with the alveolar housing and the bone volume around those teeth. The cortical plate on the mandibular canines and incisors was limited and long-term stability of the teeth was questioned.

Treatment

Orthodontics

McLaughlin dental VTO was utilized in treatment planning of the patient for estimation of necessary tooth movement in each arch quadrant. Given the limited amount of alveolar bone housing in the mandibular symphysis area and increased mandibular divergency, a comprehensive orthodontic treatment plan with extraction of teeth #5, #12, #21, and #29 was drawn up. To help achieve the planned amount of tooth movement in arch quadrants, and to control for anteroposterior (AP) and vertical anchorage, miniscrews were utilized. A single miniscrew was placed 1 mm paramedian to the midpalatal suture between the maxillary second bicuspids and maxillary first molars (1.7 × 8 mm; OrthoEasy, Forestadent, Pforzheim, Germany). A miniscrew-supported transpalatal arch design was placed to hold the maxillary first molars in AP, transverse and vertical planes. Another buccal temporary anchorage device (1.5 × 8 mm; OrthoAnchor™ System, KLS Martin Group, Jacksonville, FL, USA) was placed between the mandibular left first and second molar to support the canine retraction and midline correction.

Initially, the maxillary right canine and mandibular left lateral incisor and canine were bypassed. Mandibular left canine naturally drifted occluso-distally during the leveling and aligning stage. Following the ideal vertical positioning of the canines, the remainder of the teeth were aligned with 0.016-inch heat-activated nickel titanium (HANT) with bend-backs to maintain the incisor position. Canine and molar movements were accomplished with 0.020-inch stainless steel archwire by sliding mechanics. Before incisor retraction, the maxillary left lateral incisor was temporarily built up using composite resin, which will be placed with a veneer restoration at a later date. Space closure was accomplished on 0.019 × 0.025-inch stainless steel posted wires with active tie-backs. Miniscrews were removed when the desired canine and molar positions were achieved. Progress cephalometric and panoramic radiographs were obtained. The positioning of the mandibular incisors was deemed as acceptable as they were upright and centered in the narrow symphysis. However, for long-term stability of periodontium a referral was made to the Department of Periodontics. The case was detailed and finished with routine orthodontic procedures.

Periodontology

In order to resolve bone support around the mandibular incisors and possibly improve the long-term stability of these teeth, the periodontist decided to increase the amount of cortical bone on the site by adding bone graft to the area. Vertical incisions of the mucosa were made on the distal of teeth #23 and #26. A tunnel was created by reflecting the gum tissue from the underlying existing bone. Bone graft, comprising demineralized freeze-dried bone allograft (DFDBA) plus xenograft material, was added to the site. Simple interrupted sutures were performed to close both vertical incisions. An overview of the treatment and follow-up is presented in Figure 6.4.3.

Discussion

Ever since lateral cephalometric radiographs have been utilized in orthodontics, the area of the mandibular symphysis has received great attention. From a clinical point of view, the buccal and lingual cortical plates of the mandibular symphysis define the limits of orthodontic tooth movement that can rationally be expected. Since the cortical plates provide a physical boundary for tooth movement that cannot be exceeded without deleterious effects, they were defined as "orthodontic walls" [2]. The anatomy of the area has also served as a predictive tool for evaluation of the facial growth pattern. Growth of the mandible in an anterior direction would cause a shorter height and larger depth in the mandibular symphysis, resulting in

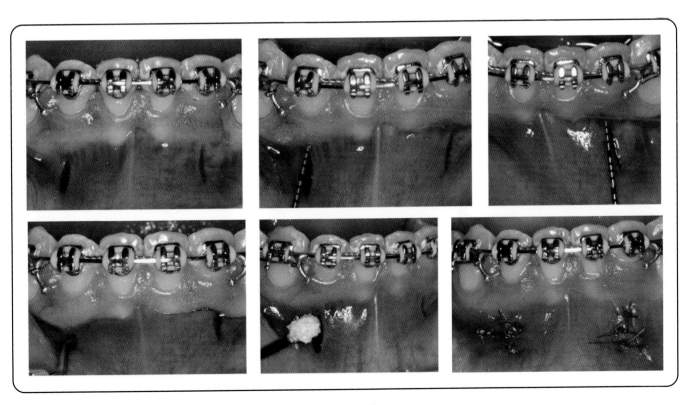

Figure 6.4.3 Intraoral photographs: tunneling and bone grafting procedure.

a smaller height to depth ratio in both males and females. Conversely, in cases of growth in a posterior direction, the symphysis would exhibit a taller height, smaller depth, and a larger ratio [3,4]. Cortical plate thickness increases in low-angle subjects and decreases in high-angle subjects [5,6]. According to Swasty et al. [6], while keeping age constant, for every one-degree increase in mandibular plane angle, the cortical bone would get thinner accordingly. According to Yamada et al. [7], as the tooth becomes more upright, or lingually inclined, the supporting alveolar bone becomes thinner. When the relationship of teeth to the anterior wall of the symphysis is considered, central incisors seem to be closer to the cortical plates in hyperdivergent facial growth patterns compared to hypodivergent patterns [4]. There is a negative correlation with the incisor mandibular plane angle (IMPA), and IMPA is lower in individuals with increased mandibular divergence [8,9]. This is a direct result of compensatory growth in hyperdivergent individuals. The increase in the anterior facial height would require the incisors to erupt to maintain overbite. As a consequence, the alveolus becomes attenuated with thinning of the width between labial and lingual walls [2].

The patient possessed many of the above-mentioned characteristics for hyperdivergent patients. The mandibular symphysis was narrower than normal, with thin buccal and lingual cortices. The challenged morphology of the alveolar bone housing made it virtually impossible for the mandibular incisors to be moved facially or lingually. In reviewing the cephalometric radiograph, an evidence-based decision was made to maintain AP position of the incisors to avoid fenestrations. Considering that there is an increased prevalence of recession for mandibular anterior areas, especially toward the end of orthodontic treatment, it was decided to proceed with the treatment before the severity of the condition was advanced [10–12]. The thin biotype and the advanced root prominence supported the proposal to to correct the alveolar housing with the use of bone graft material [13]. Therefore, a careful treatment plan was devised with no projected change in incisor position. The objective to correct the mucogingival deformities (without recession) in the mandibular anterior area was met as evidenced on the progress highlighted in the clinical and radiographic findings (Figure 6.4.4).

The patient will be carefully monitored to assure the consistency of the final findings and the favorable long-term prognosis (Figure 6.4.5).

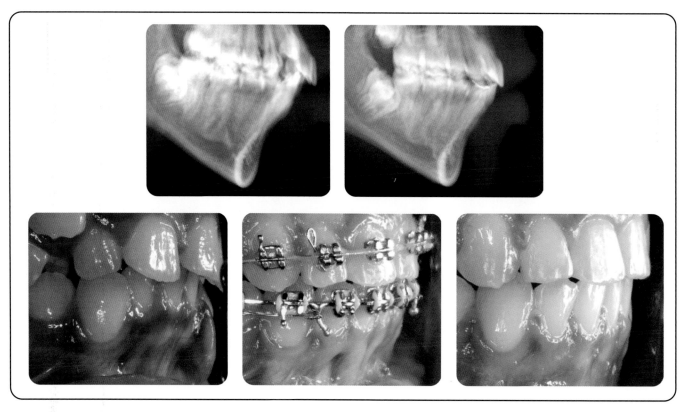

Figure 6.4.4 (Top left) Preoperative radiograph. (Top right) Postoperative radiograph. (Lower) Intraoral photographs: (left to right) preoperative; during treatment; postoperative.

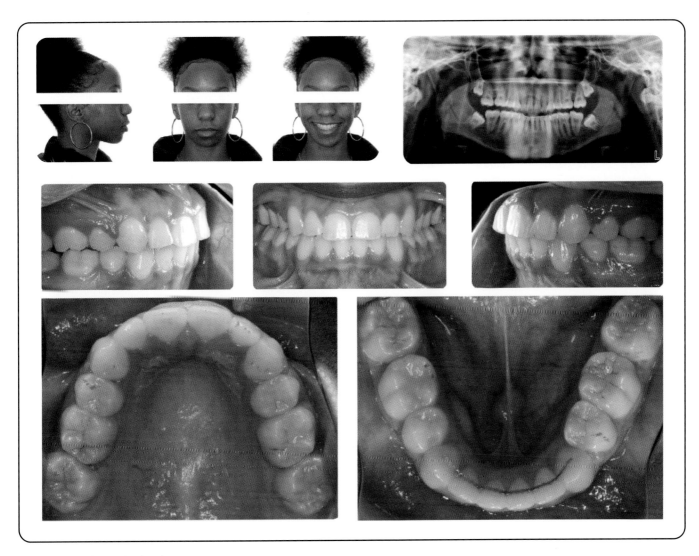

Figure 6.4.5 After orthodontic treatment.

Self-Study Questions

A. What is the influence of tooth movement on the periodontium?

B. What is the relationship between tooth alignment, oral hygiene, and periodontal disease?

C. When should gingival augmentation be considered in a child or adolescent?

D. What are types of bone graft are available and why was a combination used in this case?

E. What are the advantages and disadvantages of using a tunneling procedure in this particular situation?

Answers located at the end of the chapter.

References

1. Jepsen S, Caton JG, Albandar JM, et al. Periodontal manifestations of systemic diseases and developmental and acquired conditions: Consensus report of workgroup 3 of the 2017 World Workshop on the Classification of Periodontal and Peri-Implant Diseases and Conditions. *J Periodontol* 2018;89(Suppl 1):S237–S248.
2. Handelman CS. The anterior alveolus: its importance in limiting orthodontic treatment and its influence on the occurrence of iatrogenic sequelae. *Angle Orthod* 1996;66:95–110.
3. Aki T, Nanda RS, Currier GF, Nanda SK. Assessment of symphysis morphology as a predictor of the direction of mandibular growth. *Am J Orthod Dentofacial Orthop* 1994;106:60–69.
4. Gracco A, Luca L, Bongiorno MC, Siciliani G. Computed tomography evaluation of mandibular incisor bony support in untreated patients. *Am J Orthod Dentofacial Orthop* 2010;138:179–187.
5. Tsunori M, Mashita M, Kazutaka K. Relationship between facial types and tooth and bone characteristics of the mandible obtained by CT scanning. *Angle Orthod* 1998;68:557–562.
6. Swasty D, Lee J, Huang JC, Maki K, Gansky SA, Hatcher D, Miller AJ. Cross-sectional human mandibular morphology as assessed in vivo by cone-beam computed tomography in patients with different vertical facial dimensions. *Am J Orthod Dentofacial Orthop* (2011) 139:e377-89.
7. Yamada C, Kitai N, Kakimoto N, et al. Spatial relationships between the mandibular central incisor and associated alveolar bone in adults with mandibular prognathism. *Angle Orthod* 2007;77:766–772.
8. Gutermann C, Peltomaki T, Markic G, et al. The inclination of mandibular incisors revisited. *Angle Orthod* 2014;84:109–119.
9. Eroz UB, Ceylan I, Aydemir S. An investigation of mandibular morphology in subjects with different vertical facial patterns. *Aust Orthod J* 2000;16:16–22.
10. Renkema AM, Fudalej PS, Renkema A, et al. Development of labial gingival recessions in orthodontically treated patients. *Am J Orthod Dentofacial Orthop* 2013;143:206–212.
11. Renkema AM, Navratilova Z, Mazurova K, et al. Gingival labial recessions and the post-treatment proclination of mandibular incisors. *Eur J Orthod* 2015;37:508–513.
12. Morris JW, Campbell PM, Tadlock LP, et al. Prevalence of gingival recession after orthodontic tooth movements. *Am J Orthod Dentofacial Orthop* 2017;151:851–859.
13. Rasperini G, Acunzo R, Cannalire P, Farronato G. Influence of periodontal biotype on root surface exposure during orthodontic treatment: a preliminary study. *Int J Periodontics Restorative Dent* 2015;35:665–675.
14. Maynard J, Ochsenbein C. Mucogingival problems, prevalence and therapy in children. *J Periodontol* 1975;46:543–552.

TAKE-HOME POINTS

A. The attachment apparatus, alveolar bone, and gingiva follow the tooth during orthodontic movement due to force transmitted by the gingival fibers and periodontal fibers. However, inflammation should always be controlled to ensure that the supracrestal connective tissue remains healthy and that the crestal alveolar bone height remains at its original level. Orthodontic treatment involving intrusion of a plaque-infected tooth may shift supragingival plaque subgingivally, cause a microbial shift, infrabony pocket formation, and loss of connective tissue attachment.

B. Multiple studies have found that malaligned teeth are associated with more plaque and gingival inflammation and a greater number of filled surfaces as compared with well-aligned teeth. They also observed that the more spacing between teeth, the better the periodontal status in terms of probing depth, plaque index and gingival index, and the amount of filled surfaces. Subsequently, the fewer proximal restorations, the better the periodontal health.

C. Autogenous free gingival graft is an acceptable procedure to prevent incipient mucogingival problems from progressing. The procedure is recommended in children with less than 1 mm of keratinized gingiva, but is not necessary when the keratinized gingiva is more than 2 mm and/or attached gingiva is more than 1 mm. Maynard and Ochsenbein [14] recommend that the free gingival graft be performed prior to tooth movement.

D. Bone grafts available include xenografts, allografts, alloplasts, and autogenous. Each of them possesses key characteristics to be used in different periodontal approaches. In this particular case we used a combination of xenograft and DFDBA (allograft material) in which one has osteoconductive potential properties and the latter has been shown to have osteoinductive properties providing potential development of osteogenic cells to induce new bone formation.

E. The advantage of performing this surgery using a tunneling procedure is the minimally invasive approach with the intention of preserving the underlying integrity of the periosteum versus performing a flap surgery as in traditional guided bone regeneration surgery. It has been demonstrated that flap elevation will cause a certain degree of bone loss and that re-adaptation of the flap to its original position will cause gingival recession.

Case 5

Occlusion–Periodontology

CASE STORY

A 50-year-old Caucasian male presented and stated that he brushed twice a day and flossed occasionally and had never seen a periodontist before. The patient complained of bleeding gums on brushing and bad breath. The patient had been referred from his general dentist's office for a comprehensive periodontal evaluation.

LEARNING GOALS AND OBJECTIVES

■ Diagnose the periodontal condition properly
■ Identify whether there are possible occlusal contributing factors
■ Manage the occlusal element
■ Determine proper timing of occlusal management
■ Evaluation of the mounted diagnostic cast mounted in centric relation
■ Identification of the comorbidities associated with occlusion

Medical History

There were no significant medical conditions and the patient reported never having been hospitalized. The patient reported taking multivitamins but no other medications, and he had no known allergies.

Review of Systems

• Vital signs
  ○ Blood pressure: 140/85 mm Hg (stage 1 hypertension)
  ○ Pulse rate: 75 beats/minute (regular)
  ○ Respiratory rate: 15 breaths/minute

Social History

The patient was a nonsmoker. He did have a habit of chewing tobacco for 15 years but stopped about 10 years ago. The patient drank socially.

Extraoral Examination

There were no significant negative findings. The patient had no masses or swelling. He had a symmetrical facial appearance, with a prominent chin, and even and rounded shoulders. The temporomandibular joints (TMJs) were within normal limits.

Intraoral Examination

The soft tissues and tongue appeared normal. There was an adequate zone of keratinized gingiva, except on tooth #22. There was presence of significant local factors. There was mild gingival recession in relation to maxillary molars.

• A periodontal probing was completed (Figure 6.5.1): probing depths varied from 2 to 6 mm. Several mucogingival deformities were noted.
• The patient had partial edentulism and was missing teeth #17, #18, and #32.

Radiographic Examination

A full-mouth set of radiographs was ordered with a panoramic radiograph in order to evaluate the bone level and the TMJs via the panoramic view. Radiographs revealed that the patient had generalized bone loss with localized moderate to severe bone loss around teeth #1–3 and #14–16 (Figure 6.5.2). Distal of tooth #31 we can appreciate loss of bone due to the previous extraction of #32. Periapical radiolucency on tooth #3 was noted. Tooth #14 was overerupted with a mesial overhang. Radiographic evidence of generalized subgingival calculus was noted.

Maxillary (teeth 1–16)

	1	2	3	4	5	6	7	8	9	10	11	12	13	14	15	16
P.D.	4 4 4	9 3 5	9 3 4	4 2 3	3 3 5	5 3 5	5 2 4	4 3 5	5 2 4	5 1 5	4 1 5	5 2 6	6 2 5	5 7 9	5 1 5	4 4 4
FGM					2 2 2									2 2 2		
ATTACH	4 4 4	9 3 5	9 3 4	4 2 3	5 5 7	5 3 5	5 2 4	4 3 5	5 2 4	5 1 5	4 1 5	5 2 6	6 2 5	7 9 11	9 5 9	4 4 4
FURCA															2	
PLAQUE																
Calculus																
MGDEF																

	1	2	3	4	5	6	7	8	9	10	11	12	13	14	15	16
P.D.	4 1 7	7 1 6	6 11 5	4 1 5	5 1 5	5 1 4	5 1 4	3 1 5	5 1 4	4 1 4	5 1 5	5 1 7	7 1 4	4 2 6	7 1 6	6 3 5
FGM			4 4 4											4 4 4	4 4 4	
ATTACH	4 1 7	7 1 6	10 11 9	4 1 5	5 1 5	5 1 4	5 1 4	3 1 5	5 1 4	4 1 4	5 1 5	5 1 7	7 1 4	8 6 10	11 5 10	6 3 5
FURCA																
PLAQUE																
Calculus																
MOBILITY	2	2	2	1	1					1		1		2	2	2

Mandibular (teeth 32–17)

	32	31	30	29	28	27	26	25	24	23	22	21	20	19	18	17
MOBILITY														2		
Calculus																
PLAQUE																
FURCA		1	1													
ATTACH	3 4 4	5 4 5	4 2 5	5 2 3	3 2 3	4 2 4	3 3 3	3 3 3	3 2 4	4 2 4	4 2 4	4 2 5	6 4 4			
FGM		1 1 1														
P.D.	3 4 4	4 3 4	4 2 5	5 2 3	3 2 3	4 2 4	3 3 3	3 3 3	3 2 4	4 2 4	4 2 4	4 2 5	6 4 4			

	32	31	30	29	28	27	26	25	24	23	22	21	20	19	18	17
MGDEF																
Calculus																
PLAQUE																
FURCA		1														
ATTACH	6 3 7	9 4 6	4 2 4	3 2 4	4 4 6	6 3 9	7 2 9	8 2 5	4 2 5	5 3 5	4 2 4	4 2 4	4 2 3			
FGM		2 2 2														
P.D.	6 3 7	7 2 4	4 2 4	3 2 4	4 4 6	6 3 9	7 2 9	8 2 5	4 2 5	5 3 5	4 2 4	4 2 4	4 2 3			

Figure 6.5.1 Pretreatment periodontal charting.

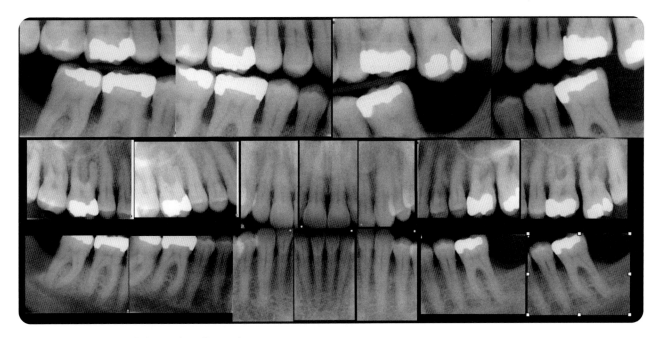

Figure 6.5.2 Pretreatment full-mouth radiographs.

Occlusion

The patient had occlusal interferences on lateral excursions on both sides. He had bilateral edge-to-edge occlusion on his posterior teeth and is a bruxist.

Diagnosis

Stage III, grade B periodontitis.

Treatment Plan

- Phase 1:
  - Oral hygiene instructions and motivational interviewing
  - Nutrition counseling
  - Interdisciplinary consults: endodontics, orthodontics, restorative
  - Generalized scaling and root planing in four quadrants
  - Reevaluation, including occlusal analysis
- Phase 2:
  - Open flap debridement with intraoperative evaluation of bone morphology with possible treatment of the osseous defects by resective or regenerative therapy
  - Occlusal management depending on the interdisciplinary consult outcomes
- Phase 3: #3 root canal therapy and further restoration
- Phase 4:
  - Occlusal guard
  - Periodontal maintenance

Figure 6.5.3 shows maxillary and mandibular occlusal views.

Discussion

When a patient presents for periodontal evaluation and diagnosis, occlusion should be examined as a routine part of the periodontal evaluation. If it is determined that occlusion may contribute to the periodontal disease, the periodontist should prepare to deal with

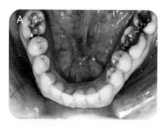
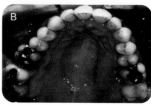

Figure 6.5.3 (A, B) Maxillary and mandibular occlusal views.

the occlusal component as part of the comprehensive periodontal treatment.

To provide guidelines about how occlusal management should be incorporated into the course of treatment, we suggest some questions to be clinically used in the treatment sequence. The role of occlusion in the etiology and progression of periodontitis as an inflammatory disease is still unclear and inconclusive. Studies show conflicting results as to whether occlusal factors are significant in the process of treatment planning [1–5].

Although most studies indicate that occlusion by itself cannot induce periodontitis, most studies recommend considering occlusal management during the course of periodontal treatment and implantology. In this case, the patient had interferences on excursion and a parafunction habit that might affect the periodontal health and progress of the periodontal disease.

The treatment chosen must address management of the occlusal component and its order within the overall treatment plan.

Self-Study Questions

A. What is the role of occlusion in periodontal health?

B. What is the effect of trauma from occlusion?

C. What are the stages of trauma from occlusion?

D. What is the relationship between occlusal trauma and periodontitis (inflammation)?

E. Should management of occlusal trauma be part of periodontal treatment?

F. How is trauma from occlusion diagnosed?

G. What are the components of a full occlusal examination?

Answers located at the end of the chapter.

References

1. Svanberg G, Lindhe J. Experimental tooth hypermobility in the dog. A methodological study. *Odontologisk Reby* 1973; 24:269–282.
2. Ericsson I, Lindhe J. Lack of effect of trauma from occlusion on the recurrence of experimental periodontitis. *J Clin Periodontol* 1977;4:115–127.
3. Polson AM, Adams RA, Zander HA. Osseous repair in the presence of active tooth hypermobility. *J Clin Periodontol* 1983;10:370–379.
4. Ericsson I, Lindhe J. Lack of significance of increased tooth mobility in experimental periodontitis. *J Periodontol* 1984;55:447-452.
5. Lindhe J, Ericsson I. The influence of trauma from occlusion on reduced but healthy periodontal tissues in dogs. *J Clin Periodontol* 1976;3:110–122.
6. Glossary of terms. *J Periodontol* 1986;57:20(Suppl 11).
7. Zander HA, Polson AM. Present status of occlusion and occlusal therapy in periodontics. *J Periodontol* 1977;48: 540–544.
8. Svanberg G, Lindhe J. Influence of trauma from occlusion on progression of experimental periodontitis in beagle dogs. *J Clin Periodontol* 1974;1:3–13.
9. Svanberg G, Lindhe J. Vascular reactions in the periodontal ligament incident to trauma from occlusion. *J Clin Periodontol* 1974;1:58–69.
10. Hallmon WW. Occlusal trauma: effect and impact on the periodontium. *Ann Periodontol* 1999;4:102–108.
11. Lobbezoo F. Topical review: new insights into the pathology and diagnosis of disorders of the temporomandibular joint. *J Orofac Pain* 2004;18:181–191.
12. Simons DC, Travell JG. *Myofascial pain and dysfunction. In: The Trigger Point Manual, 2nd edn, Vol 1. Upper Half of the Body.* Atlanta, GA: Emory University, 1998.

TAKE-HOME POINTS

A. The periodontal ligament (PDL) anchors the teeth in the bone. The periodontium has the ability to adapt, which allows the PDL to withstand some increase in occlusal forces. The role of occlusion is to maintain function, comfort, health, and stability of the dentition.

B. The effect of trauma from occlusion may contribute to more rapid periodontal destruction. As a result of adaptation, the PDL may undergo changes such as thickening. In addition there may be increased bone density and trabeculation. Once the forces exceed the adaptation limit, changes can take place in the teeth (wear and tear and/or mobility), the periodontium (PDL and bone) [6–9], or in the TMJ (pain, wear).

C. When the occlusal forces exceed the functional level of the PDL, injury may take place. The damage can be repaired if the excessive forces are eliminated or if the tooth drifts away from the forces. But if excessive occlusal forces persist, the damage may become permanent in the form of the "appearance" of angular bone loss on radiographs. In such a case, the tooth would become loose without pocket formation. This is also known as secondary trauma from occlusion.

If the excessive forces are removed, the defect will tend to heal, provided that the oral hygiene protocol is maintained [10].

D. If there is excessive force without gingival/periodontal inflammation, signs/symptoms may appear but the bone loss will not proceed at a faster rate (i.e. excessive forces alone do not cause periodontitis). If there is excessive force in the presence of gingival/periodontal inflammation, the loss of bone can occur at a relatively faster rate.

E. Absolutely! It is imperative that clinicians consider a thorough occlusal analysis as part of their consultation, diagnosis, and treatment planning.

F. To diagnose occlusal trauma, several clinical/radiographic signs and symptoms can be considered.

Clinical
- Mobility (progressive)
- Pain on chewing or percussion
- Fremitus
- Occlusal prematurities/discrepancies
- Wear facets in the presence of other clinical indicators

- Pathologic tooth migration
- Chipped or fractured tooth (teeth/roots)
- Thermal sensitivity (specially to cold)

Radiographic
- Widened PDL space
- Bone loss
- Root resorption

G. TMJ pain and symptoms may need to be checked by more than one medical specialist, such as a primary care provider, a dentist, or an ear, nose, and throat doctor, depending on symptoms. Some dentists specialize in TMJ diagnosis and treatment [11,12].

A thorough examination may involve these steps:
- Dental examination to show poor bite alignment
- Magnetic resonance imaging of the jaw area
- Feeling the joint and connecting muscles for tenderness
- Pressing around the head for areas that are sensitive or painful
- Sliding the teeth from side to side

- Watching, feeling, and listening to the jaw open and close
- X-rays to show abnormalities
- Detecting malocclusion

In conclusion, excessive and chronic occlusal forces produce adaptive changes in the morphology of the periodontium: a widened V-shaped PDL, a thickening of bone trabeculae, and bone resorption in the gingival portion of the periodontium.

Glickman introduced the concept of trauma from occlusion and the terminology of co-destruction zone. He also mentioned the buttressing bone. This bone formation occurs both in pressure as well as in tension side and both internally (marrow) or on the external surface.

If it occurs externally, it leads to cervical bulge; if it occurs internally, it will not lead to obvious change in the morphology but to an increase in the radio-opacity close to the affected PDL (thickening of the lamina dura).

Intrabony pocket formation can occur due to the interaction between bone resorption and bone formation, which is a result of traumatic occlusion.

Case 6

Periodontics–Pediatric Dentistry

CASE STORY

An 11-year-old female was brought to the Emergency Department of Boston Children's Hospital (BCH) in September 2008 for a dental injury. She had fallen off a bicycle and injured her maxillary dentition four hours prior and was sent to a local hospital for treatment. Her permanent maxillary right central incisor was extruded and the permanent maxillary left central incisor was avulsed. The emergency physician at the local hospital reimplanted the avulsed tooth immediately. The girl was then transferred to BCH for further evaluation. According to the parent's history, the extraoral dry time was approximately 15 minutes, and the tooth was not transported in any medium.

LEARNING GOALS AND OBJECTIVES

■ To be able to diagnose traumatic dental injuries and consider appropriate immediate acute and long-term dental management of such injuries

Medical History

The girl's medical history was significant for asthma and attention deficit hyperactivity disorder for which she was taking methylphenidate.

Social History

The patient was an only child and her parents were married. Both parents had a history of dental caries.

Extraoral Examination

The temporomandibular joint and mandibular ranges of motion were within normal limits. The patient had no masses or swelling in the orofacial region. Superficial abrasions were noted on the patient's forehead and upper and lower lip.

Intraoral Examination

The permanent maxillary right central incisor was extruded 2 mm and palatally luxated. The reimplanted permanent left central incisor was extruded 4 mm and labially positioned by approximately 1 mm. The gingiva surrounding both central incisors was bleeding; however, no lacerations were present.

Occlusion

There were no occlusal discrepancies or interferences.

Radiographic Examination

The radiographic examination was significant for a well-approximated root fracture in the apical third of the permanent maxillary right central incisor. The permanent left central incisor was extruded by 4 mm. Both central incisors had complete root formation (Figure 6.6.1).

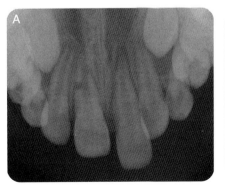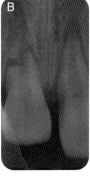

Figure 6.6.1 (A) Occlusal radiograph of maxilla. (B) Periapical radiograph.

Diagnosis

Apical root fracture of the permanent maxillary right central incisor and a partially reimplanted avulsed permanent left central incisor.

Treatment

After administering local anesthesia, the two permanent maxillary central incisors were repositioned and splinted using Ortho FlexTech wire (Reliance Orthodontic Products, Inc., Itasca, IL, USA) and light-cured composite resin (Figure 6.6.2). Postoperative instructions were given. One week after the incident, endodontic therapy was initiated on both central incisors (Figure 6.6.3). The pulpal contents were extirpated and the canals were instrumented and irrigated with sodium hypochlorite. After drying with sterile paper points, the canals were filled with calcium hydroxide paste (Pulpdent; Pulpdent Corporation of America, Watertown, MA, USA) and the

coronal access was sealed with a resin modified glass ionomer (Vitrebond).

Four weeks after the incident, the splint was removed. At eight weeks after splinting, the right central incisor was still excessively mobile. The tooth was restabilized with a new splint. Four weeks later the canals of both teeth were obturated with zinc oxide eugenol cement. The root canal of the left central incisor was obturated to the apex; the root canal of the right central incisor was obturated up to the apical root fracture site (Figure 6.6.4). At that time a periodontist was consulted to evaluate the excessive and chronic mobility of the right central incisor. After all the treatment options were considered, extraction of the right central incisor and placement of a bone graft were chosen as the preferred treatment option. Five months after the accident, the right central incisor was extracted (both apical and coronal segments) and Bio-Oss® collagen bone graft (Geistlich Pharma AG, Wolhusen, Switzerland) was placed in the socket (Figure 6.6.5). The extracted tooth was decoronated and added to the splint as a provisional pontic (Figures 6.6.6 and 6.6.7). Eight weeks after the bone graft was placed, the patient returned for an impression and the removable prosthesis was delivered shortly thereafter (Figure 6.6.8).

A radiographic examination (Figure 6.6.9) and clinical examination (Figure 6.6.10) five months after the postoperative bone graft revealed that the bone graft site was healing well.

Fourteen months after the incident, the left central incisor showed no sign of ankylosis and the probing depths were all within normal limits. The

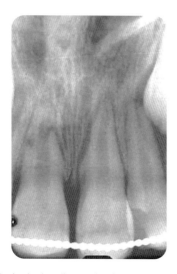

Figure 6.6.2 Periapical radiograph after splinting.

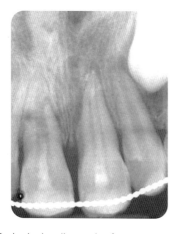

Figure 6.6.3 Periapical radiograph after root canal therapy.

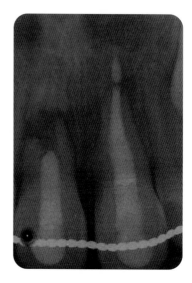

Figure 6.6.4 Periapical radiograph.

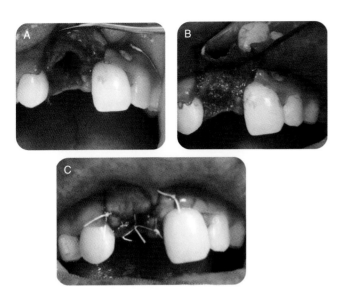

Figure 6.6.5 (A) Extraction; (B) bone graft; (C) suturing.

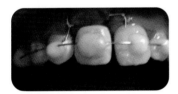

Figure 6.6.6 Temporary prostheses.

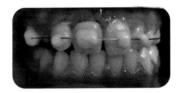

Figure 6.6.7 Postoperative view at one week.

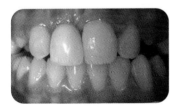

Figure 6.6.8 Temporary prosthesis.

removable prosthesis with pontic was functionally acceptable and satisfied the patient's esthetics (Figure 6.6.11).

Discussion

The primary goals for managing this patient's dental trauma include both acute as well as long-term endodontic, periodontal, and cosmetic considerations. The immediate goals included the repositioning and stabili-

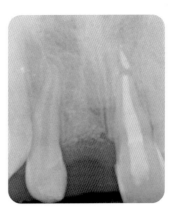

Figure 6.6.9 Five-month postoperative radiograph.

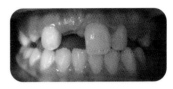

Figure 6.6.10 Five-month postoperative view.

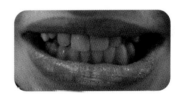

Figure 6.6.11 Fourteen-month postoperative view.

zation of the traumatized teeth. Long-term considerations included prevention of inflammatory root resorption, observation for potential ankylosis, and preservation of alveolar bone. The potential poor prognosis and possible need for extraction of both central incisors was explained to the child's parents on the day of the accident. Because of the right central incisor's failure to adequately stabilize after four months, it was extracted and a bone graft was placed. To satisfy esthetic considerations for this child, a bone graft was performed for preservation of the alveolar bone height and width. The parents were informed that a second bone graft might be needed when the child was old enough for placement of a dental implant.

Special Considerations

One week after the accident, both maxillary central incisors were filled with calcium hydroxide paste. The obturation for the maxillary right central incisor appeared to be short and may have been a contributing factor to its failure. The canal of the maxillary left central incisor was not completely obturated laterally.

Self-Study Questions

A. What are the immediate, acute dental management considerations?

1. How does the extra oral time affect the prognosis and what are the ideal transport media for an avulsed tooth?
2. What criteria would preclude reimplantation of the avulsed tooth?
3. What are the procedures for repositioning and splinting luxated permanent teeth?
4. How would you manage the soft tissue injuries?

B. Does the child's medical diagnoses affect the dental management of these injuries?

C. When and what type of radiographs should be taken?

D. Should antibiotics be prescribed, and if so which type?

E. What are the appropriate splinting times for luxations and root fractures?

F. When should endodontic intervention begin for avulsions and root fractures of permanent teeth?

G. What types of pathologic sequelae can be expected after avulsions and root fractures?

H. Is an endodontic therapy necessary for root fractures?

I. What follow-up regimen should be followed in traumatic dental cases?

J. What considerations should be taken into account if the patient in this case was six years old with open apices of the involved central incisors?

K. What is the earliest age that dental implants should be considered?

Answers located at the end of the chapter.

References

1. Fagundes NCF, Bittencourt LO, Magno MB, et al. Efficacy of Hank's balanced salt solution compared to other solutions in the preservation of the periodontal ligament. A systematic review and meta-analysis. *PLoS One* 2018;13(7):e0200467.
2. McIntyre JD, Lee JY, Trope M, Vann WF Jr. Permanent tooth replantation following avulsion: using a decision tree to achieve the best outcome. *Pediatr Dent* 2009;31(2):137–144.
3. Andersson L, Andreasen JO, Day P, et al. Guidelines for the management of traumatic dental injuries: 2. Avulsion of permanent teeth. *Pediatr Dent* 2017;39(6):412–419.
4. Flores MT, Andreasen JO, Bakland LK, et al. Guidelines for the evaluation and management of traumatic dental injuries. *Dent Traumatol* 2001;17(4):145–148.
5. Kahler B, Heithersay GS. An evidence-based appraisal of splinting luxated, avulsed and root-fractured teeth. *Dent Traumatol* 2008;24(1):2–10.
6. Diangelis AJ, Andreasen JO, Ebeleseder KA, et al. Guidelines for the management of traumatic dental injuries: 1. Fractures and luxations of permanent teeth. *Pediatr Dent* 2017;39(6):401–411.
7. Diangelis AJ, Andreasen JO, Ebeleseder KA, et al. International Association of Dental Traumatology guidelines for the management of traumatic dental injuries: 1. Fractures and luxations of permanent teeth. *Dent Traumatol* 2012;28(1):2–12.
8. Andersson L, Andreasen JO, Day P, et al. International Association of Dental Traumatology guidelines for the management of traumatic dental injuries: 2. Avulsion of permanent teeth. *Dent Traumatol* 2012;28(2):88–96.
9. Welbury R, Kinirons MJ, Day P, et al. Outcomes for root-fractured permanent incisors: a retrospective study. *Pediatr Dent* 2002;24(2):98–102.
10. Andreasen JO, Borum MK, Jacobsen HL, Andreasen FM. Replantation of 400 avulsed permanent incisors. 4. Factors related to periodontal ligament healing. *Endod Dent Traumatol* 1995;11(2):76–89.
11. Malmgren B. Ridge preservation/decoronation. *J Endod* 2013;39(3 Suppl):S67–S72.
12. Andreasen JO, Hjorting-Hansen E. Intraalveolar root fractures: radiographic and histologic study of 50 cases. *J Oral Surg* 1967;25(5):414–426.
13. NIH Osteoporosis and Related Bone Diseases National Resource Center. Osteoporosis: peak bone mass in women. http://www.niams.nih.gov/health_info/bone/osteoporosis/bone_mass.asp (accessed 3 June 2016).

TAKE-HOME POINTS

A.

1. The speed of reimplantation is essential. Immediate on-site reimplantation yields the best prognosis. If the tooth's root surface is contaminated, it is important to gently cleanse it with running water or ideal storage media if available. The tooth should be held by the crown, thus minimizing contact with the root surface that could further damage the periodontal ligament. If immediate reimplantation is not possible, it is important to place the avulsed tooth as soon as possible in Hanks balanced salt solution (HBSS), which is the ideal storage medium [1]. If HBSS is not available, milk is a good alternative storage medium [1]. The socket should be rinsed with saline prior to reimplantation.

2. Reimplantation has poor long-term prognosis if the avulsed tooth has been extraoral and dry more than 60 minutes because the periodontal ligament cells do not survive and ankylosis is inevitable. If the patient has special medical, emotional, or behavioral issues that would make essential follow-up examinations, radiographs, and/or potential treatment difficult, reimplantation may not be indicated. However, if reimplantation of a tooth with a closed apex is performed, as in this situation, the goal is to promote alveolar bone growth that will eventually encapsulate the reimplanted tooth. To reimplant a permanent tooth with an extraoral dry time of more than 60 minutes, the root should be debrided to remove the periodontal ligament with pumice prophylaxis, gauze, gentle scaling/root planing, or 3% citric acid for three minutes. The root should then be rinsed and placed in 1.23% sodium fluoride for 5–20 minutes [2,3].

3. A luxated tooth should be repositioned back into its original position using finger pressure. Local anesthesia should be used to maximize patient comfort. Teeth with more than 2 mm of mobility buccally or lingually must be stabilized with a splint to allow for optimal healing, most commonly performed with wire and composite material. The splint should be passive, flexible, without occlusal interferences, and allow for optimal oral hygiene, thus allowing optimal physiologic functional mobility, and ideal healing [4–6].

4. The gingival tissues must be allowed to heal with normal reattachment after a luxation or avulsion injury. During the reattachment process, there is a potential for ingress of bacteria via the gingival sulcus that can lead to penetration deep into the pulpal tissues with eventual devitalization [2]. Thus optimal oral hygiene, daily chlorhexidine rinses, soft diet without heavy incising, and the use of systemic antibiotics with avulsions will minimize the chances of future endodontic intervention.

B. Follow-up dental management of traumatic injuries such as avulsions requires multiple and often complex dental management. Therefore, embarking on complex dental treatment such as reimplanting an avulsed tooth in individuals with serious medical and/or behavioral issues may be contraindicated.

C. As soon as possible after the traumatic incident, several radiographic projections and angulations are recommended. The International Association of Dental Traumatology (IADT) guidelines are as follows [7]: (i) 90-degree horizontal angle with the central beam through the tooth in question; (ii) occlusal view; and (iii) lateral view from the mesial or distal aspect.

Additional radiographs should be exposed at the one-month follow-up because pulp necrosis can occur within two weeks and internal resorption within three weeks of an accident. Close follow-up is essential because inflammatory root resorption can occur quickly leading to extensive root resorption and perforation, especially in immature teeth with large pulp canals and thin dentinal walls. Additional radiographs after one month should be exposed as needed.

D. Systemic antibiotics should be administered after reimplantation for avulsed teeth. Tetracycline is the antibiotic of choice for patients older than 12 years of age (doxycycline b.i.d. for one week at the appropriate dose for patient weight and age). If the child is younger than 12 years of age, amoxicillin or penicillin should be prescribed rather than the tetracycline, which can stain calcifying teeth[3].

E. Splinting times vary depending on the type of injury [7,8]. Subluxations, extrusive luxations, and avulsions with an extraoral dry time of less than 60 minutes require splinting for two weeks. Lateral luxations, avulsions with an extraoral dry time of more than 60 minutes, root fractures (middle third), and alveolar fractures require splinting for four weeks. A root fracture in the cervical third requires splinting for up to four months. Splinting for longer than recommended and/or splinting with rigid fixation promotes ankylosis by decreasing physiologic function, which is important to allow for normal healing.

F. For a mature, closed apex tooth with an extraoral dry time of less than 60 minutes, endodontic therapy should be initiated 7–10 days after reimplantation and before the splint is removed [3]. Calcium hydroxide should be used to temporarily obturate the root canal prior to final root canal therapy. For a mature, closed apex tooth with an extraoral dry time of more than 60 minutes, endodontic therapy can be initiated prior to reimplantation or delayed to no longer than 7–10 days after replantation [3]. For root fractures, the pulp status should be monitored for at least one year [6]. If necrosis develops, endodontic therapy is usually necessary only to the fracture line where the periradicular pathology is located. Calcium hydroxide is the ideal intracanal medicament. The apical fragment usually remains vital and thus rarely exhibits periapical pathology [9]. The calcium hydroxide should be left in place for one year, followed by definitive obturation.

G. Pathologic sequelae that may result after avulsion of a closed apex tooth include inflammatory external root resorption (IRR) or replacement external root resorption (RRR). Teeth with IRR can present clinically with excessive mobility and symptoms of periradicular pathology. Teeth with RRR present with limited or no mobility, when percussed have a dull sound, and do not respond to orthodontic forces [10]. With time these teeth appear to submerge below the plane of occlusion as the alveolar bone increases in height either actively during growth or passively throughout life. Once the crown submerges significantly below the occlusal plane, one should consider decoronation of the tooth to preserve the contour of the alveolar ridge [11].

For root fractures, prognosis improves as the fracture line approaches the apex. In addition, a horizontal fracture has a more favorable prognosis than a vertical fracture, and a nondisplaced fracture is better than a displaced fracture. Healing can occur via connective tissue (periodontal ligament-like), calcified tissue (cementum-like), or bone and connective tissue. Non-healing with granulation tissue results in areas of radiographic pathology adjacent to the fracture line and requires endodontic intervention [12].

H. Pulp necrosis usually affects only the coronal fracture because the apical fragment remains vital; thus apical endodontic therapy is usually not necessary.

I. The postoperative instructions are essential and must include optimal oral hygiene with emphasis on the gingival sulcus of affected teeth and a soft diet for up to two weeks with no incising of affected teeth until the teeth are stable. Chlorhexidine oral rinses (0.12%, 15-ml swish for 30 seconds b.i.d. for one week) should be used during the initial healing period. If the status of tetanus vaccine is uncertain, the patient should be referred to a physician for evaluation. Post-trauma follow-up appointments are generally recommended at one week, one month, three months, six months, and yearly thereafter for five years [3].

J. For an avulsed permanent tooth with open apex, the goal is to promote revascularization of the pulpal tissue. If the extraoral dry time is within 60 minutes, the root surface should be covered either with Arestin (minocycline hydrochloride microspheres) or soaked in a 1% solution of doxycycline for five minutes before reimplanting the tooth. If neither is readily available, the tooth should be reimplanted as soon as possible [3].

The tooth should be monitored closely because periapical pathology and IRR can progress quickly with severe destruction of the root. Endodontic therapy should be avoided unless there is evidence of pulpal necrosis, in which case it must be initiated immediately with extirpation of the pulp contents and obturation with calcium hydroxide.

For a root-fractured tooth with an open apex, the goal is also to promote revascularization of the pulpal tissue. Immature teeth generally have a better prognosis of healing compared with mature teeth. The tooth should be monitored closely and endodontic therapy should be avoided unless there is evidence of pulpal necrosis.

K. Dental implants should be placed only after skeletal growth is complete. Up to 90% of peak bone mass is acquired by age 18 in girls and age 20 in boys [13]. Dental implant placement is recommended ideally after the indicated ages.

In the cases where dental implants have been placed in children, it has been reported that implants have been either submerged due to alveolar bone growth or displaced into the sinus. In the case of children who are still growing and in whom dental implants are being considered, the preservation of soft and hard tissue and maintenance of adequate space until the appropriate age should be evaluated. In this case since a dental implant was considered before the appropriate age, a decision was made to "preserve" the extraction socket and existing bone by placing Bio-Oss bone graft.

7

Implant Site Preparation

Case 1: Sinus Grafting: Lateral 298
*Guillaume Campard, DDS, MMSc, Emilio I. Arguello, DDS, MSc, and
Naciye G. Uzel, DMD, DMSc*

Case 2: Internal Sinus Lift Using the Crestal Window Technique 307
*Samuel Lee, DMD, DMSc, Nadeem Karimbux, DMD, MMSc, and
Y. Natalie Jeong, DMD, MA*

Case 3: Alveolar Ridge Preservation 315
Satheesh Elangovan, BDS, DSc, DMSc

Case 4: Ridge Split and Osteotome Ridge Expansion Techniques 323
Emilio I. Arguello, DDS, MSc and Daniel Kuan-te Ho, DMD, DMSc, MSc

Case 1

Sinus Grafting: Lateral

CASE STORY

A 52-year-old male presented for a consultation regarding the edentulous space in the maxillary right quadrant. His chief complaint was missing teeth on maxillary right quadrant. Figures 7.1.1 and 7.1.2 illustrate the initial clinical examination.

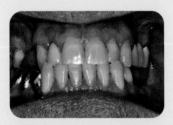

Figure 7.1.1 Facial view of the maxilla and the mandible.

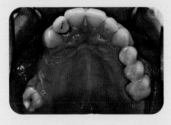

Figure 7.1.2 Occlusal view of the maxilla.

LEARNING GOALS AND OBJECTIVES

- To identify the indications for a sinus elevation
- To understand the preoperative considerations
- To be introduced to a surgical technique and biomaterial used to perform a sinus elevation

Medical History

The patient was in good health and had regular physical examinations. He did not report any allergies or sinus-related pathology.

Review of Systems

- Vital signs
  - Blood pressure: 120/65 mmHg
  - Pulse rate: 65 beats/minute (regular)

Social History

The patient did not drink alcohol and did not consume recreational drugs. He had been smoking 10 cigarettes per day for the last 25 years.

Extraoral Examination

No significant findings were noted. The patient had no masses or swelling, and no trismus. There was no palpable lymphadenopathy and the temporomandibular joints were within normal limits.

Intraoral Examination

- The soft tissues of the mouth including tongue appeared normal. The oral cancer screen was negative.
- The gingival examination revealed a generalized mild marginal erythema and a melanotic macule in the gingiva (site #5) consistent with an amalgam tattoo (Figure 7.1.2).
- A hard tissue examination was completed by the referring general dentist.
- The edentulous ridge in the maxillary right quadrant had deformities in the buccolingual and apico-coronal directions (Figure 7.1.1).
- A periodontal probing examination was carried out (Figure 7.1.3).

Buccal	---	323	---	---	---	212	322	323	323	323	323	323	---	323	---	---
Palatal	---	323	---	---	---	212	212	212	212	223	212	313	---	333	---	---

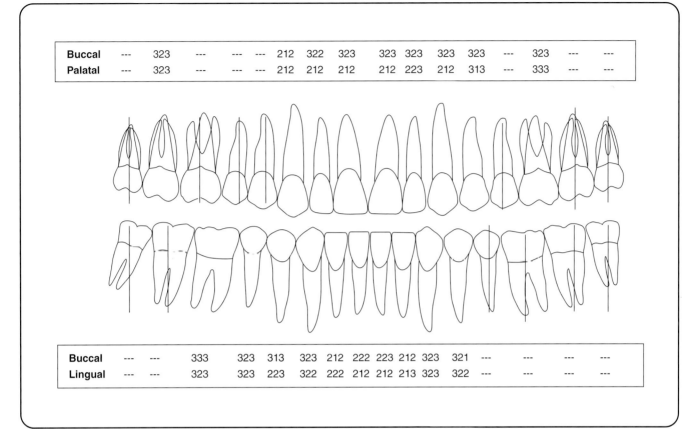

Buccal	---	---	333	323	313	323	212	222	223	212	323	321	---	---	---	---
Lingual	---	---	323	323	223	322	222	212	212	213	323	322	---	---	---	---

Figure 7.1.3 Probing pocket depth measurements.

Diagnosis
- Clinical gingival health on an intact periodontium
- Partial edentulism
- Ridge deformity (Seibert class III)

Occlusion
- Lack of posterior support
- Unprotected occlusion
- Crossbite occlusion #22 and #27

Radiographic Examination
A periapical radiograph of the right posterior maxillary sextant showed that the maxillary right sinus was pneumatized and the height of bone mesial to tooth #2 was about 1 mm (Figure 7.1.4).

Treatment Plan
Prosthodontic, endodontic, and orthodontic consultations were required to establish a comprehensive treatment plan. A cone beam computed tomography (CT) scan was ordered for the maxillary arch to obtain

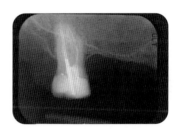

Figure 7.1.4 Radiographic evaluation: the periapical radiograph of the maxillary right quadrant shows the pneumatized sinus and the lack of bone.

further information on the anatomy and the condition of the sinus (Figure 7.1.5).

A thickening of the Schneiderian membrane was observed in the maxillary right sinus (Figure 7.1.5). A consultation with an otolaryngologist was indicated to rule out any sinus pathology. He performed a nasal endoscopy and reported a "very mild edema and erythema," diagnosing a mild sinusitis. In his opinion there were no contraindications for the sinus elevation procedure.

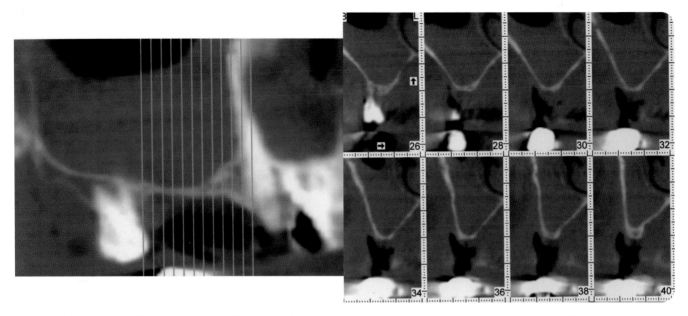

Figure 7.1.5 Cone beam CT scan of the maxillary right sinus. The Schneiderian membrane appears thickened. The residual bone height is 1 mm in sites #3 and #4.

The final treatment plan included a full-mouth prosthetic and occlusal rehabilitation, including an implant-supported fixed partial denture #3-x-5.

Treatment

The patient received oral hygiene instructions and a prophylaxis. Tooth #2 was extracted prior to the sinus elevation.

Preoperative Consultation

The medical history was reviewed. The consent form addressing the benefits and risks associated with the procedure was reviewed with the patient. Accessibility to the surgical site was clinically assessed. The CT scan showed that less than 4 mm of bone was present in the edentulous ridge area so a lateral window approach was selected to achieve 10–12 mm of bone augmentation in sites #3, #4, and #5. No evidence of the lateral branch of the posterior superior lateral artery could be seen on the CT scan (Figure 7.1.5). The following prescriptions were delivered to the patient: amoxicillin 500 mg (t.i.d. for 10 days starting 24 hours before the procedure), ibuprofen 600 mg (every four to six hours as needed for pain), and Peridex 0.12% (b.i.d.).

Sinus Elevation Procedure

A procedural sedation and analgesia nerve block and local infiltrations were achieved with lidocaine 2% (epinephrine 1:100 000) (Figure 7.1.6). A full-thickness flap was elevated in the maxilla right quadrant to

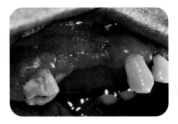

Figure 7.1.6 Preoperative condition, buccal view.

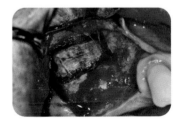

Figure 7.1.7 The lateral window is outlined with a piezotome.

expose the cortical bone of the lateral wall of the maxillary sinus. A lateral window (20 × 8 mm) was outlined with a piezotome until the Schneiderian membrane was visible (Figure 7.1.7). The Schneiderian membrane was elevated in a medial and anterior direction so that a space could be created between the Schneiderian membrane and the bony floor of the sinus. A collagenic membrane was placed in the sinus against the membrane (Figure 7.1.8). Bone grafting material, comprising a mix of rehydrated freeze-dried bone allograft (FDBA) and anorganic bovine bone mineral, was placed into the space created in the sinus

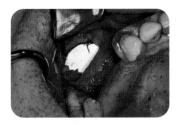

Figure 7.1.8 The Schneiderian membrane is elevated. A resorbable collagen membrane is inserted next to the Schneiderian membrane.

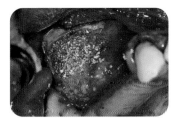

Figure 7.1.9 The bone grafting material is placed into the sinus between the Schneiderian membrane and the floor of the sinus.

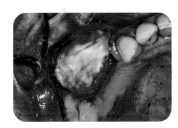

Figure 7.1.10 A collagen membrane is placed over the lateral window.

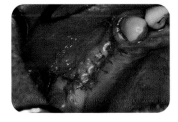

Figure 7.1.11 The flap is repositioned and sutured to achieve primary closure.

(Figure 7.1.9). A collagenic membrane was placed over the lateral window (Figure 7.1.10) and the flap was repositioned and sutured in its initial position (Figure 7.1.11). A panoramic radiograph was taken at the

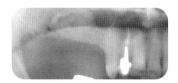

Figure 7.1.12 Panoramic radiograph the day of the procedure.

end of the surgery. The bone grafting material appeared well contained in the maxillary right sinus (Figure 7.1.12).

Discussion

Although an extensive literature reports a high predictability of sinus elevation procedures with regard to the regeneration of bone in a pneumatized maxillary sinus, this particular case presents a number of challenges that could compromise some determinants of success. One of the risk factors identified and discussed in the medical history is the smoking status of the patient, which exposes him to an elevated risk of complications. Thus an interdisciplinary approach was necessary where a well-coordinated team including the otolaryngologist and restorative dentist worked simultaneously in their respective fields in conjunction with the periodontist to provide the maximum benefit of the therapy for the patient and to evaluate and limit the risks of complications.

The surgical procedure went as planned and the patient complied with all the postoperative instructions. The patient was seen for postoperative visits at one week to remove the sutures and at three and six weeks to monitor his healing response. The allocated time for healing prior to implant placement was six months, which corresponds to the remodeling and maturation of newly formed bone and concurs with that suggested in the literature. Panoramic and periapical radiographs were taken to provide a preliminary assessment of the amount of newly formed bone present. However, a new CT scan if performed could have provided more information regarding the volume, anatomy, and irregularities of the newly formed bone. However, it was determined that the regenerated site could allow the placement of two implant fixtures, which were placed in sites #3 and #5 and would support a three-unit fixed prosthesis (FPD 3-x-5).

Self-Study Questions

A. What is the rationale for performing a sinus elevation?

B. What are the anatomic landmarks to know to perform a sinus elevation?

C. What are the techniques used?

D. Which biomaterials can be used in a sinus elevation? Is there histologic evidence of bone formation?

E. What are the determinants of success in a sinus elevation?

F. Are implants placed in a sinus elevated site as successful as implants placed in pristine bone? Does the surgical technique have an influence on the implant survival rate in the long term?

G. What are the complications associated with sinus elevations? How do you manage these complications?

Answers located at the end of the chapter.

References

1. *Mosby's Dental Dictionary*, 4th edn (ed. MJ Fehrenbach). Mosby, 2019.
2. Boyne JP, James RA. Grafting the maxillary sinus floor with autogenous marrow and bone. *J Oral Surg* 1980;38:613–616.
3. Wood RM, Moore DL. Grafting of the maxillary sinus with intraorally harvested autogenous bone prior to implant placement. *Int J Oral Maxillofac Implants* 1988;3:209–214.
4. Tatum H Jr. Maxillary and implant reconstructions. *Dent Clin North Am* 1986;30:207–229.
5. Testori T, Del Fabbro M, Weinstein R, Wallace S. (eds) *Maxillary Sinus Surgery and Alternatives in Treatment.* Chicago, IL: Quintessence, 2009.
6. Ella B, Sédarat C, Da Costa Noble R, et al. Vascular connections of the lateral wall of the sinus: surgical effect in sinus augmentation. *Int J Oral Maxillofac Implants* 2008;23:1047–1052.
7. Uschida Y, Goto M, Katsuki T, Akiyoshi T. A cadaveric study of maxillary sinus size as an aid in bone grafting of the maxillary sinus floor. *J Oral Maxillofac Surg* 1998;56:1158–1163.
8. Ella B, Da Costa Noble R, Lauverjat Y, et al. Septa within the sinus: effect on elevation of the sinus floor. *Br J Oral Maxillofac Surg* 2008;46:464–467.
9. Kim M-J, Jung U-W, Kim C-S, et al. Maxillary sinus septa: prevalence, height, location and morphology. A reformatted CT scan analysis. *J Periodontol* 2006;77:903–908.
10. Summers RB. Sinus floor elevation. *J Esthet Dent* 1998;10:164–171.
11. Jensen OT, Shulman LB, Block MS, Iacono VJ. Report of the Sinus Consensus Conference of 1996. *Int J Oral Maxillofac Implants* 1998;13(Suppl):11–32.
12. Del Fabbro M, Testori T, Francetti L, Weinstein R. Systematic review of survival rates for implants placed in the grafted maxillary sinus. *Int J Periodontics Restorative Dent* 2004;24:565–577.
13. Wallace SS, Froum SJ, Cho S-C, et al. Sinus augmentation utilizing anorganic bovine bone (Bio-Oss) with absorbable and nonabsorbable membranes placed over the lateral window: histomorphometric and clinical analyses. *Int J Periodontics Restorative Dent* 2005;25:551–559.
14. Kahnberg KE, Vannas-Löfqvist L. Sinus lift procedure using a 2-stage surgical technique: I. Clinical and radiographic report up to 5 years. *Int J Oral Maxillofac Implants* 2008;23:876–884.
15. Wallace SS, Froum SJ. Effect of maxillary sinus augmentation on the survival of endosseous dental implants. A systematic review. *Ann Periodontol* 2003;8:328–343.
16. Pjetursson BE, Tan WC, Zwahlen M, Lang NP. A systematic review of the success of sinus floor elevation and survival of implants inserted in combination with sinus floor elevation. Part I: lateral approach. *J Clin Periodontol* 2008;35(8 Suppl):216–240.
17. Boyne PJ, Lilly LC, Marx RE, et al. De novo bone induction by recombinant human bone morphogenetic protein-2 (rhBMP-2) in maxillary sinus floor augmentation. *J Oral Maxillofac Surg* 2005;63:1693–1707.
18. Boyne PJ, Marx RE, Nevins M, et al. A feasibility study evaluating rhBMP-2/absorbable collagen sponge for maxillary sinus floor augmentation. *Int J Periodontics Restorative Dent* 1997;17:11–25.
19. Valentini P, Abensur D, Densari D, et al. Histological evaluation of Bio-Oss in a 2-stage sinus floor elevation and implantation procedure. A human case report [review]. *Clin Oral Implants Res* 1998;9:59–64.
20. Coatoam GW, Krieger JT. A four-year study examining the results of indirect sinus augmentation procedures. *J Oral Implantol* 1997;23:117–127.

21. Kim DM, Nevins ML, Camelo M, et al. The efficacy of demineralized bone matrix and cancellous bone chips for maxillary sinus augmentation. *Int J Periodontics Restorative Dent* 2009;29:415–423.

22. Tarnow DP, Wallace SS, Froum SJ, et al. Histologic and clinical comparison of bilateral sinus floor elevation with and without membrane barrier placement in 12 patients. Part 3 of an ongoing prospective study. *Int J Periodontics Restorative Dent* 2000;20:117–125.

23. Torella F, Pitarch J, Cabanes G, Anitua E. Ultrasonic osteotomy for the surgical approach of the maxillary sinus: a technical note. *Int J Oral Maxillofac Implants* 1998;13:697–700.

24. Papa F, Cortese A, Maltarello MC, et al. Outcome of 50 consecutive sinus lift operations. *Br J Oral Maxillofac Surg* 2005;43:309–313.

25. Valentini P, Abensur DJ. Maxillary sinus grafting with anorganic bovine bone: a clinical report of long-term results. *Int J Oral Maxillofac Implants* 2003;18:556–560.

26. Fugazzotto PA, Vlassis J. Report of 1633 implants in 814 augmented sinus areas in function for up to 180 months. *Implant Dent* 2007;16:369–378.

27. Ferrigno N, Laureti M, Fanali S. Dental implants placement in conjunction with osteotome sinus floor elevation: a 12-year life-table analysis from a prospective study on 588 ITI implants. *Clin Oral Implants Res* 2006;17:194–205.

28. Chen L, Cha J. An 8-year retrospective study: 1,100 patients receiving 1,557 implants using the minimally invasive hydraulic sinus condensing technique. *J Periodontol* 2005;76:482–491.

29. Rosen PS, Summers R, Mellado JR, et al. The bone-added osteotome sinus floor elevation technique: multicenter retrospective report of consecutively treated patients. *Int J Oral Maxillofac Implants* 1999;14:853–858.

30. Tan WC, Lang NP, Zwahlen M, Pjetursson BR. A systematic review of the success of sinus floor elevation and survival of implants inserted in combination with sinus floor elevation. Part II: transalveolar technique [review]. *J Clin Periodontol* 2008;35(8 Suppl):241–254.

31. Tonetti MS, Hammerle CHF. Advances in bone augmentation to enable dental implant placement: Consensus Report of the Sixth European Workshop on Periodontology. *J Clin Periodontol* 2008;35(8 Suppl):168–172.

32. Krennmair G, Krainhöfner M, Schmid-Schwap M, Piehslinger E. Maxillary sinus lift for single implant-supported restorations: a clinical study. *Int J Oral Maxillofac Implants* 2007;22:351–358.

33. Khoury F. Augmentation of the sinus floor with mandibular bone block and simultaneous implantation: a 6-year clinical investigation. *Int J Oral Maxillofac Implants* 1999;14: 557–564.

34. Schwartz-Arad D, Herzberg R, Dolev E. The prevalence of surgical complications of the sinus graft procedure and their impact on implant survival. *J Periodontol* 2004;75:511–516.

35. Zijderveld SA, van den Bergh JPA, Schulten EAJM, ten Bruggenkate CM. Anatomical and surgical findings and complications in 100 consecutive maxillary sinus floor elevation procedures. *J Oral Maxillofac Surg* 2008;66: 1426–1438.

36. Fugazzotto PA, Vlassis J. A simplified classification and repair system for sinus membrane perforations. *J Periodontol* 2003;74:1534–1541.

37. Elian N, Wallace S, Cho S-C, et al. Distribution of the maxillary artery as it relates to sinus floor augmentation. *Int J Oral Maxillofac Implants* 2005;20:784–787.

TAKE-HOME POINTS

A. The absence of teeth in the posterior maxilla can become a restorative challenge when little or no alveolar bone is present. The presence of the maxillary sinus as the basis of the maxillary alveolar process can be an obstacle to the placement of an implant. In addition, sinus pneumatization, described as an enlargement of the maxillary sinus due to the aging process and as a result of the loss of maxillary teeth [1], tends to reduce the amount of bone available over time. As a consequence, there is usually a need to increase the bone volume in the posterior maxilla prior to implant placement. The goal of a sinus elevation procedure is to surgically increase the alveolar bone height by grafting bone in the floor of the maxillary sinus [2]. Evidence has shown that the imposition of an appropriate grafting material placed along the antral floor and below the Schneiderian membrane can successfully lead to viable antral bone formation and remodeling [2–4]. An implant can be placed either at the time of the sinus elevation procedure if there is sufficient native bone to stabilize the implant or at the completion of the healing response which is expected to be six to nine months, the time needed for bone formation and maturation. Such bone maturation will allow an implant to be placed with adequate primary stability, osseointegrate, and eventually be restored with high rates of success [5].

B. The maxillary sinus is an air-filled space located in the body of the maxilla. It is a pyramid with a nasal wall (its base), an anterior wall, a superior wall (the orbital floor), a lateral wall, and an inferior wall (the maxillary alveolar process). It is innervated by branches of V2 and is supplied by branches of the internal maxillary artery: the infraorbital artery, the posterior lateral artery, and the posterior superior alveolar artery that have inconsistent branches running along the lateral wall of the sinus [6]. Evaluation for the presence of these branches on CT scans is necessary prior to surgery to prevent perioperative hemorrhage if a lateral window approach is selected. The sinus drains into the nasal cavity through an ostium located in the superior aspect of its medial wall (nasal wall), about 28.5 mm above the sinus floor [7]. A sinus elevation should never obliterate the ostium so as not to compromise the sinus drainage. Septa are commonly present in the apical third of the sinus, and represent a challenge during sinus elevations. Ella et al. [8] report that 40% of patients have bony septa that can partly or totally compartmentalize the sinus. Septa are more likely to be present in the middle region of the sinus (50%) and to be highest in the medial area [9]. Radiographic examination with CT will help identify them and better evaluate the anatomic challenges faced during the procedure.

C. **There are two main approaches to performing a sinus elevation.**

1. **Crestal approach**: this technique gives access to the sinus floor through the ridge crest. Tatum [4] first described a technique involving the following sequence: flap elevation, removal of the bone until the cortical bone of the sinus floor is exposed, greenstick fracture of the cortical bone with osteotomes and burs, elevation of the Schneiderian membrane, and placement of the bone grafting material. Summers [10] described a variation of Tatum's technique called the "osteotome sinus floor elevation technique." Osteotomes of increasing diameters with concave tips are used to

relocate the existing alveolar bone apically and laterally toward the antral floor. Some bone grafting material can be added to the procedure ("bone-added osteotome sinus floor elevation technique") to decrease the risk of membrane perforation and better control the ultimate height of the grafted space.

2. **Lateral window approach**: this technique gives access through the lateral wall of the sinus [3,4]. A full-thickness flap is elevated to expose the lateral antral wall, a window is made in the bony wall using rotary or hand instruments, and then it is displaced medially. The membrane is carefully elevated, and the bone is placed in the space below the Schneiderian membrane and above the sinus floor.

D. Autografts (extraoral and intraoral), allografts (FDBA, decalcified freeze-dried bone allograft [DFDBA]), xenografts (inorganic bovine bone mineral), and alloplasts (calcium phosphate) have been used for bone grafting materials for more than 20 years. The Sinus Consensus Conference of 1996 [11] approved autogenous bone as an acceptable grafting material. Other studies have proved that bone substitutes including allografts and xenografts can be successfully used for sinus elevation [12,13]. Further evidence [14] has shown that autogenous bone is a viable option, although a higher rate of complications (including infections and bone resorption) was observed when compared with xenografts and allografts. Recent systematic reviews have shown that sinus elevation using bone substitutes alone or in combination with autogenous bone had a similar or an even better implant survival rate when compared with studies using autogenous bone only [15,16]. New materials such as bone morphogenetic protein (BMP-2) used with a collagen sponge carrier have proved their efficacy and have gained Food and Drug Administration approval for sinus elevation procedures [17,18].

A few studies have provided histologic evidence of bone formation in a grafted sinus. Histology of an explant from the maxillary sinus showed new bone formation around the implant and the xenograft particulates [19]. Another study showed evidence of bone formation when autogenous bone alone or a mix of DFDBA and autogenous bone were initially used [20].

Boyne et al. [17] and Kim et al. [21] have shown evidence of normal bone formation in an elevated sinus, respectively, when rhBMP-2 (Infuse) and demineralized bone matrix and cancellous bone chips (DynaBlast) were used as grafting material.

The placement of a membrane over the window is usually recommended to enhance bone formation [22]. Both resorbable (collagen) and nonresorbable (expandable polytetrafluoroethylene) membranes can be used, although the resorbable one is more commonly used to avoid a surgical reentry.

E. The success of a sinus elevation procedure depends on a series of parameters that include. chronologically, an uneventful surgical procedure, minimal or no postoperative pain and complications, bone formation, osseointegration of implants, and their survival under functional load.

Some determinants promoting success have been reported in the literature and include the following.
1. Absence of medical conditions (including systemic diseases, bisphosphonate therapy, and irradiation), sinus pathology, and smoking. The patient should be referred to a physician if there is any significant medical condition reported during the preoperative examination.
2. The use of rough surfaced implants as opposed to machined surface implants to enhance the survival rate [15,16].
3. The use of particulate grafts or BMP-2 as opposed to block grafts to decrease complications. However, autogenous block grafts remain a viable option [15,16].
4. The use of a membrane when a lateral window approach is selected [15,16].
5. The use of piezosurgical instruments to decrease the rate of complications at the time of osteotomy [23].
The surgeon should deliver regular postoperative instructions emphasizing the following.
1. Do not blow your nose
2. Do not sneeze
3. Do not travel by plane or scuba dive for the next 15 days

4. Do not engage in physical activity for a few days (i.e. strenuous exercise)

F. Implants placed in a sinus-elevated site have a very high rate of success (>90%), which is comparable to implants placed in pristine bone [15]. Multiple studies have proved that the lateral approach is a predictable technique and allows implant survival rates of ≥95% over the long term [24–26]. Similar results can be found when a crestal approach is used [27,28]. Nevertheless, the amount of residual bone seems to have a significant impact on the implant survival rate with this technique; a minimum of 5 mm would be necessary to achieve a high success rate [29].

Evidence has shown that there are no statistically significant differences in implant survival rates when a lateral as opposed to a crestal approach is used. A recent meta-analysis reporting on 12 020 implants placed in sinus-elevated sites with a lateral approach indicated an implant survival rate at three years of 90.1% [16], whereas the survival rate over the same period was 92.8% when a crestal approach was used [30]. If both surgical techniques are compatible with success, the Consensus Report of the Sixth European Workshop on Periodontology [31] stated that the choice of the most appropriate procedure still needed to be addressed.

G. Complications associated with sinus elevation procedures, and their management, can be divided into a number of categories.

Operative Complications
1. Perforation of the Schneiderian membrane is reported to be the most common complication and occurs on average in 19.5% [16] and in up to 58% [32] of the procedures. There is some controversy with regard to its impact on implant survival [33,34].
2. Hemorrhage at the time of osteotomy with the lateral approach is the consequence of section of a branch of the posterior lateral artery running along the lateral wall of the sinus. Zijderveld et al. [35] reported its occurrence in 2% of the cases.
3. Inadvertent implant migration in the sinus cavity and injury of the infraorbital neurovascular bundle have been rarely reported.

Postoperative Complications

1. Infection as a direct consequence of the procedure or as a result of overfill of the sinus resulting in the absence of its drainage in the nasal cavity. Infections occur in 2.9% and would be correlated with membrane perforations [16].
2. Absence of adequate bone volume: more common with autogenous bone [14].
3. Hematoma and wound dehiscence have also been reported.

Management of Perioperative Complications

1. Perforation of the Schneiderian membrane: a resorbable membrane can be placed against the Schneiderian membrane and over the perforated area. If the perforation is small, Fugazzotto advocates try not to repair it if it "folds over itself" [36]. If the perforation is large and cannot be repaired, the sinus elevation should be postponed until after complete healing of the Schneiderian membrane.
2. Hemorrhage [37]: pressure can be applied on the bleeding point with gauze until hemostasis is observed. If the severed vessel is located in a bony crypt, bone wax can be placed in it to act as a plug that encourages clot formation. One

can also inject some local anesthetic with epinephrine 1:50 000 to enhance vasoconstriction. Vessel ligature and electrocautery have also been reported, although they need to be used with caution.
3. Inadvertent implant migration: the implant should be retrieved as soon as possible. An emergency consultation with an otorhinolaryngologist should be scheduled.

Management of Postoperative Complications

1. Infections: the first choice of therapy is antibiotics and choosing the appropriate one for the specificity of the sinus infection. In this regard, Augmentin could be considered as the first choice followed by DNA gyrase inhibitors such as ofloxacin, levofloxacin, and so on. In addition, one could consider the use of broader-spectrum antibiotics such as amoxicillin or clindamycin for penicillin-allergic patients. If the infection cannot be controlled with antibiotics, removal of the bone graft might be necessary.
2. Inadequate bone volume: the clinical situation should be reevaluated. The options of placing shorter implants or performing a complementary sinus elevation can be discussed.

Case 2

Internal Sinus Lift Using the Crestal Window Technique

CASE STORY

A 32-year-old Korean female who had undergone extensive restorative treatment by her general dentist came in for an implant consultation. On examination, we determined that many of her restorations were defective and had recurrent caries. The patient's primary goal was to have fixed implant restorations to replace missing teeth #14 and #15. Figures 7.2.1 and 7.2.2 illustrate the results of the initial clinical examination.

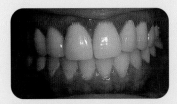

Figure 7.2.1 Facial view of the maxilla and the mandible.

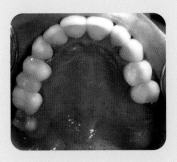

Figure 7.2.2 Occlusal view of the maxilla.

LEARNING GOALS AND OBJECTIVES

■ To identify the indications and contraindications for the crestal approach and what diagnostic information is needed to make this decision
■ To compare the advantages and disadvantages of the crestal approach
■ To evaluate the sequences of treatment (internal sinus lift with the grafts and implant completed in one treatment session vs. internal sinus lift followed by a waiting period for healing before the implant)
■ To describe the appropriate usage of Summer's osteotome, balloon, hydraulic sinus condensing, and bone condensing with drills

Medical History

The patient did not report any allergies or sinus-related pathology. She did not take any medications.

Review of Systems

• Vital signs
  ○ Blood pressure: 135/85 mmHg
  ○ Pulse rate: 65 beats/minute

Social History

The patient, who works as an emergency room nurse, reported that she was a social drinker and smoked 10 cigarettes per day. Tobacco use has been shown to "increase complication of endosseous dental implants" [1]. Therefore, the patient was advised to cease smoking at least for one month after dental implant surgery.

Extraoral Examination

The patient had no masses or swelling and no trismus. There was no palpable lymphadenopathy, and the temporomandibular joints were within normal limits.

Intraoral Examination

- The soft tissues of the mouth, including the tongue, appeared normal. The oral cancer screening was negative.
- The gingival examination revealed a generalized mild marginal erythema.
- The edentulous ridge in the maxillary left quadrant had slight deformities in the buccolingual and apico-coronal directions (Seibert class 3) (Figure 7.2.1).
- A periodontal charting was completed (Figure 7.2.3).

Occlusion

Examination showed a lack of posterior support, unprotected occlusion, and group function.

Radiographic Examination

A digital panoramic radiograph showed a pneumatized left maxillary sinus. Cross-sectional computed tomography (CT) showed about 4.1 mm of initial bone height with buccal–lingual dimension of 7.5 mm (Figure 7.2.4). There was a slight septum on the distal side of tooth #15, and the #14–15 area had a concave shape. This made a transalveolar technique preferable.

Good patency of the natural ostium of the maxillary sinus was observed on cross-section of the CT scan. This feature is important because it allows drainage of mucus and foreign material from the maxillary sinus. If this opening is obstructed, sinusitis will develop with the patient experiencing symptoms of "pressure in the sinus" [2]. CT shows that the sinus membrane was not thickened, which indicates a healthy sinus. The cavity of the maxillary sinus was clear and free of pathology.

Diagnosis

- Gingivitis-associated dental biofilm alone
- Traumatic occlusal forces

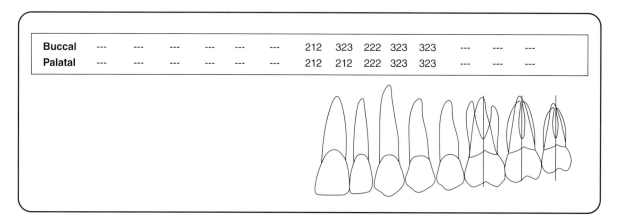

Buccal	---	---	---	---	---	---	212	323	222	323	323	---	---	---
Palatal	---	---	---	---	---	---	212	212	222	323	323	---	---	---

Figure 7.2.3 Probing pocket depth measurements of the maxillary left quadrant.

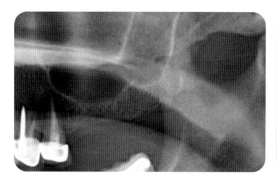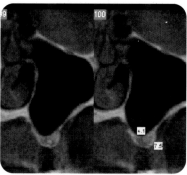

Figure 7.2.4 Cone beam CT scan of the maxillary right sinus. The Schneiderian membrane appears healthy and thin. The residual bone height is 4.1 mm in sites #14 and #15. Septum present on distal of #15 area with concave shape in #14 and #15 area, which makes transalveolar technique favorable.

- Peri-implant soft and hard tissue deficiencies (Seibert type III defect)

Treatment

Although a comprehensive treatment plan was presented to the patient to address all prosthetic needs, the patient only sought fixed implant prostheses for #14 and #15 for now.

Preoperative Consultation

The medical history was reviewed. The consent form addressing benefits and risks associated with the procedure was reviewed with the patient. She emphasized that she could not afford to be absent from her work, and that the procedure must be atraumatic. Therefore, we offered a crestal approach to reduce morbidity.

The patient received oral hygiene instructions and a prophylaxis prior to the surgical therapy. She was premedicated with amoxicillin 500 mg t.i.d., metronidazole 500 mg t.i.d., and Sudafed 30 mg [2].

Sinus Elevation Procedure

A posterior superior alveolar nerve block, greater palatine nerve block, and local infiltrations were achieved with two carpules of Septocaine 4% with epinephrine 1:100 000. A full-thickness palatal flap was elevated in the maxillary left quadrant to expose the crestal ridge of sites #14 and #15 (Figure 7.2.5). The palatal flap was used for three reasons: unilateral retraction of the flap, less postoperative discomfort (all incisions in keratinized tissue), and prevention of oral antral communication (because of the window present on the crestal aspect) [3]. In this case, a novel crestal window technique was employed using specific drill bits. The osteotomy site was marked with a pointed trephine (Figure 7.2.6). The use of a regular trephine is very technique-sensitive because it has a tendency to slide out of the intended site, whereas the pointed trephine engages the center point first, thus preventing sliding of the trephine bur from the intended site

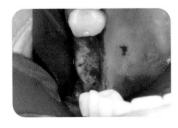

Figure 7.2.5 Full-thickness palatal flap raised on #14 and #15 site.

(Figure 7.2.6) [3]. The distance between the crest and the sinus floor was measured from cone beam CT: 1 mm was subtracted from the height of the bone and the stopper was set on an adjustable stopper and bone ejector (ASBE) trephine. This tool was used at a slow speed (30 rpm) with torque of 50 N·cm and was stopped 1 mm short of the sinus floor. When the trephine depth was close to the sinus floor, a slight tilt of the trephine was used to fracture off the bone core. After removal of this bone core, the sinus membrane could be visualized (Figure 7.2.7). Note that because the sinus floor was not flat, some parts of the floor were still intact, and manual enlargement of the sinus window was needed. A small instrument called a "mushroom elevator" was used to elevate the

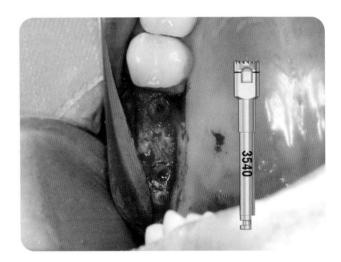

Figure 7.2.6 Pointed trephine to mark the osteotomy site.

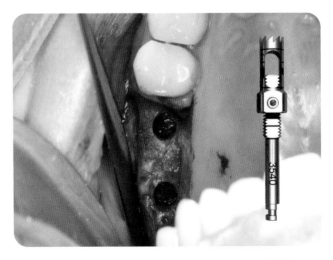

Figure 7.2.7 After the removal of bone core using ASBE trephine.

membrane (Figure 7.2.8) and pry away the remaining bone of the sinus floor (Figure 7.2.9). A bone graft, comprising rehydrated freeze-dried bone allograft (FDBA), was placed in the space created within the sinus (Figure 7.2.10). It is important to laterally condense the bone graft in order to spread it mesiodistally as well as buccolingually using the spreader instrument (Figure 7.2.11 shows before; Figure 7.2.12 shows after). About 1.5 ml of FDBA was used to graft the sinus transalveolarly. Two 5 × 10 mm EZ Plus implants (MegaGen, Englewood Cliffs, NJ, USA) were inserted on the #14 and #15 sites (Figure 7.2.13). To achieve good

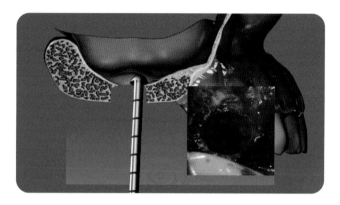

Figure 7.2.8 Mushroom elevator is used to identify and lift sinus membrane.

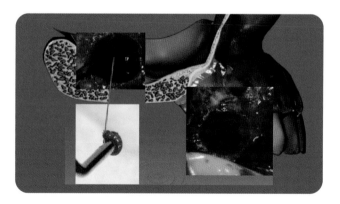

Figure 7.2.9 Mushroom elevator is used to pull out sinus floor (bone).

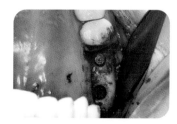

Figure 7.2.10 Bone graft (FDBA) placed.

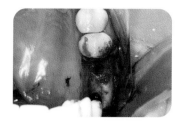

Figure 7.2.11 Use of spreader to condense bone laterally as well as mesiodistally.

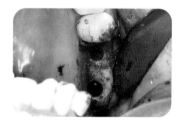

Figure 7.2.12 After use of spreader.

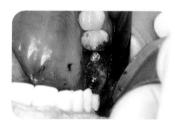

Figure 7.2.13 Two 5 × 10 mm MegaGen EZ Plus implants placed with good initial stability (45 N·cm).

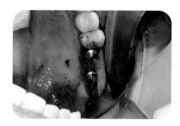

Figure 7.2.14 Healing abutment of 6 mm diameter and 3 mm height is used.

primary stability, clinicians should keep three things in mind: (i) selection of the appropriate implant (the crestal portion should be wider than the body of implant); (ii) slow insertion to expand the bone (<20 rpm); and (iii) skipping the last drill in cases of very poor-quality bone. In this case, a torque of greater than 45 N·cm was achieved, and a healing abutment was inserted, making this a one-stage surgery (Figure 7.2.14). A papillary finger flap was used to adapt the flap around the healing abutment (Figure 7.2.15). A digital panoramic scan (Figure 7.2.16) and a CT scan (Figure 7.2.17) were

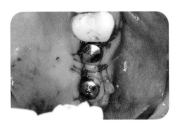

Figure 7.2.15 Papillary rotation flap used to close around healing abutment.

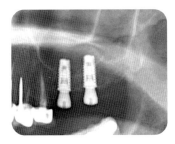

Figure 7.2.16 Panoramic radiograph after implant and sinus lift.

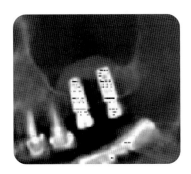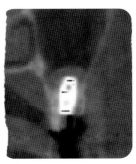

Figure 7.2.17 CT scan on the day of the procedure.

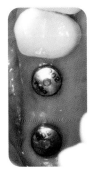

Figure 7.2.18 Healing of #14 and #15 implants with simultaneous sinus lift after six months.

taken at the end of the surgical procedure to verify the sinus membrane was intact. The bone grafting material appeared well contained in the maxillary right sinus (Figure 7.2.17). After six months, soft tissue healing was normal (Figures 7.2.18 and 7.2.19).

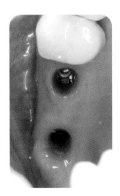

Figure 7.2.19 Removal of healing abutment from implants #14 and #15.

Discussion

Most conventional crestal approaches are blind techniques that make visualization of the Schneiderian membrane impossible [4]. Using this new crestal window technique, the membrane can be visualized and elevation of the sinus can be achieved in a more controlled fashion (see Figures 7.2.7–7.2.9). Summer's osteotome technique requires malleting, and forceful or improper malleting can lead to benign vertigo, which could become a potential medicolegal matter [5]. The crestal window technique does not use malleting and thus mitigates the patient's discomfort. Clinician confidence in the sinus procedure is increased because it is not a blind technique.

One of the main limitations of conventional crestal approaches is that they require a minimal bone height of 5 mm [6]. In contrast, the crestal window technique is easier on bone that is less than 5 mm in height. Visualization of and access to the sinus with crestal window instruments are improved if bone height to sinus floor is within 1–4 mm. If the initial stability is less than 20 N·cm or if poor bone quality is suspected, a two-stage surgery is recommended to prevent movement of the implant during the initial integration phase [7]. Conversely, excessive torque on the implant during insertion is not recommended to avoid the risk of inducing pressure necrosis of the bone, which could have occurred on the distal of #14 (Figure 7.2.20). During the surgery, the 4.3-mm drill was skipped and the final drill was 3.6 mm (for a 5-mm implant). This resulted in great initial stability, but the implant may have been overtightened and reduced blood supply to the bone surrounding the implant.

One of the most common prosthetic failures of implants is porcelain fracture. Although there are many contributing factors, the main one is poor metal design [8]. A cutback from a full-contour wax-up will

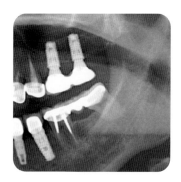

Figure 7.2.20 Digital pantograph of implants #14 and #15. Note satisfactory uniform thickness of porcelain on #14 and #15 vs. poor (too thick and irregular) on tooth #20. Also note new sinus floor (new cortical bone) formation on top of implants, and disappearance of old cortical bone.

guarantee uniform thickness of the porcelain. However, due to time constraints, many laboratory technicians use a dipping technique to wax up metal support for a porcelain-fused-to-metal (PFM) crown. This dipping wax technique results in uneven or excessive thickness of the porcelain, leading to cracks or fracture. Therefore,

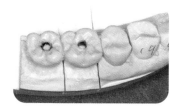

Figure 7.2.21 Full-contour wax-up to verify that technician will cut back to obtain uniform thickness of porcelain.

we recommend asking the technician specifically for a full-contour wax-up to verify that a cutback has been performed and thus guarantee uniform thickness of porcelain (Figure 7.2.21).

Radiographic evidence of successful sinus grafting can be evaluated six to nine months after the surgery. The old sinus floor will have disintegrated and a new sinus floor will be evident on a new radiograph. This represents the true morphology of any bone, i.e. medullary bone sandwiched between the cortical bones of the sinus floor and the crestal bone (Figure 7.2.20).

Self-Study Questions

A. What is the minimum bone height needed for the crestal technique?

B. What anatomic landmarks should be evaluated on a preoperative sinus CT scan?

C. What are the advantages and disadvantage of the crestal window technique, Summer's osteotome technique, the balloon sinus lift technique, the use of bone condensing drills, and the use of piezo tips?

E. How can you achieve good initial stability in the maxillary posterior bone?

F. Why is cutback technique so important in PFM fabrication?

G. What is pressure necrosis of the crestal bone, and how can you avoid it?

H. What is the radiographic evidence of successful sinus grafting?

Answers located at the end of the chapter.

References

1. Schwartz-Arad D, Samet N, Samet N, Mamlider A. Smoking and complications of endosseous dental implants. *J Periodontol* 2002;73(2):153–157.
2. Garg JN, Quinones CR. Augmentation of the maxillary sinus. A surgical technique. *Pract Periodontics Aesthet Dent* 1997;9:211–219.
3. Lee S, Kang-Lee G, Park K-B, Han T. Crestal sinus lift: a minimally invasive and systematic approach to sinus grafting. *J Implant Adv Clin Dent* 2009;1(1):75–90.
4. Chen L, Cha J. An 8-year retrospective study: 1,100 patients receiving 1,557 implants using the minimally invasive hydraulic sinus condensing technique. *J Periodontol* 2005;76:482–491.
5. Sammartino G, Mariniello M, Scaravilli MS. Benign paroxysmal positional vertigo following closed sinus floor elevation

procedure: mallet osteotome vs. screwable osteomes. A triple blind randomized controlled trial. *Clin Oral Implants Res* 2011;22:669–672.

6. Bruschi GB, Scipioni A, Calesini G, Bruschi E. Localized management of the sinus floor with simultaneous implant placement: a clinical report. *Int J Oral Maxillofac Implants* 1998;13:219–226.
7. Esposito M, Grusovin MG, Chew YS, et al. One-stage versus two-stage implant placement. A Cochrane systematic review of randomised controlled clinical trials. *Eur J Oral Implantol* 2009;2(2):91–99.
8. Cranham JC. Why porcelain breaks: ten factors to consider in the restorative process. *Dawson Acad Vistas* 2008;1:22–27.
9. Jensen OT. *The Sinus Bone Graft Book*, 2nd edn. Hanover Park, IL: Quintessence, 2006.

TAKE-HOME POINTS

A. In general, crestal (sometimes called "internal") sinus lifts need at least 5 mm of initial bone height [9]. A minimum of 5 mm of bone is necessary because clinicians must rely on bone pressure elevation of the Schneiderian membrane. In contrast to conventional crestal approaches, the crestal window technique does not require 5 mm of initial bone height [3]. More than 5 mm of bone height reduces visibility to the sinus membranes and decreases access to the sinus cavity because it hinders instruments from reaching the sinus walls. Figure 7.2.22 shows examples of 1 mm initial bone height vs. 6 mm of initial bone height. Note that visibility and access to the sinuses is much easier for 1 mm of initial bone height.

B. A CT scan should be the standard of care before performing any sinus grafting procedures. There are four anatomic landmarks that should be evaluated prior to sinus surgery: (i) patency of natural ostium, to ensure that the sinus is self-draining; (ii) thickness of the sinus membrane or any pathology associated with it (e.g. polyps, cysts, or inflammation); (iii) location of intraosseous anastomosis of the posterior superior alveolar artery; and (iv) thickness of the lateral wall, the buccal–lingual dimension of alveolar bone, and the initial bone height and quality of the alveolar bone.

C. The crestal window technique is not a blind technique. The use of an osteotome can lead to benign vertigo due to the use of a mallet [5]. Instead, the crestal window technique uses a large diamond drill, virtually eliminating any chance of benign vertigo. The use of osteotomes or other transalveolar techniques requires a minimum of 5 mm initial bone height, whereas the crestal window technique is easily achieved with only 1–4 mm of initial bone height. The use of an osteotome or other transalveolar technique relies on bone pressure elevation of the membrane and therefore it is difficult to fully elevate the buccal and palatal walls of the sinus. In

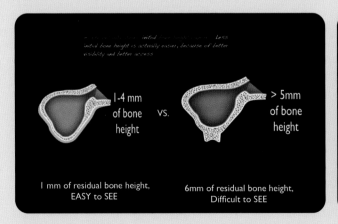
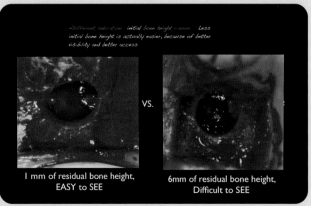

Figure 7.2.22 Crestal window technique is easier if initial bone height is less.

Table 7.2.1 Advantages and disadvantages of all internal sinus techniques.

	Minimum bone height	Visibility of sinus membrane	Access to sinus	Cost	Vertigo incidence
Crestal window	<5 mm	Very good	Very good	Moderate	None
Summer's osteotome	>5 mm	Poor	Poor	Moderate	Low
Balloon	N/A	Poor	Poor	High	None
Hydraulic sinus condensing	N/A	Good	Poor	Moderate	None
Bone condensing drills	>5 mm	Poor	Poor	Moderate	None
Piezo tips	>5 mm	Poor	Poor	High	None

contrast, the crestal window technique uses small "cobra elevators" to manually lift the buccal and palatal walls of the sinus. Advantages and disadvantages of all internal sinus techniques are listed in Table 7.2.1.

D. Three clinical tips are helpful in achieving good initial stability in posterior maxilla. First, the bone quality in the posterior maxilla is often very poor (D4 or D3). Therefore, a clinician should use a smaller drill, thus making a smaller osteotomy than he or she would in a mandibular bone. Second, selection of the implant shape is important. A wider platform than the body of an implant is essential to achieve excellent initial stability from the crestal bone. Third, slow insertion of the implant at a speed less than 20 rpm is recommended to allow the alveolar bone to expand.

E. A common complication after implant therapy is porcelain fracture. It is usually due to poor metal design in a PFM restoration, and a lack of sensation (feedback) upon biting hard substances. A uniform

thickness of porcelain is crucial to ensure the hardness of the porcelain during function. Full-contour wax-up is necessary to do cutback, and clinicians should verify this prior to casting of the metal framework [8].

F. Cortical bone (crestal bone) consists of Harversian canals that provide nutrients to osteocytes. If too much torque is applied during insertion of the implant, pressure necrosis will occur around the implant. Clinicians can avoid this by creating the proper osteotomy size to achieve 15–45 N·cm.

G. Normal morphology of any bone consists of medullary bone surrounded by cortical bone. In the case of maxillary alveolar bone, there is the sinus floor and the alveolar crest (two cortical bones). Disappearance of old sinus floor and appearance of new sinus floor indicates success. This occurs on average six to nine months after surgery depending on shape of the sinus, choice of bone graft materials, and initial bone height.

Case 3

Alveolar Ridge Preservation

CASE STORY

A 72-year-old Caucasian male presented with a chief complaint of "My front tooth broke off over the weekend." Patient was otherwise asymptomatic in relation to the site of interest at the time of initial evaluation. After hearing all the possible post-extraction replacement options, patient chose implant-supported single crown restoration as the treatment option for site #11. Patient was also missing #13 at the time of evaluation but was not interested in restoring the edentulous site.

LEARNING GOALS AND OBJECTIVES

- To understand the normal physiologic healing events following tooth extraction
- To know the indications and contraindications for alveolar ridge preservation (ARP)
- To understand the clinical procedure and materials involved in ARP

Medical History

The patient had been diagnosed with benign hypertension and hypothyroidism and was taking lisinopril and levothyroxine, respectively. Patient had osteoarthritis and took analgesics as needed. He had undergone cataract surgery in the past. On questioning, the patient reported no allergies to food or to drugs.

Review of Systems

- Vital signs
  - Blood pressure: 140/80 mmHg
  - Pulse rate: 68 beats/minute
  - Respiratory rate: 14 breaths/minute

Social History

The patient had never smoked and consumed alcohol very rarely.

Extraoral Examination

No significant findings were noted. The patient had no masses or swelling, and the temporomandibular joint was within normal limits.

Intraoral Examination

- No abnormal findings with respect to tongue, floor of mouth, palate, or buccal mucosa were observed.
- A gingival examination revealed mild marginal erythema (Figures 7.3.1 and 7.3.2).
- Periodontal charting was recorded (Figure 7.3.3).
- No mobility and no furcation involvement were noted.
- Keratinized gingival width was adequate and was 7 mm for tooth #11.
- Generalized gingival recession present but was asymptomatic.

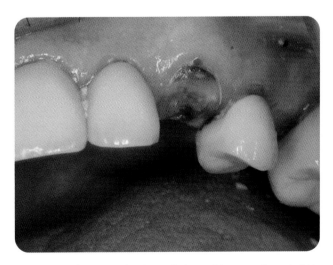

Figure 7.3.1 Preoperative frontal view of fractured tooth #11.

Occlusion

There were no occlusal discrepancies or interferences.

Radiographic Examination

Periapical radiograph of the involved area before extraction is shown in Figure 7.3.4. Normal bone levels noted interproximally between teeth and no periapical pathologies of #11 noted. Overall, hard tissues observed in the radiograph are within normal limits.

Diagnosis

The patient's history and his clinical and radiographic examinations clearly pointed to the diagnosis of fractured tooth #11 (at the gingival level) with hopeless restorative prognosis and therefore extraction was planned. Periodontally, patient was diagnosed with dental biofilm-induced gingivitis.

Treatment Plan

The treatment was planned in the following steps.
- The diagnostic phase included a comprehensive periodontal examination, radiographs, and study models.

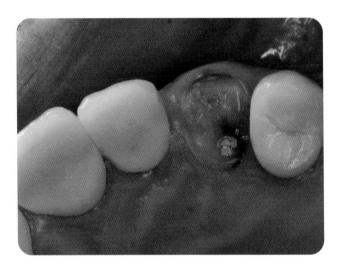

Figure 7.3.2 Preoperative occlusal view of tooth #11 fractured at the level of the gingival margin.

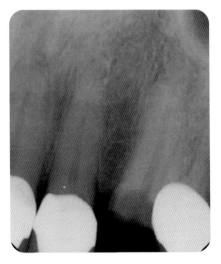

Figure 7.3.4 Preoperative periapical radiograph of fractured tooth #11.

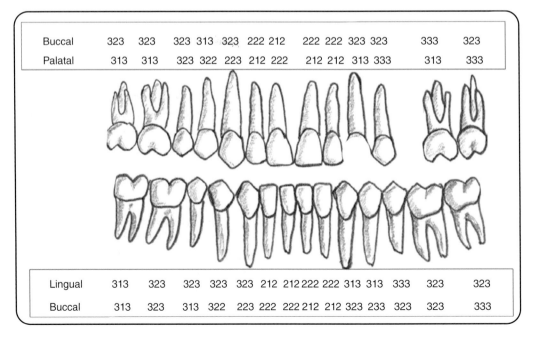

Buccal	323	323	323	313	323	222	212	222	222	323	323	333	323
Palatal	313	313	323	322	223	212	222	212	212	313	333	313	333

Lingual	313	323	323	323	323	212	212	222	222	313	313	333	323	323
Buccal	313	323	313	322	223	222	222	212	212	323	233	323	323	333

Figure 7.3.3 Probing pocket depth measurements during initial examination.

- Disease control phase included oral hygiene instruction and prophylaxis.
- Surgical phase consisted of extraction of #11 along with ARP using an allograft particulate graft and resorbable collagen membrane.
- After adequate healing of the ridge, dental implant to replace #11 will be placed in a prosthetically driven position.
- After an adequate period of osseointegration, implant #11 will be restored with a single crown.
- The patient will be placed on a periodontal recall program.

Treatment

The patient opted for a dental implant-supported single crown fixed restoration. Once the patient chose the implant option prior to extraction, the importance of ARP to the future dental implant was explained to the patient and he consented to the procedure.

Extraction of the tooth was carried out in a minimally traumatic fashion using periotomes. Once the tooth was extracted (Figure 7.3.5B), the socket was degranulated (Figure 7.3.5A) and bone grafting was performed.

Hydrated freeze-dried bone allograft (FDBA) particles were packed into the socket (Figure 7.3.5D) and a resorbable collagen membrane was used to cover the FDBA bone graft particles. The membrane was tucked underneath the buccal and palatal flaps and the flaps sutured over the membrane using interrupted and criss-cross sutures (Figure 7.3.5C,E). The patient was prescribed with a one-week course of systemic antibiotic and chlorhexidine mouthwash and was seen after two weeks for postoperative follow-up. Five months after performing ARP, the ridge volume was found to be adequate to place a dental implant of appropriate dimension (Figure 7.3.5F).

Discussion

Dental extraction is a very common procedure performed by dentists. Following single or multiple extractions, various options exist to replace the missing teeth including fixed partial dentures (if adjacent teeth are present and are good candidates as abutments), removable partial dentures, or an implant-supported prosthesis. The decision to graft the bony socket after extraction is critical and should be based on the future treatment option planned for the particular site and the

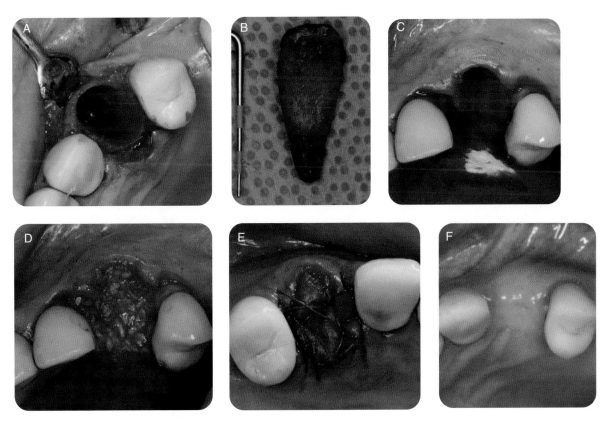

Figure 7.3.5 With minimal flap reflection, tooth #11 was extracted. Socket (#11) after tooth extraction (A) and the extracted tooth (B). Membrane was tucked underneath the palatal flap (C) and the socket packed with FDBA bone graft particles (D) and covered with a membrane and flaps sutured (E). Healed ridge five months post ARP (F).

location of the site. If an implant-supported prosthesis is planned for a particular site, maximum effort should be made to preserve the existing bone and minimize bone loss, starting with a minimally traumatic extraction procedure. Apart from bone loss that exists in a periodontally compromised tooth, the bone loss that occurs following tooth extraction will certainly impose challenges in maintaining the required bone volume for future implant placement. Inadequate bone volume will impede placement of an implant in a prosthetically driven position. ARP done at the time of extraction(s)

plays an important role in minimizing bone loss and preserving the bone (ridge) volume.

In addition, ARP allows maintenance of adequate peri-implant bone thickness, which becomes critical in maintaining peri-implant soft tissues and for the long-term success of dental implants. Another indication for ARP is in anterior sextants, where esthetics is an important consideration and bone grafting in anterior sockets can help maintain the esthetically favorable tissue bulkiness, even in cases where fixed partial dentures are planned.

Self-Study Questions

A. Describe the events involved in socket healing following tooth extraction.

B. What is the rationale for doing ARP?

C. What other terms are used to describe ARP?

D. What are the biomaterials used in ARP and what is the rationale for choosing them?

E. How would you perform the ARP procedure?

F. What are the indications and contraindications for ARP?

G. How long do you have to wait after ARP and before implant placement, and how successful are the implants placed in augmented bone?

H. What are the factors involved in the successful outcome of ARP?

I. What are the postoperative complications associated with ARP and the necessary postoperative care required after the procedure?

J. What are the drawbacks of doing ARP?

Answers located at the end of the chapter.

References

1. Araujo M, Lindhe J. The edentulous alveolar ridge. In: Lindhe J, Lang NP, Karring T (eds) *Clinical Periodontology and Implant Dentistry*, 5th edn. Oxford: Blackwell Munksgaard, 2008:57–62.
2. Pietrokovski J, Massler M. Ridge remodeling after tooth extraction in rats. *J Dent Res* 1966;46:222–231.
3. Lekovic V, Camargo PM, Klokkevold PR, et al. Preservation of alveolar bone in extraction sockets using bioabsorbable membranes. *J Periodontol* 1998;69:1044–1049.
4. Schropp L, Wenzel A, Kostopoulos L, Karring T. Bone healing and soft tissue contour changes following single-tooth extraction: a clinical and radiographic 12-month prospective study. *Int J Periodontics Restorative Dent* 2003;23: 313–323.
5. Trombelli L, Farina R, Marzola A, et al. Modeling and remodeling of human extraction sockets. *J Clin Periodontol* 2008;35:630–639.
6. Avila-Ortiz G, Elangovan S, Kramer KW, et al. Effect of alveolar ridge preservation after tooth extraction: a systematic review and meta-analysis. *J Dent Res* 2014;93(10):950–958.
7. Bassir SH, Alhareky M, Wangsrimongkol B, et al. Systematic review and meta-analysis of hard tissue outcomes of alveolar ridge preservation. *Int J Oral Maxillofac Implants* 2018;33(5):979–994.
8. Willenbacher M, Al-Nawas B, Berres M, et al. The effects of alveolar ridge preservation: a meta-analysis. *Clin Implant Dent Relat Res* 2016;18(6):1248–1268.
9. Nevins M, Camelo M, Schupbach P, et al. Human histologic evaluation of mineralized collagen bone substitute and recombinant platelet-derived growth factor-BB to create bone for implant placement in extraction socket defects at 4 and 6 months: a case series. *Int J Periodontics Restorative Dent* 2009;29:129–139.
10. Fickl S, Zuhr O, Wachtel H, et al. Dimensional changes of the alveolar ridge contour after different socket

preservation techniques. *J Clin Periodontol* 2008;35:906–913.

11. Bartee BK. Extraction site reconstruction for alveolar ridge preservation. Part 1: rationale and materials selection. *J Oral Implantol* 2001;27(4):187–193.

12. Fowler EB, Breault LG. Ridge augmentation with a folded acellular dermal matrix allograft: a case report. *J Contemp Dent Pract* 2001;2:31–40.

13. Bartee BK. Extraction site reconstruction for alveolar ridge preservation. Part 2: membrane-assisted surgical technique. *J Oral Implantol* 2001;27(4):194–197.

14. Hämmerle CH, Chen ST, Wilson TG Jr. Consensus statements and recommended clinical procedures regarding the placement of implants in extraction sockets. *Int J Oral Maxillofac Implants* 2004;19(Suppl):26–28.

15. Fugazzotto PA. Success and failure rates of osseointegrated implants in function in regenerated bone for 72 to 133 months. *Int J Oral Maxillofac Implants* 2005;20:77–83.

16. Kohal RJ, Mellas P, Hürzeler MB, et al. The effects of guided bone regeneration and grafting on implants placed into immediate extraction sockets. An experimental study in dogs. *J Periodontol* 1998;69:927–937.

TAKE-HOME POINTS

A. Tissue healing following extraction of a tooth is a highly orchestrated event ultimately leading to bone formation in the open bony socket. Soon after tooth extraction, blood clot formation occurs, leading to a seal of the open wound with blood coagulum. The platelets form a plug sealing the blood vessels that are damaged during the tooth removal process. Neutrophils and macrophages then enter the clot and clear foreign products or bacteria and make the wound sterile. The blood clot is then subsequently replaced by granulation tissue that is composed of collagenous extracellular matrix produced by the mesenchymal cells as well as blood vessels sprouting (angiogenesis) into the wound by a process called neovascularization. Mesenchymal cells from the periodontal ligament remnants or the surrounding bone enter the granulation tissue and differentiate into bone-forming osteoblasts. The osteoblasts lay down the collagen (predominantly type 1)-rich osteoid, which is mineralized to form woven bone. By a process of bone remodeling, the woven bone is then gradually replaced with mature lamellar bone and marrow. By 21 days reepithelialization begins, which will be completed in six weeks. It takes an average of six weeks for initial soft tissue and hard tissue healing to complete [1].

B. One of the key consequences of tooth extraction is alveolar ridge resorption, and this affects the future placement of implants. Studies have shown clearly that extraction of either single or multiple teeth leads to topographic changes in the alveolar ridge. It has been shown that the resorption of bone in the buccal surface is significantly more pronounced than in the palatal or lingual surface [2]. Bundle bone is a specialized hard tissue that lines the inner walls of a socket and is lost following tooth extraction. Since the buccal socket wall is inherently thinner than the palatal/lingual walls, bundle bone represents the bulk of the buccal wall. Therefore, following tooth loss the buccal wall tends to be affected more than the palatal/lingual counterparts. Without bone grafting, it has been shown that in the first six months, approximately 40–50% of the alveolar bone height and alveolar bone width will be lost [3]. Bone resorption progresses significantly faster in maxilla compared with mandible, and the degree of resorption is directly proportional to the time since the tooth was extracted.

Using subtraction radiography, researchers have shown that after extraction of the tooth, some bone loss occurs in the initial few months, with some bone gain occurring up to six months after extraction [4]. Remodeling of the bone occurs between 6 and 12 months, leading to an overall reduction in the amount of mineralized tissue. Moreover, there is considerable individual variability in the capacity to form new bone in the extraction socket [5]. Therefore it is critical to preserve as much bone as possible soon after extraction by doing ARP, which is known to minimize ridge resorption [6]. ARP at the time of extraction has the potential to reduce the need for future interventions required to augment bone (prior to dental implant placement), which are more invasive, expensive, less predictable, and time-consuming. Socket status soon after extraction can range from a complete intact socket to the loss of one or many walls (due to surgical trauma, preexisting periodontal defect, dehiscence, or previous apical surgery). Although several studies have strongly indicated the benefits of ARP at the time of extraction in all forms of post-extraction socket defects [6–8], ARP does not avoid the postoperative contour shrinkage completely [8].

C. Socket grafting, socket preservation, and ridge preservation are some of the terms used interchangeably to describe ARP.

D. ARP typically employs a scaffold to fill the socket and a barrier membrane. Scaffolds most commonly used in this procedure are particulate bone grafts. The bone grafts can range from osteogenic autogenous bone particles/chips and osteoconductive materials such as FDBA particles to osteoinductive materials such as demineralized freeze-dried bone allograft (DFDBA) particles and collagen matrix containing recombinant factors such as bone morphogenetic protein (BMP)-2. Currently, BMP-2 protein delivered in an absorbable collagen sponge (Infuse) is approved by the US Food and Drug Administration for socket preservation procedures. Apart from BMP-2, recombinant platelet-derived growth factor (PDGF)-BB has been shown to enhance bone formation in extraction sockets prior to implant placement [9]. Alloplastic materials such as hydroxyapatite, which are poor osteoconductive materials, are also available for use in ARP. Studies also indicate that bone mineral containing collagen is a favorable material for socket preservation [10].

The selection of bone graft for ARP should be based exclusively on the clinical situation and the established resorption profile of a graft material. Alloplastic materials such as dense hydroxyapatite or bioactive glass are generally used for long-term ARP (in sites where implants are not planned) because these materials are poorly osteoconductive with a low resorption capacity. In areas where implants are planned, biomaterials that allow transitional ARP with good resorption profile should be selected. Synthetic materials such as resorbable hydroxyapatite and allografts such as FDBA can be used in such clinical scenarios. For short-term ARP, DFDBA or a combination of autogenic bone with other graft materials like DFDBA can be used.

Membranes are commonly used to prevent the highly proliferating epithelial cells to enter the defect, thereby allowing the osteogenic cells to synthesize bone in and around the scaffold used. For socket preservation procedures, bioresorbable membranes such as collagen membranes (e.g. Bio-Gide, Ossix) are commonly used [11]. Collagen with different degrees of cross-linking has been shown to have different resorption profiles, providing a range of membranes for different clinical situations. Another option is to use a nonresorbable membrane such as high-density polytetrafluoroethylene membrane (e.g. Cytoplast). The extent and morphology of the defect are some of the factors that dictate the selection of nonresorbable versus resorbable membranes. Studies have shown that acellular dermal matrix allograft (e.g. AlloDerm), which is commonly used for soft tissue augmentation procedures in periodontics, can also be used as a membrane for socket preservation procedures [12].

E. In the early days, ARP was performed using hydroxyapatite in the form of root-shaped cones. Currently, socket preservation is mostly performed using particulate bone grafts and a resorbable barrier membrane. Different ARP techniques and their modifications are available and a more generic technique is described here.

Briefly, the procedure starts with minimally traumatic extraction, followed by complete debridement (curetting) of the socket and then grafting the socket with the bone graft particles. After the bone graft particles are packed into the socket, a barrier membrane is placed over the bone graft (and tucked underneath the buccal and palatal/lingual flaps) to contain or stabilize the graft particles and also to prevent epithelial ingrowth into the defect. After obtaining adequate anesthesia, a sulcular incision is made circumferentially around the tooth to be extracted in order to sever the supracrestal soft tissue attachment. The flaps can be reflected at this point to enhance access and visibility. Periotomes or physics forceps and/or tooth sectioning can be employed at this point to luxate the tooth from the socket in a minimally traumatic fashion. Once the tooth is extracted, the socket should be inspected for any remaining granulation tissue, periodontal ligament, or periapical pathologies. If the extracted tooth root(s) are close to the maxillary sinus, necessary clinical evaluation to rule out oro-antral communication should be performed. The intactness of the socket walls, especially the buccal wall which is usually thin, should be evaluated. Bone graft particles are hydrated as per instructions. Once the socket is degranulated and cleaned, well-hydrated bone graft particles are incrementally packed into the socket and gently condensed. Appropriate membrane with adequate length to cover the socket should be selected and trimmed in such a way that 3–4 mm of the membrane extends beyond the socket margin into sound host bone. The membrane is then placed over the bone graft particles, tucking it underneath the buccal and palatal/lingual flaps. The flaps are positioned to cover as much of the membrane as possible and sutured in place. Complete primary closure is not an absolute requisite for this procedure. Interrupted sutures can be placed in the two adjacent interdental papillae, and a horizontal mattress suture or a criss-cross suture can be used in the socket area (see Figure 7.3.5E). The patient will be seen after one or two weeks for the postoperative visit, during which remaining sutures will be removed [13].

F. If an implant is planned in the site that requires extraction, ARP should be an important consideration at the time of extraction. In the esthetic zone, ARP should be considered at the time of extraction, even if a fixed partial denture is planned for better esthetic outcomes at the pontic site(s).

Acute dental infection (abscess, sinus, or fistula) associated with the tooth that needs extraction is a contraindication for ARP as the failure rate of bone grafting in the presence of active bacterial infection is high. In such cases, following extraction and debridement, the patient should be placed on antibiotics for one to two weeks and after initial healing, the site can be reopened and full-fledged ridge augmentation should be performed. Another contraindication is oro-antral communication (in maxillary posterior sites), in which case the communication should be addressed and the socket allowed to heal first, prior to augmentation.

G. How long the clinician has to wait following ARP and prior to implant placement depends on various factors that include the size and shape of the socket, the biomaterials employed, the density of host bone, and the surgical skill of the operator. For example, the type of bone graft used tends to have a huge influence on the time it takes for bone regeneration to occur because different bone grafts tend to have different resorption profiles. A consensus report published by Hämmerle et al. in 2004 [14] classifies the implant placement after extraction into four types based on the length of time from extraction to implant placement. The type 4 (>16 weeks) protocol allows the placement of dental implants in clinically healed bone. With the addition of another biomaterial such as bone grafts in the extraction socket, a wait of 6–12 months is considered adequate prior to implant placement. With respect to the predictability of dental implants, studies have clearly indicated that the success rate of implants placed on grafted bone (>95%) is highly comparable with implants placed on native bone [15]. The torque required to remove dental implants placed in bone-grafted sites compared with nongrafted sites was shown to be highly comparable [16].

H.
- Case selection: both site and patient selections are important to the success of any periodontal procedure. Patients with no relevant medical conditions and a negative history of smoking tend to have better outcomes than a patient who is a chronic smoker as well as a person with uncontrolled diabetes.
- Initial socket morphology: the greater the number of walls of the socket present, the better the outcome.
- Surgical skills of the operator: minimal trauma during extraction, proper soft tissue management, and appropriate suturing to prevent membrane/graft loss are important factors.
- The type of bone graft used: autogenous versus osteoconductive versus alloplastic materials.

I.
Postoperative Complications
- Flap opening due to early loss of sutures
- Membrane loss and early loss of graft particles
- Infection

- Fibrous encapsulation and poor healing
- Injury to the neurovascular structure (if present in close proximity to the socket)

Typical Postoperative Regimen

- Antibiotic: amoxicillin 500 mg t.i.d. for seven days, or azithromycin in penicillin-allergic patients
- Pain medications: with or without codeine (as needed)
- Chlorhexidine mouth rinse (twice daily for 7–10 days)

J.

- Longer healing period is required, prior to implant placement, compared with regular extraction socket healing.
- Invasive and more technique-sensitive than extraction alone.
- May need to place the patients on a postoperative antibiotic regimen (development of antibiotic resistance).
- Additional cost associated with the use of biomaterials and antibiotics.

Case 4

Ridge Split and Osteotome Ridge Expansion Techniques

Case 4A

CASE STORY

A 53-year-old female was referred from her prosthodontist for a dental implant consultation pertaining to the patient's upper right edentulous area (Figure 7.4.1). The patient's chief complaint was the inability to properly masticate food due to the lack of multiple posterior teeth.

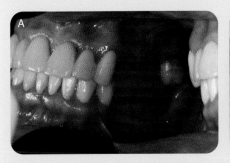 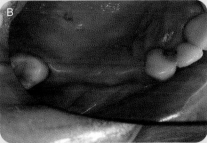 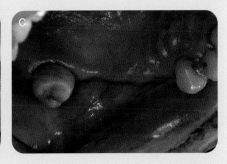

Figure 7.4.1 Preoperative clinical presentation of maxillary right quadrant: (A) buccal view; (B) occlusal view; (C) palatal view.

LEARNING GOALS AND OBJECTIVES

■ To identify the indications and rationales for ridge split
■ To understand the surgical technique for ridge split with simultaneous implant placement
■ To understand the presurgical and postsurgical considerations

Medical History

The patient's medical history was not significant. The patient was not taking any medications and denied having any allergies.

Review of Systems

• Vital signs
  o Blood pressure: 128/76 mmHg
  o Pulse rate: 68 beats/minute
  o Respiratory rate: 14 breaths/minute

Social History

The patient never smoked but occasionally drank alcohol during social events. The patient never used any recreational drugs.

Oral Hygiene Status

The patient brushed twice a day and flossed at least once a day.

Extraoral Examination

No significant findings were present.

Intraoral Examination

- Oral cancer screening was negative. Soft tissues including buccal mucosa, hard and soft palate, floor of the mouth, and tongue all appeared normal.
- There was overall an adequate amount of attached keratinized gingiva present on all remaining teeth.
- The patient had excellent oral hygiene with minimal amount of plaque accumulation and gingival inflammation.
- A full periodontal charting was completed (Figure 7.4.2).

- There was some mild clinical attachment loss with no probing depths of greater than 3 mm, no tooth mobility, and no furcation invasion.
- The patient was partially edentulous and was missing teeth #1, 3, 4, 5, 7, 12, 13, 14, 16, 17, 18, 19, 20, 29, 30, 31 and 32. All the remaining teeth were temporized.
- A Seibert class I defect was present on maxillary right quadrant.

Occlusion

The patient had Angle's class I canine occlusion. The patient was wearing maxillary and mandibular removable partial dentures for posterior occlusal support. No occlusal interferences and fremitus were detected.

Radiographic Examination

There was no evidence of periapical radiolucencies and pathologic lesions (Figure 7.4.3). With respect to edentulous sites #3, #4 and #5, preoperative computed tomography (CT) revealed mainly an insufficient horizontal ridge dimension for implant placement, although site #3 also exhibited slight bone loss in the vertical dimension (Figure 7.4.4).

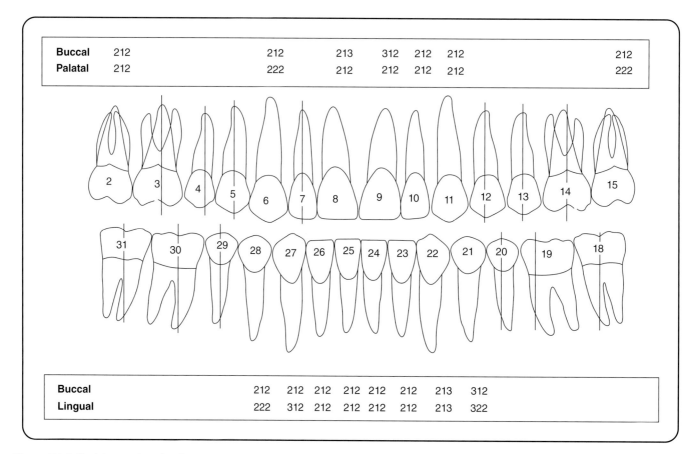

Figure 7.4.2 Probing pocket depth measurements during initial visit.

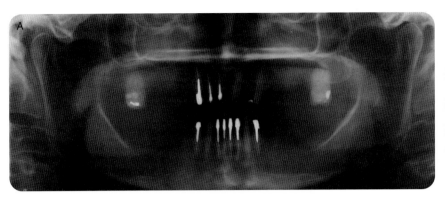
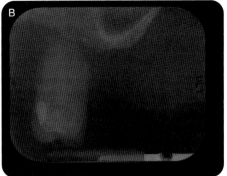

Figure 7.4.3 Preoperative radiographs: (A) panoramic radiograph; (B) periapical radiograph.

Diagnosis

A diagnosis of clinical gingival health on a reduced periodontium was given based on the clinical and radiographic examination.

Treatment Plan

Based on periodontal and prosthodontic evaluation, guided bone regeneration (GBR) using split ridge technique was recommended at edentulous sites #3, #4, and #5. After six months, a postoperative CT scan will be taken to evaluate the amount of bone generated. If adequate amount of bone is present, three implants at sites #3, #4, and #5 will be placed. Each implant will be restored with single unit crown four to six months after implant placement. Soft tissue manipulation will be done to ensure adequate amount of attached keratinized gingiva around each implant.

Treatment

The patient was encouraged to continue practicing good oral hygiene. A wax-up of edentulous sites #3, #4 and #5 was done by the prosthodontist to outline the ideal implant position and angulation.

Ridge Split Procedure

One day preoperatively, patient was given a six-day regimen of Medrol Dosepak (methylprednisolone, initial dose 24 mg/day, tapering by 4 mg/day over six days per package instructions) to reduce anticipated swelling and inflammation associated with the surgery. After achieving local anesthesia, a palatal–crestal incision was made from mesial of #2 to distal of #6 with intrasulcular incisions around #2 and #6. No vertical incisions were made. A full-thickness flap was raised using periosteal elevators to expose the native bone. Clinically, there was generally about 2–3 mm ridge width present at the crest at edentulous sites #3, #4, and #5 (Figure 7.4.5A). To preserve as much crestal bone as possible, ridge split was initiated by using a sharp no. 15 blade. Specifically, mid-crestal bone was first scored using the no. 15 blade to delineate the line of split. Then the no. 15 blade was used as a "chisel" in combination with a mallet to start the split. As shown in Figure 7.4.5B, the no. 15 blade was inserted apically to about 6–7 mm between the buccal and palatal plates. Caution was taken to avoid breaking the sinus floor while splitting the ridge. Chisel was then used to continue the split to push the two cortical plates buccal and palatally (Figure 7.4.5C). Figure 7.4.5D shows the ridge after the split. To widen and maintain the split at the crest of the ridge, surgical screws were used to push the buccal cortical plate buccally, resulting in about 3–4 mm crestal split between the two cortical plates (Figure 7.4.5E). A few tenting screws were then inserted through the buccal cortical plate to maintain the space for augmenting bone on the buccal aspect of the resorbed ridge (Figure 7.4.5F). A mixture of freeze-dried bone allograft (FDBA) and Bio-Oss was packed on the buccal aspect of the ridge defect as well as between the two split cortical plates. A bioresorbable barrier membrane was used (Figure 7.4.5G). The buccal flap was advanced coronally to allow for tension-free primary closure. The surgical site was then sutured with a few horizontal mattress and multiple single interrupted sutures (Figure 7.4.5H,I). Hemostasis was achieved and postoperative instructions and ice pack were given to the patient. Amoxicillin (500 mg t.i.d. for seven days), chlorhexidine 0.12% mouthwash (b.i.d. for seven days), and ibuprofen (800 mg every six hours as needed) were prescribed.

Sutures were removed two weeks postoperatively, and soft tissues at the surgical site were healing well with no signs of infection (Figure 7.4.5J). Two months

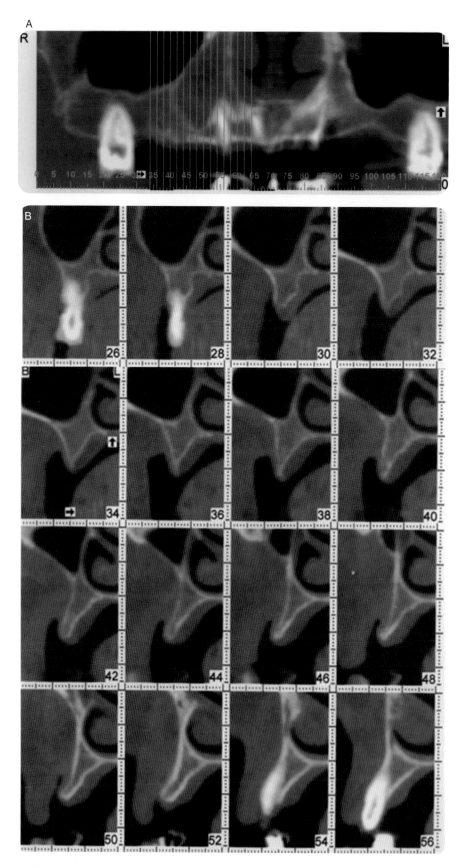

Figure 7.4.4 Preoperative CT scan of maxillary right quadrant: (A) panoramic view; (B) lateral slice cross-sectional view of edentulous sites #3, #4, and #5.

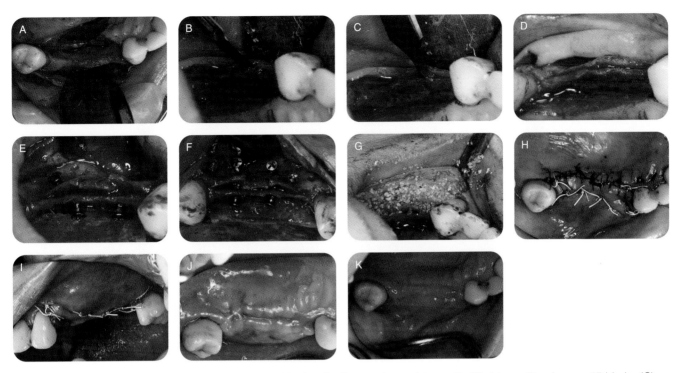

Figure 7.4.5 Ridge split at sites #3, #4, and #5: (A) residual native bone prior to ridge split; (B) ridge split using no. 15 blade; (C) ridge split using chisel; (D) ridge after the split; (E) surgical screws used to increase and maintain the split between buccal and palatal plates; (F) tenting screws used on the buccal aspect of the ridge to maintain space for buccal ridge augmentation; (G) bone grafting materials and barrier membrane in place; (H) occlusal view of primary closure of the surgical site; (I) buccal view of primary closure of the surgical site; (J) two-week postoperative surgical site; (K) two-month postoperative surgical site.

postoperatively, the surgical site appeared healthy and clinically there was evidence of augmentation at sites #3, #4, and #5 (Figure 7.4.5K). The area was temporized with a fixed provisional prosthesis.

A CT scan was taken six months postoperatively with the patient wearing the radiographic stent indicating the proposed ideal implant position. The CT showed a tremendous amount of bony augmentation, on

average 5 mm, on the buccal aspect of the previously resorbed alveolar ridge (Figure 7.4.6).

Clinically, there was a significant amount of bone regenerated at the ridge split area six months after ridge augmentation (Figure 7.4.7A,B). Three Straumann tissue level implants 4.1 × 10 mm RN, 4.1 × 10 mm RN, and 4.8 × 10 mm WN were placed at sites #3, #4, and #5, respectively (Figure 7.4.7C–F).

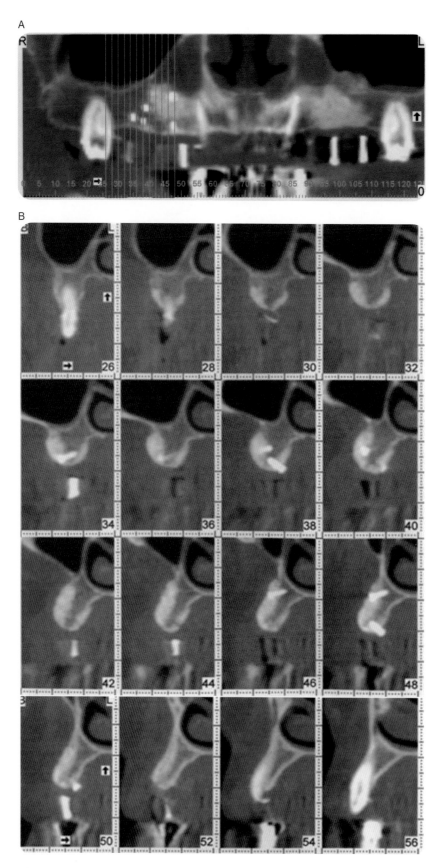

Figure 7.4.6 Postoperative CT scan of maxillary right quadrant: (A) panoramic view; (B) lateral slice cross-sectional view of edentulous sites #3, #4, and #5.

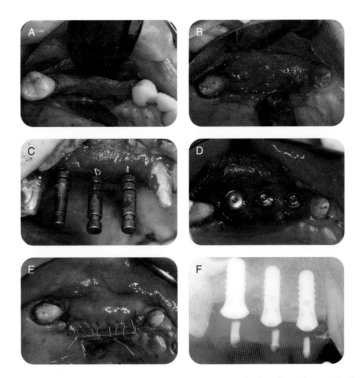

Figure 7.4.7 Ridge augmented site and implant placement: (A) pre-augmented alveolar ridge; (B) alveolar ridge six months after augmentation; (C) implant guide pins showing implant position at sites #3, #4, and #5; (D) implant placement in alveolar ridge; (E) occlusal view of primary closure of the surgical site; (F) periapical radiograph showing implant placement in alveolar ridge.

Case 4B

CASE STORY

The patient was a 48-year-old woman who was referred by the prosthodontist for evaluation for an implant placement on #9; the tooth had been extracted two years ago. There was an existing ridge deformity and the referring clinician had been worried that there was insufficient bone in the buccolingual direction for an implant placement. The patient's chief complaint was to have the tooth replaced with an implant and a single crown and restore the maxillary anterior sextant with single ceramo-metal crowns. Figure 7.4.8 illustrates the clinical situation at the first periodontal examination.

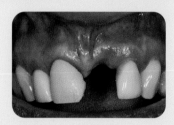

Figures 7.4.8 Preoperative view.

LEARNING GOALS AND OBJECTIVES

- To identify the indications and rationale for osteotome ridge expansion
- To understand the surgical technique for ridge expansion with simultaneous implant placement
- To understand the presurgical and postsurgical considerations

Medical History

The patient was healthy and received a medical examination every year. She did not take medications and did not report any allergies or any medical problems.

Review of Systems

- Vital signs
  - Blood pressure: 125/75 mmHg
  - Pulse rate: 60 beats/minute (regular)

Social History

The patient did not drink alcohol; she did not smoke and denied using recreational drugs.

Extraoral Examination

No significant findings were noted. The patient had no masses or swelling and the temporomandibular joints were within normal limits.

Intraoral Examination

- The soft tissues of the mouth appeared normal and the oral cancer screen was negative.
- The gingival examination in the maxillary anterior sextant revealed a thick and flat periodontium with localized mild marginal erythema, rolled margins, and blunted papillae (Figure 7.4.8).
- A hard tissue examination had been completed by the prosthodontist, who had found enough sound tooth structure available for the prosthetic restoration of teeth #7, #8, #10 and #11.
- A periodontal examination was completed by the periodontist and all probing depths were within normal limits of 2–3 mm and clinical attachment level <2 mm. with no bleeding on probing.
- The edentulous ridge on site #9 had a ridge deformity in the buccolingual direction (Seibert class I).

Occlusion

The canine and molar relationships were Angle class I. There was a posterior group function in lateral excursion, anterior guidance in protrusion, and 1 mm of overbite with 2 mm of overjet in the anterior sextant. No fremitus or interferences detected.

Radiographic Examination

There was no evidence of periapical radiolucencies or horizontal or vertical bone loss, and the lamina dura was visible and continuous (Figure 7.4.9).

Diagnosis

A diagnosis of clinical gingival health on an intact periodontium was given based on the clinical and radiographic examination.

Treatment Plan

Periodontal, prosthodontic, endodontic evaluations were performed to assess the restorability of the teeth. The

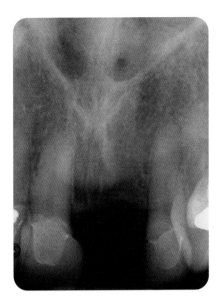

Figure 7.4.9 Preoperative radiograph.

multidisciplinary team deemed the teeth restorable with ceramo-metal crowns and without endodontic treatment for teeth #7, #8, and #10, a ridge augmentation procedure for edentulous area of #9 followed by single tooth replacement for #9 with an implant-retained ceramo-metal crown.

Treatment

The patient received oral hygiene instructions and prophylaxis. A wax-up of the anterior sextant was performed by the prosthodontist as well as fabrication of a surgical guide.

Preoperative Consultation

The medical history was reviewed. Clinical and radiographic examinations were performed. The amount of remaining native bone was determined by bone sounding after local infiltration of anesthesia in the edentulous area of #9. Alternatively, a CT scan could have been taken to more accurately determine the existing bone dimensions. It was determined that the existing bucco-lingual dimension of the edentulous ridge was approximately 4 mm in width and sufficient to place a 4-mm implant fixture with a simultaneous ridge augmentation procedure or ridge expansion. A consent form addressing benefits and risks associated with the procedure was reviewed with the patient. The following preoperative prescriptions were delivered to the patient: amoxicillin 500 mg (t.i.d. for seven days starting the night prior to procedure), ibuprofen 600 mg (every four to six hours, as needed for pain), and Peridex 0.12% (b.i.d.).

Ridge Expansion Procedure

Anesthesia of the maxillary anterior sextant was achieved by local infiltration of lidocaine 2% (epinephrine 1:100 000). A surgical incision was made on the palatal–crestal edentulous ridge of #9 with a vertical releasing incision on the mesiobuccal line angle of #10 and a vertical releasing incision preserving the papillae along the frenum on the mesiobuccal line angle of edentulous #9 (see outline in Figure 7.4.10).

A full-thickness flap elevation was done to expose the crestal bone and the surgical guide was placed to determine the optimum prosthetic implant position, which guided the initial 2-mm twist drill to final length for the initial implant osteotomy (Figure 7.4.11).

After the initial osteotomy of 2 mm, the remaining bony wall from the buccal aspect was about 1 mm and from the palatal aspect about 1.5 mm in thickness; because the desired implant fixture was 4 mm in diameter, two drilling sequences for the final osteotomy needed to be performed; however, if performed, the risk of a full dehiscence or complete destruction of any of the remaining bony walls was evident. Thus, a 2.5-mm tapered osteotome was inserted into the 2-mm osteotomy and tapped to final length (Figure 7.4.12A). Although there was a fenestration on the apical extent on the buccal side due to normal ridge concavity, the coronal bony wall remained intact. A 3-mm tapered osteotome was then inserted and tapped to final length, followed by a 3.5-mm osteotome, also tapped to final length (Figure 7.4.12B). A 4.2 × 10 mm implant

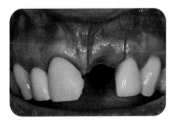

Figure 7.4.10 Incision design.

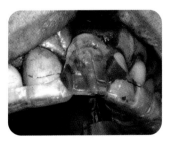

Figure 7.4.11 The full-thickness flap reflection with the surgical guide in place and the 2-mm twist drill in the correct prosthetic position.

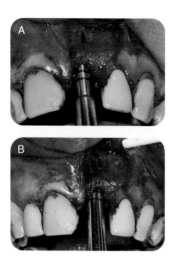

Figure 7.4.12 (A, B) The sequential osteotome expansion.

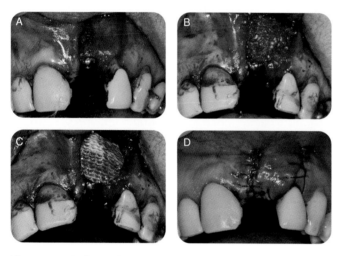

Figure 7.4.13 Steps followed after osteotome expansion was completed: (A) implant placement; (B) FDBA placement; (C) collagen membrane adapted; (D) primary closure and suturing.

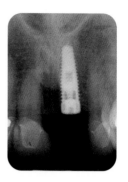

Figure 7.4.14 Postoperative radiograph.

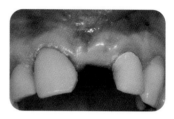

Figure 7.4.15 Healing response six months postoperatively.

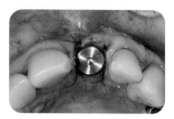

Figure 7.4.16 Implant exposure and healing abutment by means of an apically repositioned flap.

fixture was then placed into the expanded osteotomy to 35 N·cm torque with primary stability (Figure 7.4.13A). A freeze-dried bone allograft (FDBA) was placed on the buccal aspect in order to cover the existing fenestration and to augment the remaining buccal bone (Figure 7.4.13B). A resorbable cross-linked bovine collagen membrane was placed over the bone graft (Figure 7.4.13C). A tension-free flap was repositioned and secured in placed with sutures, obtaining primary closure (Figure 7.4.13D). A radiograph was taken to verify the position of the implant fixture (Figure 7.4.14). Full clearance in area of #9 of the transitional removable prosthesis was created in order to avoid any pressure on the surgical site.

Postoperative instructions including oral hygiene were delivered and an ice pack was placed against the patient's lip.

The patient was seen for a postoperative consultation at 14 days for suture removal and at one, three, and six months (Figure 7.4.15). After six months of healing and osseointegration, implant was exposed on a stage 2 procedure using an apically repositioned flap procedure where implant stability was tested and a healing abutment was placed (Figure 7.4.16).

After four weeks, the healing abutment was replaced by a final prosthetic ceramic abutment on implant #9 torqued at 35 N·cm, and adjacent #7, #8, and #10 were prepared for a final single-unit crown restoration (Figure 7.4.17). Two weeks later the final restorations on these teeth were delivered and the final restorations for all mandibular anterior teeth completed (Figure 7.4.18).

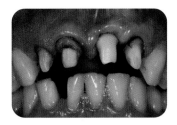

Figure 7.4.17 Placement of a full ceramic esthetic abutment on implant #9 and final preparation of teeth #7, #8, and #10.

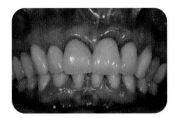

Figure 7.4.18 Final delivery of permanent restorations and completion of the case.

Discussion

A clinician can choose from a variety of treatment modalities to provide dental implant therapy for alveolar ridge deformities. With respect to the cases presented here, the choices for treatment may include a guided bone regeneration (GBR) procedure and a subsequent implant placement or implant placement with simultaneous bone grafting of the remaining bony walls or implant surfaces, among others. Ultimately, the choice of treatment relies on the amount of native bone remaining as well as the clinical expertise of the clinician. In Case 4A, a ridge split technique was performed without simultaneous implant placement due to a considerable amount of buccal concavity at the edentulous site and the amount of bone remaining on the crest of the alveolar ridge (2–3 mm), which was insufficient to obtain implant stability. A ridge split technique was used in conjunction with a bone graft anticipating the native bone to provide containment and stability of the bone grafting material as well as supply osteogenic cells for bone regeneration (see Question B for advantages of ridge split procedure).

In contrast, in Case 4B the amount of native bone remaining was sufficient to provide primary stability of

the implant; in this case osteotome expansion allowed the preservation of the buccal and palatal native bone that otherwise would have been drilled away if a standard implant placement protocol was followed. Although the bone expansion allowed for the preservation of the native bone, the remaining buccal wall was thinner than the suggested 1.5–2 mm outlined in the literature and thus the need for bone graft material in order to increase the buccal bone width was evident.

When discussing the specifics of each approach, one could argue the use of different instrumentation to achieve the desired goal; for instance, in Case 4A, a no. 15 blade was used as a chisel in conjunction with light tapping with a mallet to initiate the split and preserve as much bone as possible. Alternatively, one could have used bone chisels, piezosurgical tips, or a bone saw. However, it is necessary to keep in mind that the thinner the bone cutting instrument, the better preservation of the native bone is attained. In Case 4B, the initial 2-mm twist drill was used to initiate the osteotomy followed by sequential use of the osteotome; conversely, one could have considered the use of slightly tapered bone expanders or threaded and noncutting drill bits of different diameters that attach to a handpiece or hand ratchet. One could argue that tapping of the osteotome at the time of expansion could be more traumatic for the patient and the bone itself compared with use of expanding bits, although according to the literature both are equally successful; in either case the direction of travel of the osteotome or expanding bit is critical since the implant will follow this path.

Like other GBR surgeries, the success of a ridge split or expansion procedure depends on (i) the medical status of the patient for an optimal host response, (ii) the availability of osteogenic cells from the surgical site, (iii) the vascularity of the surgical site, (iv) the stability and turnover rate of the bone graft materials, (v) epithelial exclusion through a barrier membrane, and (vi) the soft tissue management to achieve primary closure. Factors that would lead to less favorable results include infection, absence of primary closure, sloughing of flap edges with soft tissue dehiscence, loss of bone graft materials, and lack of implant stability if implants are simultaneously placed [1,2].

Self-Study Questions

A. What is the purpose of ridge split and osteotome ridge expansion?

B. What are the advantages and indications for performing ridge split or ridge expansion?

C. What are the disadvantages, limitations, and complications associated with ridge split and ridge expansion procedures?

D. Describe Seibert's classification system for alveolar ridge defect.

E. How are ridge split and osteotome ridge expansions performed?

F. What are the criteria for performing ridge split and osteotome ridge expansion?

Answers located at the end of the chapter.

ACKNOWLEDGMENT

Special thanks to Dr. Jacob Pourati for his contribution to this chapter.

References

1. Coatoam GW, Mariotti A. The segmental ridge-split procedure. *J Periodontol* 2003;74(5):757–770.
2. Machtei EE. The effect of membrane exposure on the outcome of regenerative procedures in humans: a meta-analysis. *J Periodontol* 2001;72(4):512–516.
3. Donos N, Mardas N, Chadha V. Clinical outcomes of implants following lateral bone augmentation: systematic assessment of available options (barrier membranes, bone grafts, split osteotomy). *J Clin Periodontol* 2008;35(8 Suppl):173–202.
4. Tonetti MS, Hämmerle CH; European Workshop on Periodontology Group C. Advances in bone augmentation to enable dental implant placement: Consensus Report of the Sixth European Workshop on Periodontology. *J Clin Periodontol* 2008;35(8 Suppl):168–172.
5. Peñarrocha M, Pérez H, Garciá A, Guarinos J. Benign paroxysmal positional vertigo as a complication of osteotome expansion of the maxillary alveolar ridge. *J Oral Maxillofac Surg* 2001;59(1):106–107.
6. Kaplan DM, Attal U, Kraus M. Bilateral benign paroxysmal positional vertigo following a tooth implantation. *J Laryngol Otol* 2003;117(4):312–313.
7. Flanagan D. Labyrinthine concussion and positional vertigo after osteotome site preparation. *Implant Dent* 2004;13(2):129–132.
8. Seibert JS. Reconstruction of deformed, partially edentulous ridges, using full thickness onlay grafts. Part I. Technique and wound healing. *Compend Contin Educ Dent* 1983;4(5):437–453.
9. Rambla-Ferrer J, Peñarrocha-Diago M, Guarinos-Carbó J. Analysis of the use of expansion osteotomes for the creation of implant beds. Technical contributions and review of the literature. *Med Oral Patol Oral Cir Bucal* 2006;11(3):E267–271.

TAKE-HOME POINTS

A. Both ridge split and osteotome ridge expansion procedures are surgical approaches used to augment atrophic edentulous alveolar ridges in order to generate adequate amount of bone for implant placement (see previous chapters for discussion of other types of bone grafting procedures).

Ridge split is usually performed over a larger span of the edentulous area rather than a single tooth site. In ridge split, implants can be placed either concomitant with the procedure or at a later time, depending on the size of the ridge defect, the presence of implant primary stability, and the appropriateness of the anticipated implant angulation.

In osteotome ridge expansion, an implant is usually placed simultaneously with ridge expansion, as the implant is needed to maintain the expansion. In both cases the bone is subject to fractures or micro-fractures; the traumatic events will initiate a bone healing response and the preservation of as much native bone as possible will aid the availability of osteoprogenitor cells for regeneration of the defect and the added bone graft material.

B. Among the factors for a predictable ridge split procedure for alveolar ridge augmentation is the concept that the bone grafting material is placed in a well-contained, "four-wall" defect between two cortical bony plates. This four-wall defect will also provide a sufficient number of osteogenic cells for bone regeneration [3,4].

Ridge split and ridge expansion techniques allow simultaneous implant placement in an atrophic alveolar ridge that otherwise would not have been possible. Note that the ridge expansion technique is almost always done with simultaneous implant placement.

Unlike onlay bone grafting procedures, ridge split and ridge expansion procedures do not require a second surgical site to harvest a block of autogenous bone. Hence, these procedures reduce the morbidities associated with bone harvesting.

Comparing this technique to a procedure where an implant is placed over a thin shell of cortical plate or bony dehiscence that requires additional bone grafting, ridge split and ridge expansion techniques are more advantageous because a minimal amount of bone is lost during the procedures. Oftentimes, a lesser amount of bone grafting materials is required during simultaneous implant placement.

C. Performing a ridge split or ridge expansion procedure produces a traumatic event in the bone and thus, depending on the surgical experience of the clinician and the quality of the patient's bone, splitting or expanding the alveolar ridge may sometimes result in unintentional fracture or displacement of cortical plate(s) which may lead to bone necrosis of the displaced segment. In certain areas of the

mandible where the cortical bone is denser with lower plasticity and the alveolar ridge too thin (usually <3 mm), a ridge split procedure represents a higher risk and may not be recommended. In addition, tapping on the alveolar ridge using a surgical mallet may be unpleasant for the patient. An uncontrolled force applied during these procedures could damage anatomic structures such as nerves, arteries and facial spaces, among others, so caution most be exercised and therefore site and case selection are important. Typically, osteotome ridge expansion is not recommended in the mandible, so alternative expansion techniques should be considered, such as the use of expansion bits as outlined in the discussion. Although chisels could be used for a mandibular ridge split, when addressing a surgical site in the mandible one should also consider alternative instrumentation.

Other side effects that patients may develop as a result of these procedures and which have been reported in the literature include postoperative nausea, vomiting, and dizziness. In more serious situations, patients may develop benign paroxysmal positional vertigo and labyrinthine concussion due to traumatic percussion from tapping [5–7]. These complications are self-limiting and usually last for several days to a week. Finally, local paresthesias, transitional or permanent could occur due to the nature of the instrumentation and the damage to nerves that are in close proximity to the surgical site.

D. Seibert's classification of alveolar ridge defect [8] is as follows.

- Class I defect: buccolingual loss of tissue with normal ridge height in apico-coronal dimension.
- Class II defect: apico-coronal loss of tissue with normal ridge width in buccolingual dimension.
- Class III defect: combined buccolingual and apico-coronal loss of tissue resulting in loss of normal ridge height and width.

E.
Ridge Split
The operator should make a soft tissue incision slightly palatal or lingual to mid-crest where the ridge will be split. After raising a full-thickness flap and

removing all the soft tissue tags, the operator will determine the extent of the alveolar ridge defect. Should the defect qualify for ridge split, the procedure can then be started. First, use a sharp chisel or a no. 15 blade to score a line along the crest of the alveolar ridge. The score line should come no closer than 2 mm from the adjacent teeth [1]. Deepen the entire score line to about 3 mm by using a surgical mallet to gently tap on the flat end of the chisel. Continue to deepen the entire score line until desired depth has been reached. Alternatively, the score line can be made by using piezosurgical tips. Piezosurgery offers ease in making the initial score line; however, about 1 mm of crestal bone will be lost when using piezosurgery because the piezosurgical cutting tip is itself about 1 mm in thickness. Depending on the preference of the clinician, bony vertical releases at the two ends of the crestal bony incision/split line can then be made. Gently separate the two cortical plates of the split ridge as much as possible by twisting the chisel while preventing fracture of the bony plates to maintain bone vitality. If the surgical site allows for the simultaneous placement of the implant, prepare the implant osteotomy utilizing the drilling sequence that best fits the split to the desired diameter and length. However, if only a bone-grafting procedure is desired, place the bone grafting material between the two cortical plates. On some occasions surgical screws can be used in a buccopalatal/buccolingual direction to maintain the space created between the two cortical plates. A membrane barrier may be used prior to closure of the flaps. It is crucial to achieve tension-free primary closure to ensure optimal bone grafting results.

Ridge Expansion with Osteotomes

Ridge expansion is usually performed in conjunction with implant placement and is similar to performing osteotome sinus elevation [9]. After full-thickness flap elevation is achieved, a surgical guide is used to determine the optimal position of the implant fixture; then, a 2-mm twist drill is used to final length to obtain the initial implant osteotomy.

After the initial osteotomy of 2 mm, it is necessary to determine the amount of residual buccal and palatal bone and the diameter of the desired implant fixture, accounting for an optimal buccal and palatal bone width of 1.5–2 mm prior to final insertion of the implant. Insert and tap into a final length a 2.5-mm osteotome, remove, and then repeat the procedure with the 3-mm osteotome; continue the same sequence until the final diameter of the desired implant fixture minus 0.5 mm has been achieved. Place implant and ensure primary stability. If any of the remaining bony walls are less than 1.5–2 mm in width, place a bone graft material on the bony surface, cover it with a barrier membrane, and ensure tension-free primary flap closure or proceed with stage 1 implant.

F.

Ridge Split

- It can be done for individual sites in the mandible or maxilla.
- A minimum of 3 mm of existing bone is needed.
- Usually performed in large edentulous areas, but can be done for single-tooth edentulous sites as long as the split is kept at 2 mm from the adjacent teeth.
- Beware of the limitations outlined in Question C.

Ridge Expansion

- It can be done for individual or multiple implant sites.
- A minimum of 4 mm of existing native bone is needed.
- Limited to maxillary sites when utilizing osteotomes. However, if performing expansion in mandibular edentulous sites, consider use of expansion bits instead of osteotomes as previously described.
- Beware of the limitations outlined in Question C.

8

Dental Implants

Case 1: Conventional Implant Placement 338
Samuel Koo, DDS, MS

Case 2: Immediate Implant Placement 345
Mohamed A. Maksoud, DMD

Case 3: Sinus Lift and Immediate Implant Placement 350
Samuel Lee, DMD, DMSc, Nadeem Karimbux, DMD, MMSc, Ningyuan Sun, B.D.S, Ph.D,
and Irina F. Dragan, DDS, DMD, MS

Case 4: Implant Rehabilitation for Missing Adjacent Teeth in the Maxillary Esthetic Zone 357
Panos Papaspyridakos, DDS, PhD, MS, Behshid Bahraini, DDS, MS,
Aikaterini Papathanasiou, DDM, DMD, and Wael Att, DDS, PhD, Dr Med Dent

Case 5: Combination of Implant Single Crowns and Porcelain Veneers in the Esthetic Zone 365
Aikaterini Papathanasiou, DDM, DMD, Rayyan A. Alfirdous, BDS, MS, BMS-MS,
Dip ABOP, Abiar Alwael, DDS, MS, Panos Papaspyridakos, DDS, PhD, MS, and Wael Att,
DDS, PhD, Dr Med Dent

Case 1

Conventional Implant Placement

CASE STORY

A 38-year-old Caucasian male presented with a chief complaint of "I need a cleaning and also I have a tooth missing." The patient had not had a teeth cleaning in three years (Figure 8.1.1), and tooth #19 had been extracted elsewhere 18 months ago (Figure 8.1.2) due to extensive caries (Figure 8.1.3). The patient claimed to brush his teeth two to three times daily. He flossed once a day but denies use of any mouth rinse.

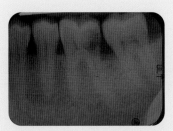

Figure 8.1.3 Tooth #19 was extracted due to large distal caries.

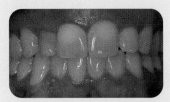

Figure 8.1.1 Preoperative frontal view.

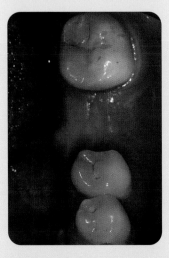

Figure 8.1.2 Missing mandibular first molar area.

LEARNING GOALS AND OBJECTIVES

- To understand the indications of implant treatment
- To interpret radiographic examinations for implant surgical planning
- To understand the sequence of conventional implant therapy

Medical History

The patient was prehypertensive but had no other significant medical problems and no known allergies. Occasionally the patient took diphenhydramine hydrochloride (Benadryl) for seasonal allergy.

Review of Systems

- Vital signs
  - Blood pressure: 138/86 mmHg
  - Pulse rate: 67 beats/minute (regular)

Social History

The patient was a social drinker (three to four glasses per weekend). Currently he did not smoke, but he had a history of social smoking for one year during college.

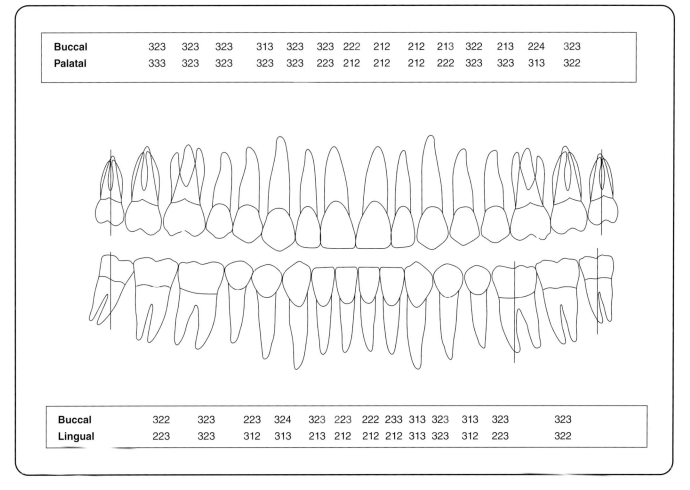

Buccal	323	323	323	313	323	323	222	212	212	213	322	213	224	323
Palatal	333	323	323	323	323	223	212	212	212	222	323	323	313	322

Buccal	322	323	223	324	323	223	222	233	313	323	313	323	323
Lingual	223	323	312	313	213	212	212	212	313	323	312	223	322

Figure 8.1.4 Probing pocket depth measurements.

Extraoral Examination
No significant findings were noted. The patient had no masses or swelling and the temporomandibular joint was within normal limits.

Intraoral Examination
- There was no lymphadenopathy and oral cancer screen was negative.
- There was an adequate band of attached gingiva. Stippling was present.
- A hard tissue and soft tissue examination was completed (Figures 8.1.4–8.1.6).

Occlusion
The patient presented normal molar relationship and no interference in excursive movements (Figure 8.1.7).

Radiographic Examination
No caries or significant crestal bone loss were seen on examination of the bitewing radiographs (Figure 8.1.8).

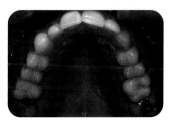

Figure 8.1.5 Occlusal view of the maxillary arch.

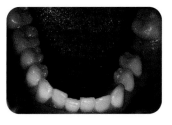

Figure 8.1.6 Occlusal view of the mandibular arch.

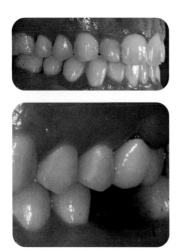

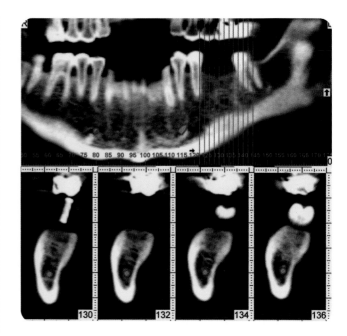

Figure 8.1.7 Normal molar occlusal relationship.

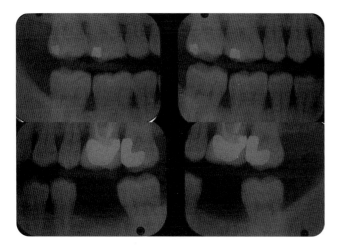

Figure 8.1.8 Bitewing radiographs depicting the interproximal bone levels.

A computed tomography (CT) image (Figure 8.1.9) revealed the presence of available bone >15 mm in height and sufficient width for wide-diameter implant placement. Therefore no bone graft was necessary for implant placement (Figure 8.1.9).

Diagnosis

The patient had partial edentulism and was diagnosed as American Dental Association (ADA) type I due to gingivitis.

Treatment Plan

The treatment plan for this patient included an initial phase of scaling with polishing and implant-supported porcelain-fused-to-metal (PFM) crown for the area of #19.

Figure 8.1.9 CT images reveal sufficient bone available for implant placement without bone graft. Radiographic guide is placed at the site of implant surgery for planning.

Treatment

After the consult and diagnostic phase, the patient received initial therapy of scaling and polishing. The patient was able to maintain good oral hygiene in follow-up visits. Study models of maxillary and mandibular arch were fabricated to evaluate adequate spacing of area #19. The mesiodistal space of missing molar #19 area was compatible with the contralateral molar. A radiographic template was fabricated before sending the patient for CT evaluation. The CT revealed adequate quantity of bone and healing of extraction site with normal pattern of trabeculation.

The patient refused the alternative treatment option of a three-unit fixed partial denture (FPD) #18-x-20 because the virgin abutment teeth would require preparation. A step-by-step description of implant therapy was discussed including possible complications. A consent form was obtained prior to the procedure.

On the day of the procedure, the patient's blood pressure was measured and it was in a similar range of hypertensive level as the initial visit. Local infiltration anesthesia was given in the surgical area with lidocaine 2% (epinephrine 1:100 000). A full-thickness flap was raised after midcrestal incision. A surgical template was used to guide sequential drilling with copious irrigation to prepare the site for implant placement (Figure 8.1.10). One-stage implant of 4.8 × 10 mm and a wide neck

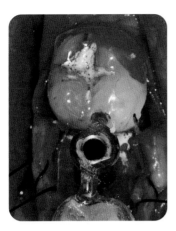

Figure 8.1.10 A surgical template was used to guide angulations of drills.

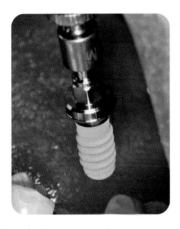

Figure 8.1.11 A wide-diameter implant was placed in the molar region.

platform for prosthesis connection was placed (Figure 8.1.11). The implant was clinically stable and a short healing abutment was screwed in (Figures 8.1.12 and 8.1.13). A periapical radiograph confirmed appropriate implant angulation and a safe distance from the inferior alveolar nerve. Flaps were sutured for primary closure. Minimum bleeding was observed before the patient left. Postoperative instructions were given. The patient received prescriptions for pain medication and an oral rinse.

One week later, sutures were removed and soft tissue was healing normally. Minimum postoperative discomfort was reported.

The prosthetic phase of the case was initiated two months after the surgery. An impression coping was attached for closed final impression using polyether. An appropriate shade was selected for porcelain fabrication. The favorable implant position allowed for selection of a prefabricated straight abutment (Figure 8.1.14).

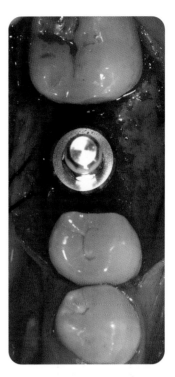

Figure 8.1.12 Implant placed in the molar area with appropriate angulation and distance from adjacent teeth.

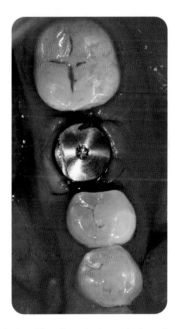

Figure 8.1.13 A short healing abutment placed and sutured for primary closure.

Four weeks after the final impression, final implant-supported PFM was cemented (Figure 8.1.15). A periapical radiograph was taken as a baseline for future reference. Oral hygiene instruction was reinforced and the patient was scheduled for recall

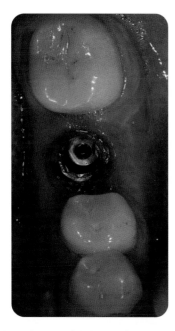

Figure 8.1.14 A straight prefabricated final abutment was used for restoration.

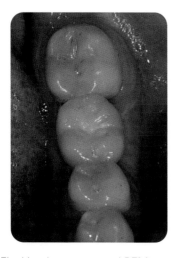

Figure 8.1.15 Final implant-supported PFM was delivered.

visit every six months. A radiograph was exposed at the first six-month follow-up (Figure 8.1.16).

Discussion

Implant-supported restorations have become routine treatment in dental practice with predictable outcomes and a high success rate [1]. However, the prevention aspect should be emphasized with patients so loss of tooth due to caries or periodontal disease may be minimized. Effective oral home care including fluoride with periodic professional visits is crucial for appropriate prevention and early detection of oral disease.

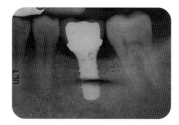

Figure 8.1.16 Postoperative periapical radiograph.

The initial therapy of oral prophylaxis and compliance with oral home care is an important factor before considering implant therapy [2]. Once the implant option is chosen, study models and radiographic images are used as part of the planning. The planning should be done with the final outcome in mind. Various radiographic examinations may be prescribed, such as conventional two-dimensional panoramic or CT, which has the advantage of three-dimensional analysis of anatomic structures with minimum distortion [3]. When the radiographic template has the appropriate angulation, the same device may be used as a surgical template. If incorrect angulation is detected in the radiograph, appropriate modification should be made before the surgery.

In radiographic analysis, important anatomic structures should be identified. Ideally in the maxilla, implants should not penetrate the maxillary sinus space. In the mandible, the apex of implants should be 2 mm away from the inferior alveolar nerve or the mental foramen. Convergence of roots should also be evaluated, especially in patients with a history of orthodontic treatment, to avoid damaging root structures during implant placement. Implant diameter is selected to give appropriate support and emergence profile for the size of the crown. However, there should be a space of approximately 2 mm from implant to root surface [4].

Once the implant is placed, a certain period of time is necessary for healing and osseointegration. Branemark et al. [5] originally suggested a healing time of four months for the mandible and six months for the maxilla. Recent advances in bone biology and implant designing have allowed a shortening of the waiting time from implant placement and final delivery of crown with predictable results [6]. In limited cases, it is also possible to extract the tooth, place the implant, and restore it all in the same day [7].

After final delivery of the restoration, the patient should be in strict recall protocol for professional oral hygiene and radiographic reevaluation.

Self-Study Questions

A. Is there any age limitation to place a dental implant?

B. What kind of radiographs could be ordered for an implant case planning?

C. What are the advantages and disadvantages of implant treatment compared with conventional FPD?

D. What is the difference between the one-stage and two-stage implant approach?

E. What are the possible postoperative complications in the short and long term?

Answers located at the end of the chapter.

References

1. Adell R, Eriksson B, Lekholm U, et al. Long-term follow-up study of osseointegrated implants in the treatment of totally edentulous jaws. *Int J Oral Maxillofac Implants* 1990;5:347–359.
2. Wennström JL, Ekestubbe A, Gröndahl K, et al. Oral rehabilitation with implant-supported fixed partial dentures in periodontitis-susceptible subjects. A 5-year prospective study. *J Clin Periodontol* 2004;31:713–724.
3. Harris D, Buser D, Dula K, et al. E.A.O. guidelines for the use of diagnostic imaging in implant dentistry. A consensus workshop organized by the European Association for Osseointegration in Trinity College Dublin. *Clin Oral Implants Res* 2002;13:566–570.
4. Buser D, Martin W, Belser UC. Optimizing esthetics for implant restorations in the anterior maxilla: anatomic and surgical considerations. *Int J Oral Maxillofac Implants* 2004;19(Suppl):43–61.
5. Branemark PI, Hansson BO, Adell R, et al. Osseointegrated implants in the treatment of the edentulous jaw. Experience from a 10-year period. *Scand J Plast Reconstr Surg Suppl* 1977;16:1–132.
6. Bornstein MM, Schmid B, Belser UC, et al. Early loading of non-submerged titanium implants with a sandblasted and acid-etched surface. 5-year results of a prospective study in partially edentulous patients. *Clin Oral Implants Res* 2005;16:631–638.
7. Misch CE, Hahn J, Judy KW, et al. Workshop guidelines on immediate loading in implant dentistry. Immediate Function Consensus Conference. *J Oral Implantol* 2004;30:283–288.
8. Op Heij DG, Opdebeeck H, van Steenberghe D, Quirynen M. Age as compromising factor for implant insertion. *Periodontol 2000* 2003;33:172–184.
9. Park SH, Wang HL. Implant reversible complications: classification and treatments. *Implant Dent* 2005;14:211–220.

TAKE-HOME POINTS

A. There is no upper age limit for implant placement as long as the patient fulfills the prerequisites for general surgery. However, an implant placed in a young patient may work as an ankylosed structure and interfere with the growth of facial bones [8]. In general, growth spurt occurs at the age of 12 years for girls and 14 for boys. However, craniofacial/skeletal growth may continue further, and individual variation may account for differences of up to six years. Therefore the chronological age is not sufficient to estimate growth cessation. A more reliable test would be superimposing tracings of cephalometric radiographs taken at least six months apart and determining the growth cessation.

B. Bitewing, periapical, and panoramic radiographs are the most common radiographic techniques in the dental setting. Bitewing is not appropriate for implant planning because it only shows a limited range of the crestal bone area. A periapical radiograph may be used in limited cases, but it may fail to show anatomic sites such as the maxillary sinus and inferior alveolar nerve. Panoramic radiograph has the advantage of showing a large area, but it has greater distortion than a periapical radiograph. Because it is a superimposed two-dimensional image, bone width cannot be determined. The CT scan is the ideal radiograph for planning since it is a three-dimensional image with minimum distortion. CT images can also be applied to software to fabricate computer-generated surgical templates.

C. The greatest advantage of a dental implant is that the preparation of neighboring teeth is avoided. The physiologic stimulation to the alveolar bone through the dental implant also prevents further bone loss. In cases where distal abutment is absent, a dental implant may be the only alternative to deliver a fixed prosthesis option. However, treatment length for an implant may be longer compared with conventional FPD, and patients may reject the idea of having surgical intervention, especially when it requires the additional steps of bone grafting.

D. Traditionally, implants were designed to be closed with the soft tissue at the time of implant placement. After a period of healing, implants would be uncovered by placing a healing abutment at the second stage. This two-stage approach would require a second surgical intervention and further waiting time for soft tissue maturation.

Other implants are designed with a longer neck; therefore soft tissue would be adapted around it instead of covering the implant at the time of placement. This one-stage approach eliminates the necessity of a second surgical intervention to expose the implant. Two-stage designed implants can be used as one-stage approach by inserting a healing abutment at the time of implant placement.

E. Some of the intraoperative surgical-related complications are as follows [9]:
- Damage of adjacent teeth
- Lack of primary stability
- Hemorrhage
- Nerve injury
- Penetration of sinus floor
- Fracture of mandible

Careful planning and knowledge of anatomy are important to avoid these types of complications. Minor complications such as a small perforation of sinus floor may not require removal of implants, and antibiotics and a decongestant may help to avoid complications. Complications such as nerve injury and fracture of the mandible require immediate removal of implant, and further treatment should be considered.

The postoperative surgical-related complications are as follows:
- Incision line opening
- Prolonged pain
- Fistula and abscess
- Peri-implantitis

Even if sutures loosen earlier than expected, the site may not require resuturing. If pain persists longer than usual, the dentist should suspect overheating during drilling preparation or carefully evaluate for possible anatomic injuries. Abscess and fistula may occur when cover screws become loose. Debridement of the implant surface in conjunction with an antibiotic may be necessary in cases of infection; implant removal may even be indicated in more advanced peri-implantitis.

Case 2

Immediate Implant Placement

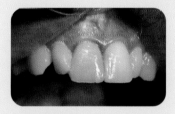
Medical History

There were no significant medical problems; however, the patient reported an allergy to penicillin. She had no known medical illnesses and exercised regularly. On questioning, the patient stated that she took no medications except for birth control pills.

Review of Systems

• Vital signs
  o Blood pressure: 118/75 mmHg
  o Pulse rate: 76 beats/minute (regular)
  o Respiratory rate: 15 breaths/minute

Social History

The patient did not drink alcohol and did not smoke (B).

Extraoral Examination

No significant findings were noted. The patient had no masses or swelling, and the temporomandibular joint was within normal limits.

Intraoral Examination

• The soft tissues of the intraoral mucosa, gingiva, palate, and tongue appeared normal.
• The gingival examination revealed a normal gingival architecture including the gingival margins and interdental papillae.
• Moderate mobility was noticed on tooth #8 with an enamel fracture line extending to the gingival margin.
• Mild tenderness to apical percussion was noted.

Occlusion

The patient demonstrated class I occlusion with slight drifting of the two central incisors buccal and downward. The interincisal relationship showed an overbite with no occlusal discrepancies or interferences (C).

Radiographic Examination

A single periapical film was ordered. On radiographic examination it was determined that tooth #8 had undergone endodontic treatment and loss of the tooth structure of the crown was evident. No periapical radiolucency was seen (Figure 8.2.2).

Diagnosis

After reviewing the history and completing the clinical and radiographic examination, a differential diagnosis was generated.

Treatment Plan

The treatment plan comprised extraction of tooth #8 followed by immediate implant insertion (D) and a temporary crown. Following the osseointegration period, a permanent crown can be fabricated (E).

Treatment

Anesthesia was achieved via infiltration buccal and lingual for the purpose of hemostasis and analgesia. Tooth #8 was extracted atraumatically. During the extraction the crown separated from the root due to a horizontal tooth fracture (Figure 8.2.3). The root was retrieved using small elevators and periotomes to preserve the integrity of the extraction socket walls (Figure 8.2.4). Following the extraction the socket was

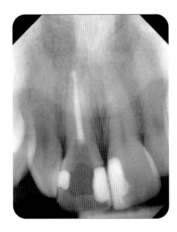

Figure 8.2.2 A periapical radiograph of the maxillary anteriors.

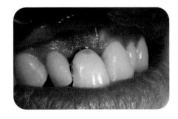

Figure 8.2.3 Preoperative view of tooth #8.

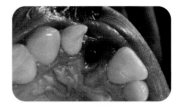

Figure 8.2.4 View following the extraction.

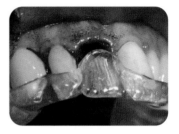

Figure 8.2.5 The surgical guide.

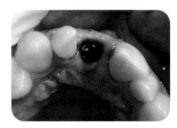

Figure 8.2.6 Implant placed.

examined and showed no granulation tissue. Using consecutive drills, the implant osteotomy was completed utilizing the surgical stent as a guide (Figure 8.2.5). The osteotomy was planned to be approximately 2 mm beyond the apical portion of the extraction socket and 2–3 mm subgingivally (Figure 8.2.6). The implant was torqued to 35 N·cm and a periapical film was taken that showed a good position of the implant in relation to the neighboring teeth and good clearance from the incisive foramen and the floor of the nasal sinuses (Figure 8.2.7). A temporary abutment was placed and restored with a provisional crown (Figure 8.2.8). Incisal occlusion was adjusted to avoid excessive forces on the implant crown, and the patient was advised to avoid biting on hard objects. Postoperative instructions were given. The patient tolerated the procedure very well. She was alert with no signs of distress upon dismissal (F).

Discussion

In this case the patient was conscious of the abnormal changes that had occurred in her dentition following trauma. Early diagnosis and treatment impact the

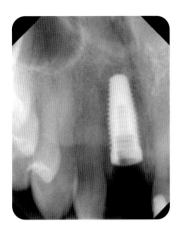

Figure 8.2.7 Postoperative radiograph.

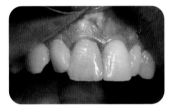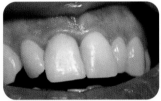

Figure 8.2.8 Preoperative and postoperative view of tooth #8.

treatment outcome. If no treatment was rendered, an infection could eventually develop that would alter the treatment plan. Antibiotics would have to be prescribed followed by a follow-up visit to determine the best treatment options based on the extent of the infection and the amount of remaining bone to host an implant with or without the need for bone augmentation.

Another treatment option would be an extraction followed by the fabrication of a fixed or removable prosthesis.

The initial stability of the immediate implant placement is crucial for the subsequent survival of the implant. This can only be accomplished by placement of the implant beyond the apical portion of the extraction socket and torqued as recommended by the implant manufacturer. An atraumatic extraction will aid in the preservation of the bone to host the implant. Finally, the placement of the implant and the provisional crown subgingivally will help preserve the interdental papillae for the best esthetic results.

Although acceptable and predictable results can be achieved when immediate implants are placed into extraction sockets, there are risk factors which should be considered at the time of treatment planning. Gingival recession on the buccal aspect of the immediate implant is a common risk factor and is related to the thickness of the buccal plate, fenestration or dehiscence and thin gingival biotype. The decision to place immediate implants into fresh extraction sockets has to be determined based on the integrity of the buccal plate on a cone beam image or with bone sounding of the extraction walls after tooth removal. Other factors that should be considered are height of the smile line, infection at the site, bone height at the adjacent teeth, restorative status of adjacent teeth, patient esthetic requirements, and overall patient health. Delayed implant placement, extraction socket augmentation, or other restorative options should be discussed as alternatives.

Self-Study Questions

A. List the local reasons why patients might present with discolored teeth. What questions in a dental history might help you begin to form a differential diagnosis?

B. What effects can smoking have on dental implants?

C. Can occlusal discrepancies and parafunctional habits be responsible for tooth fracture?

D. What are the factors to consider when recommending immediate implants?

E. What other treatment options should be considered in this case?

F. What are the possible complications associated with immediate implant placement in the anterior region?

G. What are the risk factors to be considered when treatment planning an immediate implant placement?

Answers located at the end of the chapter.

References

1. Chung EM, Sung EC. Dental management of chemoradiation patients. *J Calif Dent Assoc* 2006;34:735–742.
2. Kidd EA, Joyston-Bechal S, Smith MM. Staining of residual caries under freshly-packed amalgam restorations exposed amalgam to tea/chlorhexidine in vitro. *Int Dent J* 1990;40:219–224.
3. Billings RJ, Berkowitz RJ, Watson G. *Teeth. Pediatrics* 2004;113(4 Suppl):1120–1127.
4. Doyle SL, Hodges JS, Pesun IJ, et al. Factors affecting outcomes for single implants and endodontic restorations. *J Endod* 2007;33:399–402.
5. Proceedings of the Fourth International Team for Implantology (ITI) Consensus Conference, August 2008, Stuttgart, Germany. *Int J Oral Maxillofac Implants* 2009;24(Suppl):39–65.
6. Udoye CI, Jafarzadeh H. Cracked tooth syndrome: characteristics and distribution among adults in a Nigerian teaching hospital. *J Endod* 2009;35:334–336.
7. Cohen S, Berman LH, Blanco L, et al. A demographic analysis of vertical root fractures. *J Endod* 2006;32:1160–1163.
8. Thompson BA, Blount BW, Krumholz TS. Treatment approaches to bruxism. *Am Fam Physician* 1994;49:1617–1622.
9. De Rouck T, Collys K, Cosyn J. Single-tooth replacement in the anterior maxilla by means of immediate implantation and provisionalization: a review. *Int J Oral Maxillofac Implants* 2008;23:897–904.
10. Kan JYK, Rungcharassaeng K, Lozada J. Immediate placement and provisionalization of maxillary anterior single implants: 1-year prospective study. *Int J Oral Maxillofac Implants* 2003;18:31–39.
11. Casado PL, Donner M, Pascarelli B, et al. Immediate dental implant failure associated with nasopalatine duct cyst. *Implant Dent* 2008;17:169–175.
12. Casap N, Zeltser C, Wexler A, et al. Immediate placement of dental implants into debrided infected dentoalveolar sockets. *J Oral Maxillofac Surg* 2007;65:384–392.
13. Artzi Z, Nemcovsky CE, Bitlitum I, Segal P. Displacement of the incisive foramen in conjunction with implant placement in the anterior maxilla without jeopardizing vitality of nasopalatine nerve and vessels: a novel surgical approach. *Clin Oral Implants Res* 2000;11:505–510.
14. Razavi T, Palmer RM, Davies J, et al. Accuracy of measuring the cortical bone thickness adjacent to dental implants using cone beam computed tomography. *Clin Oral Implants Res* 2010;21:718–725.
15. Luo Z, Zeng R, Chen Z. Single implants in the esthetic zone: analysis of recent peri-implant soft tissue alterations and patient satisfaction. A photographic study. *Int J Oral Maxillofac Implants* 2011;26:578–586.

TAKE-HOME POINTS

A.

- **Foods/drinks**: coffee, tea, colas, wines, and certain fruits and vegetables (e.g. apples and potatoes) can stain teeth.
- **Tobacco use**: smoking or chewing tobacco can stain teeth.
- **Poor dental hygiene**: inadequate brushing and flossing to remove plaque and stain-producing substances like coffee and tobacco can cause tooth discoloration.
- **Disease**: treatments for certain conditions can also affect tooth color. For example, head and neck radiation and chemotherapy can cause teeth discoloration [1]. In addition, certain infections in pregnant mothers can cause tooth discoloration in the infant by affecting enamel development.
- **Medications**: the antibiotics tetracycline and doxycycline are known to discolor teeth when given to children whose teeth are still developing (<8 years of age). Mouth rinses and washes containing chlorhexidine and cetylpyridinium chloride can also stain teeth. Antihistamines (e.g. Benadryl), antipsychotic drugs, and drugs for high blood pressure also cause teeth discoloration.
- **Dental materials**: amalgam restorations can stain teeth a gray-black color [2].
- **Age**: as people age, the outer layer of enamel gets worn away revealing the natural yellow color of dentin.
- **Genetics**: some people have naturally brighter or thicker enamel than others.
- **Environment**: excessive fluoride from either environmental sources (naturally high fluoride levels in water) or excessive use (fluoride applications, rinses, toothpaste, and fluoride supplements taken by mouth) can cause teeth discoloration [3].
- **Trauma**: for example, damage from a fall can disturb enamel formation in young children whose teeth are still developing. Trauma can also cause discoloration to adult teeth due to internal bleeding.

B. There is an increased risk of peri-implantitis in smokers compared with nonsmokers. Studies have shown the survival rate of implants in smokers to be 73% [4]. The deleterious effects include impaired wound healing, reduced collagen production, impaired fibroblast function, reduced peripheral circulation, and compromised function of the neutrophils and macrophages. Heavy smokers are not good candidates for dental implants; light to medium smokers should be informed of the increased risk of peri-implantitis and implant failure [5].

C. Porcelain fracture associated with an implant-supported metal ceramic crown, or fixed partial denture occurs at a higher rate than in tooth-supported restorations, according to the literature [6]. There is a significantly higher risk of porcelain fracture in patients with bruxism habits when the patient has no protective occlusal device. In addition, parafunctional habits have resulted in vertical loss of the peri-implant bone [7,8].

D. Immediate anterior implants should be considered in cases where the configuration of the extraction is still intact and no pathology exists. The implant length should be selected 3 mm longer than the extraction socket so it will integrate into the bone beyond the apical portion for primary stability.

Subcrestal placement should be considered in anticipation of bone remodeling following the placement of the prosthesis. A bone graft should be considered to fill in the gap between the walls of the extraction socket and the implant body with the use of a membrane [9,10].

E. A fixed or removable prosthesis can be considered; however, the advantages and disadvantages of each option should be discussed with the patient.

F.
- Infection can occur due to possible preexisting pathology in the socket [11,12]
- Nerve damage to the incisive foramen [13]
- Iatrogenic damage to neighboring teeth
- Interproximal bone loss followed by loss of the interdental papillae
- Primary wound closure

G.
- Height of the smile line
- Bone height at the adjacent teeth
- Restorative status of adjacent teeth
- Patient esthetic requirements
- Patient overall health

Case 3

Sinus Lift and Immediate Implant Placement

A 43-year-old female patient was referred by an endodontist. The endodontist had diagnosed a root fracture for tooth #3 and suggested restoring the area by placing an implant after sinus grafting. The patient mentioned that she needed to return to Korea once her husband finished his work in the USA, so the treatment needed to be finished in eight months. In addition, the patient preferred to have a limited number of surgical procedures. Figure 8.3.1 shows the initial clinical and radiographic presentation.

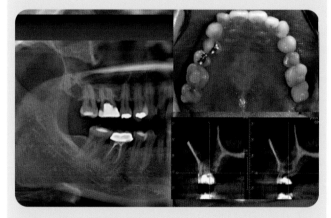

Figure 8.3.1 Initial clinical and radiographic presentation: fracture of tooth #3 after endodontic attempt; slightly thickened maxillary sinus membrane due to irritation from tooth #3.

LEARNING GOALS AND OBJECTIVES

- Understand the decision-making process for performing a simultaneous (one-visit) sinus lift/extraction and immediate implant placement
- Discuss the indications/contraindications for a sinus lift/extraction/immediate placement:
  - To learn how to perform a sinus lift from a molar extraction socket
  - To learn how to place an immediate dental implant at the time of the extraction/sinus lift

Medical History

The patient was in good health, and her last physical checkup was within six months before the presentation to the periodontal office.

Review of Systems

- Vital signs
  - Blood pressure: 107/65 mmHg
  - Pulse rate: 60 beats/minute (regular)

Social History

The patient did not drink alcohol or smoke.

Extraoral Examination

No significant findings were noted. The patient has no masses or swelling, and no trismus. There was no palpable lymphadenopathy and the temporomandibular joints were within normal limits.

Intraoral Examination

- The soft tissues of the mouth including tongue appear normal. Oral cancer screening was negative.
- The gingival examination revealed a generalized mild marginal erythema with no significant probing depths except area #3 (Figure 8.3.2).
- A hard tissue examination was completed by the referring endodontist.
- The patient had moderate pain on biting (tooth #3) and a tooth fracture was suspected (see Figure 8.3.1).

Occlusion

Canine guidance, deep bite, and a mild curve of Spee. Opposing occlusion is natural teeth.

Radiographic Examination

A digital panoramic radiograph (Figure 8.3.1) shows a temporary filling material in the pulp chamber of tooth #3. The cone beam computed tomography (CT) showed mild inflammation of the sinus membrane. There was 4 mm initial bone height from crestal bone to sinus floor (Figure 8.3.1).

Treatment

The patient received oral hygiene instructions and a prophylaxis. She was premedicated with amoxicillin 500 mg t.i.d., metronidazole 500 mg t.i.d., and Sudafed 30 mg.

Preoperative Consultation

The medical history was reviewed. The consent form addressing benefits and risks associated with the procedure was reviewed with the patient. The patient was seeking a fixed restoration so implant was recommended. Because the maxillary sinus floor was only 5 mm from the alveolar crest, a sinus grafting procedure was recommended. However, due to limited time available and upcoming travel plans, the patient requested that restoration be placed within one year.

Sinus Elevation Procedure

A posterior superior alveolar nerve block and local infiltrations were achieved with Septocaine (4% with epinephrine 1:100 000). Atraumatic extraction of tooth #3 was done, preserving buccal plate (Figures 8.3.3 and 8.3.4). A blunt-ended Glick instrument was used to probe around the socket to obtain a mental three-dimensional "view" of the socket and to ensure there were no major dehiscences or fenestrations. Several methods could be used to achieve the internal sinus lift (osteotome; vertical approach and/or crestal approach). In this case a pointed trephine bur was used to mark the location of the future implant (Figure 8.3.5). The adjustable stopper and bone ejector (ASBE) trephine was used, with the stopper set 1 mm short of the sinus floor (Figure 8.3.6). This ensures that the sharp teeth of the ASBE trephine do not penetrate the Schneiderian membrane. A slow speed is recommended to induce fracture of the bone core (Figure 8.3.7). Location and trephine should be verified again to ensure that the implant is placed in the center of the extraction socket (Figure 8.3.8). The bone core should be removed after use of the elevator to fracture it off the sinus floor (Figure 8.3.9). A flat-ended diamond drill was used to

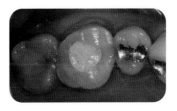

Figure 8.3.3 Preoperative view prior to extraction.

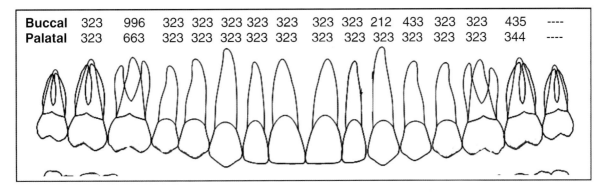

| Buccal | 323 | 996 | 323 | 323 | 323 | 323 | 323 | 323 | 323 | 212 | 433 | 323 | 323 | 435 | ---- |
| Palatal | 323 | 663 | 323 | 323 | 323 | 323 | 323 | 323 | 323 | 323 | 323 | 323 | 323 | 344 | ---- |

Figure 8.3.2 Periodontal charting at the initial consult.

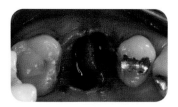

Figure 8.3.4 After extraction, note preservation of buccal plate.

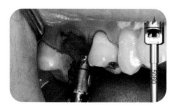

Figure 8.3.5 Pointed trephine to mark implant location precisely.

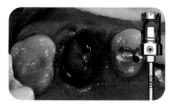

Figure 8.3.6 ASBE trephine to go 1 mm below estimated sinus floor.

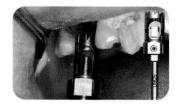

Figure 8.3.7 Slow speed is used with ASBE trephine.

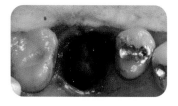

Figure 8.3.8 After ASBE trephine.

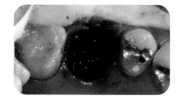

Figure 8.3.9 Bone core removed.

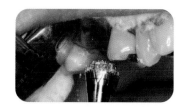

Figure 8.3.10 Flat diamond bur to expose sinus membrane.

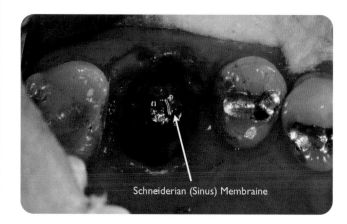

Schneiderian (Sinus) Membraine

Figure 8.3.11 Sinus membrane exposed.

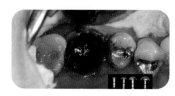

Figure 8.3.12 Series of mushroom elevators used to detach and elevate sinus membrane.

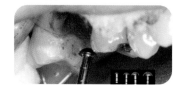

Figure 8.3.13 Mushroom elevators are also used to make crestal window larger by pulling sinus floor away from membrane.

grind away the sinus floor without perforating the Schneiderian membrane (Figure 8.3.10). Cold saline should be used to clean the socket, visualizing the Schneiderian membrane. The cold temperature reduces blood flow to the socket, thereby improving visibility of the crestal window (Figure 8.3.11). A series of mushroom elevators were used to elevate the sinus membrane (Figure 8.3.12) as well as pry away bony tips from the sinus floor, thus further enlarging the crestal window (Figure 8.3.13). A Cobra instrument was used to further elevate the sinus membrane (Figure 8.3.14), but this

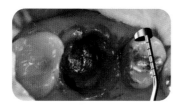

Figure 8.3.14 Cobra instrument is used to further elevate the sinus membrane.

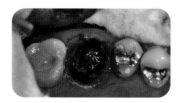

Figure 8.3.15 Movement of sinus membrane is verified to check if membrane perforation has occurred.

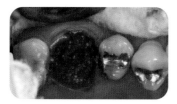

Figure 8.3.16 FDBA is introduced to sinus window as well as to socket.

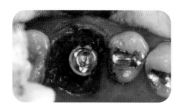

Figure 8.3.17 Implant, MegaGen Rescue 6.5 × 10 mm is placed slowly.

step can usually be skipped if the sinus membrane is thick (white color). The patient was asked to breathe in and out via her nose to verify that the membrane was not torn (Figure 8.3.15). An intact membrane moves up and down, whereas expelled air can be detected with a perforated membrane. Then, 1.5 ml of freeze-dried bone allograft (FDBA) was packed into the sinus and around the socket (Figure 8.3.16). A wide-diameter implant (MegaGen Rescue Implant 6.5 × 10 mm) was inserted slowly with good initial stability (>20 N·cm) (Figure 8.3.17). If poor initial stability is achieved, then a greater diameter implant insertion is recommended (e.g. 7.0 or 7.5 mm). A super-wide diameter healing abutment is used to seal the socket (Figure 8.3.18) to retain the bone graft material and to achieve primary closure.

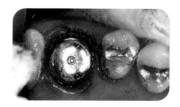

Figure 8.3.18 An 8-03 healing abutment is placed to seal the socket and retain bone graft material.

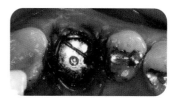

Figure 8.3.19 A 4-0 gut suture is used to further tighten and seal the socket to prevent loss of blood clot and bone graft materials.

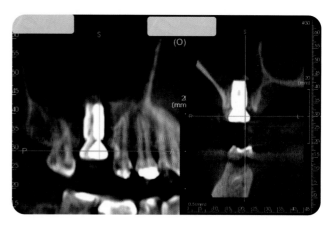

Figure 8.3.20 Postoperative CT scan showing bone graft intact under the Schneiderian membrane.

Simple interrupted sutures or continuous locking sutures are recommended with 4-0 gut chromic to further tighten and seal the socket (Figure 8.3.19). A postoperative radiograph should be taken to verify that bone graft material is retained below the Schneiderian membrane (Figure 8.3.20).

Discussion

As mentioned earlier, most crestal approaches are "blind" techniques. In contrast, this technique is not a blind technique [1]. It is especially useful in extraction of multirooted teeth, because elevation of the sinus can be achieved via the socket without laying any flap.

The average buccolingual dimension of a molar tooth is 11 mm. Therefore, the crestal approach can be done with a 5- to 6-mm window via the septum of the molar socket [2–7]. Trephine is used to cut septal bone 1 mm below the sinus wall. Slow speed (<30 rpm) and a twist of ASBE trephine when close to the sinus floor are recommended to help to fracture the septal bone away from the sinus floor. Slow speed increases friction between the bone core and inner side of the ASBE trephine, thus inducing fracture of bone. The ASBE trephine has an inner shank that can be used to expel bone core from the trephine. If the septal bone does not come out with the ASBE trephine and stays intact as in this case (Figure 8.3.8), induction of septal fracture is done with a narrow luxator or thin elevator. After removal of this bone core, flat diamond drill is used. The flat diamond drill has a large surface area at the tip of the bur, and thus creates less pressure on the Schneiderian membrane (P = F/A). As emphasized earlier, this technique is *not* a blind technique, and manual elevation is done with mini instruments with the aid of magnification (loupes).

In contrast to the conventional recommendation of a two-stage approach when the initial bone height is less than 5 mm, this unique technique shortens treatment time by six to eight months and reduces the multiple numbers of surgeries for our patients (Table 8.3.1) [3,4]. No flap is raised, and therefore patients do really well postoperatively without any pain, swelling, or bruising. Case selection is critical in these cases. Clinicians need to select cases that have low initial bone height

(1–5 mm) with wide buccolingual bone (>9 mm). If there are periapical lesions, or fracture of the buccal bone during extractions, two-stage approaches are recommended (bone graft first, sinus lift and implant later). Clinicians should strive for primary stability and not overtorque the implant. Also, care should be taken not to displace the implant into the sinus.

Initial stability is achieved with very minimal bone to implant contact. Occasionally (<10% of cases) the implant might lose stability as bone heals and therefore a monthly checkup is recommended. A dental no. 5 explorer is used on the screw hole of the healing abutment and a light shake determines the stability of an implant. If any mobility is suspected (usually in the first month after surgery), the implant is rotated out counterclockwise, and a 1-mm larger diameter implant is placed after degranulating the osteotomy site. The same healing abutment is replaced. This procedure usually takes less than three minutes, and there is no associated postoperative discomfort. This ensures that the implant will integrate well.

The use of super-large healing abutments (8–10 mm in diameter) can achieve primary closure in large extraction sockets without raising any flap. If a small gap of less than 2 mm is still present, suturing with 4-0 chromic gut is recommended. If a gap of more than 2 mm is present, collagen tape can be used around this gap, or a semilunar coronally positioned flap can be elevated to close the gap (Figures 8.3.21 and 8.3.22). This super-large healing abutment prepares the gingiva for an appropriate emergence profile for molar restoration.

Table 8.3.1 Comparison of crestal window technique with conventional two-stage approach.

Timeline	Conventional two-stage approach	Crestal window technique immediately after extraction
First surgery (4–6 months)	Extraction and ridge preservation	Extraction, sinus grafting, implant placement, ridge preservation, and one-stage surgery (healing abutment)
Second surgery (4–6 months)	Sinus grafting	Already done on first surgery
Third surgery (4–6 months)	Implant placement	Already done on first surgery
Fourth surgery (3 weeks)	Second-stage surgery	Already done on first surgery

This technique shortens treatment time threefold, and reduces multiple numbers of surgeries to patients. Therefore this is a less traumatic approach for patients needing an implant in the pneumatized posterior maxilla. Despite the fact that multiple procedures are performed simultaneously, not all clinicians might be comfortable with this approach.

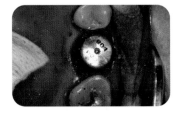

Figure 8.3.21 Palatal flap is opened even with a super-wide diameter healing abutment.

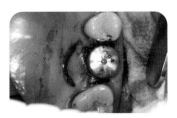

Figure 8.3.22 Semilunar coronally positioned flap used to close the palatal gap.

Self-Study Questions

A. What are the advantages of using the internal sinus lift (in this case the crestal window technique) in an extraction socket?

B. What speed is recommended when using ASBE trephine and why?

C. Which bony (wall) is the most important bone to preserve in an extraction?

D. If good initial stability of an implant is not achieved, which protocol should be followed?

E. What is the recommended postoperative follow-up with crestal window technique in an extraction socket?

F. If the gap between a super-large healing abutment and the gingival margin still exists, what are the three techniques discussed that can be used to achieve good primary closure?

G. What are two clinical advantages of using a super-large healing abutment?

H. What are the contraindications to performing a sinus lift/extraction immediate implant placement? How will one manage possible complications (perforated Schneiderian membrane, no primary stability, etc.)?

Answers located at the end of the chapter.

References

1. Lee S, Kang-Lee G, Park K-B, Han T. Crestal sinus lift: a minimally invasive and systematic approach to sinus grafting. *J Implant Adv Clin Dent* 2009;1(1):75–90.
2. Boyne PJ, James RA. Grafting of the maxillary sinus floor with autogenous marrow and bone. *J Oral Surg* 1980;38:613–616.
3. Misch CE. Maxillary sinus augmentation for endosteal implants: organized alternative treatment plans. *Int J Oral Implant* 1987;4:49–58.
4. Garg JN, Quinones CR Augmentation of the maxillary sinus. A surgical technique. *Pract Periodontics Aesthet Dent* 1997;9:211–219.
5. Summers RB. The osteotome technique: part 3. Less invasive methods of the elevating the sinus floors. *Compendium* 1994;15:698, 700, 702–704.
6. Summers RB. The osteotome technique: part 2. The ridge expansion osteotomy (REO) procedure. *Compendium* 1994;15:422, 424, 426.
7. Summers RB. A new concept in maxillary implant surgery: the osteotome technique. *Compendium* 1994;15:152, 154–156, 158.
8. Bori JE. A new sinus lift procedure: Sa-4/'O'. *Dent Implantol Update* 1991;2:33–37.
9. Smiler DG. The sinus lift graft: basic technique and variations. *Pract Periodontics Aesthet Dent* 1997;9:885–893.
10. Bruschi GB, Scipioni A, Calesini G, Bruschi E. Localize management of the sinus floor with simultaneous implant placement: a clinical report. *Int J Oral Maxillofac Implants* 1998;13:219–226.
11. Toffler M. Site development in the posterior maxilla using osteocompression and apical alveolar displacement. *Compend Contin Educ Dent* 2001;22:775–784.
12. Fugazzotto PA, De PS. Sinus floor augmentation at the time of maxillary molar extraction: success and failure rates of 137 implants in function for up to 3 years. *J Periodontol* 2002;73:39–44.
13. Winter AA, Pollack AS, Odrich RB. Placement of implants in the severely atrophic posterior maxilla using localized management of the sinus floor: a preliminary study. *Int J Oral Maxillofac Implants* 2002;17:687–695.
14. Soltan M, Smiler DG. Antral membrane balloon elevation. *J Oral Implantol* 2005;31:85–90.
15. Chen L, Cha J. An 8-year retrospective study: 1,100 patients receiving 1,557 implants using the minimally invasive hydraulic sinus condensing technique. *J Periodontol* 2005;76:482–491.
16. Wallace SS, Froum SJ. Effect of maxillary sinus augmentation on the survival of endosseous dental implants. A systematic review. *Ann Periodontol* 2003;8:328–343.
17. Yamada J, Park H. Internal sinus manipulation (ISM) procedure: a technical report. *Clin Implant Dent Relat Res* 2007;9(3):128–135.
18. Lee S, Lee G. Minimally invasive sinus grafting with autogenous bone. *Implant Tribune* 2008;3(2).
19. Petrie C, Williams JL. Comparative evaluation of implant designs: influence of diameter, length, and taper on strains in the alveolar crest. A three-dimensional finite-element analysis. *Clin Oral Implant Res* 2005;16:486–494.
20. Davarpanah M, Martinez H, Kebir M, et al. Wide diameter implants: new concepts. *Int J Periodontics Restorative Dent* 2001;21:149–159.
21. Degidi M, Piatelli A, Iezzi G, Carinci F. Wide-diameter implant: analysis of clinical outcome of 304 fixtures. *J Periodontol* 2007;78:52–58.

TAKE-HOME POINTS

A. The crestal window technique is a minimally invasive procedure, and the clinician is able to lift sinus in a predictable manner because it is not a blind technique. Because there is no flap elevation in an extraction socket, and because the socket is sealed by the implant, the patient experiences less postoperative pain. In addition, sinus lift, socket grafting, implant placement, and the one-stage approach are all done in one visit, reducing treatment time threefold compared with conventional techniques (see Table 8.3.1) [1–10].

B. Slow speed of less than 30 rpm is recommended for the ASBE trephine. Slow speed increases friction between bone core and the trephine, increasing the chance of bone core fracture from the sinus floor. Slow speed eliminates the need to use irrigation (to reduce bone heating), and thus patient comfort can be increased and visibility improved compared with high speed, which requires irrigation (1000 rpm) [11–13].

C. The buccal plate is composed of bundle bone. It is the weakest bone in an extraction socket. Therefore, preservation of buccal bone is important in immediate implant placement. No elevator should be used directly on buccal bone, and care should be taken not to fracture this thin bone.

D. If the stability of an implant is less than 10 N·cm, then a 0.5-mm larger diameter implant should be placed to increase initial stability. If an implant undergoes any micromovement, it will not integrate with bone and will be surrounded by granulation tissues. However, if buccal bone is thin and the distance from buccal plate to implant is less than 2 mm, a larger-diameter implant should not be placed. Instead, a two-stage approach with healing cap is recommended, or the open membrane technique should be used to cover the socket.

E. Initial stability decreases as bone remodels, and is weakest during the third week. Therefore, the first month checkup of these implants is crucial to check mobility. Remember that initial stability in this technique is achieved by only thin cortical bone of the sinus floor [14]. If any movement of an implant is suspected, it should be removed by counterclockwise rotation, and replaced with a 1-mm larger diameter implant. This ensures no embarrassment and surprises six months later.

F.
1. Semilunar coronally repositioned flap (Figures 8.3.21 and 8.3.22)
2. Apply CollaTape around the healing abutment
3. Suture with 4-0 chromic gut if gap is <2 mm

G. Super-large healing abutment (8–10 mm in diameter) is useful in sealing the extraction site. This technique preserves a zone of keratinized tissue and reduces patient morbidity [15–17]. It also molds tissue to achieve an appropriate emergence profile for molar restorations.

H. The contraindications for performing a sinus lift/extraction/immediate implant placement include sinus pathology, lack of buccal bone or palatal bone, and the presence of pus in a socket [18].

Small torn sinus membrane (<4 mm) can be patched with collagen membrane if access is possible. If not, lateral window can be performed to gain better access to the torn membrane, and it can be patched with collagen membrane. If the tear is greater than 7 mm, the procedure should be avoided and retried in three months [19–21].

In cases of lack of initial stability ("spinner"), a larger implant can be used to achieve better initial stability. If a larger implant cannot be used, the implant should be submerged and an open membrane technique should be employed with nonresorbable membrane. If the implant rocks mesiodistally or buccolingually, just bone grafting (socket preservation) should be employed.

Case 4

Implant Rehabilitation for Missing Adjacent Teeth in the Maxillary Esthetic Zone

A 49-year-old African American patient presented for consultation. Her chief complaint was "I want to fix my smile, I am missing my two front teeth." This patient had lost her two maxillary central incisors 11 years ago. On clinical and radiographic examination, no significant finding except minor gingival recession were observed (Figure 8.4.1). The patient reported that she did not visit her dentist regularly. She occasionally used dental floss and brushed her teeth twice daily.

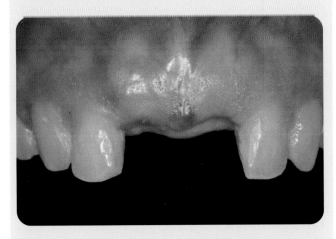

Figure 8.4.1 Preoperative presentation (frontal view).

Medical History

The patient was healthy and the medical history was not contributory.

Review of Systems

- Vital signs
  - Blood pressure: 120/75 mmHg
  - Pulse rate: 88 beats/minute (regular)
  - Respiratory rate: 16 breaths/minute

Social History

The patient did not drink alcohol and did not smoke.

Extraoral Examination

No significant findings were noted. The patient had no masses or swelling and the temporomandibular joints

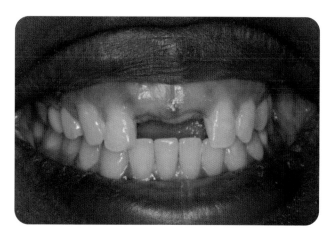

Figure 8.4.2 High smile line.

were within normal limits. There was no facial asymmetry and her lymph nodes were normal on palpation. A high smile line was noted, making the treatment of this case very challenging (Figure 8.4.2).

Intraoral Examination

- Oral cancer screening was negative.
- Soft tissue examination including tongue and floor of the mouth were within normal limits.
- Periodontal examination revealed pocket depths in the range of 2–3 mm.
- Localized areas of gingival inflammation were noted.
- Evaluation of the alveolar ridge in the areas #8 and #9 revealed minor horizontal and vertical resorption of bone (Figure 8.4.3).

Occlusion

Facial midline was coincident with dental midline with 3-mm overjet and 2-mm overbite. Maximum mouth opening was 45 mm and there were no occlusal discrepancies or interferences.

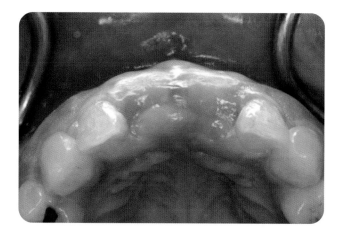

Figure 8.4.3 Preoperative presentation (occlusal view).

Radiographic Examination

Periapical radiographs of the upper anterior teeth were ordered (Figure 8.4.4). Radiographic examination revealed normal crestal bone levels. Previous amalgam restorations on #2, #12, and #15 were observed.

Diagnosis

American Academy of Periodontology (AAP) diagnosis was localized mild gingivitis. Partial edentulism was also diagnosed as class IV Kennedy classification.

Treatment Plan

An initial phase of therapy including oral prophylaxis and oral hygiene instructions to eliminate gingival inflammation was scheduled. Restoration of the missing anterior teeth with dental implants or a four-unit fixed dental prosthesis (FDP) was discussed. However, she did not want to damage her natural teeth and a removable interim prosthesis was not acceptable due to her social activity. After discussing all the options, the patient elected for treatment with dental implants.

Treatment

During the initial phase therapy, a removable Essix retainer was used to provisionalize the patient. Cone beam computed tomography (CBCT) was performed for presurgical evaluation and three-dimensional implant positioning. Intraoral digital scanning was also performed with an intraoral scanner (TRIOS; 3Shape, Copenhagen, Denmark) and the generated Standard Tesselation Language (STL) file was saved. The STL file from the intraoral scanning and the DICOM (Digital

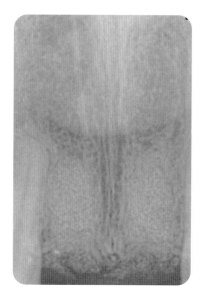

Figure 8.4.4 Initial radiograph.

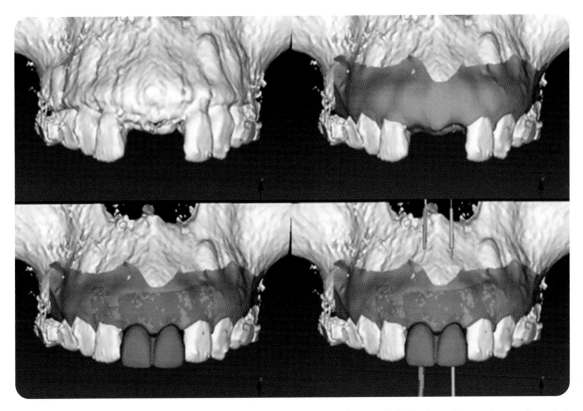

Figure 8.4.5 Digital implant planning after import of all files into planning software. STL file from intraoral scanning of the partially edentulous patient superimposed on the DICOM file and the STL file from scanned wax-up.

Imaging and Communication in Medicine) file generated from the CBCT scanning were imported into a commercially available planning software (Nobel Clinician; Nobel Biocare, Kloten, Switzerland) and superimposed for digital implant planning (Figure 8.4.5) [1].

After digital implant planning was completed, a stereolithographic surgical template was fabricated and two implants were planned to replace the two missing maxillary central incisors (Figure 8.4.6).

On the day of implant placement, after obtaining profound anesthesia at the surgical site using local anesthetic solution, osteotomy drilling was performed through the surgical template guided by the metal sleeves. After osteotomy preparation, two moderately rough surface dental implants (NP Nobel Replace Conical Connection; Nobel Biocare) were placed in a flapless approach with tissue punches (Figure 8.4.7). Implant

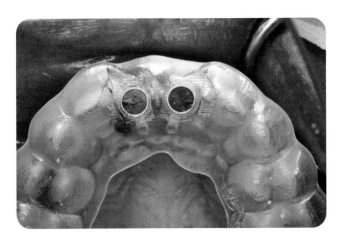

Figure 8.4.6 Stereolithographic surgical template in place (occlusal view).

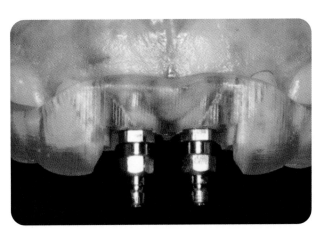

Figure 8.4.7 Implant placement in an ideal prosthetically driven position with a flapless approach due to sufficient keratinized mucosa.

stability reached 15 N·cm and the decision was made not to immediately load the implants. Short healing abutments were placed and implants were left submerged after sling sutures were placed (Figure 8.4.8). After an uneventful healing period of three months, the patient presented for second-stage surgery (Figure 8.4.9).

At the second-stage surgery, provisional implant-supported screw-retained single crowns were delivered, followed by peri-implant soft tissue conditioning for a period of three months. After three months of soft tissue conditioning and changes in the contours of the provisional restorations, the patient presented for final impression (Figure 8.4.10).

In order to transfer the emergence profile digitally, a new technique of digital scanning was introduced (Figure 8.4.11). At the impression appointment, the provisional implant-supported screw-retained single crowns were digitally scanned both intraorally (first scan) and extraorally (second scan). Additionally, scan bodies

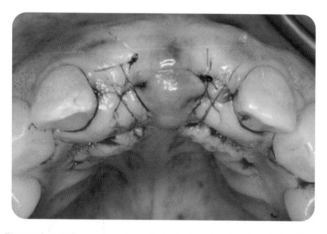

Figure 8.4.8 Postoperative clinical situation (occlusal view).

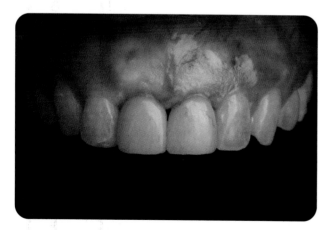

Figure 8.4.9 Fixed provisionalization with provisional implant-supported screw-retained single crowns inserted immediately after second-stage surgery.

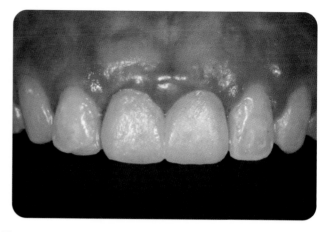

Figure 8.4.10 Provisional implant-supported screw-retained single crowns after three months of soft tissue conditioning.

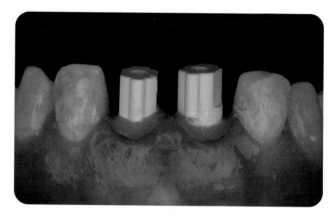

Figure 8.4.11 Scan bodies prior to intraoral digital impression.

were placed intraorally, and an implant-level digital impression was taken (third scan). The three STL files derived from the triple digital scanning were imported into CAD software and superimposed into one file that contained all the information from the implant three-dimensional position, prosthesis contours as well as the transmucosal part of the peri-implant soft tissues (Figure 8.4.12).

Subsequently, monolithic zirconia screw-retained single crowns were CAD designed in commercially available CAD software (Exocad) (Figure 8.4.13). The single crowns were milled in monolithic zirconia. After staining and sintering, titanium inserts were bonded on the monolithic zirconia crowns and the single crowns were tried in intraorally. Once fit and esthetics were confirmed clinically, the crowns were torqued at 35 N·cm (Figures 8.4.14–8.4.16).

The patient was satisfied with the esthetic and functional outcome and was enrolled on a six-month recall program. Under complete digital workflow, the definitive zirconia single crowns met the esthetic expectations of the patient (Figure 8.4.17).

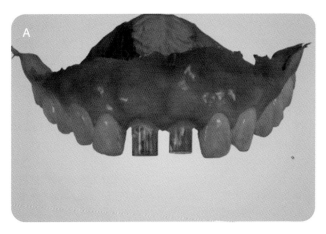
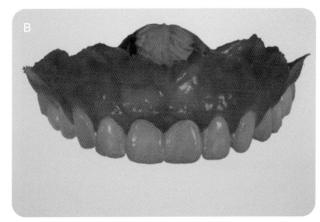

Figure 8.4.12 (A, B) STL file from intraoral digital impression.

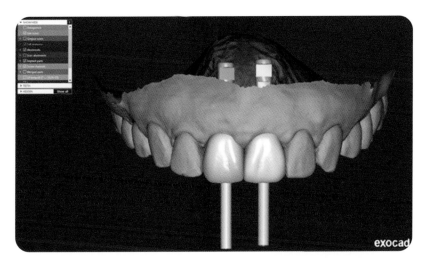

Figure 8.4.13 CAD design of final crowns after superimposition of the three STL files from the intraoral and extraoral digital scans.

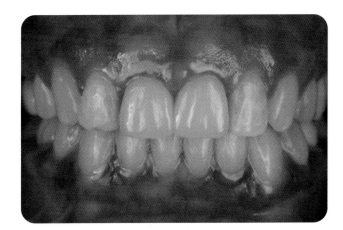

Figure 8.4.14 Definitive crowns delivery (frontal view).

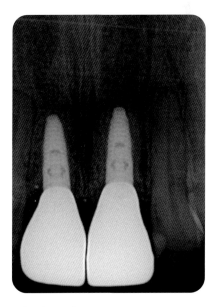

Figure 8.4.15 Radiograph.

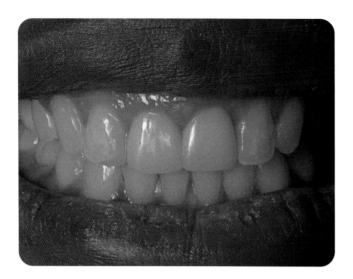

Figure 8.4.16 Smile.

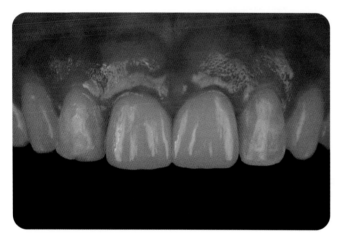

Figure 8.4.17 Clinical outcome after one year.

Discussion

Case selection and accurate three-dimensional implant positioning are of utmost importance since there is a high risk for esthetic complications [1]. In this case, digital implant planning and guided implant placement with a stereolithographic template ensured correct three-dimensional implant placement and management of the soft tissue profile around the dental implant during the fixed provisionalization. A stable and esthetic outcome was maintained at one-year clinical follow-up with great patient satisfaction. Undercontouring the transmucosal part of the provisional crown during healing is crucial for the soft tissue conditioning and may prevent gingival apical recession. Conventional loading was done because of the absence of high primary stability after placement.

The applications of digital technology in implant dentistry have transformed the field [1–10]. Digital imaging with CBCT and digital planning software with computer-guided implant placement have enabled clinicians to use available bone optimally for implant support. Additionally, the need for extensive grafting procedures is reduced, simultaneously allowing prosthodontically driven implant placement. A flapless technique may be possible with the guidance of a CAD/CAM surgical template generated from preoperative virtual implant planning, and CAD/CAM prosthodontic rehabilitation using a digital workflow. Digital impressions improve patient comfort and satisfaction, reduce costs, and can also be a powerful patient education tool. A complete digital workflow is a reality for single crowns and short-span FDPs, but not yet for full-arch prostheses. Currently, for full-arch implant rehabilitation, a combination of conventional and digital workflow is necessary [2,3].

Self-Study Questions

A. How is digital implant planning performed?

B. What are the benefits of guided implant placement?

C. How predictable is the digital impression?

D. What is the digital workflow?

E. How predictable is the use of CAD/CAM technology in implant prosthodontics?

F. What are the recent advances and/or new techniques in digital workflow?

Answers located at the end of the chapter.

ACKNOWLEDGMENT

The authors would like to thank Mr. Yukio Kudara for his laboratory expertise during the treatment of the patient.

References

1. Papaspyridakos P, Tarnow DP, Eckert SE, Weber HP. Replacing six missing adjacent teeth in the anterior maxilla with implant prostheses: a case series. *Compend Contin Educ Dent* 2018;39:e1–e4.
2. Joda T, Brägger U. Patient-centered outcomes comparing digital and conventional implant impression procedures: a randomized crossover trial. *Clin Oral Implants Res* 2016;27:e185–e189.
3. Papaspyridakos P, Chen YW, Gonzalez-Gusmao I, Att W. Complete digital workflow in prosthesis prototype fabrication for complete-arch implant rehabilitation: a technique. *J Prosthet Dent* 2019;122:189–192.
4. Monaco C, Ragazzini N, Scheda L, Evangelisti E. A fully digital approach to replicate functional and aesthetic parameters in implant-supported full-arch rehabilitation. *J Prosthodont Res* 2018;62:383–385.
5. Papaspyridakos P, Kang K, DeFuria C, et al. Digital workflow in full-arch implant rehabilitation with segmented minimally veneered monolithic zirconia fixed dental prostheses: 2-year clinical follow-up. *J Esthet Restor Dent* 2018;30:5–13.
6. Chochlidakis KM, Papaspyridakos P, Geminiani A, et al. Digital versus conventional impressions for fixed prosthodontics: a systematic review and meta-analysis. *J Prosthet Dent* 2016;116:184–190.
7. Wöhrle PS. Predictably replacing maxillary incisors with implants using 3-D planning and guided implant surgery. *Compend Contin Educ Dent* 2014;35:758–762.
8. Monaco C, Evangelisti E, Scotti R, et al. A fully digital approach to replicate peri-implant soft tissue contours and emergence profile in the esthetic zone. *Clin Oral Implants Res* 2016;27:1511–1514.
9. Tahmaseb A, Wismeijer D, Coucke W, Derksen W. Computer technology applications in surgical implant dentistry: a systematic review. *Int J Oral Maxillofac Implants* 2014;29(Suppl):25–42.
10. Papaspyridakos P, Chen CJ, Gallucci GO, et al. Accuracy of implant impressions for partially and completely edentulous patients: a systematic review. *Int J Oral Maxillofac Implants* 2014;29:836–845.
11. Lin WS, Harris BT, Elathamna EN, et al. Effect of implant divergence on the accuracy of definitive casts created from traditional and digital implant-level impressions: an in vitro comparative study. *Int J Oral Maxillofac Implants* 2015;30:102–109.
12. Basaki K, Alkumru H, De Souza G, Finer Y. Accuracy of digital vs conventional implant impression approach: a three-dimensional comparative in vitro analysis. *Int J Oral Maxillofac Implants* 2017;32:792–799.
13. Chew AA, Esguerra RJ, Teoh KH, et al. Three-dimensional accuracy of digital implant impressions: effects of different scanners and implant level. *Int J Oral Maxillofac Implants* 2017;32:70–80.
14. Papaspyridakos P, Gallucci GO, Chen CJ, et al. Digital versus conventional implant impressions for edentulous patients: accuracy outcomes. *Clin Oral Implants Res* 2016;27:465–472.
15. Amin S, Weber HP, Finkelman M, et al. Digital versus conventional full-arch implant impressions: a comparative study. *Clin Oral Implants Res* 2017;28:1360–1367.
16. Vandenweghe S, Vervack V, Dierens M, De Bruyn H. Accuracy of digital impressions of multiple dental implants: an in-vitro study. *Clin Oral Implants Res* 2017;28:648–653.
17. Joda T, Ferrari M, Brägger U. Monolithic implant-supported lithium disilicate (LS2) crowns in a complete digital workflow: a prospective clinical trial with a 2-year follow-up. *Clin Implant Dent Relat Res* 2017;19:505–511.
18. Joda T, Brägger U. Time-efficiency analysis of the treatment with monolithic implant crowns in a digital workflow: a randomized controlled trial. *Clin Oral Implants Res* 2016;27:1401–1406.
19. Schepke U, Meijer HJ, Kerdijk W, Cune MS. Digital versus analog complete-arch impressions for single-unit premolar implant crowns: operating time and patient preference. *J Prosthet Dent* 2015;114:403–406.
20. Peñarrocha-Diago M, Balaguer-Martí JC, Peñarrocha-Oltra D, et al. A combined digital and stereophotogrammetric technique for rehabilitation with immediate loading of complete-arch, implant-supported prostheses: a randomized controlled pilot clinical trial. *J Prosthet Dent* 2017;118:596–603.

TAKE-HOME POINTS

A. The DICOM file resulting from the CBCT examination is loaded into virtual implant planning software for implant treatment planning. The DICOM file acquired from the CBCT scan is superimposed with an STL file of the partially edentulous patient. This STL file is acquired from a digital impression with an intraoral scanner (IOS) of the partially edentulous patient. The superimposition of the intraoral surface STL data, acquired using IOS, and the radiographic CBCT data leads to an unprecedented wealth of information for the clinician to plan, execute, and rehabilitate the patient [5,7,8]. The digital planning software provides many treatment planning advantages for evaluating potential sites for implant placement. Anatomic limitations, such as nerve proximity or sinus floor pneumatization and alveolar ridge deficiencies, are identified and the need for guided bone augmentation is assessed preoperatively. The computer software advantages range from allowing an accurate measurement of ridge dimensions to virtual implant placement and abutment evaluation prior to guided implant placement [1–10]. Digital wax-ups can be made with the digital planning software; alternatively, digital scanning of the physical wax-up is possible, for additional superimposition to the CBCT data.

B. After digital implant planning, the clinician can perform guided surgery with surgical templates. Digitally planned template-guided implant placement represents one of the advances in implant dentistry, and provides great benefits when planning and executing implant surgery, including its minimally invasive nature, prosthodontically driven implant placement, predictability, and reduced time required for definitive rehabilitation. The benefits of flapless implant placement include reduced healing times, fewer changes in crestal bone levels, less bleeding, and minimal postoperative discomfort and swelling [9].

C. Intraoral digital impressions are gaining popularity. The splinted, open tray impression represents the gold standard according to the literature. The digital impression will create an STL file that can be used in either a digital or conventional workflow for the fabrication of the final implant prosthesis. Digital impressions are acquired by use of an IOS to produce an STL file. This STL file is used to generate either a physical cast (stereolithography, three-dimensional printing, milling) or a digital cast for a complete digital workflow [11–20].

With regard to the accuracy of digital versus conventional implant impressions for partially edentulous patients, recent studies have shown that digital impressions achieved a similar level of accuracy to splinted conventional impressions [11–13]. Equivalent comparisons for fully edentulous patients have found the same results. Comparative studies are currently emerging showing that full-arch digital implant impressions (with TRIOS, Omnicam, and True Definition scanner) display

the same or even better accuracy as the conventional ones [14–16].

D. There is a tendency in the medical and dental fields to reduce treatment time and simplify procedures in order to improve patient acceptance and enhance satisfaction while maintaining long-term predictability of treatment outcomes. Digital workflow and CAD/CAM technology in implant prosthodontics has helped to simplify a number of steps of fixed implant rehabilitation. The digital workflow can be complete or combined with conventional workflow [3,16–20].

E. When designing a single-unit or short-span screw-retained implant-fixed prosthesis, CAD/CAM technology offers the possibility for a complete digital workflow [2,3,5,18–20]. This technique pertains to a milled implant prosthesis that will be cemented to a titanium insert with resin cement before delivery or to custom abutment with a cement-retained crown. It is well documented for single crowns. It can also be used for short-span three-unit FDPs. The milled superstructure is cemented to a titanium insert (Ti-base) and the whole assembly is screw retained to the implant level. During a complete digital workflow, the cast is not necessary since the superstructure and the Ti-base can be cemented without a cast or even intraorally. Further research is needed to evaluate the outcome and the amount of tolerable deviation of implant position by this technique.

F. Digitally planned, template-guided implant surgery has gained increased popularity. It has been proposed that implant three-dimensional planning software should be used in every case whether or not it will be coupled with template-guided surgery. Planning and visualizing the implant surgery prior to performing the actual procedure has great advantages. A complete digital workflow is a reality for single crowns and short-span implant FDPs, but not yet for full-arch prostheses. Currently, for full-arch implant rehabilitation, a combination of conventional and digital workflow is necessary. However, considerable advances are currently being made in virtual articulation, virtual facebow, and printed cast fabrication and articulation so that a complete digital workflow for full-arch implant rehabilitation will soon be a reality.

Case 5

Combination of Implant Single Crowns and Porcelain Veneers in the Esthetic Zone

CASE STORY

A 21-year-old Caucasian female presented with a chief complaint of "I don't like the spaces between my teeth. I need to close the spaces." The patient had congenitally missing maxillary lateral incisors and she had undergone thorough orthodontic treatment for several years (Figures 8.5.1 and 8.5.2). The patient had an orthodontic retainer with attached denture teeth #7 and #10 for esthetic purposes and to prevent post-orthodontic tooth movement. Additionally, the patient had inadequate bone thickness in the areas of #7 and #10. The patient visited her dentist for regular recalls and she had very good oral hygiene.

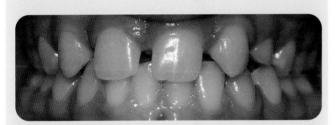

Figure 8.5.1 Initial pre-orthodontics presentation.

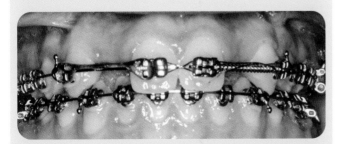

Figure 8.5.2 Final teeth position presentation prior to orthodontics debonding.

Medical History

The patient's medical history revealed no significant general conditions or allergies.

Review of Systems

• Vital signs
  ○ Blood pressure: 117/70 mmHg
  ○ Pulse rate: 54 beats/minute (regular)
  ○ Respiratory rate: 15 breaths/minute (regular)

Social History

The patient did not smoke and only drank alcohol occasionally (three drinks per week).

Extraoral Examination

The examination showed compromised esthetics due to her missing maxillary laterals and diastemas between her maxillary anterior teeth. No other significant findings were noted. The temporomandibular joint was within normal limits and her lymph nodes were normal on palpation.

Intraoral Examination

• Oral cancer screening was negative.
• Soft tissue examination including floor of the mouth and tongue was within normal limits.

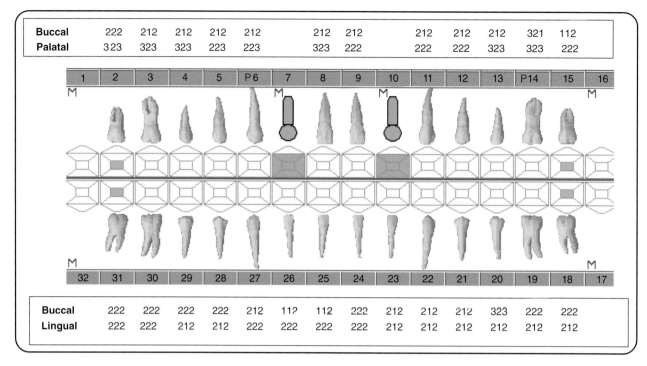

	1	2	3	4	5	P6	7	8	9	10	11	12	13	P14	15	16
Buccal		222	212	212	212	212		212	212		212	212	212	321	112	
Palatal		323	323	323	223	223		323	222		222	222	323	323	222	

	32	31	30	29	28	27	26	25	24	23	22	21	20	19	18	17
Buccal		222	222	222	222	212	112	112	222	212	212	212	323	222	222	
Lingual		222	222	212	212	222	222	222	222	212	212	212	212	212	212	

Figure 8.5.3   Probing pocket depth measurements during the initial preoperative visit.

- Periodontal examination revealed pocket depths between 1 and 3 mm (Figure 8.5.3).
- Localized areas of gingival inflammation were noted.
- Gingival recession on teeth #5 and #12.
- Seibert class I in edentulous area of #7 and #10 with inadequate bone thickness.
- Inadequate bone thickness of the alveolar ridge in the areas #7 and #10.
- Existing composite restorations on teeth #2, #15, #18 and #31. No caries was detected.

Occlusion

Facial midline was slightly cant. No occlusal discrepancies or interferences were noted.

Radiographic Examination

Radiographic examination (Figure 8.5.4) revealed short roots for teeth #8 and #9 and normal bone levels overall. There was a slight loss of bone noted in the crestal bone height at teeth #7 and #10. The cone beam computed tomography (CT) evaluation revealed inadequate facial/buccal bone thickness for implant placement in the areas #7 and #10.

Diagnosis

American Academy of Periodontology (AAP) diagnosis of plaque-induced mild localized gingivitis with mucogingival conditions and deformities on edentulous ridge.

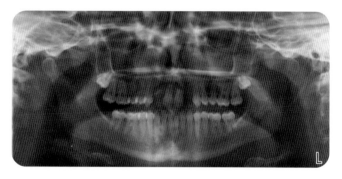

Figure 8.5.4   Initial panoramic radiograph (post orthodontics).

Treatment Plan

The treatment plan for this patient consisted of initial phase therapy that included oral prophylaxis with oral hygiene instructions and guided bone regeneration (GBR) procedure to address the bone deficiency prior to implant placements on #7 and #10. All different restorative treatment options concerning her missing laterals and diastema closure were discussed and it was decided that the combination of implants and porcelain veneers would give the patient optimum esthetics and function while using a minimally invasive approach.

Treatment

After the comprehensive examination and the diagnostic work-up, the placement of two implants on teeth #7 and #10 and porcelain veneers on #6, #8, #9, and #11 was selected for esthetic purposes.

The initial phase therapy included oral prophylaxis and oral hygiene instructions to address localized gingival inflammation. This was followed by a GBR procedure to augment the buccal deficiency of the alveolar ridge and facilitate implant placement on #7 and #10. The goals of surgery were the horizontal and potential vertical augmentation of the crestal ridge. Intrasulcular incisions were made on the buccal and palatal from teeth #5–8 and #9–12. A mid-crestal, slightly palatal incision was made in the edentulous area of #6–8 and #9–11. Full-thickness elevations were made past the mucogingival junction. The osseous crest was decorticated with a carbide round bur. Then 1.0 ml of freeze-dried bone allograft (MinerOss; BioHorizons, Birmingham, AL, USA) was hydrated and placed in the defect. A membrane (DynaMatrix; Citagenix, Laval, Quebec, Canada) was then adapted over the area and graft material. An additional GBR procedure was performed for area #7 in the same way for contour augmentation. After four months of adequate bone healing, Straumann dental implants were placed in #7 and #10 with simultaneous bone grafting at both sites (Figure 8.5.5).

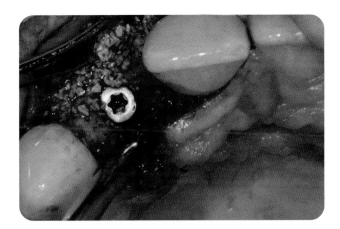

Figure 8.5.5   Implant placement with simultaneous bone grafting for tooth #7.

After a three-month period allowing for osseointegration (Figure 8.5.6), second-stage surgery was performed to expose the implants and provisional implant crowns were fabricated to create the proper soft tissue contour. Soft tissue conditioning in esthetic areas may take time; hence a maturation period of several weeks is needed, and this was accomplished by modifying the temporary implant crown to gain more papillae.

Veneer preparations were done for teeth #6, #8, #9, and #11 followed by final impression of prepared teeth and implants (Figure 8.5.7). The final impression was taken using customized impression copings to ensure the accurate transfer of the emergence profile, created during provisionalization, to the master cast (Figure 8.5.8). The final rehabilitation consisted of implant-level screw-retained porcelain-layered zirconia single crowns on #7 and #10 and lithium disilicate glass ceramic porcelain veneers on teeth #6, #8, #9, and #11 (Figures 8.5.9 and 8.5.10). The patient was very happy with the esthetic and functional outcome of her dental treatment (Figure 8.5.11).

Discussion

This prosthetic treatment option solved the esthetic and restorative problems arising from congenitally missing lateral incisors (#7 and #10) and misaligned teeth in the esthetic zone. Proper provisionalization ensured the biologic, functional, and esthetic outcome of the final implant crowns. The resulting prosthesis achieved the esthetic expectations of the patient.

Treatment sequence is key when handling esthetically challenging cases in the maxillary esthetic zone. It becomes even more challenging when a combination of implant- and tooth-supported restorations are needed for the rehabilitation. Comprehensive diagnostic work-up prior to initiation of treatment is essential and the final outcome can be visualized with wax-up and mock-up try-in.

In this case with bilaterally missing lateral incisors, the first step is orthodontic positioning of the teeth

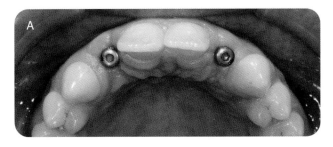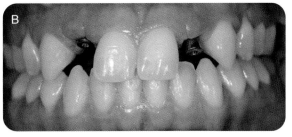

Figure 8.5.6 (A, B) After three-month healing period of implant placement at #7 and #10 (occlusal and frontal views).

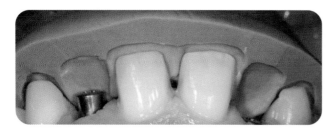

Figure 8.5.7   Veneer preparations for teeth #6, #8, #9 and #11. A PVS key is used to confirm appropriate reduction.

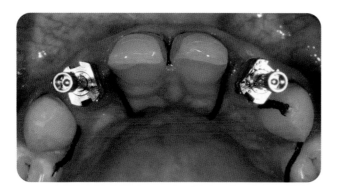

Figure 8.5.8   Final impression of veneer-prepared teeth #6, #8, #9, and #11 and implants #7 and #10 with customized impression copings.

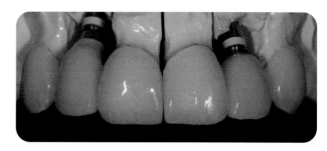

Figure 8.5.9   Porcelain veneers and implant restorations on the master cast.

ideally prior to implant placement. Prosthetically driven implant placement follows after mock-up try-in to confirm esthetics and phonetics. After implant osseointegration, implant-fixed provisionalization is the next step in order to condition the soft tissues.

Once the tissue contours and gingival zeniths have been achieved harmoniously, then the preparation of the teeth follows with impressions for both implant- and tooth-supported restorations. At the insertion appointment, the porcelain veneers must be cemented first, followed by insertion of the implant-supported single crowns. A pleasant esthetic and functional outcome was achieved after implementation of the aforementioned protocol.

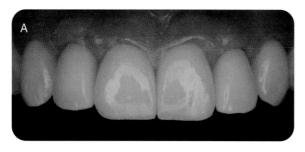

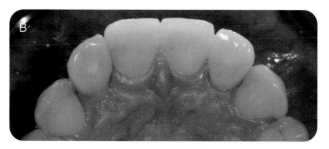

Figure 8.5.10 (A, B) Postoperative frontal and occlusal views.

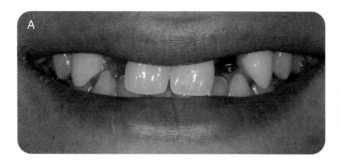

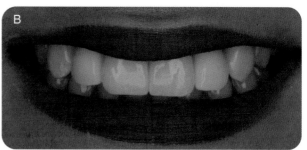

Figure 8.5.11   Preoperative (A) and postoperative (B) comparison of smile.

Self-Study Questions

A. How often do congenitally missing laterals occur and how do they affect the patient?

B. Which are the treatment options for congenitally missing lateral incisors?

C. What are the contraindications for implant restorations when replacing congenitally missing laterals?

D. How can the completion of growth be determined for individual patients?

E. What materials are usually used for porcelain veneers?

F. What is the cementation procedure sequence for porcelain veneers?

Answers located at the end of the chapter.

ACKNOWLEDGMENT
The authors would like to thank Oral Design for its laboratory expertise during the treatment of the patient.

References

1. Rakhshan V. Congenitally missing teeth (hypodontia): a review of the literature concerning the etiology, prevalence, risk factors, patterns and treatment. *Dent Res J (Isfahan)* 2015;12(1):1–13.
2. Behr M, Proff P, Leitzmann M, et al. Survey of congenitally missing teeth in orthodontic patients in Eastern Bavaria. *Eur J Orthod* 2011;33:32–36.
3. Kinzer GA, Kokich VO. Managing congenitally missing lateral incisors. Part I: canine substitution. *J Esthet Restor Dent* 2005;17(1):5–10.
4. Kinzer GA, Kokich VO. Managing congenitally missing lateral incisors. Part II: tooth-supported restorations. *J Esthet Restor Dent* 2005;17(2):76–84.
5. Kinzer GA, Kokich VO. Managing congenitally missing lateral incisors. Part III: single-tooth implants. *J Esthet Restor Dent* 2005;17(4):202–210.
6. Krassnig M, Fickl S. Congenitally missing lateral incisors: a comparison between restorative, implant, and orthodontic approaches. *Dent Clin North Am* 2011;55(2):283–299.
7. Schliephake H, Sicilia A, Al Nawas B, et al. Drugs and diseases: summary and consensus statements of Group 1. The 5th EAO Consensus Conference 2018. *Clin Oral Implants Res* 2018;29(Suppl 18):93–99.
8. Zachrisson BU, Mjör IA. Remodeling of teeth by grinding. *Am J Orthod* 1975;68:545–553.
9. Fudalej P, Kokich VG, Leroux B. Determining the cessation of vertical growth of the craniofacial structures to facilitate placement of single-tooth implants. *Am J Orthod Dentofacial Orthop* 2007;131(Suppl 4):S59–S67.
10. Kokich VG. Managing orthodontic-restorative treatment for the adolescent patient. In: McNamara JA, Brudon WL (eds) *Orthodontics and Dentofacial Orthopedics*. Ann Arbor, MI: Needham Press, 2001:423–452.
11. Baccetti T, Franchi L, McNamara JA. The cervical maturation (CVM) method for the assessment of optimal treatment timing in dentofacial orthopedics. *Semin Orthod* 2005;11(3):119–129.
12. Spear F, Mathews D, Kokich VG. Interdisciplinary management of single tooth implants. *Semin Orthod* 1997;3:45–72.
13. Kokich VG. Maxillary lateral incisor implants: planning with the aid of orthodontics. *Int J Oral Maxillofac Surg* 2004;62:48–56.
14. Rotoli BT, Lima DANL, Pini NP, et al. Porcelain veneers as an alternative for esthetic treatment: clinical report. *Oper Dent* 2013;38(5):459–466.
15. Magne P, Belser UC. Novel porcelain laminate preparation approach driven by a diagnostic mock-up. *J Esthet Restor Dent* 2004;16(1):7–16; discussion 17–18.
16. Donovan TE. Factors essential for successful all-ceramic restorations. *J Am Dent Assoc* 2008;139(Suppl):14S–18S.
17. McLaren EA, Whiteman YY. Ceramics: rationale for material selection. *Compend Contin Educ Dent* 2010;31(9):666–668, 670, 672 passim; quiz 680, 700.
18. Soares CJ, Soares PV, Pereira JC, Fonseca RB. Surface treatment protocols in the cementation process of ceramic and laboratory-processed composite restorations: a literature review. *J Esthet Restor Dent* 2005;17(4):224–235.
19. Giordano R, McLaren EA. Ceramics overview: classification by microstructure and processing methods. *Compend Contin Educ Dent* 2010;31(9):682–684, 686, 688 passim; quiz 698, 700.
20. Della Bona A, Kelly JR. The clinical success of all-ceramic restoration. *J Am Dent Assoc* 2008;139(Suppl):8S–13S.
21. Layton D, Walton T. An up to 16-year prospective study of 304 porcelain veneers. *Int J Prosthodont* 2007;20(4):389–396.
22. Fradeani M, Redemagni M, Corrado M. Porcelain laminate veneers: 6- to 12-year clinical evaluation. A retro-

spective study. *Int J Periodontics Restorative Dent* 2005; 25(1):9–17.

23. Sá TCM, Figueiredo de Carvalho MF, de Sá JCM, et al. Esthetic rehabilitation of anterior teeth with different thicknesses of porcelain laminate veneers: an 8-year follow-up clinical evaluation. *Eur J Dent* 2018;12(4):590–593.

24. Morita RK, Hayashida MF, Pupo YM, et al. Minimally invasive laminate veneers: clinical aspects in treatment planning and cementation procedures. *Case Rep Dent* 2016; 2016:1839793.

25. Magne P, Cascione D. Influence of post-etching cleaning and connecting porcelain on the microtensile bond strength of composite resin to feldspathic porcelain. *J Prosthet Dent* 2006;96(5):354–361.

26. Canay S, Hersek N, Ertan A. Effect of different acid treatments on a porcelain surface. *J Oral Rehabil* 2001;28(1):95–101.

TAKE-HOME POINTS

A. Maxillary lateral incisors are most probably considered the most common bilateral missing teeth, followed by the mandibular second premolar [1]. Patients with missing teeth usually face challenges associated with appearance, malocclusion, and periodontal condition. Furthermore, patients with congenitally missing laterals may have esthetic concerns and low self-esteem, inadequate pronunciation, and compromised bone growth in the specific area and function [1,2]. A multidisciplinary approach with lengthy and costly dental treatment is usually needed when treating these clinical cases[1,2].

B. Maxillary lateral incisors are often congenitally missing and dental professionals have to choose among different treatment options. The available restorative treatment options for this type of clinical cases are canine substitution (lateralization of the canine), single implant restoration, resin-bonded fixed partial denture (Maryland bridge), cantilevered fixed partial denture, and fixed partial denture [3–6]. The factors which need to be examined prior to selecting the treatment of choice include the patient's occlusal scheme, available restorative space, adjacent teeth condition and position, and patient's esthetic expectations. Interdisciplinary treatment planning and detailed evaluation of all these criteria are important when treating these cases [3–6]. Furthermore, the age of the patient should be taken into account when considering the implant restorative option. Incomplete facial growth is a contraindication for implant placement [5]. One of the concerns when replacing a congenitally

missing lateral incisor with an implant is the inadequate bone thickness of the alveolar ridge. Because of the fact that the permanent lateral incisor does not erupt, the osseous ridge is usually underdeveloped [5]. Ideally, the treatment of choice should be the most conservative approach that will fulfill the esthetic and functional demands and provide long-term success [4,5].

C. Replacing congenitally missing laterals with single implant restorations is the most conservative approach as it does not involve any tooth preparation. However, implants are not recommended for medically compromised patients, patients taking medication for osteoporosis, patients whose facial growth is incomplete, when there is restorative space limitation, and when there is inadequate bone [5–7]. It is recommended that patients with missing laterals be monitored from an early age for optimal site development [5,6]. In many cases, a bone graft is recommended prior to implant placement or simultaneously in order to enhance alveolar ridge thickness [5,6]. Furthermore, the amount of interradicular and coronal space is also critical for implant placement. Radiographic evaluation and a conventional diagnostic or digital wax-up, respectively, will assist in evaluating the available space for implant restoration. In general, the lateral coronal space width is 5–7 mm, while the interradicular minimum distance is 5 mm for a small implant [5,6].

D. Generally, craniofacial growth continues until the age of 17 years for females and until age 21 years for males [5–9]. A method for evaluating a patient's individual growth pattern involves comparing hand/wrist radiographs [5,6]. Nonetheless, the completion of facial growth cannot be determined by hand/wrist radiographs. The most commonly used method for assessing facial growth involves the comparison of lateral cephalometric radiographs taken 6–12 months apart [5,10]. This technique was introduced by Baccetti et al. and evaluates cervical vertebral maturation (CVM) [6,11]. Evaluation of CVM by noticeable changes in the vertebral body through superimposition of lateral cephalometric radiographs is the most accurate technique for assessing the cessation of facial growth [9,12,13]. Facial growth can be considered complete if the nasion to menton distance is stable within one year [6]. In addition, in cases where implants are planned, it is important to confirm facial growth completion by confirming deep concavities on the second, third, and fourth cervical vertebrae, and a greater height (vertical) than length (horizontal) of the vertebral bodies [6].

E. The materials indicated for porcelain laminate veneers are feldspathic porcelain or hot-pressed glass ceramic [14]. Because of their properties, they can mimic the translucency and opacity of the natural dentition while the associated tooth preparation can be minimally invasive [14–18]. Despite the fact that feldspathic porcelain has a flexural strength of around 60–70 MPa [14,19], feldspathic porcelain veneers are very conservative restorations with excellent esthetic outcome and long-term results. Based on the literature, feldspathic veneers have high survival rates of 93% at 10–11 years and can reach 91–94.4% at 12 years [20–22].

F. The internal surface of feldspathic porcelain veneers is first etched with 10% hydrofluoric acid for 20 seconds or 9% hydrofluoric acid for 90 seconds, and then washed and air-dried [23,24]. The use of 37% phosphoric acid for one minute is recommended for cleaning the internal surface of the restorations and removing the insoluble silica-fluoride salts prior to silanization [24–26]. The surface is then silanized for one minute with silane coupling agent. A thin layer of adhesive is applied and air-thinned.

Simultaneously, the surface of the prepared tooth is etched with 37% phosphoric acid for 20 seconds, rinsed and air-dried (without overdrying). A thin layer of adhesive agent is then applied and air-thinned. With regard to the polymerization of the bonding agent, opinions vary as to whether light curing should be recommended [14,24].

Light curing resin cement is placed on the internal surface of the veneer, positioned on the tooth, and light activated initially for one to two seconds. After removal of excess cement, the cement is light cured for 40 seconds from the palatal and facial directions. It is critical that the veneer cementation is done under proper isolation.

9

Preventive Periodontal Therapy

Case 1: Plaque Removal 374
Paul A. Levi Jr., DMD and Luca Gobbato, DDS, MS

Case 1

Plaque Removal

CASE STORY

A 55-year-old Caucasian male, a plumber by trade, presented with a chief complaint of "I know that my teeth are bad, and I want them fixed" (Figures 9.1.1 and 9.1.2).

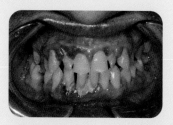

Figure 9.1.1 Initial presentation on examination.

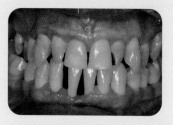

Figure 9.1.2 One year following plaque control instruction and scaling and root planing.

LEARNING GOALS AND OBJECTIVES

- To understand that the behavioral motivation of a patient, to be consistent and thorough with biofilm removal, is of paramount importance in successful dental therapy, and that no matter how thorough scaling and root planing therapy is done, it is the *daily* removal of biofilm by the patient that sustains the professional therapy
- To know that the removal of the etiologic agents can lead to healing with repair of the periodontium and sometimes even to regeneration
- To learn various techniques of behavioral motivation and of plaque removal

Medical History

The patient had no significant past medical problems other than stage 3, grade B periodontitis. He reported no allergies, no present medical illnesses, and stated that he was taking no medications. He had not had a general physical examination for several years.

Dental History

Over the past several years, the patient had noticed blood on his toothbrush and in his saliva whenever he brushed his teeth, and he stated that his wife complained that he had bad breath. The patient claimed to brush his teeth only once or twice a week because he did not like the taste of blood. He did not use dental floss or any other means of interproximal plaque control. He used mouthwash occasionally. His most recent visit to the dentist had been "several" years ago for "some fillings."

Review of Systems

- Vital signs
  - Blood pressure: 120/65 mmHg
  - Pulse rate: 72 beats/minute (regular)
  - Respiratory rate: 15 breaths/minute

Social History

The patient did not drink alcohol. He had smoked cigarettes since he was age 23 and currently smoked half a pack (10 cigarettes) daily.

Extraoral Examination

No significant findings were noted. The patient had no masses or swelling, and the temporomandibular joint was within normal limits.

Intraoral Examination

- Plaque control techniques were observed and were inadequate for complete plaque removal.
- The soft tissues of the mouth, apart from the gingiva, appeared normal.

- The gingival examination revealed severe marginal erythema, with rolled margins and edematous, bulbous, and spongy papillae (Figure 9.1.1).
- A dental examination revealed cervical and interproximal smooth surface caries.
- A periodontal probing examination was completed (Figure 9.1.3).

Occlusion

There were no occlusal discrepancies or interferences. There were no parafunctional problems, and there was no significant attrition.

Radiographic Examination

A full-mouth series of periapical radiographs revealed calculus, caries, defective restorations, evidence of 25–85% angular bone loss, loss of crestal–septal density, and a root tip with root canal therapy on tooth #29. Figure 9.1.4 shows the patient's mandibular anterior periapical radiographs before treatment and Figure 9.1.5 shows the radiographs one year post treatment.

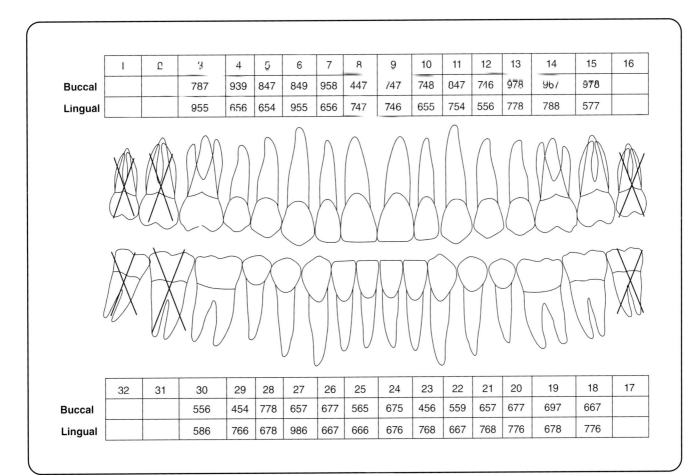

	1	2	3	4	5	6	7	8	9	10	11	12	13	14	15	16
Buccal			787	939	847	849	958	447	747	748	847	716	978	967	978	
Lingual			955	656	654	955	656	747	746	655	754	556	778	788	577	

	32	31	30	29	28	27	26	25	24	23	22	21	20	19	18	17
Buccal			556	454	778	657	677	565	675	456	559	657	677	697	667	
Lingual			586	766	678	986	667	666	676	768	667	768	776	678	776	

Figure 9.1.3 Probing pocket depth measurements.

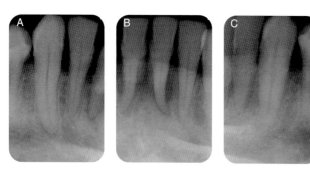

Figure 9.1.4 (A–C) Periapical preoperative radiographs depicting the interproximal bone levels.

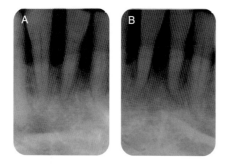

Figure 9.1.5 (A, B) Periapical postoperative radiographs depicting the interproximal bone levels.

Diagnosis

1. Generalized stage 3, grade B periodontitis
2. Dental caries and fractured teeth
3. Missing teeth
4. Defective restorations

Treatment Plan

1. General physical examination (the patient had not had a recent physical examination)
2. Phase 1: disease control therapy:
   a. Plaque control instruction (PCI) and gross debridement
   b. Continued PCI with scaling and root planing (SRP)
   c. Caries control, extraction of nontreatable teeth
   d. Periodontal reevaluation
3. Phase 2: surgical pocket-reducing therapy as needed (resective or regenerative) and periodontal reevaluation
4. Phase 3: restorative treatment (as planned)
5. Maintenance therapy:
   a. PCI and SRP every three months or as indicated
   b. Periodic periodontal reevaluation
   c. Periodic restorative reevaluation

Treatment

At the outset of the initial treatment visit, the patient was instructed in the Bass intrasulcular technique of brushing and dental tape for interproximal cleaning [1,2]. In addition, interproximal brushes and gauze bandage were used for the proximal surfaces (Figure 9.1.6). Following PCI, a gross debridement was performed using hand curettes and power instrumentation without local anesthetic. Before the end of the appointment, plaque removal techniques were again reviewed.

At the second appointment, PCI was reviewed at the beginning of the appointment, and scaling, root planing, and polishing were performed using local anesthetic.

Hygiene therapy visits (PCI and SRP) were performed at two-week intervals for three months. After the first three months, PCI and SRP were continued at five-week intervals. After one year of treatment the patient had achieved greatly improved home care techniques and consistency. There was significant resolution of the inflammation and reduced pocketing (see Figure 9.1.2).

Postoperative radiographs of the mandibular anterior teeth at one year revealed apparent bone fill associated with tooth #24 (see Figure 9.1.5).

Discussion

Periodontitis, as seen in this patient, is a chronic infection caused by dysbiotic bacterial communities and likely eukaryotic viruses [3]. This plaque-induced inflammatory disease is initiated by the waste products of periodontal pathogens; these organisms possess a glycocalyx that allows them to adhere to the tooth surface at and apical to the gingival crevice.

The treatment and prevention of periodontitis involves four main factors:

1. That the patient is *motivated* to perform daily home care techniques
2. That the patient is *taught, knows, and performs* appropriate plaque removal techniques
3. That the patient is able to *access* the tooth exposed to oral fluids in order to perform the correct techniques
4. That the patient *is encouraged to seek* professional dental hygiene therapy regularly. The interval will depend on the patient's susceptibility to dental diseases, and the degree of disease present at the time of the visit, which will be determined by the clinician.

The theory of plaque removal from teeth is a basic principle of physics: "Two objects cannot occupy the same place at the same time and the object of the greater mass will displace the object of the lesser mass." Plaque removal is a displacement process, not an abrasive process. Thus, scrubbing one's teeth is not only unnecessary, but is often harmful due to friction. If toothbrush bristle tips are moving across a tooth in a scrub motion on the cervical third of the tooth, abrasion

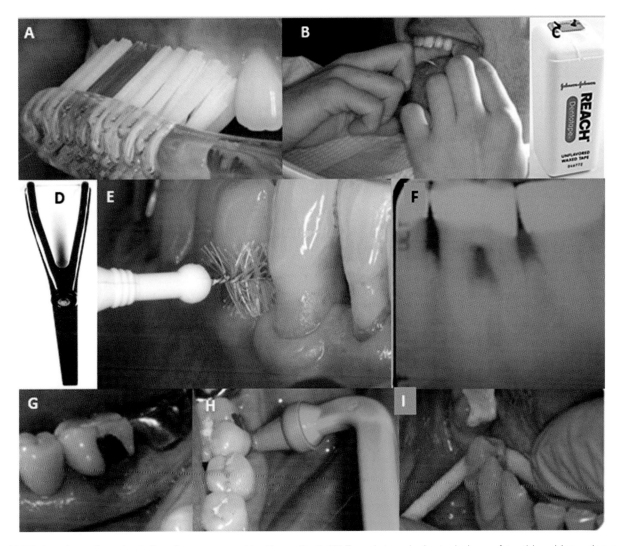

Figure 9.1.6 A variety of methods for plaque removal by the patient: (A) Bass intrasulcular technique of toothbrushing using a straight-cut multi-tufted nylon bristle toothbrush; (B) dental tape using an adapted horizontal technique; (C) dental tape; (D) floss holder; (E) interproximal brush; (F) radiographic furcation involvement; (G) furcation involvement; (H) rubber tip in facial furcation; (I) use of gauze bandage to clean proximal surfaces of teeth next to an edentulous area.

of the teeth and gingiva can occur. On the tooth, noncarious cervical lesions can be created (toothbrush wear). Additionally, the bristle tips cannot access the gingival crevice to remove subgingival plaque, and with a thin phenotype, gingival recession can occur.

The technique shown to the patient was an intrasulcular technique of brushing, the *stationary bristle tip [Bass] technique* [1,4,5]. This technique involves using a multi-tufted nylon toothbrush with bristle diameters of 0.18 mm. Brushing begins with the most posterior tooth in the arch. The brush head is angled slightly toward the gingival crevice (approximately 45–70 degrees). The brush head is placed approximately at the middle of the clinical crown (at the maximum convexity) and adequate pressure is applied against the tooth to allow the bristle

tips to enter the gingival sulcus and to maintain the tips *stationary* on the tooth surface within the gingival crevice. The handle of the brush is moved in a *short* back-and-forth (3–4 mm) motion for two to three seconds, which is then repeated three to four times in each location. The patient should concentrate on feeling the toothbrush bristles in the gingival crevice. We recommend that the patient begin on the facial aspect of the most posterior tooth in any quadrant and move anteriorly overlapping the bristle placement, once crossing the midline then moving posteriorly and ending on the facial aspect of the most posterior tooth in the opposite quadrant. The patient will continue on to the lingual surfaces of the teeth in a like manner until ending back at the beginning. The opposite arch is cleaned in the same manner. With a power brush, the same technique is used *without moving the handle in a vibratory motion*.

For interproximal plaque control, we recommended dental tape, rubber tip, and interproximal brushes. The technique for dental tape was to anchor the tape on the ring finger, to use the index finger and thumb to adapt the tape in a "C" fashion around the tooth to ensure the line angles are cleansed, and to use a buccolingual–apico-occlusal movement of the tape with firm lateral pressure against the tooth surface, similar to the method people use to dry their back with a towel. The tape is placed subgingivally until the base of the sulcus is reached with lateral pressure. There should be *no* apical pressure against the epithelial attachment, only lateral pressure against the proximal surface of the tooth and the line angles. All mesial and distal surfaces are to be cleaned in this fashion [2].

We recommended a rubber tip be used from the facial to the lingual and vice versa for interproximal pockets that cannot be accessed by the dental tape, where there are subgingival tooth concavities, where the papilla are edematous, where pockets exceed 4 mm, and where there are accessible furcation involvements. The rubber tip is also effective when used to displace plaque from furcations. The interproximal brush is effective supragingivally and when there are tooth concavities or class 2 or 3 furcation involvements (see Chapter 4).

Other interproximal plaque control devices include bridge threaders to carry the dental tape interproximally where contacts are not open. Balsa wood triangular interdental devices, which simulate a rubber tip, are difficult to use. Moist gauze bandage strips (5 cm wide by 25 cm long) are recommended for cleaning the proximal surfaces of teeth next to edentulous areas.

Other brush-type devices are single-tufted brushes to enter furcations and end-tuft brushes to remove plaque on the distal of posterior teeth next to an edentulous area, especially if there are furcations exposed (see Figure 9.1.6).

Self-Study Questions

A. When in a treatment plan should plaque control therapy (plaque control instruction, scaling, root planing and polishing) be instituted?

B. How frequently should patients clean (brush, floss, etc.) their teeth?

C. Why is it recommended to concentrate on brushing and flossing (taping) techniques, and what is the concern about "random" brushing?

D. Why use an intrasulcular technique, and what is the advantage of dental tape?

E. Why is an angle of the toothbrush bristles to the tooth of 45–70 degrees recommended over the classic 45 degrees?

F. Why place the toothbrush bristles primarily on the clinical crown of the tooth and forced into the gingival crevice and not half on the tooth and half on the gingiva?

G. Why should brushing begin posteriorly and not at the midline?

H. Why should the toothbrush technique be repeated two to three times in each location?

I. How often should PCI be done and why?

J. Why do PCI at the outset of the appointment and not following the debridement?

K. How can smoking mask the signs of gingival inflammation and mislead the clinician and patient?

L. How is it possible to achieve regeneration from excellent plaque removal by a patient and comprehensive root debridement (root planing)?

M. Why were all the pockets not resolved?

N. What questions should be asked in cases where the gingivitis or periodontitis does not resolve?

Answers located at the end of the chapter.

References

1. Ausenda F, Jeong N, Arsenault P, et al. The effect of the Bass intrasulcular toothbrushing technique on the reduction of gingival inflammation: a randomized clinical trial. *J Evid Based Dent Pract* 2019;19:106–114.
2. Basali DH *The effect of instructed dental flossing on interdental gingival bleeding: a randomized controlled clinical trial. Master's Thesis, Department of Periodontology*, Tufts University School of Dental Medicine, 2019.
3. Armitage G. A brief history of periodontics in the United States of America: pioneers and thought-leaders of the past, and current challenges. *Periodontol 2000* 2020;82:12–25.
4. Bass CC. The optimum characteristics of dental floss for personal oral hygiene. *Dent Items Interest* 1948;70:921–934.
5. Levi PA, Rudy R, Jeong N, Coleman DK. *The Non-Surgical Control of Periodontal Diseases: A Comprehensive Handbook*. Berlin, Heidelberg: Springer-Verlag, 2016.
6. Rosenberg ES, Evian CI, Listgarten MA. The composition of the subgingival microbiota after periodontal therapy. *J Periodontol* 1981;52:435–441.
7. Bergström J, Preber H. The influence of cigarette smoking on the development of experimental gingivitis. *J Periodontal Res* 1986;21:668–676.
8. Bergström J, Floderus-Myrhed B. Co-twin control study of the relationship between smoking and some periodontal disease factors. *Community Dent Oral Epidemiol* 1983;11:113–116.
9. Preber H, Bergström J. Occurrence of gingival bleeding in smoker and non-smoker patients. *Acta Odontol Scand* 1985;43:315–320.
10. Bergström J. Cigarette smoking as risk factor in chronic periodontal disease. *Community Dent Oral Epidemiol* 1989;17:245–247.
11. Bergström J. Oral hygiene compliance and gingivitis expression in cigarette smokers. *Scand J Dent Res* 1990;98:497–503.
12. Johnson GK, Hill M. Cigarette smoking and the periodontal patient [review]. *J Periodontol* 2004;75:196–209.
13. Papapanou PN. Periodontal diseases: epidemiology [review]. *Ann Periodontol* 1996;1:1–36.
14. Tonetti MS. Cigarette smoking and periodontal diseases: etiology and management of disease [review]. *Ann Periodontol.* 1998;3:88–101.
15. Stambaugh RV, Dragoo M, Smith DM, Carasali L. The limits of subgingival scaling. *Int J Periodontics Restorative Dent* 1981;1:30–41.

TAKE-HOME POINTS

A. Plaque control therapy should be the *first* therapy on the definitive treatment plan sequence following these steps:

- Any medical consultations that need to be done where treatment could negatively affect the patient's health.
- All dental consultations have been done that might affect whether or not a tooth should be retained.
- Any emergency therapy that is needed to eliminate pain or acute infection, or replace an avulsed tooth in the esthetic zone.
- Any emergency caries control to prevent an irreversible pulpitis.
- Any emergency extraction of an extremely mobile and nontreatable tooth.

B. Because plaque generally matures in one to three days, the ideal frequency for a patient to remove all plaque (biofilm) from all tooth surfaces to preserve health is at least once daily. That said, however, it depends on the patient's susceptibility to dental caries and/or periodontal or peri-implant infections (gingivitis, periodontitis, peri-implant mucositis, or peri-implantitis). Clearly, if the patient has a high caries rate, shows significant gingival inflammation, and/or exhibits evidence of attachment loss caused by present or past periodontitis, thorough plaque removal should be done twice a day. If the patient has malposed teeth where there is a high likelihood of food collection, if they exhibit oral malodor or "feel" their teeth are not clean, the removal of food debris and plaque is indicated more than once daily.

C. Plaque is generally invisible to patients and to us when we are cleaning our teeth. Subgingival plaque is always invisible even if a plaque-disclosing preparation is used. Even with them, it is virtually impossible for a patient to see interproximally and to see the lingual surfaces of most teeth. The disclosing preparations used by the patient to detect unremoved plaque show the surfaces of the teeth most easily cleaned and not the hard-to-clean surfaces, and can lead to a false sense of security.

Cleaning plaque from teeth is a bit like trying to paint a wall without missing any area when blind-folded. Like painting a wall, once the techniques are learned, they are not difficult; however, unlike painting a wall, we cannot see plaque that is missed. Therefore, brushing and flossing techniques need to be done with concentration. That means thinking as one is doing plaque removal techniques: "Do I feel the toothbrush bristles in the gum crevice? Am I keeping the toothbrush bristle tips stationary on the tooth at the gum crevice and not scrubbing? Am I overlapping strokes so as not to miss an area? Am I adapting the dental tape to the tooth surface and moving it up and down (apically occlusally) and not sawing it into the gum? Am I using adequate pressure with the dental tape horizontally against the tooth?" Not concentrating on techniques can lead to a rote repetitive situation where plaque can remain on the teeth following home care, which might cause caries, gingival inflammation and attachment loss, and perhaps abrade the gingiva or the teeth.

D. In 1948, C.C. Bass [4], a physician from Louisiana, wrote in the *Louisiana Medical Journal* that a brushing technique that used a soft multi-tufted nylon toothbrush and an intrasulcular technique of brushing was preferable to the techniques taught in those days. In the days prior to Dr. Bass and for many years thereafter, the brushing technique that was advocated was a Stillman or Charter (sweeping) technique or Fones (scrubbing) technique. The Stillman and Charter techniques recommended the use of an extra-hard natural bristle toothbrush. Bass stated that the biofilm from the bacterial cells that caused gingival inflammation was attached to the tooth subgingivally and would not be removed with the other techniques.

Dental tape is wider than dental floss. Although it is made of the same nylon filaments as dental floss, there are a greater number of them. Its benefit over dental floss is that dental tape covers a greater surface area of the tooth, and there is increased frictional grip to the tooth with dental tape than with dental floss. The frictional grip is important because it provides the patient with control and lessens the risk of cutting the gingiva or harming the epithelial attachment. As the tape is made of the same

filaments as floss, it is not thicker but is wider. Most dental tape tends to shred or tear less than dental floss.

E. An angle of 45–70 degrees of the toothbrush bristles to the tooth will access *all* gingival crevices, whereas a 45-degree angle frequently does not allow the toothbrush bristles to access the gingival crevice on the lingual of the mandibular posterior teeth, because the bristle tips are prevented from reaching the gingival crevice by the occlusal surface. The cervical lingual of the mandibular teeth is a very common area for gingival/periodontal infection. That said, it is not recommended to explain an "angle" to a patient because many people do not understand angles and can become confused about what to do. With the intrasulcular technique of brushing, when the patient feels the bristles enter the gum crevice, their angulation must be correct. Thus, the suggestion is to recommend that the patient angle the brush bristle tips toward the gum crevice.

F. The patient should ensure the bristles engage the tooth on the facial or lingual surface roughly in the middle (at the maximum convexity) and then press the bristles firmly against the tooth until they "feel" the bristles *enter* the gum crevice. Then if using a hand (nonpower) brush, they should move the handle in short strokes (3–5 mm) back and forth with sufficient pressure to maintain the bristle tips at the gum crevice stationary and connected with the tooth. This technique avoids scrubbing and toothbrush abrasion of the gingiva and the tooth. The stationary bristle tip technique (Bass) differs only slightly from what Dr. Bass taught, as it avoids talking about a 45-degree angle, and suggests that the bristles be entirely on the tooth and not half on the tooth and half on the gingiva as with the modified Bass technique. The reasons for not using the statement "half on the tooth and half on the gingiva" is because dental biofilm, the primary cause of caries or periodontal disease, resides on the tooth, and it is best not to confuse the patient by inferring that brushing the gums is important for gingival health. Brushing the gingiva can cause more harm than good and can lead to gingival recession in a thin periodontal phenotype or ulceration of the gingiva due to epithelial and connective tissue abrasion.

G. Since the patient cannot see plaque on their teeth, it is easy to incompletely remove the plaque. By starting with the most posterior tooth and moving anteriorly with overlapping strokes, it is less likely to miss an area.

H. Since the toothbrush bristle tips splay apart, repeating the brushing technique three to four times in the same area will help prevent the subgingival tooth surface from not being cleaned.

I. The need for PCI depends on the patient's abilities with a toothbrush, dental tape (floss), and other recommended plaque removal aids. From a physical therapy viewpoint, it is imperative that a patient demonstrate brushing and flossing (taping) techniques at the outset of their initial comprehensive examination. Frequently, we find that a patient who seemingly has excellent plaque control and who shows no signs of gingival inflammation is scrubbing the teeth and is likely in time to cause cervical abrasion and gingival recession. Part of a comprehensive examination is knowing the patient's dental hygiene techniques. We cannot rely on the patient to describe it to us any more than a golf coach can rely on a client's description of how the golf club is swung.

J. Instruction in plaque removal techniques (PCI) should be done at each visit for hygiene therapy regardless of whether the visit is a periodic maintenance appointment or part of initial phase therapy including SRP [6] and regardless of how much plaque we can see because we cannot visualize subgingival and interproximal plaque. It should be done at the inception of the visit and if necessary repeated at the end. It should be done *before* local anesthesia is used (topical or injectable) because all the intrasulcular brushing techniques rely on the patient's proprioception, which will be lost following anesthesia. For a patient with natural teeth or with implants, the key to oral and general health is controlling the biofilm on the tooth or implant. This must be primarily done by the patient because plaque can mature in as little as 24 hours, and it is the

patient's responsibility to achieve and preserve dental health and our responsibility to be their coaches and assist them in removing what cannot be removed with a brush, dental tape (floss), and other aids. We have always been taught to do the most important things first, so always begin with a dental hygiene technique review. If the patient's plaque control is unacceptable and the patient is being seen for a visit other than hygiene therapy, PCI should be instituted at the outset of that appointment and before local anesthesia is administered.

K. Smoking appears to reduce the clinical signs of inflammation with plaque accumulation [7].
- Clinical studies show that smokers exhibit less inflammation than nonsmokers [8–11].
- Although the signs of inflammation appear less in smokers than in nonsmokers, the preponderance of studies show that smoking is a major risk factor for periodontitis and that periodontitis is more prevalent and more severe in smokers than nonsmokers [12–14].

L. Periodontal regeneration (see Chapter 4) can occur when the conditions for healing are present. Regeneration might occur on occasion with "nonsurgical" periodontal therapy, as in the following situations.
- The tooth is thoroughly debrided of biofilm and calculus, and has been thoroughly root planed to remove bacterial toxins.
- There is an adequate blood supply.
- The infrabony defect is narrow and generally has three walls and one tooth surface.
- There is an adequate surface area of periodontal ligament exposed inside the infrabony defect as a result of instrumentation.
- The patient is performing an excellent level of supragingival and subgingival plaque control.
- The patient is systemically healthy and is a nonsmoker.

M. If pockets do not resolve, it is likely that not all the calculus was removed from the tooth surface, the patient is not following the prescribed plaque removal techniques or their frequency, or that the pocket depth precluded the patient's access with daily hygiene techniques. Stambaugh and Dragoo [15] stated that it was unlikely in pockets ≥5 mm to do complete root debridement and calculus removal. Patients with a thick phenotype and pockets ≥5 mm are less likely to resolve than patients with a thin phenotype.

N. When gingival or peri-implant inflammation does not resolve, it is important to determine the etiology.

- **Is the patient concordant with their home care, and do they use the correct techniques?** If patients are not consistent with brushing and taping (flossing), then continue to explain that they have disease and only they can eliminate it with thorough and consistent plaque removal. If the patient is consistent, however, on observing the techniques and plaque is not being removed, work on techniques and emphasize the need to concentrate on techniques and not to do them by rote.
- **Are there any systemic factors preventing normal healing?** Assess when the patient last had a general physical examination. If it has been over two years or if there is a suspected systemic problem and it has not been diagnosed, consult the patient's physician.

- **Does the patient use tobacco products?** If so and the patient wishes to eliminate the tobacco habit, offer a tobacco cessation program or refer the person to their physician or to an ongoing tobacco cessation program.
- **Is there detectable subgingival calculus?** If so, redo the SRP. Repeated subgingival SRP when the patient initially presents with deep pockets and heavy calculus is necessary in most instances.
- **Are there pockets that cannot be accessed for complete daily plaque control?** If so, explain pocket-reducing surgical therapy and initiate therapy or refer the patient to a periodontist for diagnosis and therapy.

Never give up and write off a patient as noncompliant and never compliant. Sometimes it takes years; however, many patients will eventually see the value in correct and consistent plaque control techniques. When we remain silent as a result of inadequate plaque control, nobody will benefit. The patient's dental health will deteriorate, the work we do for the patient will deteriorate, and our self-esteem will also deteriorate. If we continue the mantra of emphasizing excellence in home care, we have done all that is possible to assure that our patients will receive the best treatment we can provide.

INDEX

A

abrasion 254
accessory pulpal canals 54
acellular dermal matrix (ADM) 229, 230, 232, 234, 243, 245
Actisite 96, 98, 99
acute dental infection 321
adalimumab 73
adapted horizontal technique 377
adjunctive systemic antibiotics 104–106
  advantages 104
  periodontal infections, treatment of 109
adjustable stopper and bone ejector (ASBE) trephine 309, 351, 352, 354
ADM *see* acellular dermal matrix (ADM)
advanced glycation end products (AGEs) 63
adverse pregnancy outcomes 69
aggressive periodontitis 30–33, 43
alloderm 228–233
allografts
  extraction socket, placement in 205
  intrabony defects treatment by 164–167
  for mucogingival therapy 228–233
alloplast 171, 195
alloplastic materials 187
  hydroxyapatite (HA) 185
  intrabony defects treatment by 181–183
alveolar bone loss 41
alveolar ridge preservation 315–322
alveoloplasty 266
amoxicillin 36, 103, 107, 112, 244, 294, 300, 325, 331
angular bone loss 77, 78
ankyloglossia 239
apical foramen communication 255
Arestin 96, 98–100, 294
Atridox 94, 96, 98, 99
autogenous free gingival graft 282

autografts 171, 194
  limitations 171, 195
azithromycin 29

B

bacterial biofilms 96
bacterial effect 255
bacterial plaque 160
Bass intrasulcular technique of toothbrushing 14, 147, 249, 250, 377
β-Tricalcium phosphate (β-TCP) 185
bioactive glasses (bio-glasses) 185
Biolase (Er,Cr:YSGG) 118
biologic width 134, 135, 137, 180
  definition of 130
  invasion of 265–266
biomarkers 41, 69, 71, 72
Bio-Oss® collagen bone graft 290, 295, 325
bisphosphonates 194
bitewing radiographs 80, 81, 229
bleeding on probing (BOP) 102
blunt-ended Glick instrument 351
bone-added osteotome sinus floor elevation technique 304
bone allograft 195
bone graft 279, 282, 290, 291, 310, 317, 335, 370
  alloplasts for 185
  for ARP 320, 321
  materials 304
  for ridge augmentation 196
bone loss 142
bone morphogenetic protein (BMP)-2 179, 304
bone remodeling 319
bone resorption progresses 319
Bruno's technique 212
bruxism 76, 149, 255
buccal flap 230, 231, 325

buccal furcation groove   55
buccal radicular groove   54
buccal temporary anchorage device   278
bundle bone   319

C

calcium hydroxide   294
calcium sulfate   185
cancellous bone chips (DynaBlast)   305
canine exposure   271, 272
carbon dioxide laser surgery   240
cardiac pacemakers   90
cardiovascular disease   68–69, 71
cavitation   90
Cavitron   50, 53, 116
cementoenamel junction (CEJ)   28, 38, 52
centric occlusion   260
cephalometric radiograph   278
ceramo-metal crowns   331
cervical enamel projection (CEP)   49, 50, 52, 53, 161
cervical vertebral maturation (CVM)   371
chemical irritation   254
chisel   325, 333
chlorhexidine   96, 148, 209, 237
chlorhexidine oral rinses   294
chronic periodontal disease   154
chronic periodontitis   38–44, 46, 105, 112
civatte bodies   21
clinical attachment level (CAL)   38
clinical attachment loss (CAL)   16
closed eruption technique   272, 274
cobra elevators   314
Cobra instrument   352, 353
collagenic membrane   300, 301
colloid bodies   21
computed tomography   80, 340
cone-beam computed tomography (CBCT)   77–78, 80–82, 273, 274
connective tissue grafts   206–212
    crown margins   211
    implant collar   211
    inadequate attached gingiva with recession   211
    indications for   210
    keratinized/attached gingiva   207, 210, 220
    lingual recession   211
    postoperative follow-up   210
    postoperative instructions   209
    prescriptions   209
    probing pocket depth/recession measurements   207
    progressive recession   211
    root coverage and ridge augmentation   212
    root preparation   208–209
    root wear/erosion/cervical abrasion   211
    SCTG, treatment with   211
    suturing   209
    techniques of   211–213
    teeth with gingival recession   210
    teeth without gingival recession   210
    Zucchelli technique   208
connective tissue growth factor   28
conventional crestal approaches   311
conventional implant placement   338–342
    intraoperative surgical-related complications   344
    postoperative surgical-related complications   344
conventional periodontal therapy   118
coronally positioned flap   203
corticosteroid   18
craniofacial growth   370
crestal approach   304
crestal sinus lifts   313
crestal window technique   311, 313, 314, 356
    with conventional two-stage approach   354
    internal sinus lift   307–312
critical probing depth   91
crown lengthening   130–132, 134, 186, 265
    contraindication   135
    final cast post and core   132
    full-thickness flap   131
    gingivectomy   131
    indication   135
    orthodontic extrusion   137
    ostectomy   131
    osteoplasty   131
    permanent FPD   132
    submarginal incisions   131
    surgical crown lengthening   136–137
    temporary FPD   132
cyclosporine   25, 27

D

decalcified freeze-dried bone allograft (DFDBA)   171
demineralized freeze-dried bone allograft (DFDBA)   171, 279, 320
dental biofilm-induced gingivitis   87, 88, 316
dental implant replacement
    extraction of tooth   176
    flapless extraction and grafting   176
    growth factor-enhanced therapy   176
dental implants   295
    conventional implant placement   338–342
    immediate implant placement   345–347
    implant rehabilitation for missing adjacent teeth in maxillary esthetic zone   357–362
    implant single crowns and porcelain veneers in esthetic zone   365–368
    sinus lift and immediate implant placement   350–354
dental plaque   7
dental plaque-induced gingivitis   12–14, 126
dental rehabilitation   265

dental tape   377, 380
dentinal tubules   255
dentogingival junction   134
Depakote   23
desquamative gingivitis (DG)   18, 20
    characterization of   20
    symptoms of   20
developmental depressions   55
developments in diagnostics   73–78
dexamethasone elixir   20
DG see desquamative gingivitis (DG)
diabetes   63, 68, 71, 194
digital subtraction   80
Dilantin   23
distal furcation   259
distal wedge procedure   140, 143
disuse atrophy   77
double papilla flap   203
doxycycline   209
drug-influenced gingival enlargement   27
    clinical characteristics of   27
    definition of   27
    treatment of   29
dysesthesia   144

E

early-onset periodontitis see molar/incisor pattern
    periodontitis
edentulous alveolar ridge   10
electrosurgery   240
Elyzol   96, 99, 100
enamel matrix derivative (EMD)   36
enamel pearls   52, 53, 161
endodontically treated teeth   266–267
endodontic–periodontal lesions   82–83
endodontics   149, 248–257, 294, 295
epithelio-connective tissue palatal pedicle graft   223
equine hydroxyapatite and collagen (eHAC)   179
erosive/erythematous lichen planus   21
Er:YAG laser   123
erythema   2, 21
esthetic crown lengthening   135, 266
esthetic plastic periodontal therapy   10
examination and diagnosis   2–5
    aggressive periodontitis   30–33
    chronic periodontitis   38–44
    dental plaque-induced gingivitis   12–14
    developments in diagnostics   73–78
    gingival enlargement   23–25
    local anatomic factors, to periodontal disease   48–50
    non-plaque-induced gingivitis   14, 17–22
    oral–systemic links   57–64
    periodontal charting   4
external bevel gingivectomy   122, 123, 125, 126

F

familial aggregation   46
FDBA see freeze-dried bone allograft (FDBA)
feldspathic porcelain   371
ferrule, lack of   266
fiberotomy   239, 241
fibroblast growth factor (FGF)-2   179
fixed partial denture (FPD)   130, 132, 340
flap osseous surgery   138–144
flap sloughing   197
fluocinonide gel   20
Fones (scrubbing) technique   380
free gingival graft   214–218, 220, 221, 226–228
    advantages of   222
    connective tissue as   224, 225
    contraindications   222
    disadvantages of   222
    root coverage with   225
free gingival margin (FGM)   38
freeze-dried bone allograft (FDBA)   167, 176, 191, 300,
        310, 332, 353
fremitus   261
frenectomy   235–237
frenum   239
full-and partial-thickness rotated palatal flaps   204
full-thickness buccal flap   50, 157
full-thickness flap   131, 140, 325, 331
full-thickness lingual flaps   50
full-thickness mucoperiosteal flap   148
functional crown lengthening   134–135
furcation entrances, size of   53
furcation invasion   160
    classification systems of   55–56
    definition of   55
    Glickman classification for   55
    Hamp classification for   55
    Tarnow and Fletcher classification for   56
furcations   55
    definition of   152
    in lateral canal   255
    occlusal trauma   161
    predisposing anatomic factors   161
    primary factors for   160
    treatment of   156–158, 162–163

G

GBR see guided bone regeneration (GBR)
generalized gingival edema   2
generalized gingival erythema   17
generalized severe chronic periodontitis   116
generalized subgingival calculus   284
gingival bleeding   27
gingival enlargement   23–25, 135
    biologic origins for   28

gingival enlargement (*cont'd*)
  drug-influenced gingival enlargement   27, 29
  phenytoin-associated   24
  probing depth   27–28
gingival inflammation   27
gingival recession   38, 101, 200, 220, 243, 244, 347
  Miller Classification System of   201
  submarginal metal strips in   221
  teeth with   210
  teeth without   210
gingivectomy   24, 120–123, 131, 142
  case study   120–123
  contraindications to   125
  crown lengthening   131
  definition of   125
  indications for   125
gingivitis   258
  clinical signs of   16
gingivoplasty   24, 122, 126
  indications for   125
Glickman's furcation classification   8, 55, 152, 156, 160
Gracey curettes   90, 115
growth factors, intrabony defects treatment
      by   174–177
GTR *see* guided tissue regeneration (GTR)
guided bone regeneration (GBR)   150, 188–191, 193, 325,
      333, 366
  bone materials for   194–195
  complications of   196
  contraindications for   194
  management of complications   196–197
  nonresorbable membranes   194
  preoperative consultation   190
  procedure   190–191
  resorbable membranes   194
guided tissue regeneration (GTR)   36, 149, 162, 167,
      169
  bone materials   171–172
  complications in   173
  management of complication   173
  nonresorbable membranes in   170
  perioperative   172
  postoperative   172
  preoperative   172
  procedure   166–167
  resorbable membranes in   170
gum diseases   2

H
Hamp classification, for furcation invasion   55, 152
hand and automated instrumentation
  cardiac pacemakers   90
  case study   86–88
  Gracey curettes   90

hand *vs.* powered mechanical instruments   87,
      88, 91
  magnetorestrictive ultrasonic scalers   90
  piezoelectric ultrasonic scalers   90
  sickle scalers   90
  sonic scalers   90
hand instruments   116
Hanks balanced salt solution (HBSS)   293
healthy architecture, definition of   140
hemisection   152
hemostasis   237, 325
hereditary gingival fibromatosis (HGF)   27
horizontal furcation classification   160
horizontal ridge augmentation   196
hydrated freeze-dried bone allograft (FDBA)
      particles   317
hydroxyapatite   320
hyperkeratosis   261

I
ibuprofen   122, 244, 300, 325, 331
immediate anterior implants   349
immediate implant placement   345–347
implant rehabilitation for missing adjacent teeth in
      maxillary esthetic zone   357–362
implant single crowns and porcelain veneers in esthetic
      zone   365–368
implant site preparation
  alveolar ridge preservation   315–322
  internal sinus lift, crestal window
      technique   307–312
  ridge expansion techniques   330–333
  ridge split techniques   323–329
  sinus grafting, lateral   298–301
incisor mandibular plane angle (IMPA)   280
infection   144, 173, 197
infectious pathway   70
inflammatory external root resorption (IRR)   294, 295
inflammatory pathway   70
inflammatory reaction   173, 197
infrabony osseous defect   143
interarch space, lack of   266
interdisciplinary treatment, periodontics
  endodontics   248–257
  occlusion–periodontology   284–286
  orthodontics   268–272, 276–281
  pediatric dentistry   289–291
  prosthodontics   260–263
intermediate bifurcation ridges   54
internal bevel approach   29
internal bevel gingivectomy   126
internal sinus lift, crestal window technique   307–314
intrabony defects treatment
  by allografts   164–167

by alloplastic materials   181–183
by growth factors   174–177
intrabony pocket formation   288
intraoral digital impressions   364
intraoral radiographs   81
inverse bevel distal wedge technique   126

K
Kennedy classification   267
keratinized gingiva   8, 15, 49, 135, 143, 210, 215, 282

L
LANAP (Nd:YAG)   118
Langer's technique   212
Lares (Er:YAG)   118
laser-assisted surgery   127
laser gingivectomy   123
lasers in periodontology
    benefits of   118
    case study   114–117
    Er:YAG laser   115, 116
laser (light amplification by stimulated emission of
    radiation) therapy   96, 239–240
lateral cephalogram   270
lateral cephalometric radiographs   371
laterally positioned flap   203
lateral window approach   304
lichen planus (LP)   18, 21–22
    characteristic histopathology of   21
    classifications of   21
    clinical manifestations of   21
    etiology of   21
lidocaine   130
local anatomic factors, to periodontal disease   48–50
local drug delivery   92–94
    Actisite   98, 99
    Arestin   98–99, 99–100
    Atridox   98, 99
    case study   92–94
    Elyzol   99, 100
    tetracycline derivatives   96
    tetracyclines   96
localized aggressive periodontitis see molar/incisor
    pattern periodontitis
localized mild vertical bone loss   92
localized prepubertal/juvenile periodontitis see molar/
    incisor pattern periodontitis
localized tooth-related factor   186
luxated tooth   293

M
magnetorestrictive ultrasonic scalers   90
mandibular left sextant   115, 117
mandibular lingual frenectomy   239

using carbon dioxide laser surgery   240
mandibular molars   55
marginal gingiva   210
maxillary labial frenectomy   237
maxillary lateral incisors   370
maxillary molars   55
maxillary sinus   304
mechanical debridement   97
MegaGen EZ Plus implants   310
membrane exposure   173, 196–197
mesalamine   73
mesial and distal root concavities   53
metronidazole (MTZ)   29, 36, 96, 103, 106, 107, 112
Michel's medium   18
mild gingival inflammation   201
mild marginal erythema   30
mild sinusitis   299
Miller classification system   201, 225
minimally invasive coronally advanced flap
    techniques   242–245
minimum inhibitory concentration (MIC)   106
mobile teeth   144
modified Bass technique   380
modified Stillman's technique   14
molar/incisor pattern grade C periodontitis   35, 37
molar/incisor pattern periodontitis
    definition of   35
    microbiomes of   36
    prevalence of   35–36
    treatment of   36
monolithic zirconia screw-retained single crowns   360
motrin   209
mucogingival anatomy   8
mucogingival defects   58, 174
    definition of   220
    treatment of   220
mucogingival surgical therapy   220
mucogingival therapy
    allografts (alloderm) for mucogingival
        therapy   228–233
    connective tissue grafts   206–212
    free gingival grafts   214–218
    frenectomy   235–237
    minimally invasive coronally advanced flap
        techniques   242–245
    pedicle flaps   200–201
    vestibuloplasty   235–237
mucous membrane pemphigoid   20
mushroom elevator   309, 310, 252

N
Nabers probe   7, 148
necrotizing gingivitis, systemic antibiotics for   106
nerve paresthesia   144

nickel allergic contact stomatitis 123
nickel titanium wires 270
nifedipine 27
non-plaque-induced gingivitis 14, 17–22
nonresorbable membranes 170
  for guided bone regeneration 194
  guided tissue regeneration 170
nonsurgical periodontal therapy
  hand and automated instrumentation 86–88
  lasers in periodontology 114–117
  local drug delivery 92–94
  systemic antibiotics 101–109
nontraumatic brushing technique 230

O
obesity 70, 72
occlusal orthosis 261
occlusal trauma 10, 161, 287–288
  definition of 172
  first-degree 172
  second-degree 172
occlusion–periodontology 284–286
odontoplasty 131
open membrane technique 356
open wound 108
oral health-related quality of life (OHRQoL) 109
oral–systemic links 57–64
orthodontic extrusion 137
orthodontic intrusion 266
orthodontics 161, 268–272, 276–281, 278–279
orthodontic treatment 272, 277, 282
orthodontic treatment-induced gingival
    enlargement 123
orthodontic walls 279
osseous recontouring 143
osseous resective surgery 144
ostectomy 131, 143
osteoplasty 143
osteotome sinus floor elevation technique. 304
osteotomy 311, 346

P
pain 101
palatal flap 354
palato-gingival grooves 54
panoramic radiograph 80, 81, 269, 270, 278, 344
papillary finger flap 310
papillary rotation flap 311
partial edentulism 358
pediatric dentistry 289–291
pedicle flaps 200–201, 205, 212
  contraindications for 204
  incision 203
  indications for 204

  rotation of 204
  sutured to recipient site 204
penicillin 294
periapical periodontitis 259
periapical radiographs 79, 83, 229
Peridex 122, 300
peri-implantitis 10, 348
PerioChip 96
periodontal chart, components of 15
periodontal diseases
  dental plaque 7
  environmental factor 6–7
  mucogingival deformity 8
  pathogenesis of 6, 7
  pathologic migration 8
  susceptible host 6
periodontal lesions 256
periodontal ligament (PDL) 261, 287
periodontal phenotype 43
periodontal plastic surgery 212, 220
periodontal regeneration 381
periodontics
  endodontics 248–257
  orthodontics 268–272, 276–281
  pediatric dentistry 289–291
  prosthodontics 260–263
periodontitis 28, 44, 46, 92–94, 97, 258, 376
  adverse pregnancy outcomes 69
  cardiovascular disease and 68–69
  classification of 9
  with deep pockets 258
  definition of 41, 67
  diabetes and 63, 68
  diagnosis of 43
  molar/incisor pattern 35
  obesity 70, 72
  rheumatoid arthritis (RA) 69–72
  systemic antibiotics for 105–107
  treatment and prevention of 376
periodontitis stage III, localized, grade C 42–43
periodontology 279
phenytoin 27
phenytoin-induced gingival enlargement 23, 24, 125
photodynamic light therapy 96
piezoelectric ultrasonic scalers 90
piezosurgery 336
piezotome 300
plaque control instruction (PCI) 376, 381
plaque control techniques 60, 145, 249, 375, 379
plaque-induced gingivitis with gingival enlarge-
    ment 120, 122
plaque-induced mild localized gingivitis with mucogingi-
    val conditions 366
plaque removal 374–378

platelet-derived growth factor (PDGF)   180
polymers   185
porcelain fracture   311, 349
porcelain-fused-to-metal (PFM) crown   312, 340
porcelain veneers in esthetic zone   365–368
pregnancy   71
preprosthetic hard tissue and soft tissue crown
      lengthening   128–132
preventive periodontal therapy   374–378
primary endodontic lesion   259
primary periodontal lesion   256
primary pulpal lesions   256
probing depth   27, 28
progressive periodontal disease   220
prosthodontics   260–263
proximal contact relation   52
pseudo-pocket   28
pulpal infection   256
pulpal inflammation   254
pulpal necrosis   259
pulpal–periodontal lesion   256
pulpitis   256
pulp necrosis   294

R
radiography   81
recombinant human bone morphogenetic protein 2
      (rhBMP-2)   172
recombinant human platelet-derived growth factor BB
      (rhPDGF-BB)   158, 172, 176, 179, 180, 195
red complex   96
regeneration, definition of   169
regenerative therapy
      allografts, intrabony defects treatment by   164–167
      alloplastic materials, intrabony defects treatment
         by   181–183
      furcations, treatment of   156–158
      growth factors, intrabony defects treatment
         by   174–177
      guided bone regeneration   188–191
replacement external root resorption (RRR)   294
rescue therapy   100
resective periodontal therapy
      flap osseous surgery   138–144
      gingivectomy   120–123
      preprosthetic hard tissue and soft tissue crown
         lengthening   128–132
      root resection   145–150
residual root sensitivity   144
resorbable membranes   170
      for guided bone regeneration   194
      guided tissue regeneration   170
restorative considerations   54–55
reticular lichen planus   21

rheumatoid arthritis (RA)   69–72
ridge expansion techniques   330–337
ridge expansion with osteotomes   336
ridge split technique   323–329, 333–336
root amputation   150, 152
root canal therapy   256, 286, 290
root concavity   52, 161
root divergence   53
root fracture   294
root fusion   53
root proximity   52
root resection   145–150, 152, 162
      contraindications for   152
      indications for   152
      maxillary and mandibular molars   153
root trunk length   54
rotated palatal pedicle graft   204

S
scaling and root planing (SRP)   36, 40, 91, 103, 147,
      148, 170
Schneiderian membrane   299–301, 303, 313, 352
SCTG see subepithelial connective tissue graft (SCTG)
Seibert classification   193, 335
semilunar coronally positioned flap   354
sequential osteotome expansion   332
short clinical crown   266
sickle scalers   90, 115
sinus elevation procedure   300–301, 305, 309–311,
      351–353
      crestal approach   304
      lateral window approach   304
      management of complications   306
      operative complications   305
      postoperative complications   306
sinus grafting, lateral   298–301
sinus pneumatization   303
small torn sinus membrane   356
sonic scalers   90
split-thickness flap   230
stage III grade B periodontitis   49, 286
stage III grade C periodontitis   32
Standard Tesselation Language (STL) file   358
stationary bristle tip technique   377
Stillman/Charter (sweeping) technique   380
Straumann dental implants   367
subcrestal placement   349
subepithelial connective tissue graft (SCTG)   208, 211, 212,
      220, 221
subgingival biofilm   108
subgingival calculus   38, 102, 115, 382
subgingival plaque   379
subgingival scaling and root planing (SRP)   94, 97, 98
sublingual edema   197

submarginal incisions   131
subpapillary continuous sling suturing method   230, 231
subpapillary suturing technique   244
supportive periodontal therapy (SPT)   37
supracrestal fiberotomy   239
supragingival calculus   38, 102
surgical crown lengthening   136–137
systemic antibiotics   33, 170, 196, 293–294
    benefits of   113
    case study   101–109
    evidence for   105
    for necrotizing gingivitis   106
    prophylactic use of   108
    risks in   104
    timing of antibiotic administration   107–108

T
tamsulosin   73
Tarnow and Fletcher classification, for furcation
    invasion   56
temporomandibular joint disorder (TMD)   261
tetracycline   36, 96, 157, 293–294
tetracycline derivatives   96
thermal injury   254
thin biotype   201, 210, 239, 280
Tooth Slooth®   254
transalveolar technique   313
trauma, due to surgery   274

trephine   309, 354
tunneling procedure   230, 279, 283
type I gingivitis   229

U
ulcerated lichen planus   21
ultrasonic-powered mechanical instrument   115
ultrasonic scalers   90
universal curettes   90

V
veneer preparations   367, 368
vertical dimension of occlusion (VDO)   265, 266
vertical furcation classification   160
vertical root fracture   81–82, 161
vestibular incision subperiosteal tunnel access (VISTA)
    approach   243, 244, 246
vestibuloplasty   235–237, 239, 240
vicodin   209

W
wound healing   127, 179, 180

X
xenograft   171, 195

Z
Zucchelli technique   208
Zyprexa   23